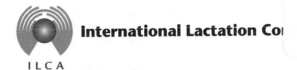

International Lactation Co

M000197781

ILCA

CORE CURRICULUM FOR LACTATION CONSULTANT PRACTICE

SECOND EDITION

Edited by

Rebecca Mannel, BS, IBCLC
Lactation Center Coordinator and Clinical Instructor
OU Medical Center and OU Health Sciences Center
Oklahoma City, Oklahoma

Patricia J. Martens, IBCLC, PhD
Director, Manitoba Centre for Health Policy
Associate Professor, Department of Community Health Sciences
Faculty of Medicine
University of Manitoba
Winnipeg, Canada

Marsha Walker, RN, IBCLC
Executive Director, National Alliance for Breastfeeding Advocacy
Research, Education, and Legal Branch
Weston, Massachusetts

JONES AND BARTLETT PUBLISHERS
Sudbury, Massachusetts
BOSTON   TORONTO   LONDON   SINGAPORE

World Headquarters

Jones and Bartlett Publishers
40 Tall Pine Drive
Sudbury, MA 01776
978-443-5000
info@jbpub.com
www.jbpub.com

Jones and Bartlett Publishers Canada
6339 Ormindale Way
Mississauga, Ontario L5V 1J2
Canada

Jones and Bartlett Publishers
International
Barb House, Barb Mews
London W6 7PA
United Kingdom

Jones and Bartlett's books and products are available through most bookstores and online booksellers. To contact Jones and Bartlett Publishers directly, call 800-832-0034, fax 978-443-8000, or visit our website www.jbpub.com.

The authors, editor, and publisher have made every effort to provide accurate information. However, they are not responsible for errors, omissions, or for any outcomes related to the use of the contents of this book and take no responsibility for the use of the products and procedures described. Treatments and side effects described in this book may not be applicable to all people; likewise, some people may require a dose or experience a side effect that is not described herein. Drugs and medical devices are discussed that may have limited availability controlled by the Food and Drug Administration (FDA) for use only in a research study or clinical trial. Research, clinical practice, and government regulations often change the accepted standard in this field. When consideration is being given to use of any drug in the clinical setting, the health care provider or reader is responsible for determining FDA status of the drug, reading the package insert, and reviewing prescribing information for the most up-to-date recommendations on dose, precautions, and contraindications, and determining the appropriate usage for the product. This is especially important in the case of drugs that are new or seldom used.

Production Credits

Executive Editor: Kevin Sullivan
Production Director: Amy Rose
Acquisitions Editor: Emily Ekle
Associate Editor: Amy Sibley
Editorial Assistant: Patricia Donnelly
Associate Production Editor: Jamie Chase
Senior Marketing Manager: Katrina Gosek
Associate Marketing Manager: Rebecca Wasley

Manufacturing and Inventory Coordinator: Amy Bacus
Composition: Auburn Associates, Inc.
Cover Design: Kate Ternullo
Cover Image: © "The Visitors" by R.C. Gorman (1932–2005). The Gorman Estate
Cover Image: © Jeffrey Schmieg/ShutterStock, Inc.
Printing and Binding: Malloy, Inc.
Cover Printing: Malloy, Inc.

Library of Congress Cataloging-in-Publication Data

Core curriculum for lactation consultant practice / International Lactation Consultant Association; edited by Rebecca Mannel, Patricia J. Martens, and Marsha Walker.—2nd ed.
   p.; cm.
   Includes bibliographical references and index.
   ISBN-13: 978-0-7637-4503-5
   ISBN-10: 0-7637-4503-0
   1. Breastfeeding—Examinations, questions, etc. 2. Lactation—Examinations, questions, etc. 3. Breastfeeding—Outlines, syllabi, etc. 4. Lactation—Outlines, syllabi, etc. I. Mannel, Rebecca. II. Martens, Patricia J. III. Walker, Marsha.
IV. International Lactation Consultant Association.
   [DNLM: 1. Breast Feeding. 2. Lactation. 3. Mothers—education.   WS 125 C797 2007]
   RJ216.C657 2007
   649'.33076—dc22
6048   2006036707
Printed in the United States of America
11 10 09 08 07   10 9 8 7 6 5 4 3 2 1

CONTENTS

Acknowledgments

The revision of the Second Edition of ILCA's *Core Curriculum for Lactation Consultant Practice* has truly been a collaborative undertaking. Our editorial team wishes to extend our sincere gratitude to all of the chapter authors whose diligence and expertise enabled the association to update the information in this text. A special thanks also goes to the ILCA office team of Amber Maxa, Natalie Porterfield, and Jim Smith for their invaluable assistance and support. This Second Edition could not have materialized without their team effort. We also wish to acknowledge the Jones and Bartlett staff for their patience and support and the ILCA Board of Directors for their vision and action to ensure that this revision took place.

On a personal note, we wish to thank our families for their encouragement and support. A project of this magnitude takes a great deal of time away from your family. Thank you to our husbands, Robert Mannel, Gary Martens, and Hap Walker for keeping our families intact and functioning! Lastly, we acknowledge all of our hard-working peers in lactation who keep us motivated to continue to strengthen our profession through publications such as the *Core Curriculum*.

Rebecca Mannel
Patricia J. Martens
Marsha Walker

PREFACE

With the vast amount of information available about breastfeeding and human lactation, it is challenging to reflect key concepts in a single core text. As the editors of the *Core Curriculum for Lactation Consultant Practice*, Second Edition we envision this as a practical, succinct, and user-friendly resource for lactation consultants and other healthcare providers.

First and foremost, this text serves as a guide for aspiring lactation consultants as they study for the certification exam administered by the International Board of Lactation Consultant Examiners (IBLCE). Its content is patterned after the exam blueprint and encompasses all required topic areas. Use of this guide will help exam candidates assess their level of knowledge, experience, and expertise in order to develop an effective study plan. A unique feature of the book is a mapping plan that cross reference topics found in the IBLCE exam blueprint with relevant information found in particular chapters. This information allows users to easily locate topics of specific interest in a quick reference format.

This text is also designed to be used as a resource for practicing lactation consultants as well as for development of educational programs. The core curriculum content, along with its hundreds of citations, represents the knowledge base required to practice the profession of lactation consulting. In addition to its use as a valuable reference, it can be a source for staff development training, orientation of new staff, and as a resource when designing a curriculum for aspiring lactation consultants. Because this book will be utilized by a wide variety of healthcare providers, the editors chose the American Medical Association style of referencing.

Used in conjunction with lactation textbooks, the reader will find this core curriculum invaluable in devising an effective study plan. The authors who participated in the creation of this resource provide a wealth of knowledge and expertise, resulting in information being available in one convenient location.

We hope that this text will be helpful to all who use it and that ultimately it benefits all the mothers, babies, and families with whom we interact in our lactation consultant roles.

Rebecca Mannel, BS, IBCLC
Lactation Center Coordinator and
    Clinical Instructor
OU Medical Center and OU Health
    Sciences Center
Oklahoma City, Oklahoma

Patricia J. Martens, IBCLC, PhD
Director, Manitoba Centre for
    Health Policy
Associate Professor, Department of
    Community Health
    Sciences, Faculty of Medicine
University of Manitoba
Winnipeg, Canada

Marsha Walker, RN, IBCLC
Executive Director, National
    Alliance for Breastfeeding Advocacy
Research, Education, and Legal Branch
Weston, Massachusetts

CONTRIBUTORS

Gini Baker, RN, MPH, IBCLC
Perinatal Health Programs Coordinator
University of California San Diego, College
of Extended Studies
San Diego, California

Priscilla G. Bornmann, JD
McKinley & Bornmann, P.L.C.,
Alexandria, Virginia

Karin Cadwell, PhD, FAAN, RN, IBCLC
The Healthy Children Project
East Sandwich, Massachusetts

Ann M. Calandro, BSN, RNC, IBCLC
Piedmont Medical Center
Rock Hill, South Carolina

Cathy Carothers, BLA, IBCLC
Co-Director
Every Mother, Inc.,
Greenville, Mississippi

Suzanne Cox, AM, RN, RM, IBCLC
Private Practice Lactation Consultant
Tasmania, Australia

Melissa Cross, RN, IBCLC
Saint Luke's Hospital
Kansas City, Missouri

Marie Davis, RN, IBCLC
Kaiser Permanente Riverside, Retired
Riverside, California

Sara Gill, PhD, RN, IBCLC
Associate Professor, Family Nursing
University of Texas Health Science Center,
School of Nursing
San Antonio, Texas

Elsa Regina Justo Giugliani, MD, PhD,
IBCLC
Federal University of Rio Grande do Sul
Porto Alegre, Brazil

Joy Heads, OAM, RN, RM, MHPEd, IBCLC
Lactation Consultant
Royal Hospital for Women
South Eastern Sydney Illawarra Area
    Health Service
New South Wales, Australia

Kay Hoover, MEd, IBCLC
The Pennsylvania State University
University Park, Pennsylvania

Vergie Hughes, RN, MS, IBCLC
Inova Learning Network
Fairfax, Virginia

Kathleen Kendall-Tackett, PhD, IBCLC
Family Research Laboratory
University of New Hampshire
Durham, New Hampshire

Karen Kerkoff Gromada, MSN, RN, IBCLC
Lead Lactation Consultant Educator
TriHealth Hospitals
Cincinnati, Ohio

Mary Grace Lanese, RN, BSN, IBCLC
Saint Luke's Hospital
Kansas City, Missouri

Judith Lauwers, BA, IBCLC
Education Coordinator
International Lactation Consultant
    Association
Chalfont, Pennsylvania

Rebecca Mannel, BS, IBCLC
Lactation Center Coordinator and Clinical
    Instructor
OU Medical Center and OU Health
    Sciences Center
Oklahoma City, Oklahoma

Lisa Marasco, MA, IBCLC
Santa Barbara County Public Health
    Department
Nutrition Services/WIC
Santa Barbara, California

Patricia J. Martens, IBCLC, PhD
Director, Manitoba Centre for Health Policy
Associate Professor, Department of
    Community Health Sciences
Faculty of Medicine
University of Manitoba
Winnipeg, Canada

Nancy Mohrbacher, IBCLC
Co-author, *The Breastfeeding Answer Book*
Arlington Heights, Illinois

Frank J. Nice, RPh, DPA, CPHP
National Institutes of Health
Bethesda, Maryland

Sallie Page-Goertz, MN, CPNP, IBCLC
Clinical Assistant Professor
Pediatrics
Kansas University School of Medicine
Kansas City, Kansas

Judith Rogers, OTR/L
Pregnancy & Parenting Equipment
    Specialist
Through the Looking Glass (National
    Resource Center for Parents with
    Disabilities)
Berkeley, California

Carol A. Ryan, MSN, RN, IBCLC
Georgetown University Hospital
Washington, DC

Michelle Scott, MA, RD/LD, CSP, IBCLC
Wellspring Nutrition and Lactation
  Services
Mason, New Hampshire

Noreen Siebenaler, MSN, RN, IBCLC
Lactation Consultant
Kaweah Delta District Hospital
Maternal Child Services
Visalia, California

Angela Smith, RN, RM, BA, IBCLC
Post Natal Nursing Unit Manager KGV
Royal Prince Alfred Hospital
Sydney, Australia

Linda J. Smith, BSE, FACCE, IBCLC
Director
Bright Future Lactation Resource Centre
  Ltd
Dayton, Ohio

Amy Spangler, MN, RN, IBCLC
President
Amy's Babies
Atlanta, Georgia

Virginia Thorly, OAM, DipEd, MA, IBCLC
Private Practice Lactation Consultant
Queensland, Australia

Mary Rose Tully, MPH, IBCLC
Center for Infant/Young Child
  Feeding/Care
Maternal Child Health, School of Public
  Health
University of North Carolina
Chapel Hill, North Carolina

Cynthia Turner-Maffei, MA, IBCLC
Faculty
Healthy Children Project, Inc.
East Sandwich, Massachusetts

Marsha Walker, RN, IBCLC
Executive Director, National Alliance for
  Breastfeeding Advocacy
Research, Education, and Legal Branch
Weston, Massachusetts

Catherine Watson Genna, BS, IBCLC
Private Practice Lactation Consultant
Woodhaven, New York

Barbara Wilson-Clay, BSEd, IBCLC
Private Practice Lactation Consultant
Manchaca, Texas

Contributors to First Edition:

Genevieve Becker, IBCLC, MSc, Reg Nutr

Thomas W. Hale, RPh, PhD

Heather Jackson, RGON, RM, MA, IBCLC

Chele Marmet, BS, MA, IBCLC

JoAnne Scott, MA, IBCLC

Ellen Shell, IBCLC

Ruth Worgan, RN, CM, C&FH, IBCLC

MAP OF THE CORE CURRICULUM CHAPTERS

The following table is a "road map" of the objectives and standards in the IBLCE Exam cross referenced to coverage of that topic in this book. Use it as a guide to explore each discipline in depth according to the perspective provided in relevant chapters.

Discipline	Chapters
A. Maternal and infant ANATOMY Includes: breast and nipple structure and development; blood, lymph, innervation, mammary tissue; infant oral anatomy and reflexes; assessment; anatomical variations.	12, 13, 14, 15, 23, 26, 29, 36, 39
B. Maternal and infant normal PHYSIOLOGY and ENDOCRINOLOGY Includes: hormones; lactogenesis; endocrine/autocrine control of milk supply; induced lactation; fertility; infant hepatic, pancreatic and renal function; metabolism; effect of complementary feeds; digestion and GI tract; voiding and stooling patterns.	12, 14, 15, 25, 26, 27, 28, 29, 30, 32, 36, 37, 38, 39
C. Maternal and infant normal NUTRITION and BIOCHEMISTRY Includes: breast milk synthesis and composition; milk components, function, and effect on baby; comparison with other	14, 16, 17, 18, 20, 26, 27, 28, 30, 39

(continues)

Discipline	Chapters
products/milks; feeding patterns and intake over time; variations of maternal diet; ritual and traditional foods; introduction of solids.	
D. Maternal and infant IMMUNOLOGY and INFECTIOUS DISEASE Includes: antibodies and other immune factors; cross-infection; bacteria and viruses in milk; allergies and food sensitivity; long-term protective factors.	16, 19, 20, 26, 33, 38, Appendix C
E. Maternal and infant PATHOLOGY Includes: acute/chronic abnormalities and diseases (both local and systemic); breast and nipple problems and pathology; endocrine pathology; mother/child physical and neurological disabilities; congenital abnormalities; oral pathology; neurological immaturity; failure to thrive; hyperbilirubinemia and hypoglycemia; impact of pathology on breastfeeding.	13, 15, 20, 23, 26, 27, 28, 29, 30, 34, 35, 36, 37, 39, 40
F. Maternal and infant PHARMACOLOGY and TOXICOLOGY Includes: environmental contaminants; maternal use of medication, over-the-counter preparations, effects of social or recreational drugs on the infant, on milk composition, and on lactation; galactagogues/suppressants; effects of medications used in labor; contraceptives; complementary therapies.	1, 21, 22, 32, 34, 36, 37, 38, 40
G. PSYCHOLOGY, SOCIOLOGY, and ANTHROPOLOGY Includes: counseling and adult education skills; grief, postnatal depression and psychosis; effect of socio-economic, lifestyle, and employment issues on breastfeeding; maternal-infant relationship; maternal role adaptation; parenting skills; sleep patterns; cultural beliefs and practices; family; support systems; domestic violence; mothers with special needs, such as adolescents and migrants.	1, 3, 4, 5, 6, 7, 23, 25, 26, 27, 28, 29, 30, 32, 34, 35, 37

(continues)

Chronological Periods	**Chapters**
• Preconception	17, 21, 22, 35, 38
• Prenatal	6, 15, 16, 17, 19, 20, 21, 22, 27, 35, 38
• Labor and Birth (Perinatal)	5, 15, 17, 19, 24, 25, 27, 28, 30, 34, 35
• Prematurity	15, 17, 19, 21, 26, 27, 30, 37
• 0–2 Days	5, 7, 15, 17, 18, 19,20, 21, 22, 24, 25, 27, 28, 29, 30, 31, 34, 35, 36, 37, 38
• 3–14 Days	5, 6, 7, 15, 17, 18, 19, 20, 21, 22, 27, 28, 29, 30, 31, 34, 35, 36, 37, 38, 39, 40
• 15–28 Days	5, 6, 7, 17,18, 19, 20, 21, 22, 27, 28, 29, 30, 34, 35, 36, 37, 38, 39, 40
• 1–3 Months	5, 6, 7, 17, 18, 19, 20, 21, 22, 27, 28, 29, 32, 35, 36, 37, 38, 40
• 4–6 Months	5, 6, 7, 17, 18, 19, 20, 21, 22, 27, 28, 29, 32, 35, 36, 38, 40
• 7–12 Months	5, 6, 7, 17, 18, 19, 20, 21, 22, 27, 28, 29, 32, 35, 36, 38
• 12 Months and Older	7, 17, 19, 20, 27, 28, 29, 32, 36
• General Principles	2, 3, 4, 5, 7, 8, 9, 13, 16, 17, 19, 27, 28, 31, 33, 35

Profession of
Lactation Consulting

Promotion and Support

The Code of Ethics for International Board Certified Lactation Consultants: Ethical Practice

JoAnne Scott, MA, IBCLC
Revised by Ann M. Calandro, BSN, RNC, IBCLC

OBJECTIVES

- Define the purpose of the Code of Ethics for the International Board Certified Lactation Consultant (IBCLC) from the International Board of Lactation Consultant Examiners (IBLCE).
- Discuss each tenet as it relates to lactation consultant practice.
- Describe when and how to report violations of the Code of Ethics.

Introduction

The purpose of the Code of Ethics is to provide guidance to the IBCLC in professional practice and conduct. By virtue of seeking and using this credential, the IBCLC and any candidate seeking certification whose application has been approved by the IBLCE has accepted these obligations to herself or himself, the client, colleagues, society, and the profession. According to the Code of Ethics, "The International Board Certified Lactation Consultant shall act in a manner that safeguards the interests of individual clients, justifies public trust in her/his competence, and enhances the reputation of the profession." The IBCLC credential is a conditional privilege that can be revocable for cause.

The preamble to the Code states that the IBCLC is personally accountable for her/his practice and, in the exercise of professional accountability, must:

1. Tenet 1. "Provide professional services with objectivity and with respect for the unique needs and values of individuals."

    a. In practice, the IBCLC will strive to focus on the problem as presented by the client and will attempt to resolve the problem in a professional manner to the satisfaction of the client, regardless of whether that outcome is the same outcome that the IBCLC would have chosen for himself or herself. IBCLCs may work in many settings. The Code of Ethics applies to lactation consultants in hospital, home, or health office settings.

    b. The mother must be involved in the decision-making process.

        i. For example, a mother might choose not to breastfeed exclusively or may choose to wean completely before the child is one year of age.

        ii. As long as the mother has been made aware of the advantages to herself and to her child of exclusive breastfeeding for the first six months and for continuing human milk in the child's diet until he or she reaches a minimum of one year of age, it is the mother's decision how she will breastfeed.

    c. The IBCLC will collaborate with the mother to help her achieve her personal breastfeeding goals.

2. Tenet 2. "Avoid discrimination against other individuals on the basis of race, creed, religion, gender, sexual preference, age, and national origin."

    a. In practical terms, the IBCLC will provide the same skilled level of help to individuals whose circumstances or lifestyles he or she may disagree with as she does to those with whom he or she agrees.

    b. The IBCLC will make every attempt to understand the client's goals, especially when they are expressed in an idiom, custom, or context with which the IBCLC is unfamiliar or uncomfortable.

        i. For example, when consulted by a lesbian couple who wish to induce lactation in the non-biological parent, the IBCLC—who might find a homosexual lifestyle unacceptable—will provide the same competent care as he or she would to a heterosexual couple.

        ii. If the IBCLC realizes that his or her own values make giving competent care to a client difficult, then the IBCLC should make every effort to refer the client to another IBCLC who does not feel conflicted about caring for the client.

3. Tenet 3. "Fulfill professional commitments in good faith."

    a. Once a commitment has been made to help a particular client, to give a presentation, or to perform any other professional service, the IBCLC will make every effort to honor and fulfill that commitment.

4. Tenet 4. "Conduct herself/himself with honesty, integrity, and fairness."

    a. The IBCLC will abide by his or her word, will make his or her best effort to serve a client once accepted, will charge a fair price for services according to community standards, and will facilitate the client's best interests even if those interests do not coincide with the best interests of the IBCLC. IBCLCs who work in health care settings that charge for their services should encourage their institution to charge fees that are consistent with community standards. If possible, a sliding scale fee could be charged for those women who have no health coverage or financial means to pay for services, so that lactation care would be available for all women and children.

    i. For example, the IBCLC will schedule sufficient time to investigate a client's problems thoroughly and will refrain from "quick fixes," although he or she might be pressured by an employer to see more clients in a given period of time.

    ii. The IBCLC will recognize the value of being courteous, respectful, and allowing sufficient time to listen attentively to clients.

    iii. The IBCLC will assess the mother-baby dyad, recommend a plan of care, modify the plan after collaboration, and communicate the plan orally and in writing with the mother and the health care provider.

5. Tenet 5. "Remain free of conflict of interest while fulfilling the objectives and maintaining the integrity of the lactation consultant profession."

    a. The IBCLC who earns part of his or her livelihood from the rental or sale of breastfeeding aids and devices must remain aware of the conflict of interest that encourages recommending such aids when they are not necessary in order to solve particular breastfeeding problems.

        i. A common example would be breast pumps, the use of which can help to preserve breastfeeding when the mother and baby must be separated but which are not needed by every lactating mother.

        ii. Lactation consultants employed by hospitals should refrain from referring mothers to themselves if they also have a private practice. If possible, the mother should have a list of community lactation consultants from which to choose.

        iii. If possible, mothers should be given a choice, rather than having only one brand of breast pump and lactation device available.

        iv. Another example would be supplemental feeding devices that enable the baby to be supplemented at the breast; while the use of these devices certainly can be appropriate in certain circumstances, they should never substitute for careful investigation of the causes of and correction for inadequate infant weight gain.

    b. For example, the IBCLC might consider whether an inexpensive feeding tube and syringe would be just as effective in short-term feeding supplementation as an expensive manufactured feeding system.

6. Tenet 6. "Maintain confidentiality."

    a. IBCLCs have a duty to maintain confidentiality of the client, and abide by the health information privacy legislation or regulation in their country. For example, they must abide by the Health Insurance Portability and Accountability Act regulations in the United States.

    b. Lactation consultants employed in hospitals should follow their institution's policy on confidentiality and refrain from discussing identifiable details in public places (i.e., elevator, hallway).

    c. Sharing case studies with colleagues is a legitimate method of learning; however, IBCLCs must be very careful to disguise all details that could serve to identify the individual clients. Referrals, with the permission of the client, are acceptable in cases where another IBCLC may have more experience and knowledge of a particular breastfeeding problem.

    d. The number of details that need to be suppressed might vary depending on the audience with whom one intends to share the case.

      i. For example, if an IBCLC practices in a small community, details such as the baby's age, gender, and ethnic origin might be sufficient for the client to be identified by other health care providers in the community.

      ii. Those details would not need to be altered if the presentation were done in a large metropolis or at a conference at a distant location.

      iii. IBCLCs should be particularly careful to obtain permission before sharing cases on Internet lactation consultant Web sites, because these are in the public domain.

      iv. It is recommended that permission to share information be incorporated into the IBCLC's routine intake form.

7. Tenet 7. "Base his/her practice on scientific principles, and on current research and information."

    a. This principle is termed *evidence-based practice* or *research-based practice.*

    b. The IBCLC must be careful not to base parts of his or her practice on common assumptions but rather to substantiate recommendations with published, peer-reviewed literature and scientific evidence wherever possible.

    c. A corollary to this principle is that he or she must make reasonable efforts to remain up-to-date with published research and information.

    d. Where published, substantiating, scientific, medical, and/or technical information does not (yet) exist but the IBCLC has clinical experience relevant to the issue at hand, the client should be informed.

8. Tenet 8. "Take responsibility and accept accountability for personal competence in practice."

    a. Keeping current with the latest published information and research is a part of accountability for personal competence in practice.

    b. It is part of one's obligation to clients, the public, and the profession to remain current, because lactation research is ever expanding.

    c. Taking responsibility for personal competence includes understanding research tools and terminology, and developing the ability to distinguish properly designed research from faulty research.

    d. This responsibility includes acquiring clinical skills as well as knowledge.

    e. Competence involves taking the time to study with skilled practitioners, colleagues, and mentors in order to learn "hands-on" skills that cannot easily be taught by the written word.

    f. The IBLCE recommends that IBCLCs obtain professional liability insurance. In most countries, liability insurance is provided by the hospital/clinic where an IBCLC works. For private practice IBCLCs, insurance is available in many countries. It is important to pursue obtaining professional liability insurance and to obtain it if at all possible. Some IBCLCs report that their regional lactation consultant associations have arranged to obtain group rates for IBCLCs in their area. Hospital-employed lactation consultants should also maintain their own liability insurance and not rely on "blanket" liability coverage from their employer.

9. Tenet 9. "Recognize, and exercise professional judgment within, the limits of her/his qualifications. This principle includes seeking counsel and making referrals to appropriate providers."

    a. Unless the IBCLC has other health professional qualifications and is legally entitled to act within the parameters of those qualifications, he or she must keep a clear distinction in mind at all times between the "mechanical" management of breastfeeding problems, such as latch and positioning and medical management of breastfeeding, such as prescribing herbs or medications, which is beyond the parameters of their qualifications. These parameters may vary worldwide. For example, in the United States, IBCLCs who are *not* physicians, advanced practice nurses with prescribing privileges, or nurse midwives may *not* "prescribe" herbs or medications of any sort to mothers. It is acceptable to discuss the use of such herbs or medications and to share information about these herbs or medications, but the mother must be counseled to contact her health care provider before obtaining or using such herbs or medications.

    b. The IBCLC will refer to the International Lactation Consultant Association's "Standards of Practice for International Board Certified Lactation Consultants" for guidance in practice (see Appendix A).

        i. For example, the IBCLC is within his or her scope of practice to become concerned at excessive infant weight loss or inadequate weight gain, but he or she is not qualified to recommend a specific brand of infant formula for immediate supplementation. The IBCLC's role would be to inform the appropriate primary health care provider of concerns and to help the mother maintain the breastfeeding relationship while supplementing the baby and working to increase the maternal milk supply.

        ii. Another example would be when the IBCLC suspects a fungal infection on the mother's nipples because of clinical symptoms and a predisposing history. The IBCLC cannot make a diagnosis. The IBCLC can inform the client of what is suspected, but clinically relevant information should be forwarded to the client's primary health care provider for medical review and follow-up.

   iii. If clinical concerns involve both mother and baby and each has a different primary health care provider, a copy of the report should be sent to both.

   iv. Documentation must be done correctly, thoroughly, and in a timely way.

   v. It is the responsibility of the IBCLC to understand how to document legally.

     1. For example, all documentation must be done in ink rather than with a pencil that could be erased.

     2. It is never acceptable to change or "white out" information after documentation; however, if it is found to be incorrect, the information may be marked through and initialed by the IBCLC.

     3. When an IBCLC uses electronic charting, it is important to abide by the regulations of the institution where he or she works. Changes or additions to electronic charting in a home setting also should be noted if they are made. This is for the protection of the IBCLC.

   vi. A court of law cannot protect the IBCLC who does not document because as far as the law is concerned, if it was not documented, it was not done.

  c. When the IBCLC encounters puzzling aspects of a case that appear to be non-medical in nature, he or she should confer with colleagues for additional perspectives or research information about the problem in current literature.

  d. Where in the judgment of the IBCLC, either member of the client pair would benefit from consultation with another allied health care provider (for example, a physical therapist, or dietitian), the IBCLC should include this suggestion in the report to the primary health care provider along with names of practitioners of these specialties whom the IBCLC has found to be clinically skillful and supportive of breastfeeding.

10. Tenet 10. "Inform the public and colleagues of her/his services by using factual information. An International Board Certified Lactation Consultant will not advertise in a false or misleading manner."

  a. An IBCLC will not allow descriptions of his or her services to imply unrealistic outcomes or fees.

   i. For example, not all breastfeeding problems can be solved with good information and instruction, and to imply that seeking the services of a particular practitioner will ensure success is false.

   ii. To advertise fees that would cover only a standard 15 or 30 minute visit is misleading because most consultations take an hour or longer.

   iii. Lactation consultants employed in a hospital or clinic setting should check that their services are accurately marketed by the institution.

11. Tenet 11. "Provide sufficient information to enable clients to make informed decisions."
    a. It is the duty of the IBCLC to provide the client with all information that is relevant to the purpose of his or her consultation, taking into account the client's ability to understand and absorb information at this time.
        i. For example, a mother might make the decision not to continue breastfeeding because the actions needed to resolve the problem will require more time and energy than she is realistically willing to give.
        ii. The IBCLC might have made a different personal decision under similar circumstances, but the temptation to minimize difficulties and withhold factual information in order to encourage the mother to persevere must be resisted.
        iii. If barriers to communication exist between the IBCLC and the client because of significant differences in formal education, culture, or language, it is the IBCLC's duty to work even harder to communicate the full range of options in a clear, simple, and unambiguous manner. If interpreter services are available, they should be utilized as the first choice in interpreting. Interpreter services are more likely to interpret in an unbiased manner and to interpret information more completely than would a friend or family member.
        iv. Institutional barriers regarding what can be said to breastfeeding patients should be addressed. Some hospital cultures and health providers may try to restrict certain breastfeeding information given to their patients.
12. Tenet 12. "Provide information about appropriate products in a manner that is neither false nor misleading."
    a. The ethical advocacy of breastfeeding aids and devices for the IBCLC consists of these tools' appropriateness to solve breastfeeding problems or to make life easier for the breastfeeding mother.
    b. To recommend the use of a product and then to sell or rent it to the client might be a practical necessity, but it gives the appearance of a conflict of interest.
    c. IBCLCs who engage in commercial promotion of these items must be especially careful not to recommend products in ambiguous situations but rather to discuss their pros and cons and to make it completely clear when a less expensive product will serve the purpose just as well as a more expensive one.
        i. For example, when an IBCLC recommends spoon or cup feeding to a baby who needs to be supplemented, he or she should show the parents inexpensive medicine spoons and mention cups that the parents might already have at home as well as showing relatively expensive, specialized cups and soft, flexible spoons with one-way valves. The IBCLC should always allow the parents to make their own decisions about which tool they choose to use.

    d. IBCLCs who teach mothers how to use a product have the responsibility to provide follow-up care with the mother to ensure that the product is effective and useful.

        i. For example, if an IBCLC teaches a mother to use a nipple shield to assist her baby with latching either in the hospital or after hospital discharge, it is important to stay in contact with the mother who is breastfeeding with the shield in place, to ensure that the baby is obtaining sufficient milk and is growing appropriately.

13. Tenet 13. "Permit use of her/his name for the purpose of certifying that lactation consultant services have been rendered only if she/he provided those services."

    a. An IBCLC who employs or supervises uncertified people who work with breastfeeding mothers and babies cannot allow clients, other health care providers, or third-party reimbursement agencies to assume that these uncertified practitioners are board certified lactation consultants.

    b. In order to protect the credential, the IBCLC must make it routinely and abundantly clear that those individuals who have provided services are not International Board Certified Lactation Consultants certified by the IBLCE.

14. Tenet 14. "Present professional qualifications and credentials accurately, using "IBCLC" only when certification is current and authorized by the IBLCE, and complying with all requirements when seeking initial or continued certification from the IBLCE. The lactation consultant is subject to disciplinary action for aiding another person in violating any IBLCE requirements or aiding another person in violating any IBLCE requirements or aiding another person in representing herself/himself as an IBCLC when she/he is not."

    a. Continuing to represent oneself as an IBCLC after certification has lapsed, or permitting oneself to be described or advertised as such, is in breach of copyright and will be grounds for denying eligibility if the person should ever seek to certify again.

    b. Use of terms such as *IBCLC candidate* or *student IBCLC* are potentially misleading to the public and also can only be grounds for denying eligibility should certification ever be sought.

    c. False or misleading statements or information or incorrect reporting of practice hours on applications for initial candidacy will result in eligibility being denied, disciplinary action being imposed, or revocation of certification if discovered after the applicant has passed the exam.

    d. False or misleading statements on applications for recertification are also grounds for de-certification.

    e. The IBCLC who allows the public to assume that he or she has other health care credentials when he or she does not (for example, nursing or midwifery) is also in breach of this tenet of the Code of Ethics.

f. If an IBCLC has knowledge that another is representing himself or herself as an IBCLC when that person is not currently certified, and does not report this to the IBLCE, this is a violation of the code.

15. Tenet 15. "Report to an appropriate person or authority when it appears that the health or safety of colleagues is at risk, as such circumstances may compromise standards of practice and care."

   a. Knowingly permitting a colleague to continue to practice as an IBCLC when that person's health or safety is at risk, and whose condition might compromise client care, endangers not only the mothers and babies whose welfare is our primary duty but also endangers the reputation of the credential.

      i. For example, if a colleague is engaging in substance abuse, although that person might seem to avoid substance use when on duty, judgment might be impaired and the individual might use the substance when seeing clients if the IBCLC is under unusual stress.

      ii. It is the duty of the IBCLC to bring such situations to the attention of appropriate authorities.

16. Tenet 16. "Refuse any gift, favor, or hospitality from patients or clients currently in her/his care which might be interpreted as seeking to exert influence to obtain preferential consideration."

   a. This statement in the code is not meant to direct IBCLCs to refuse small token gifts of appreciation from clients, which are customary in many cultures. Hospital-based IBCLCs are required to abide by their institution's guidelines for accepting gifts. Some hospitals do not allow employees to accept any gifts, and other hospitals place a limit on types of gifts and amounts of gifts that are deemed to be acceptable.

   b. The tenet is intended to alert IBCLCs to the possibility that judgment can be influenced by gifts or contributions.

      i. For example, an IBCLC who owns a business or makes decisions about which products will be carried by the health care institution in which he or she is employed is in a position to be influenced by such favors to carry certain products for sale to mothers and to exclude other products.

      ii. Favors might influence which products are selected to be used in connection with lactation research and which products are mentioned in published results.

   c. The IBCLC must be careful to avoid the appearance of a conflict of interest.

17. Tenet 17. "Disclose any financial or other conflicts of interest in relevant organizations providing goods or services. Ensure that professional judgment is not influenced by any commercial considerations."

   a. For example, an IBCLC who is employed by a health care facility might also be engaged in private practice.

   b. Referral in his or her employee capacity to the private practice, without disclosing the connection, would violate this principle of the Code of Ethics.

   c. An IBCLC who receives a stipend, honorarium, or grant from an organization that has commercial ties to lactation should disclose this connection before presenting or publishing, if relevant.

18. Tenet 18. "Present substantiated information and interpret controversial information without personal bias, recognizing that legitimate differences of opinion exist."

   a. The IBCLC should present substantiated evidence-based information to clients and colleagues whenever possible.

   b. Clinical experience and new information that is not yet substantiated might have valuable bearing on the issue at hand and should be presented without personal bias and with courtesy and respect for differing opinions.

   c. Sometimes collegial behavior and courtesy to other members of one's profession can be problematic, especially when there are strong differences of opinion.

   d. Courtesy toward colleagues is expected both in person and in public forums such as Internet sites.

   e. While noncollegial behavior is seldom a factual basis for a violation of the Code of Ethics, the IBCLC is reminded that public arguments discredit all parties and jeopardize public trust and the profession itself.

19. Tenet 19. "Withdraw voluntarily from professional practice if she/he has engaged in any substance abuse that could affect her/his practice; has been adjudged by a court to be mentally incompetent; or has a physical, emotional or mental disability that affects her/his practice in a manner that could harm the client."

   a. Colleagues might need to help an IBCLC to realize that he or she is breaching this tenet of the code because substance abuse, mental incompetence, or physical, emotional, or mental disability can impair the IBCLC's capacity to realize that he or she could harm mothers and babies.

   b. Voluntary surrender of the credential will cause the Board of Examiners to look favorably upon resumption of its use once the disability has been ameliorated.

20. Tenet 20. "Obtain maternal consent to photograph, audiotape, or videotape a mother and/or her infant(s) for educational or professional purposes."

   a. Such consent should be obtained in writing, dated and should clearly limit the use of the material to professional audiences.

   b. The material to which consent has been given should be described on the consent document. IBCLCs are advised to develop standard consent forms and to have the content of such forms reviewed by an attorney or legal expert.

   c. The employed (as opposed to the self-employed) IBCLC is advised to obtain the consent of the employer, as well.

    d. Most hospitals have "consent to photograph" forms available that employees are required to use.

    e. Unauthorized use of photographs or using them for an audience other than the permission for use was granted constitutes invasion of privacy.

21. Tenet 21. "Submit to disciplinary action under the following circumstances: If convicted of a crime under the laws of the practitioner's country which is a felony or a misdemeanor, an essential element of which is dishonesty, and which is related to the practice of lactation consulting; if disciplined by a national, state, province, or local government or authority, and at least one of the grounds for the discipline is the same or substantially equivalent to these principles; if committed an act of misfeasance or malfeasance which is directly related to the practice of the profession as determined by a court of competent jurisdiction, a licensing board, or an agency of a governmental body; or if violated a principle set forth in the *Code of Ethics for International Board Certified Lactation Consultants* which was in force at the time of the violation."

    a. Any IBCLC who is convicted of a crime involving dishonesty that is related to IBCLC practice is required to report this conviction to the IBLCE.

    b. Any IBCLC who has been disciplined by a governmental agency, a licensing board, or a court for an act that is a crime, or is a violation of a tenet, or that results in the loss of the IBCLC's license, is required to report to the IBLCE the action taken by the governmental agency, the licensing board, or the court.

    c. Colleagues might need to remind an IBCLC of this duty, or to report such a conviction or disciplinary action to the chair of the Ethics and Discipline Committee if a voluntary report is not made by the individual concerned.

    d. An IBCLC who has first-hand knowledge about another IBCLC's violation of a tenet is required to file an Ethics and Discipline Complaint describing the violation if the IBCLC involved fails to change his or her conduct in compliance with the requirements of the Code of Ethics after being advised of the infraction.

    e. If an IBCLC Board Member or Staff Member receives a written certificate from the clerk of any court with valid jurisdiction stating that an IBLCE Certificant or Applicant has been convicted of a crime, the IBLCE will suspend the convicted person's IBLCE certification until a determination (after a hearing) can be made by the Ethics and Discipline Committee.

    f. Violations that take place before the relevant tenet was adopted do not constitute grounds for disciplinary action.

22. Tenet 22. "Accept the obligation to protect society and the profession by upholding the *Code of Ethics for International Board Certified Lactation Consultants* and by reporting alleged violations of the Code through the defined review process of the IBLCE."

a. It is the IBCLC's duty not only to adhere to the principles of the Code of Ethics himself/herself but also to bring violations on the part of other certificants to the attention of the IBLCE.

b. A careful and thorough investigation will follow and will provide the accused party (respondent) with every opportunity to respond in a professional and legally defensible manner.

c. Only signed, written complaints will be considered.

d. The person against whom the complaint has been brought (respondent) will receive a copy of the complaint and will be notified of the name of the complainant as well as the tenets that were allegedly violated.

e. The IBCLC should encourage others, such as members of the supervising and coordinating professions, and employers and clients who have direct knowledge of violations, to report as well.

f. A profession that does not police itself forfeits the public's trust.

g. Complaints should be mailed to:
   i. Chair, Ethics and Discipline Committee
   International Board of Lactation Consultant Examiners
   7245 Arlington Blvd., Suite 200
   Falls Church, Virginia 22042-3217 USA

h. E-mail questions should be sent to: ethics@iblce.org. The IBLCE staff cannot answer hypothetical questions.

i. Complaint forms can be downloaded from the IBLCE Web site (http://www.iblce.org).

23. Tenet 23. "Require and obtain consent to share clinical concerns and information with the medical practitioner or other primary health care provider before initiating a consultation."

a. For the IBCLC in private practice or who works in an outpatient clinic, language giving consent to share clinical concerns and information with the physician or other primary health care provider should be incorporated into routine intake forms and signed by the client before the consultation begins.
   i. For employed IBCLCs, such consent is usually incorporated into admitting forms in health care facilities.
   ii. Entries made in patient charts, routinely reviewed by the primary health care provider, should be sufficient except in emergency situations.
   iii. IBCLCs who are in private practice are advised to secure a legal review of consent language and, for their own safety, to decline consulting with clients who refuse to sign such consent or who refuse to list a primary health care provider.
   iv. Unless the IBCLC is also a primary health care provider, the IBCLC endangers himself or herself as well as the client by practicing without medical review.

v. These statements apply to an IBCLC conducting a consultation, and not when engaged in assisting a woman who chooses a breast pump or instructing a woman in how to maintain lactation when she returns to work.

vi. Refuse to consult with a client who asks the IBCLC to keep secrets from the health care provider.

24. Tenet 24. "Adhere to those provisions of the *International Code of Marketing of Breast-milk Substitutes,* and subsequent WHA resolutions, which pertain to health workers." (See Appendix B.)

a. Portions of the International Code that apply to health workers include the following:

i. Do not give free samples of breast milk substitutes to parents or other relatives of a new baby. (If it is determined during a consultation that an infant is not thriving, must be fed, and breast milk is unavailable, then it is acceptable practice for the IBCLC to supply emergency supplementation at that time in conjunction with the infant's primary care provider.)

ii. Do not promote such products in health care facilities.

iii. Do not accept gifts from manufacturers or distributors of such products, and do not accept samples for personal use.

b. If item a is part of the job description for IBCLCs, discuss with the employer the possibility of delegating this task to others, because the employer may not be aware of the IBCLC's obligations to uphold the World Health Organization Code. Hospital employees may have the option to conscientiously object to this practice and to sign a form stating their objection to giving out infant formula or commercial bags or samples.

c. It is acceptable to attend in-services in health care settings in order to be informed about products and to share information, as long as food and gifts are not accepted by the IBCLC.

d. The IBCLC is expected to take every opportunity to educate coworkers, supervisors, and administrators about the detrimental effects of marketing breast milk substitutes to consumers.

25. Tenet 25. "Understand, recognize, respect, and acknowledge intellectual property rights, including but not limited to copyrights (which apply to written material, photographs, slides, illustrations, etc.), trademarks, service marks, and patents."

a. The IBCLC will not use materials developed by others in ways that may violate their intellectual property rights unless he or she has received written permission to use materials such as handouts, educational programs, artwork, or slides.

b. Even if the material does not have a copyright mark, it belongs to the author, photographer, or artist and cannot be used without permission.

c. Give credit to authors in presentations when discussing their published work.

    d. Seek accurate educational materials for which the author has given permission to freely copy and distribute for educational purposes.

    e. Rather than copying valuable educational copyrighted articles, share links to Web sites so that participants can research and read these articles themselves.

Conclusion

The Code of Ethics is a non-negotiable standard for every IBCLC. All IBCLCs should be familiar with the 25 Tenets of the Code, and should refer to the Code in making practice decisions. The Ethics and Discipline committee convenes twice a year to discuss signed complaints. As of September 2006, two complaints have led to revocation of certification, one complaint has led to a public reprimand of an IBCLC, five complaints have led to private reprimands, and 20 complaints have been dismissed. Even if the case was dismissed, these IBCLCs experienced worry and concern during the disciplinary process. In many cases, poor communication and the client feeling disrespected caused the complaint to be issued. Had the IBCLC paid careful attention to his or her client, listened attentively, and used effective communication techniques, most likely there would have been no complaint filed. Because ethics are so important to IBCLCs, the Board of Directors approved a recommendation that education in ethics be required for recertification by Continuing Education Recognition Points (CERPs). Five hours of Category E CERPs are required to be part of the 75 CERP hour totals every five years for those IBCLCs recertifying by CERPs.

    Lactation consultants take ethics seriously. It is an honor to be a member of a profession that protects breastfeeding and respects the rights of mothers and babies.

References

Anonymous. Standards for privacy of individually identifiable health information: final rule. In: *HIPAA: Health Insurance Portability and Accountability Act* (under Security Tab) (2002, August 14). Available at: http://www.hipaa.org/. Accessed September 4, 2006.

International Board Certified Lactation Consultant Examiners (IBLCE). *Code of Ethics*. Available at: http://www.iblce.org. Accessed September 4, 2006.

International Lactation Consultant Association (ILCA). *Standards of Practice*. Available at: http://ilca.org. Accessed September 4, 2006.

World Health Organization (WHO). *International Code of Marketing of Breast-milk Substitutes* (1981). Available at: http://www.who.int/nutrition/publications/code_english.pdf. Accessed September 4, 2006.

International Initiatives to Promote, Protect, and Support Breastfeeding

Karin Cadwell, PhD, FAAN, RN, IBCLC

OBJECTIVE

- Discuss international statements and documents that are used as tools to protect, promote, and support breastfeeding.

Introduction

Alarmed over the unnecessary deaths related to the industry-created bottle-feeding culture, two agencies of the United Nations, the World Health Organization (WHO) and the United Nations Children's Fund (UNICEF), held an international meeting in 1979 concerning infant and young child feeding. The ultimate result was the creation of the International Code of Marketing of Breast-milk Substitutes. The International Code of Marketing and subsequent resolutions have been approved in the World Health Assembly. This document and others strive to replace the commercial barriers to breastfeeding with protection for a health-related behavior that is in danger of extinction. In 2002, WHO and UNICEF jointly endorsed the Global Strategy for Infant and Young Child Feeding, which builds on successful programs of the past.

"Malnutrition has been responsible, directly or indirectly, for 60% of the 10.9 million deaths annually among children under five. Well over two-thirds of these deaths, which are often associated with inappropriate feeding practices, occur during the first year of life. No more than 35% of infants worldwide are exclusively breastfed during the first four months of life; complementary feeding frequently begins too early or too late, and foods are often nutritionally inadequate and unsafe. Malnourished children who survive are more frequently sick and suffer the life-long consequences of impaired development. Rising incidences of overweight and obesity in children are also a matter of serious concern. Because poor feeding practices are a major threat to social and economic development, they are among the most serious obstacles to attaining and maintaining health that face this age group" (World Health Organization, 2003, p. 5).

I. The Global Strategy for Infant and Young Child Feeding

A. The Global Strategy for Infant and Young Child Feeding was jointly endorsed in 2002 by WHO and UNICEF. This publication renewed the commitment of these organizations to continuing joint efforts including the Baby-Friendly Hospital Initiative™ (BFHI), the International Code of Marketing of Breast-milk Substitutes, and the Innocenti Declaration on the Protection, Promotion and Support of Breastfeeding. The Global Strategy urges countries to "formulate, implement, monitor and evaluate a comprehensive national policy on infant and young child feeding," and includes "ensuring sufficient maternity leave to promote exclusive breastfeeding."

B. According to the Global Strategy, appropriate infant and young child feeding practices include:

- Exclusive breastfeeding for six months.

- Timely initiation of nutritionally adequate and safe complementary foods while continuing breastfeeding up to two years or beyond.

- Appropriate feeding of infants and young children living in especially difficult circumstances (low-birth-weight infants, infants of human immunodeficiency virus (HIV)-positive mothers, infants in emergency situations, malnourished infants, etc.).

C. The strategy calls for action in the following areas:

- "All governments should develop and implement a comprehensive policy on infant and young child feeding, in the context of national policies for nutrition, child and reproductive health, and poverty reduction.

- All mothers should have access to skilled support to initiate and sustain exclusive breastfeeding for six months, and ensure the timely introduction of adequate and safe complementary foods with continued breastfeeding up to two years or beyond.

- Health care workers should be empowered to provide effective feeding counseling, and their services should be extended in the community by trained lay or peer counselors.

- Governments should review progress in national implementation of the International Code of Marketing of Breast-milk Substitutes, and consider new legislation or additional measures as needed to protect families from adverse commercial influences.

- Governments should enact imaginative legislation protecting the breastfeeding rights of working women and establishing means for its enforcement in accordance with international labor standards."

The strategy specifies not only responsibilities of governments, but also of international organizations, nongovernmental organizations (NGOs), and other concerned parties. It engages all relevant stakeholders and provides a framework for accelerated action, linking relevant intervention areas and using resources available in a variety of sectors.

II. The International Code of Marketing of Breast-milk Substitutes

A. Doubts and pressures about "not enough milk" have been cleverly communicated to mothers by manufacturers of breast milk substitutes, feeding bottles, and teats.

B. WHO and UNICEF drafted the Code of Marketing of Breast-milk Substitutes, which was adopted by the World Health Assembly (WHA) in May 1981. An international recommendation, the Code is put into effect at the national level. According to the International Baby Food Action Network (IBFAN), by 1998 over 116 countries had taken some action to implement the International Code and over half the world's population now live in countries where laws are in place that broadly incorporate its main provisions.

C. The IBFAN set up the International Code Documentation Centre (ICDC) with the task of keeping track of code compliance both by governments and by companies. IBFAN's work also includes:

- Networking with partners around the world in a spirit of solidarity for mutual support and empowerment.

- Advocacy for the International Code and Resolutions in national and international measures.

- Capacity building and Code training courses for NGOs, consumers, and policy makers in all parts of the world.

- Monitoring the state of implementation of and compliance with the International Code and Resolutions.

- Awareness-raising through publications, the media, and grassroots outreach.

- Coordinating manufacturer campaigns (such as the Nestlé boycott).

- Policy development on food standards, maternity legislation, emergency relief, and HIV.

D. Further resolutions have clarified and strengthened the Code, including a statement that member states "ensure that there are no donations of free or subsidized supplies of breast milk substitutes and other products" covered by the Code. This resolution forbids health care facilities to accept free or low-cost supplies.

E. The 1996 WHA Resolution urged member states to "ensure that complementary foods are not marketed for or used in ways that undermine exclusive and sustained breastfeeding."

F. The scope of the Code applies to the marketing and practices related to:

- Breast milk substitutes, including infant formula; other milk products, foods, and beverages, including bottle-fed complementary foods, when marketed or otherwise represented to be suitable, with or without modification, for use as a partial or total replacement of breast milk.
- Feeding bottles and teats.
- The quality, availability, and information concerning the use of products mentioned above.

G. Promotion to the public and the health care system of products covered by the Code:

- There should be no advertising or other form of promotion (such as free samples or gifts of articles or utensils) to the general public of products within the scope of the Code. There should be no promotion to health care workers as a means of indirect promotion to the public.
- The Code also charges governments with the responsibility to "ensure that objective and consistent information is provided on infant and young child feeding."
- Covered are the planning, provision, design, and dissemination of information or their control.

H. There is a gray area between information and promotion that may be easily crossed by manufacturers and cast doubt on a woman's ability to breastfeed.

I. Labeling is also covered under the Code.

Labels should offer information about the appropriate use of the product in a way that does not discourage breastfeeding. The label should be clear and understandable, using appropriate language, with no pictures of infants. Some countries also require the age recommended for introduction of particular infant foods, as well as certain health claims (such as the use of the word "hypoallergenic").

J. Definitions of terms used in the Code.

- *Breast milk substitute* means any food being marketed or otherwise represented as a partial or total replacement for breast milk, whether or not suitable for that purpose.
- *Infant formula* means a breast milk substitute formulated industrially in accordance with applicable Codex Alimentarius standards, to satisfy the normal nutritional requirements of infants up to between four and six months of age, and adapted to their physiological characteristics. Infant formula can also be prepared at home, in which case it is described as *home-prepared.*
- *Complementary food* means any food, whether manufactured or locally prepared, that is suitable as a complement to breast milk or to infant formula, when either becomes insufficient to satisfy the nutritional requirements of the infant. Such food is also commonly called weaning food or breast milk supplement.

III. Relevant Parts of World Health Assembly Resolutions

A. WHA 39.28: "Any food or drink given before complementary feeding is nutritionally required may interfere with the initiation or maintenance of breastfeeding and therefore should neither be promoted nor encouraged for use by infants during this period; The practice being introduced in some countries of providing infants with specially formulated milks (so-called follow-up milks) is not necessary."

B. WHA 47.5: Member States are urged to "foster appropriate complementary feeding from the age of about six months."

C. WHA 49.15: Member States are urged to "ensure that complementary foods are not marketed for or used in ways that undermine exclusive and sustained breastfeeding."

D. At the 58th World Health Assembly (May 2005), results of the joint Food and Agriculture Organization (FAO)/(WHO) expert meeting on *Enterobacter sakazakii* and other microorganisms in powdered infant formula, which had been held in 2004, were brought forward. The expert meeting concluded that intrinsic contamination of powdered infant formula with *E. sakazakii and Salmonella* had been a cause of infection and illness, including severe disease in infants, particularly preterm, low-birth-weight, or immunocompromised infants, and could lead to serious developmental sequelae and death. There was recognition of the need for parents and caregivers to be fully informed of evidence-based public health risks of intrinsic contamination of powdered infant formula and the potential for introduced contamination, and the need for safe preparation, handling, and storage of prepared infant formula. The WHA urged Member States:

1. "to continue to protect, promote and support exclusive breastfeeding for six months as a global public health recommendation, taking into account the findings of the WHO Expert Consultation on optimal duration of exclusive breastfeeding, and to provide for continued breastfeeding up to two years of age or beyond, by implementing fully the WHO global strategy on infant and young-child feeding that encourages the formulation of a comprehensive national policy, including where appropriate a legal framework to promote maternity leave and a supportive environment for six months' exclusive breastfeeding, a detailed plan of action to implement, monitor and evaluate the policy, and allocation of adequate resources for this process;

2. to ensure that nutrition and health claims are not permitted for breast-milk substitutes, except where specifically provided for in national legislation;

3. to ensure that clinicians and other health-care personnel, community health workers and families, parents and other caregivers, particularly of infants at high risk, are provided with enough information and training by health-care providers, in a timely manner on the preparation, use and handling of

powdered infant formula in order to minimize health hazards; are informed that powdered infant formula may contain pathogenic microorganisms and must be prepared and used appropriately; and, where applicable, that this information is conveyed through an explicit warning on packaging;

4. to ensure that financial support and other incentives for programs and health professionals working in infant and young-child health do not create conflicts of interest;

5. to ensure that research on infant and young-child feeding, which may form the basis for public policies, always contains a declaration relating to conflicts of interest and is subject to independent peer review;

6. to work closely with relevant entities, including manufacturers, to continue to reduce the concentration and prevalence of pathogens, including *Enterobacter sakazakii,* in powdered infant formula;

7. to continue to ensure that manufacturers adhere to Codex Alimentarius or national food standards and regulations;

8. to ensure policy coherence at national levels by stimulating collaboration between health authorities, food regulators and food standard-setting bodies;

9. to participate actively and constructively in the work of the Codex Alimentarius Commission;

10. to ensure that all national agencies involved in defining national positions on public health issues for use in all relevant international forums, including the Codex Alimentarius Commission, have a common and consistent understanding of health policies adopted by the Health Assembly, and to promote these policies."

IV. The Baby-Friendly Hospital Initiative™

A. The BFHI was designed to rid hospitals of their dependence on breast milk substitutes and to encourage maternity services to be supportive of breastfeeding.

B. Launched in June 1991 at a meeting of the International Pediatric Association in Ankara, Turkey, by WHO and UNICEF, the global initiative is aimed at promoting the adoption of the "Ten Steps to Successful Breastfeeding" (see below) in hospitals worldwide.

C. The BFHI is designed to remove hospital barriers to breastfeeding by creating a supportive environment with trained and knowledgeable health care workers.

D. The 10 steps to successful breastfeeding:

1. Have a written breastfeeding policy that is routinely communicated to all health care staff.

2. Train all health care staff in skills necessary to implement this policy.

3. Inform all pregnant women about the benefits and management of breastfeeding.

4. Help mothers initiate breastfeeding within a half hour (one hour in the United States) of birth.

5. Show mothers how to breastfeed and how to maintain lactation even if they should be separated from their infants.

6. Give newborn infants no food or drink other than breast milk unless medically indicated.

7. Practice rooming-in: enable mothers and infants to remain together 24 hours a day.

8. Encourage breastfeeding on demand.

9. Give no artificial teats or pacifiers (also called dummies or soothers) to breastfeeding infants.

10. Foster the establishment of breastfeeding support groups and refer mothers to them upon discharge from the hospital or clinic.

V. The FAO/WHO International Conference on Nutrition

A. The FAO/WHO International Conference on Nutrition was held in Rome, Italy in December 1992, and signatories adopted the World Declaration on Nutrition and the Plan of Action for Nutrition. Article 19 of the World Declaration on Nutrition pledged "to reduce substantially within this decade social and other impediments to optimal breastfeeding."

B. The plan of action endorsed breastfeeding under sections on preventing and managing infectious diseases and preventing and controlling specific micronutrient deficiencies. The action also called for the promotion of breastfeeding by governments by providing maximum support for women to breastfeed.

VI. The Innocenti Declaration

A. The Innocenti Declaration was adopted at a meeting sponsored jointly by UNICEF, WHO, the United States Agency for International Development, and the Swedish International Development Authority in Florence, Italy in August 1990. The Innocenti Declaration calls for concrete actions for governments to take by 1995.

B. Attainment of Innocenti goals requires, in many countries, the reinforcement of a "breastfeeding culture" and the vigorous defense against incursions of a "bottle-feeding culture."

C. Operational targets: All national governments by the year 1995 should have:

1. Appointed a national breastfeeding coordinator of appropriate authority and established a multisector national breastfeeding committee composed of representatives from relevant governmental departments, nongovernmental organizations, and health professional associations.

2. Ensured that every facility providing maternity services fully practices all 10 of the Ten Steps to Successful Breastfeeding set out in the joint WHO/UNICEF statement, "Protecting, promoting and supporting breastfeeding: the special role of maternity services."

3. Taken action to implement the principles and aim of all articles of the International Code of Marketing of Breast-milk Substitutes and subsequent relevant WHA resolutions in their entirety.

4. Enacted imaginative legislation protecting the breastfeeding rights of working women and established means for its enforcement.

D. All international organizations were called upon by the Innocenti Declaration to:

- Draw up action strategies for protecting, promoting, and supporting breastfeeding, including global monitoring of the evaluation of their strategies.

- Support national situation analyses and surveys and the development of national goals and targets for action.

- Encourage and support national authorities in planning, implementing, monitoring, and evaluating their breastfeeding policies.

E. The Innocenti Declaration was adopted by the World Summit for Children in September 1990 and by the 45th World Health Assembly in May 1992 in Resolution WHA 45.34.

VII. Innocenti + 15

A. The targets of the 1990 Innocenti Declaration and the 2002 Global Strategy for Infant and Young Child Feeding remain the foundation for action. While remarkable progress has been made, much more needs to be done.

B. Innocenti + 15 issued this Call for Action so that all parties:

- "Empower women in their own right, and as mothers and providers of breastfeeding support and information to other women.

- Support breastfeeding as the norm for feeding infants and young children.

- Highlight the risks of artificial feeding and the implications for health and development throughout the life course.

- Ensure the health and nutritional status of women throughout all stages of life.

- Protect breastfeeding in emergencies, including by supporting uninterrupted breastfeeding and appropriate complementary feeding, and avoiding general distribution of breast-milk substitutes.

- Implement the HIV and Infant Feeding–Framework for Priority Action, including protecting, promoting and supporting breastfeeding for the general population while providing counseling and support for HIV-positive women."

C. All governments were called upon to:

- "Establish or strengthen national infant and young child feeding and breastfeeding authorities, coordinating committees and oversight groups that are free from commercial influence and other conflicts of interest.

- Revitalize the Baby-Friendly Hospital Initiative™ (BFHI), maintaining the Global Criteria as the minimum requirement for all facilities, expanding the Initiative's application to include maternity, neonatal and child health services and community-based support for lactating women and caregivers of young children.

- Implement all provisions of the International Code of Marketing of Breast-Milk Substitutes and subsequent relevant World Health Assembly resolutions in their entirety as a minimum requirement, and establish sustainable enforcement mechanisms to prevent and/or address non-compliance.

- Adopt maternity protection legislation and other measures that facilitate six months of exclusive breastfeeding for women employed in all sectors, with urgent attention to the non-formal sector.

- Ensure that appropriate guidelines and skill acquisition regarding infant and young child feeding are included in both pre-service and in-service training of all health care staff, to enable them to implement infant and young child feeding policies and to provide a high standard of breastfeeding management and counseling to support mothers to practice optimal breastfeeding and complementary feeding.

- Ensure that all mothers are aware of their rights and have access to support, information and counseling in breastfeeding and complementary feeding from health workers and peer groups.

- Establish sustainable systems for monitoring infant and young child feeding patterns and trends and use this information for advocacy and programming.

- Encourage the media to provide positive images of optimal infant and young child feeding, to support breastfeeding as the norm, and to participate in social mobilization activities such as World Breastfeeding Week.

- Take measures to protect populations, especially pregnant and breastfeeding mothers, from environmental contaminants and chemical residues.

- Identify and allocate sufficient resources to fully implement actions called for in the Global Strategy for Infant and Young Child Feeding.

- Monitor progress in appropriate infant and young child feeding practices and report periodically, including as provided in the Convention on the Rights of the Child."

D. All manufacturers and distributors of products within the scope of the International Code were called upon to:

- "Ensure full compliance with all provisions of the International Code and subsequent relevant World Health Assembly resolutions in all countries, independently of any other measures taken to implement the Code.

- Ensure that all processed foods for infants and young children meet applicable Codex Alimentarius standards."

VIII. The International Baby Food Action Network

A. IBFAN was created at the WHO/UNICEF Meeting on Infant and Young Child Feeding, which took place in Geneva, Switzerland in October 1979.

B. By the end of the meeting, representatives from six of the NGOs attending decided to form the IBFAN.

C. One of IBFAN's objectives was to monitor the marketing practices of the industry around the world and to share and publicize the information gathered.

D. The group also stated that "there should be an international code of marketing of infant formula and other products used as breast milk substitutes."

E. IBFAN has also set up the ICDC with the task of keeping track of code compliance both by governments and by companies.

IX. WHO Global Data Bank on Breastfeeding

A. The WHO Global Data Bank on Breastfeeding is maintained in the Nutrition Unit of WHO in Geneva. Information from national and regional surveys and studies is pooled that deals specifically with breastfeeding prevalence and duration.

B. Reports are prepared on breastfeeding trends in countries for which data are available. Every effort is made to achieve worldwide coverage.

X. Pontificiae Academiae Scientiarum Documenta 28

A. The Pontifical Academy of Sciences and the Royal Society held a Working Group on: Breastfeeding: Science and Society on May 11–13, 1995, at the Vatican.

B. The meeting was part of an overall study on population and resources.

C. Pope Pius XII had urged Catholic mothers to nourish their children themselves. Pope John Paul II emphasized that "mothers need time, information and support in order to breastfeed; no one can substitute for the mother in this natural activity."

XI. Protection, promotion and support of breastfeeding in Europe: a blueprint for action (Developed and written by participants of the project: Promotion of Breastfeeding in Europe.)

Under six headings, the document, *"Protection, promotion and support of breastfeeding in Europe: a blueprint for action"* intends that its application will achieve a Europe-wide improvement in breastfeeding practices and rates (initiation, exclusivity, and duration); more parents who are confident, empowered and satisfied with their breastfeeding experience; and health care workers with improved skills and greater job satisfaction.

References

Division of Child Health and Development. Evidence for the ten steps to successful breastfeeding. Geneva: World Health Organization; 1998.

European Union. EU Project on Promotion of Breastfeeding in Europe. Protection, promotion and support of breastfeeding in Europe: a blueprint for action. European Commission, Directorate Public Health and Risk Assessment, Luxembourg; 2004. Available at: http://europa.eu.int/comm/health/ph_projects/2002/promotion/promotion_2002_18_en.htm. Accessed November 13, 2006.

Innocenti Declaration 2005 On Infant and Young Child Feeding. 2005. Available at: http://innocenti15.net/declaration.pdf.pdf. Accessed November 13, 2006.

Nutrition Unit, Division of Food and Nutrition. The International Code of Marketing of Breastmilk Substitutes: A Common Review and Evaluation Framework. Geneva: World Health Organization; 1997.

Pontificia Academia Scientiarum. Working Group on: Breastfeeding: Science and society. Citta Del Vaticano: Pontificia Academia Scientiarum; 1996.

Sokol EJ. *The Code Handbook: A Guide to Implementing the International Code of Marketing of Breastmilk Substitutes*. Penang, Malaysia: International Code Documentation Centre, 1997.

World Health Organization. *World Health Organization Global Strategy for Infant and Young Child Feeding*. Geneva: WHO; 2003.

Suggested Readings

Armstrong HC, Sokol E. The international code of marketing of breastmilk substitutes: What it means for mothers and babies world-wide. Raleigh, NC: International Lactation Consultant Association; 1994.

Baby Friendly Hospital Initiative: Learning to be Baby Friendly (video). Sandwich, MA: Baby-Friendly, USA.

Breaking the rules: Stretching the rules 2004. A worldwide report on violations of the WHO/UNICEF International Code of Marketing of Breastmilk Substitutes. Geneva: IBFAN. Available at: http://www.ibfan.org/english/codewatch/btr04/btr04contents. html. Accessed November 13, 2006.

Chetley A, Allain A. *Protecting infant health: A health worker's guide to the International Code of Marketing of Breastmilk Substitutes.* 9th ed. Geneva: IBFAN; 1998.

Complying with the code? A manufacturers' and distributors' guide to the code. Penang, Malaysia: IBFAN; 1998.

Department of Health and Human Services (DHHS). Healthy People 2010. Washington, DC: Public Health Service: National Health Promotion and Disease Prevention Objectives; 2000. Available at: http://www.healthypeople.gov/. Accessed November 13, 2006.

Global Strategy for Infant and Young Child Feeding. WHO and UNICEF jointly developed the Global Strategy for Infant and Young Child Feeding, whose aim is to improve—through optimal feeding—the nutritional status, growth and development, health, and thus the very survival of infants and young children. Geneva: WHO; 2003.

Hospital self appraisal tool: Promoting breastfeeding in health facilities: A short course for administrators and policy-makers. Geneva: UNICEF and WHO; Dec 2004. Available at: http://www.unicef.org/spanish/nutrition/files/December2004 BFHISectCE9.pdf. Accessed November 13, 2006.

Innocenti Declaration on the Protection, Promotion, and Support of Breastfeeding in the 1990s Global Initiative. WHO/UNICEF-sponsored meeting, Florence, Italy, 1990; Innocenti+15 was held in Florence, Italy 2005.

International Baby Food Action Network (IBFAN). Penang, Malaysia. Available at: http:ifban.org. Accessed November 13, 2006.

Richter J. *Engineering of consent: Uncovering corporate PR.* Dorset, UK: The Corner House; 1998.

Salisbury L, Blackwell AG. Petition to Alleviate Domestic Infant Formula Misuse and Provide Informed Infant Feeding Choice. Public Advocates, Inc., 1535 Mission St., San Francisco, CA 94103; 1981.

Sethi SP. *Multinational corporations and the impact of public advocacy on corporate strategy: Nestlé and the infant formula controversy.* Norwell, MA: Kluwer Academic Publishers; 1994.

Shuber S. *The international code of marketing of breastmilk substitutes: An international measure to protect and promote breastfeeding.* Cambridge, MA: Kluwer Law International; 1998.

Sokol EJ. The *Code Handbook: A Guide to Implementing the International Code of Marketing of Breastmilk Substitutes.* Penang, Malasia: International Code Documentation Center/IBFAN; 1997.

The Infant Feeding Action Coalition (INFACT) Canada. WBW Action Kit. Available at: http://www.infactcanada.ca/. Accessed November 13, 2006.

United Nations Conventions: Convention on the Elimination of All Forms of Discrimination Against Women; Convention on the Rights of the Child; International Labor Organization Convention on Maternity Protection; International Convention on Economic, Social, and Cultural Rights; World Breastfeeding Week. Available at: http://www.un.org. Accessed November 13, 2006.

United States Department of Agriculture. Nutrition action themes for the United States: A report in response to the international conference on nutrition. Center for Nutrition & Policy Promotion, USDA 1120 20th St, NW, Suite 200, North Lobby, Washington, DC 20036.

World Alliance for Breastfeeding Action (WABA). P.O. Box 1200, 10850 Penang, Malaysia 60.4.6584816. FAX: 60.4.6572655.

World Breastfeeding Week (WBW). WBW Action Folder. La Leche League, International. 1400 N. Meacham Rd., Schaumburg, IL 60173; telephone (847) 519-7730. Available at: http://www.lllusa.org/index.php. Accessed November 13, 2006.

World Breastfeeding Week (WBW). WBW Action Pack. International Lactation Consultant Association (ILCA). 1500 Sunday Dr., Suite 102, Raleigh, NC 27607; telephone (919) 787-5181.

World Alliance for Breastfeeding Action (WABA). Protecting breastfeeding: Making the code work. World Breastfeeding Week Action Folder, 1994 and 2006. Available at: http://www.waba.org.my/. Accessed November 13, 2006.

World Health Organization. *Evidence for the Ten Steps to Successful Breastfeeding.* Geneva: WHO; 1998.

World Health Organization (WHO). *International Code of Marketing of Breast-milk Substitutes.* Geneva; 1981.

World Health Organization (WHO). *The International Code of Marketing of Breast-milk Substitutes: A common review and evaluation framework.* Geneva: WHO; 1997.

World Health Organization (WHO). *Marketing & Dissemination.* Avenue Appia 20, CH1211-Genève 17, Switzerland.

World Health Organization and Wellstart International. *Promoting Breast-Feeding in Health Facilities: A Short Course for Administrators and Policy-Makers.* Geneva: WHO; 1996.

World Health Organization (WHO) and United Nations Children's Fund (UNICEF). *Protecting, Promoting, and Supporting Breastfeeding. The Special Role of Maternity Services.* Geneva: WHO/UNICEF; 1989.

World Health Organization (WHO). *World Health Organization Global Strategy on Infant and Young Child Feeding.* Geneva: WHO; 2003.

COMMUNICATION AND COUNSELING SKILLS

Judith Lauwers, BA, IBCLC

OBJECTIVES

- Identify principles of adult learning that lead to the empowerment of mothers.
- Describe the relative importance of the three components of communication and how to strengthen the message that is sent.
- Describe the counseling process and strategies for meeting the mother's needs for emotional support, understanding, and action.
- Discuss the relative roles of the consultant and the mother in guiding and leading counseling methods and the appropriate use of each method.
- Demonstrate a variety of guiding skills that will elicit information from and provide support to the mother.
- Implement effective problem solving and follow-up within the context of consulting.
- Recognize the needs of grieving parents and strategies for providing support.

Introduction

Effective counseling skills and communication techniques are essential tools of the lactation consultant. Use of these skills provides mothers with the support and teaching that will help them develop confidence in their mothering and breastfeeding. The degree to which mothers are helped by support and advice from a lactation consultant is determined in large part by the lactation consultant's attitude and approach. Adult learners need to perceive themselves as having control over their outcomes. Therefore, an approach that establishes a partnership between the mother and lactation consultant will foster the mother's learning and growth. This approach also increases the likelihood of the mother complying with her lactation consultant's advice. New mothers and those who are breastfeeding for the first time are vulnerable to messages and impressions that compromise their self-confidence. An awareness of effective body language and voice tone will assist the lactation consultant in creating an atmosphere in which the mother feels empowered and self-confident. Choice of positive words and phrases also contributes to an effective learning climate. Providing emotional support to mothers is pivotal to helping them feel confident and empowered in their breastfeeding. Learning how to listen attentively and respond with sensitivity and validation will increase the mother's sense of value and control. It is important that the lactation consultant gather sufficient information and insights during a consultation before engaging in problem solving. Use of the counseling skills presented in this chapter will optimize the lactation consultant's effectiveness with mothers and contribute to meaningful interactions. They can be considered as part of the lactation consultant's toolbox, to be pulled out as each situation warrants.

I. Principles of Adult Learning

A. The adult learner expects frankness and honesty.

   1. Health care providers have a responsibility to give parents the information they need to make informed decisions (Northouse, 1985).

   2. Educating parents empowers them to become informed health care consumers and to make responsible choices.

   3. The fear of creating guilt if a mother chooses not to breastfeed should not be allowed to compromise the parents' right to evidence-based facts.

   4. Trust parents to learn about the health consequences of not breastfeeding, and to make an informed decision about infant feeding.

B. The adult learner is an active participant in the learning process (Knowles, 1980).

   1. Planning is done mutually between the consultant and the mother.

   2. Self-direction, self-reliance, and risk taking are encouraged.

   3. The mother develops problem-solving skills.

   4. The mother takes ownership for the plan and is responsible for the outcome.

   5. The mother evaluates her own learning and takes necessary action.

C. An effective learning climate creates a positive impression.

   1. Display self-confidence, an ability to relate to people, a sense of humor, enthusiasm, and informality.

   2. Respect the learner and be willing to be flexible and to adapt.

   3. Be neat, clean, and wear tasteful attire.

   4. Maintain positive body language, frequent eye contact, a strong voice, and carefully pronounced words.

   5. Maintain a strong knowledge base and demonstrate a desire to share knowledge.

6. Use humor and laughter to enhance learning (Ziv, 1983).
   a. It reduces tension and anxiety, and increases productivity.
   b. It stimulates divergent thinking and increases the mother's willingness to look at a situation in a new way.
   c. It stimulates and integrates the right and left hemispheres of the brain so that learning is at its highest level.

D. Every encounter is individualized to accommodate the particular mother and baby.

   1. Recognize the abilities of every mother and baby and let them set the pace.

   2. Respect the mother's background and tap into it.

   3. Assess the mother's learning needs and her readiness to learn before engaging in problem solving.
      a. Capitalize on the "teachable moment" that will maximize her ability to learn and process information.
      b. Consider the mother's physical comfort, confidence level, emotional state, and the health of the mother and baby in determining the teachable moment.
      c. Use the mother's language style and imagery, and match her intensity and sense of humor.

   4. Make sure every intervention is focused and justified.

   5. Tailor suggestions and actions to the mother's responses.

   6. Provide appropriate written materials.

E. Learning takes place at three levels.

   1. Tell me and I may remember.
      a. Sharing information verbally is the lowest level of learning.
      b. Verbal instruction is appropriate when visual or interactive reinforcement is not needed.
      c. Example: discussion of contraception or nutrition.

   2. Show me and I may understand.
      a. Adding visual reinforcement to verbal instruction increases the level of learning.
      b. This is appropriate when interactive reinforcement is not needed.
      c. Example: use of a cloth breast to demonstrate latch on.

   3. Involve me and I may master.
      a. Engaging the learner to participate actively in the learning process produces the highest level of learning.
      b. The combination of verbal and visual reinforcement demonstrates whether the mother has mastered the technique being taught.
      c. Example: demonstration of the use of a breast pump with the mother giving a return demonstration.

II. Components of Communication

A. Communication requires two basic elements: the delivery and the reception of a message.

B. The way in which a message is received depends on a combination of three factors: the spoken message, tone of voice, and body language (DeVito, 1989).

C. The words the speaker uses account for 7% of the message received.

   1. Avoid negative terminology and imagery that undermine the mother's self-confidence.

   2. Avoid words that imply success or failure, adequacy or inadequacy.

   3. Avoid words that imply the mother is doing or saying something wrong.
      a. The conjunction *but* negates the first half of a thought and can be replaced with the word *and* as in, "You are holding your baby in a good position, (but) *and* if you turn him slightly you will find that he can get an even better latch."
      b. The verb *should* implies judgment and can be avoided by rephrasing. Instead of, *You should feed your baby whenever he wants*, rephrase to, *When you feed your baby whenever he wants, you will be meeting his needs.*

   4. Select words and phrases that correct inappropriate practices without compromising the mother's self-confidence.

   5. Avoid sending mixed messages; be certain that the words create the desired effect.

   6. Supplement verbal messages with demonstrations, visual aids, and written instructions to strengthen understanding.

D. Voice tone accounts for 38% of the message received.

   1. Manner of speech can create a warm, friendly, humorous atmosphere.

   2. Use a moderate volume (not too loud or too low).

   3. Use a moderate rate of speech (not too fast or too slow).

   4. Use a moderate pitch, and guard against your voice becoming higher-pitched when you are angry or excited.

E. Body language accounts for 55% of the message received.

   1. It is based on the behavioral patterns of nonverbal communication and includes all body movements (Fast, 1970).
      a. It ranges from a very deliberate to an unconscious movement or posture.
      b. It may vary culturally or cut across cultural barriers and needs to reflect the client population.

   2. A smile adds to a warm and inviting atmosphere, puts mothers at ease, and elicits a smile from the mother.

3. Eyes are the most important component of body language.
   a. Eye contact conveys a desire to communicate and establishes a warm, caring, and inviting climate.
   b. Eye contact serves as a powerful tool for influencing others.
   c. Try to maintain eye contact at least 85% of the time.
   d. Failure to establish eye contact sends a negative message.

4. A relaxed and comfortable posture creates a warm and inviting climate.
   a. Sit or stand squarely with both feet flat on the floor.
   b. Rest the arms at one's side, or on one's knees when sitting.
   c. Open body posture shows an openness to communicate on a meaningful level; crossing the arms or legs conveys disinterest and emotional distance.
   d. Combining open posture with leaning forward further conveys interest in engaging the mother.

5. Altitude and distance can either enhance or detract from a message.
   a. Establish a comfortable position—not too far away or too close—using the mother's reactions as a guide. Standing or sitting too close invades another's personal space (their comfort zone). Standing or sitting too far away conveys a message of being too busy or uninterested.
   b. Height in relation to another person conveys who possesses the greatest importance or control. A position equal to or below the mother puts her in control and leads to greater self-reliance and empowerment.

6. Touch can convey warmth, caring, and encouragement.
   a. It must come at the right moment and in the right context.
   b. Ask permission before touching the mother's breasts or her baby.

7. Learn to read the body language of mothers.
   a. Observe and respond to the mother's reactions and body language.
   b. Be alert for nonverbal messages the mother sends and watch for signs of physical discomfort.

III. The Counseling Process

A. The goal of counseling is to fulfill the mother's needs for emotional support, physical comfort, understanding, and action (Brammer, 1973).
   1. Give the mother the support that is needed to develop confidence.
   2. Encourage the mother to express herself.
   3. Educate and problem-solve with the mother.
   4. Help the mother develop self-sufficiency and satisfaction.

B. Personality and attitude are important to the counseling process.
   1. Knowledge of people's attitudes provides insight into understanding and predicting their behavior.

2. Personal experience and other sources of information can change attitude.

3. A warm and caring attitude shows deep and genuine concern and empathy.
   a. Openness to disclosing feelings and thoughts encourages trust and openness in the mother when done appropriately.
   b. Acknowledging the mother's individuality and worth, without judgment, gives the mother freedom to be herself.
   c. Clear, accurate communication reduces confusion and frustration.
   d. Flexibility helps the consultant respond appropriately to the mother at different stages in the counseling process.

4. Ineffective communication skills may transmit an attitude of disinterest or emotional distance.

5. A noncommittal attitude about breastfeeding by health care workers may unintentionally promote the use of artificial baby milk.

C. Effective counseling helps to meet the mother's needs for emotional support.

1. Listen to what the mother is not saying; look for her underlying message.

2. Send the message that you genuinely care about her well-being and concerns.

3. Provide a sense of security that encourages her to verbalize feelings and anxieties.

4. Praise her actions and validate her feelings, emotions, and concerns.

5. Help her arrive at a state where she can take in information and problem-solve.

D. The counseling process can be hindered when the mother has physical discomfort. The mother may be too uncomfortable to listen and learn. Help her relieve discomfort before proceeding with educating and problem solving.

E. The desired outcome of a consultation is for the mother to understand and take positive action.

1. She needs to understand herself and her feelings to clearly define and understand the problem and its cause and to understand her options in resolving the problem.

2. Meeting these needs will help her make informed choices and assume responsibility for her actions. She will gain satisfaction in knowing she is actively working on the problem.

IV. Methods of Counseling

A. Counseling involves three distinct methods: guiding, leading, and follow-up (Brammer, 1973).

B. The process of guiding will help you genuinely listen to the mother and empathize with her through understanding her feelings, goals, and other factors that influence her actions.

1. Begin with guiding and continue to use it throughout the contact.

2. The guiding process provides emotional support to the mother.
    a. It transmits a message of acceptance and concern.
    b. It encourages her to express her ideas and concerns openly.
    c. It helps her *hear* what you are saying.

3. The guiding process is characterized by limited direction from the counselor.
    a. The mother is encouraged to do most of the talking.
    b. You listen most of the time to gather necessary information and insights.
    c. Careful listening helps you hear what the mother is *not* saying.

C. The leading method requires a more active role by the consultant in directing the conversation.

    1. It helps you and the mother see the situation more clearly.

    2. It helps the mother who is unable to solve a problem.

    3. It helps define options that will lead to a plan of action.

    4. It enables you and the mother to form a problem-solving partnership.

D. Follow-up is essential to the counseling process.

    1. It determines how and when to plan the next contact.

    2. It identifies what preparation is needed for the next contact.

    3. It analyzes the efficacy of the contact.

    4. It indicates whether your suggestions have been useful.

    5. It identifies the mother's need for further support or assistance.

    6. It lets the mother know how concerned you are in helping her.

V. Skills in the Guiding Method

A. Counseling skills in the Guiding Method encourage the mother to continue talking freely and promote her active participation in the discussion.

B. *Listening skills* reinforce what is said, clarify the mother's statements, show acceptance of her situation, and encourage her to arrive at solutions.

    1. *Attending* is the lowest level of listening.
        a. You listen passively to indicate that you are paying attention.
        b. Examples of attending include: eye contact, open posture, calm gestures, a silent pause, or saying, *Yes* or *Mmm*.

    2. *Active listening*, also called reflective listening, paraphrases what you believe the mother meant.
        a. Shows acceptance of the mother's viewpoint.
        b. Encourages a response from the mother.
        c. Clarifies the message so that the mother can reflect on it.

3. *Empathetic listening* goes beyond merely reflecting words.
   a. You listen with the intent to understand emotionally and intellectually.
   b. You rephrase both the content and the feeling of what she said.
   c. It helps the mother know if she sent the intended message.
C. *Facilitating skills* actively encourage the mother to give more information and define her situation better.
   1. They focus on specific concerns and pinpoint issues and feelings to explore.
   2. *Clarifying* helps to make a point clear, as in, *Do you mean that your nipples hurt only when . . .*
   3. *Asking open-ended questions* is a useful skill for gathering information.
      a. It is a question that cannot be answered by a simple "yes" or "no."
      b. The question begins with *who, what, when, where, why, how, how much,* or *how often.*
      c. Instead of asking, *Does your baby nurse often enough?* ask, *How many times does she nurse in 24 hours?*
   4. *Interpreting* takes active listening one step farther to empathetic listening.
      a. You interpret what was said rather than merely restating it.
      b. It enables the mother to process your interpretation and to agree or disagree.
      c. It describes the emotion that is being expressed, as in, *You're worried that your baby is not getting enough milk.*
   5. *Focusing* pursues a topic that is helpful to explore or condenses several points.
      a. Selects one particular point to repeat.
      b. Useful when the mother gets into an unrelated topic.
      c. Example: "Tell me more about . . ."
   6. *Summarizing* highlights and reinforces important information.
      a. Restates the plan of action.
      b. Reassures the mother that the consultant has been tuned into her.
      c. Helps you know that you understood the mother.
      d. Most effective when done by the mother, as in, *We talked about several things to try; which will work best for you?*
D. *Influencing skills* instill a positive outlook in the mother and encourage her to continue to seek help.
   1. *Reassuring* helps a mother see that her situation is normal and assures her that her situation will improve, as in, *Your breasts will feel more comfortable after the initial fullness goes down.*
   2. *Building hope* helps the mother see how her feelings relate to her situation.
      a. Encourages her to talk about her feelings.
      b. Helps relieve tension.
      c. Encourages her to take positive action.

    d. Example: *I'm glad your mother could join us. Maybe if you are patient with her, she will begin to be more supportive now that she has a better understanding of breastfeeding.*

  3. *Identifying strengths* helps the mother focus on her positive qualities and those of her baby.

    a. Counteracts negative factors.

    b. Encourages the mother to persevere.

    c. Encourages the mother to develop and rely on her own resources.

    d. Helps her to recall enjoyable memories.

    e. Example: *You did that really well!*

VI. Skills in the Leading Method

A. Skills in the leading method place more responsibility for the direction of the discussion on the consultant.

B. The goal is to understand a problem and develop a plan of action.

  1. It is used when the mother is unable to solve a problem.

  2. It provides additional resources to lead the mother toward a solution.

  3. Gather enough information so your problem solving is not premature or incorrect.

  4. Take time to gain the mother's trust and clarify the situation before problem solving.

  5. Give parents proper information at the appropriate time.

C. *Informing* explains how something functions and the reasons behind it.

  1. Correct misconceptions or mismanagement with sensitivity.

  2. Suggest appropriate resources to help them grow as parents.

  3. Provide anticipatory guidance at times when retention will be high and decision making will occur.

  4. Encourage initial learning before delivery so postpartum teaching can focus on reinforcement.

  5. Example: *When your baby suckles, it stimulates the nerve endings, and in turn signals milk production. Therefore . . .*

D. *Problem solving* is accomplished by forming a partnership between the mother and consultant.

  1. Form your first *hunch* (a hunch refers to an idea or a hypothesis) based on information and impressions you gained.

  2. Look for additional factors that will confirm the hunch.

  3. Test the hunch by suggesting what the problem might be.

4. If the mother rejects the hunch, explore alternative hunches with the use of guiding skills to gain further insights and information.

5. When the hunch is confirmed, develop a *plan of action* with the mother.

6. Use a nonassertive approach to encourage the mother to be active in problem solving.

7. Limit suggestions to two or three actions to avoid overwhelming the mother.

8. Ask the mother to summarize the plan in order to demonstrate her understanding.

9. Set a time limit on the actions to be taken, and follow up to learn whether the plan worked or whether further suggestions are needed.

VII. Skills in Follow-Up

A. Follow-up is an ongoing process and should be done after every contact. The urgency of the situation will determine how soon and how frequent follow-up is necessary.

B. Evaluating the session.

1. Determine how effective the contact was and whether the mother's needs were met.

2. Assess the use of appropriate counseling skills.

3. Evaluate the information and advice given to the mother.

4. Evaluate the method of documentation.

C. Arranging the next contact.

1. Let the mother know what follow-up to expect, when the contact will occur, and who will initiate it.

2. Determine any additional information or assistance that is needed.

3. Leave the door open for the mother to contact you when needed.

4. Make appropriate referrals to other health care professionals and community resources.

5. Arrange frequent contact during the early weeks postpartum, either personally or through referral to a support group.

D. Researching outside sources.

1. Accessing information and resources helps you grow as a lactation consultant and provides further input and a fresh outlook on a problem.

2. Seek support and advice from colleagues.

E. Renewing the counseling process.

1. The counseling process begins anew with each successive contact.

2. Begin with guiding skills and progress to leading skills and further follow-up as needed.

VIII. Counseling a Mother Who is Grieving

A. Parents who lose a baby progress through several stages of grief before their loss is resolved (Figure 3-1).

1. They need time and privacy with their family immediately after the loss to begin the grieving process.

2. Talking about her feelings will help the mother through the grief process.

3. Resolution could take as long as two years, depending on the amount of support and understanding the parents receive.

4. Mothers who had been nursing or expressing milk for their babies can be further comforted in knowing they gave their babies the best possible care.

5. Donating milk that may help save another baby's life can be a part of the mother's emotional healing.

6. Talking with other parents who have had similar experiences can help their perspective.

7. Counseling is available through local clergy and social service organizations.

B. Appropriate counseling techniques, insight into the mother's emotions, and sincere empathy will help you approach the situation confident in your ability to comfort the mother.

1. Reflect back to the mother how you imagine she must feel, as in "You must be heartbroken," or, "I can't imagine the loss you feel."

2. Acknowledge her baby's importance by asking his name and using it during conversations.

3. Let her know you will be glad to listen, assuring her that you do not want to invade her privacy.

4. Help parents assert their rights to hold or see their baby after he dies, take pictures, and keep the identification bracelet as mementos.

5. You may wish to attend the funeral if you have cared for the mother and baby.

C. Parents of high-risk infants may experience a similar grief process.

1. They may avoid contact with other parents who have healthy babies.

2. They may avoid involvement with their baby to protect themselves from becoming attached to a baby they may lose.

3. Such feelings usually subside after they accept their baby's condition.

4. Parents also grieve when it is necessary to transfer their infant to another facility.

5. Encourage parents to seek support, both in the hospital and within their community.

Figure 3-1 Sequence of the grief process. *Source:* Lauwers J and Swisher A, *Counseling the Nursing Mother: A Lactation Consultant's Guide, Third Edition,* Jones and Bartlett Publishers, 2005.

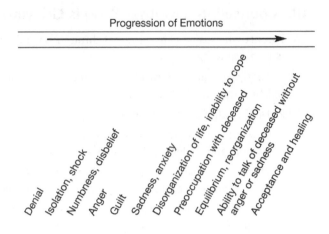

References

Brammer LM. *The Helping Relationship.* Upper Saddle River, NY: Prentice Hall; 1973.

DeVito JA. *The Interpersonal Communication Book.* 5th ed. New York: Harper & Rowe; 1989.

Fast J. *Body Language.* New York: Pocket Books; 1970.

Knowles M. *The Modern Practice of Adult Education from Pedagogy to Androgogy.* Chicago: Follett Publishing; 1980.

Northouse PG. *Health Communication: A Handbook for Health Professionals.* Englewood Cliffs, NJ: Prentice-Hall; 1985.

Ziv A. The influence of humorous atmosphere on divergent thinking. *Contemp Edu Psychol.* 1983;9:413–421.

Suggested Readings

Ellis D, Livingstone VH, Hewat RJ. Assisting the breastfeeding mother: a problem-solving process. *J Hum Lact.* 1993;9:89–93.

Fletcher D, Harris H. The implementation of the HOT program at the Royal Women's Hospital. *Breastfeed Rev.* 2000;8:19–23.

Isselman M, Deubner LS, Hartman M. A nutrition counseling workshop: integrating counseling psychology into nutrition practice. *J Am Diet Assoc.* 1993;93:324–326.

Lauwers J, Swisher A. *Counseling the Nursing Mother: A Lactation Consultant's Guide Third Edition.* Sudbury, MA: Jones and Bartlett Publishers; 2005.

THE PARENTAL ROLE

Marsha Walker, RN, IBCLC
Revised by Judith Lauwers, BA, IBCLC

OBJECTIVES

- Describe parents' role in the health care system.
- Identify factors in parent-infant bonding and attachment.
- Describe the common emotions of new parents and recognize signs of inadequate coping.
- Recognize signs of a history of sexual abuse.
- Discuss postpartum sexual adjustments and family planning options.
- Describe breastfeeding in the context of a major life change and alternative family styles.
- Identify support systems for mothers.

Introduction

Parenting roles and family relationships are influenced by social, cultural, and historical factors. Parents share many of the same goals across cultures but differ in how they approach meeting them. Some cultures place a strong emphasis on family and group identity. Others value individuality and independence. Childrearing attitudes and recommendations have changed over the years, as have the roles of men and women. Mothers and fathers often are challenged with balancing multiple roles while promoting the optimal development of their children. Articles and books contain conflicting information and advice that can be confusing for both parents and children. Parents who are in nuclear families have lost the modeling and influence of the extended family in their learning and practicing for the parental role. Any number of family configurations can be found, from the traditional married man and woman with the man as the major breadwinner to blended families through divorce and remarriage, to single mothers with children. Families living in poverty face significant parenting challenges and barriers. As hospital stays shorten, families are geographically spread out, and economic factors force women into employment after short maternity leaves, educational needs for new parents have burgeoned. The lactation consultant is in a unique position to both assist with breastfeeding and to offer valuable support to new families.

I. Parents' Roles in the Health Care System

A. Become active health care consumers who are informed and responsible decision makers regarding their care and the care of their baby.

B. Express concerns and preferences in a courteous manner.

C. Reinforce positive aspects of their care.

D. Carry through on an agreed plan of care and accept the consequences of their actions.

E. Allow reports and follow-up from the lactation consultant to their physicians for coordination of care.

II. Acquiring the Parental Role

A. Stages of parental role acquisition (Bocar & Moore, 1987)

1. *Anticipatory:* The anticipatory stage occurs before delivery and is a time when parents begin learning about their new roles. They read, talk with their own parents, ask questions of other family members and parents, and attend classes.

2. *Formal:* The formal stage begins after delivery. Parents create the "perfect parent" image or an idealized version of parenting. They are interested in mastering practical child care skills. They may lack self-confidence and become easily overwhelmed and confused by conflicting information. New parents need concrete demonstrations and suggestions as well as acknowledgment that they are the experts on their own baby. Once they develop confidence in their ability to meet their baby's basic needs, they progress to the informal stage.

3. *Informal:* During the informal stage, parents begin interacting with their peers and have other informal interactions. They begin to relax the more rigid rules and directions used to acquire the caretaking behaviors.

4. *Personal:* The personal stage is when parents modify their practices and evolve their own unique parenting styles.

B. Parents who follow rigid "baby training" programs that prescribe scheduled feedings, limited contact, and specified sleep periods find it difficult to move beyond the formal stage of parenting.

1. Upwardly mobile, career-minded professionals are drawn to such programs.

2. There are concerns about the psychological outcome of children left to "cry it out" (Aney, 1998). Some infants demonstrate detachment, depression, eating issues, and self-stimulating and self-soothing behaviors (Webb, 2003; Williams, 1998, 1999).

3. Low milk supply, low infant weight gain, or the baby rejecting the breast may result (Aney, 1998; Moody, 2002).

4. These babies are at risk for attachment problems; babies who are left to "cry it out" might sleep through the night after abandoning hope of being parented in the evening and might experience despair.

5. With reflective listening, you can be accepting of parents without endorsing their practices. A nonjudgmental approach creates a climate where parents can question their approach and be open to alternatives.

C. The term *maternal role attainment*, first described by Rubin (1967a, 1967b), describes the phases of taking in, taking hold, and letting go as characteristic of the behavior of new mothers.

D. Anticipatory guidance and active involvement in the pregnancy and birth enhance role acquisition (Freed, Fraley & Schanler, 1992; Gamble & Morse, 1992; Jordan & Wall, 1990).

III. Attachment and Bonding

A. Infant-to-parent attachment

1. Attachment is viewed as a behavioral system (Bowlby, 1969).
   a. Infant attachment or signaling behaviors such as cooing, smiling, and crying initiate and maintain contact between the mother and infant.
   b. A secure attachment helps the infant develop a sense of security that was described by Erikson (1950) as basic trust.
   c. The first six months of life are considered a sensitive period when the infant develops a trusting relationship with the caregiver.
   d. Parents should watch their baby and respond to approach behaviors and feeding cues.
   e. Keeping mothers and babies together and avoiding unnecessary separations will enhance bonding and attachment.

2. Ainsworth et al. (1978) described three general patterns of infant-to-parent attachment: avoidant, ambivalent, and secure.
   a. Avoidant infants show little distress during separation, treat a stranger the same way as the mother, and avoid proximity or interaction with the mother during a reunion after separation.
   b. Ambivalent infants resist contact with a stranger and might be angry or resistant to the mother upon reunion following a separation; once contact with the mother is initiated, the infant seeks to maintain it.
   c. Securely attached infants seek proximity and contact with the mother (especially during reunions) but also explore the environment.

3. Parental sensitivity and responsiveness may be key indicators of a parent's attachment to his or her infant and can affect the infant's subsequent attachment to the parent (Graham, 1993).

    a. Mothers who are sensitive and responsive to the infant's needs during the early months and who promptly meet the infant's needs foster the development of secure attachment relationships.

    b. Mothers who fail to respond to their infants or respond inappropriately foster the development of avoidant or ambivalent attachments.

  4. Secure infant-to-parent attachments at age 12 to 18 months are related to the child's adaptive problem-solving ability at two years of age and to social competence at age three.

B. Parent-to-infant attachment

  1. Parents begin to form attachments to the baby in utero, and their interaction during the early weeks is a get-acquainted process.

  2. Parental, situational, and infant factors are related to the development of a parent's attachment to the infant.

    a. Early contact and bonding behaviors have been suggested as being important during the early hours following birth; Klaus and Kennell (1982) describe a sensitive period following birth as being important in establishing attachment; while humans are capable of adaptation and growth in this area, the concept might be of special importance to mothers who are at risk of developing maladaptive parent-child relationships.

    b. Attachment behaviors of all women are enhanced by keeping mothers and babies together in a rooming-in environment; this may be especially relevant to low-income or indigent women.

    c. If there are discrepancies between what parents had fantasized their baby would be like and the reality of their child, parents might be delayed in their attachment progress.

  3. The temperament of an infant has a great effect on parental feelings of competence and interactions.

    a. Compatibility can have an effect on parenting behaviors.

    b. Infants who are difficult to console or whose needs are difficult to meet might have parents who feel it is a challenge to develop quality interactions.

    c. When parents perceive their efforts as successful in meeting the needs of their infants, they perceive themselves as competent and effective caregivers.

  4. Father's interaction with baby.

    a. Father-to-infant attachment is enhanced by his presence at the birth and extended contact with his infant during the newborn period (Sears & Gotsch, 2003).

    b. Fathers have unique ways of interacting with their infants, frequently called *engrossment* in the early period.

    c. Fathers learn their role through society's definitions, experience with their own fathers, and pressure from family members and other men.

    d. The father often feels as though he has lost his mate, because she seems immersed in the care of the baby.

    e. Fathers experience a hormonal response to their babies' cries, with a rise in prolactin and testosterone levels (Fleming et al., 2002).

    f. Fathers benefit from learning about infant cues and responsiveness in order to recognize what is normal and how to interact with their young infants (Delight et al., 1991).

IV. Emotional Adjustments Postpartum

A. Maternal postpartum mood changes are usually mild and self-limiting.

    1. There is disagreement in the literature as to whether postpartum psychological complications are unique to the postpartum period or are symptoms of an underlying disorder that is triggered by childbirth.

    2. Possible causes include hormonal adjustments, chemical imbalances, a genetic predisposition, poor ego development, low self-esteem, poor interpersonal relationships, and the perception of the inability to meet others' needs.

B. "Baby blues"

    1. As many as 50% to 80% of postpartum women experience a period of emotional distress beginning two to three days after delivery.

    2. Baby blues are characterized by feelings of ambivalence, tearfulness, sadness, insomnia, anxiety, irritability, poor concentration, and lack of self-confidence.

    3. Baby blues are more common in women with their first baby. A disappointing birth experience, poor nutrition, and a fussy baby increase feelings of sadness.

    4. If the baby blues last more than two weeks, these feelings indicate that the mother may be depressed (Kendall-Tackett, 2001).

    5. Emotional support, practical help, realistic expectations, and interaction with other new mothers can minimize baby blues.

    6. If baby blues progress to depression or psychosis, recognize your limitations and when to refer.

C. Postpartum depression

    1. A small number of women become clinically depressed starting two to six weeks after delivery and lasting for several months. This postpartum depression is thought to occur in 10% to 20% of new mothers, but in certain high-risk groups can be as high as 50%.

    2. Risk factors for postpartum depression include: single mother; low socioeconomic level; limited education; pregnancy or health complications; and personal or family history of depression; difficult birth experience; immune system alterations; history of trauma or abuse; and a lack of social support (Beck, 1998; Misri, 2002).

    3. Postpartum depression is characterized by mood changes, feelings of sadness, loss of pleasure, poor concentration, low self-esteem, guilt at failing as a mother and wife, sleep disturbances, and fatigue.

4. Red flags for postpartum depression in a mother include:
    a. Lacks confidence in her ability to breastfeed.
    b. Lacks tolerance for family members and others.
    c. Feels hopeless, unable to cope, and not in control over her life.
    d. Feels detached from her baby and does not call her baby by name.
    e. Describes vague physical complaints.

5. Premature weaning is more frequent among depressed women (Cooper et al., 1993).

6. Women who are clinically depressed for several months require professional help beyond the role of the International Board Certified Lactation Consultant.
    a. They should be encouraged to contact their physician for a referral to a professional therapist.
    b. If medications are prescribed, they must be checked for compatibility with breastfeeding, though most antidepressant medications are compatible with breastfeeding.

D. Postpartum psychosis

1. Postpartum psychosis, characterized by severe changes in emotions and behavior, is rare and occurs in 1 to 2 of every 1000 women (Gale & Harlow, 2003; Gold, 1995).

2. Red flags for postpartum psychosis in a mother include:
    a. Hallucinations or delusions.
    b. Loss of control, rational thought, and social functioning.
    c. Bizarre or violent behavior.
    d. Threats of harm to herself or to her baby.
    e. Suicide attempts (Oates, 2003).
    f. Decreased communication and marital discord.
    g. Inadequate parenting and behavioral problems with other children.

3. If severe enough, postpartum psychosis might result in hospitalization, medications, and psychiatric counseling. The lactation consultant is an important member of her health care team.
    a. Help secure a breast pump if the mother and baby are separated.
    b. Serve as a resource for information about medications and breastfeeding.
    c. Help the mother maintain breastfeeding and to relactate or wean if necessary.

V. Sexual Abuse Survivors

A. As many as one in three women will be sexually assaulted in their lifetime.

1. The incidence ranges from 7% to 36% of women (Finkelhor, 1994).

2. Sexual abuse affects functioning of at least 20% of adult survivors (Briere & Runtz, 1991).

B. Pregnancy and childbirth are often times that remind survivors of past sexual abuse.

1. These events may cause the memory to surface for the first time.

2. Mothers may experience flashbacks, depression, anger, a loss of control, powerlessness, and a sense of confusion about relationships.

C. Memories, flashbacks, and feelings may interfere with a woman's ability to breastfeed (Kendall-Tackett, 1998).

1. The mother may have difficulty dealing with the intimacy of breastfeeding and prefer to pump milk and feed the expressed milk with a bottle.

2. Breastfeeding at night, in a darkened room, in a bed, or with others around may be difficult or impossible.

a. Exploring choices of breastfeeding times and places can avoid situational flashbacks or unpleasant feelings.

b. The mother may be able to breastfeed during the day if someone else handles the nighttime feedings.

3. The mother may be comfortable nursing a young baby but have difficulty with an older baby who smiles and plays at the breast.

a. Offer information about typical older baby behavior at the breast.

b. Emphasize the functional role of the breasts as opposed to the sexual role.

D. Warning signs that may indicate a history of abuse include late prenatal care, substance abuse, mental health concerns, eating disorders, poor compliance with self-care, and sexual dysfunction.

VI. Postpartum Sexual Adjustments

A. Sexuality and intercourse

1. Many physicians recommend waiting to resume sexual relations until after the six-week checkup; not all couples will need to wait for that period, however.

2. Adjustments in routine

a. Having a baby interferes with freedom and sexual spontaneity, and some fathers may resent the attention the baby receives.

b. Some women might feel tired, "touched out," or too overwhelmed to concentrate on sexual needs.

c. Nursing the baby immediately before bedtime and taking advantage of moments alone during naptime can provide the parents with an opportunity for intimacy.

d. Other forms of intimacy and variations in techniques or routines can be explored during this time.

3. Physical adjustments

a. Kegel exercises will help with general toning and facilitate entrance in intercourse.

b. Vaginal dryness caused by hormone changes may cause some physical discomfort when first resuming sexual intercourse. The mother can relieve her discomfort with an artificial lubricant.

      c. Some women find that their breasts are very sensitive to touch or not sensitive at all.

      d. Adjustments in positioning can help alleviate physical discomfort caused by a painful incision or full breasts.

      e. Oxytocin released during orgasm may cause the breasts to leak. Feeding the baby or expressing milk beforehand reduces leakage during lovemaking.

      f. Experiencing increased sensuality when breastfeeding is a result of oxytocin release and is a normal response for many women.

B. Amenorrhea and ovulation

    1. During the immediate postpartum period and for varying lengths of time thereafter, the breastfeeding mother experiences amenorrhea or the absence of the menses.

      a. Return of menses is dependent on factors such as exclusive breastfeeding, nighttime breastfeeding, short intervals between breastfeedings, and duration of feeds; the average time to menses for women following these practices is around 14 months (Kippley, 1987; Kippley & Kippley, 1972).

        i. The return of menses in a breastfeeding mother occurs at three months for 9% to 30% of mothers, and at six months for 19% to 53% of mothers.

        ii. Some women do not resume their cycles until after weaning has occurred.

      b. Some women experience scanty show before their true cycles resume.

      c. The menstrual cycle absence can be followed by anovulatory cycles (absent egg release).

      d. Menstruation causes no significant changes in the composition of the mother's milk but may change the taste of her milk and cause the baby to be fussy or refuse to nurse.

    2. Suppression of ovulation is associated with levels of growth hormone, leutinizing hormone, follicle-stimulating hormone, and estrogen (McNeilly, 1993).

    3. The most important factor in suppression of ovulation during lactation is the early establishment of frequent and strong suckling by the baby (McNeilly, 1993; Tay, Glasier, & McNeilly, 1996).

    4. Factors in the length of amenorrhea and infertility include:

      a. Breastfeeding frequency and short intervals between feedings (Gray et al., 1993).

      b. Duration of feedings (Diaz et al., 1991; Gellen, 1992; McNeilly, Tay, & Glaiser, 1994; Vestermark et al., 1994).

      c. Nighttime feedings (Vestermark et al., 1994).

      d. Absence of supplemental foods in the baby's diet (Diaz et al., 1992).

    5. Women can become pregnant while they are breastfeeding and have a number of family planning options.

VII. Contraception

A. Natural family planning methods rely on fertility awareness to prevent or space pregnancies. These methods include calendar, basal body temperature, cervical mucous, and symptothermal.

B. Lactational amenorrhea method offers pregnancy protection during the first six months postpartum (Kennedy et al., 1998; Labbok et al., 1997). The risk of pregnancy during this time is less than 1%. Three conditions must exist. If any one of these conditions is not met, backup contraception is needed. The conditions are:

1. The mother's menses have not yet returned.

2. The baby is breastfed around the clock and receives no other foods or pacifiers.

3. The baby is younger than six months of age.

C. Hormonal contraceptives (ABM, 2005)

1. Generally, breastfeeding women should use non-estrogen contraceptive methods.
   a. Those that contain both estrogen and progesterone appear to cause the most difficulty in lactating women, especially in the early postpartum period before lactation is well established.
   b. Estrogen has the risk of reducing milk quantity and can also pass into the milk (Kelsey, 1996; Koetsawang, 1987).

2. Oral contraceptives have been in use for more than 40 years. Two types are on the market today: a combined estrogen/progestin pill and a progestin-only formulation.
   a. Breastfeeding women usually use the progestin-only pill in the early phase of breastfeeding (the first six months).
   b. Progestin-only oral contraceptives do not appear to interfere with milk production, and therefore are acceptable during lactation (Bjarnadottir et al., 2001; Dunson et al., 1993; Kelsey, 1996; Speroff, 1992–1993). However, women should not use this method before six weeks postpartum.

3. Intrauterine devices (IUDs) prevent a fertilized egg from implanting (Williams, 2003).
   a. The non-hormonal IUD does not seem to have any effect on lactation (Koetsawang, 1987).
   b. The progesterone-releasing IUD has been associated with a slight decrease in milk volume (Kelsey, 1996).
   c. Women are at a higher risk of expulsion of the IUD during the early breastfeeding period because of the uterine contractions caused by suckling.

4. The vaginal ring is a hormone-releasing ring a woman can self-insert. Effectiveness, milk production, and infant growth with a progesterone-releasing ring are similar to IUD use (Sivin et al., 1997).

5. Levonorgestrel (Norplant®) is a flexible, plastic progestin implant that is inserted surgically under the skin of the upper arm. It slowly releases progesterone for up to five years.
   a. Half of women continue to ovulate and half have it removed due to unpleasant side effects.
   b. Norplant is not currently available in the United States.

6. Depo-Provera® is a progestin injection given every three months, with infertility lasting up to one year.
   a. When administered immediately postpartum, an impaired milk supply may result, though one clinical study showed no impact on lactation (Danli et al., 2000).
   b. Mothers should delay use of Depo-Provera for six weeks until lactation is well established.

7. The "patch" delivers estrogen and progesterone through the skin into the bloodstream and is about as effective as combination oral contraceptives.

8. Spermicidals prevent pregnancy by destroying sperm before it can reach and fertilize an egg. Vaginal spermicides are 69% to 89% effective and are used after the cervix has closed. There are no side effects or contraindications while breastfeeding.

D. Barrier methods

1. Condoms have about a 14% failure rate (Williams, 2003).
   a. A male condom is a thin latex or silicone sheath that covers the male penis. The male condom combined with foam is an effective contraceptive.
   b. A female condom is a thin polyurethane sheath with soft rings that fit over the cervix and part of the perineum and labia during intercourse. The female condom does not require fitting by a health care professional.

2. A diaphragm must be refitted after each pregnancy.

3. A cervical cap is placed over the cervix.

E. Sterilization

1. Bilateral tubal ligation ties the fallopian tubes in the woman. There is no evidence that it hampers milk production.

2. Vasectomy severs the vas deferens in the man, the main duct through which sperm travel during ejaculation.

VIII. Siblings and Breastfeeding

A. Each child needs time and understanding to prepare for and adjust to the arrival of a new sibling. Planning time each day where the mother's total attention is devoted to the older sibling will help the adjustment.

B. Tandem nursing (breastfeeding of 2 or more children of different ages).

1. The new baby takes precedence over the toddler, with access to both breasts before the toddler nurses.

2. If a mother wishes to wean the older sibling, she can wean in a gradual manner by substituting activities for nursings, and feeding the new baby when the older child is either not present or is occupied with other things.

3. Some mothers reserve time each day for the older sibling to nurse in order to provide special time together.

C. Accommodating a sibling during feedings.

1. Nurse where there is ample room to read a book or play simple games. Using the football hold will free the mother's hand for cuddling the older child.

2. A child who has previously weaned might show renewed interest in breastfeeding when he or she sees the new baby at the breast. This renewed interest in breastfeeding is usually temporary. The sibling may simply be curious about the taste of the milk, so expressing some into a cup may satisfy this curiosity.

IX. Family Lifestyle

A. The mother's ability to adapt her lifestyle to motherhood will depend on her emotional well-being, her physical recovery, her maturity, and the support she receives from family and friends.

B. Women in the United States with unwanted pregnancies are less likely to initiate or continue breastfeeding than women with intended pregnancies (Taylor & Cabral, 2002).

C. Single mothers

1. In the United States, 34% of births in 2002 were to unmarried women (CDC, 2003).

2. A woman may have sole responsibility of her baby because of a choice to remain single, separation or divorce, the death of the spouse, or a situation that requires the baby's father to be away from home for extended periods.

   a. She may live alone, with a partner or roommate, or with family members.
   b. She may have multiple responsibilities of work, school, household chores, and parenting.
   c. She may have little privacy or support for what she is doing.
   d. Emotional stress and demands for dealing with divorce, separation, or loss of a spouse may result in missed feedings and lowered milk production.
   e. Single mothers who are divorced or in the process of divorcing may have custody or visitation issues that impact separations and breastfeeding.

3. The lactation consultant's role is to be familiar with community resources for single mothers and to find ways to meet the mother's and baby's needs while preserving breastfeeding.

D. Adolescent mothers

1. Many pregnant teenagers elect to keep their babies, and about 17% go on to have a second child within 3 years (NCHS, 2001).

2. Teens have a higher incidence of preterm, low-birth-weight infants, stillbirths, and neonatal death than do post-adolescent mothers (March of Dimes, 2002).

3. Adolescents are physically and psychologically capable of breastfeeding.

4. Breastfeeding rates are lower for teen mothers than adults, partly because of lack of knowledge (Dewan et al., 2002).
   a. They typically choose to breastfeed because it is good for the baby and because of the closeness of the relationship.
   b. Some choose to breastfeed because it gives them some control over the situation.
   c. Those who have a dependent relationship with their mothers are less likely to breastfeed.

5. Teens who are the most likely to breastfeed:
   a. Older teens who are exposed to other breastfeeding mothers and/or prenatal breastfeeding education.
   b. Older teens who are married and no longer in school during their pregnancy (Lizarraga et al., 1992)
   c. Teens who see other women breastfeed and who were breastfed as babies (Lefler, 2000).

6. Adolescent mothers want to be treated as adults.
   a. They respond poorly to lecturing, advice-giving, mandates, and patronizing discussions or actions.
   b. They respond best to sincere, consistent, and honest support.
   c. They respond best to interactive learning and the right to refuse to participate if they feel threatened.
   d. They learn best in an environment that is nonjudgmental, fun, and supportive of their decisions.

7. An adolescent mother faces unique challenges.
   a. Poor nutrition and inadequate prenatal care.
   b. A mother who opposes breastfeeding or creates a power struggle.
   c. Difficulty seeing beyond her own needs.
   d. Unresolved issues about her sexuality and concerns about modesty.
   e. Resentment toward the baby and parenting because it interferes with her social life.
   f. The need to return to school within as little as two weeks after delivery, and to plan breastfeeding or milk expression around breaks and classes.

8. Adolescent mothers need a strong information and support system.
   a. An adolescent mother needs a trusting relationship with her mother, grandmother, partner, or pregnancy coordinator (Dykes et al., 2003).

  b. Other family members, especially the teen's mother, might need information about breastfeeding and can be provided with ideas for supporting it.

  c. Peer counselors are a valuable addition to the support for teen mothers.

  d. One prenatal program resulted in 97.6% wanting to breastfeed and 82.8% breastfeeding at discharge (Greenwood & Littlejohn, 2002).

  e. Staff in the hospital can encourage adolescent mothers to room in with their baby, invite interaction between the mother and baby, and treat the mother in an adult manner, giving options and including her in decision making.

  f. Teachers may need help in understanding that breastfeeding is not being used as an excuse to miss classes.

E. Co-sleeping

  1. Co-sleeping refers to the infant sleeping in close social and/or physical contact with a committed caregiver.

    a. Parent–child co-sleeping provides physical protection for the infant against cold and extends the duration of breastfeeding (McKenna, 1986; McKenna et al., 1993).

    b. Parents should be educated about risks and benefits of co-sleeping and unsafe co-sleeping practices and make their own informed decision (ABM, 2006).

    c. The American Academy of Pediatrics (AAP) recommends that mothers and infants sleep in proximity to each other to facilitate breastfeeding (AAP, 2005; Blair et al., 1999).

  2. Bedsharing refers to the infant sharing a bed with a committed caregiver.

    a. Bedsharing is controversial because of concern for the baby's safety (AAP 2005).

    b. Bedsharing between parents and their babies is widely practiced (McCoy et al., 2004; Willinger et al., 2003). The baby should not share a bed with anyone other than a parent.

    c. Parents need to know safe bedsharing practices (Jenni et al., 2005; McKenna & McDade, 2005).

    d. Smothering is strongly linked to alcohol and drug use by bed partners.

    e. No research has yet shown a risk to the baby from a sober, nonsmoking, breastfeeding mother on a safe surface.

    f. Recommendations about bedsharing are different for the sober, nonsmoking, breastfeeding mother on a safe surface with her infant (see Section E4 to E6).

  3. Bedsharing may have potential health benefits for babies.

    a. Incidence of Sudden Infant Death Syndrome is decreasing at the same time as bedsharing is increasing (Arnestad et al., 2001).

    b. Increased sensory contact and close proximity with the mother have potential for behavioral and physiological changes in the infant (Ball, 2003).

    c. Bedsharing breastfeeding mothers have heightened sensitivity and responsivity to their infants.

d. Bedsharing breastfeeding mothers and infants have increased interactions and arousals, face-to-face body orientations, increased breastfeeding, increased heart rate, increased infant body temperatures, increased movements and awakenings, and less deep sleep (Goto et al., 1999).

4. Bedsharing safety requires a safe environment (Blair et al., 1999; Fleming et al., 1996; Hauck et al., 2003; Kemp et al., 2000; Nakamura, Wond, & Danello, 1999).

5. Potentially unsafe practices related to bed sharing/co-sleeping (ABM, 2006; AAP 2005) include:
   a. Environmental smoke exposure and maternal smoking.
   b. Sharing sofas, couches, or daybeds with infants.
   c. Sharing waterbeds or the use of soft bedding materials.
   d. Sharing beds with adjacent spaces that could trap an infant.
   e. Placement of the infant in the adult bed in the prone or side position.
   f. The use of alcohol or mind-altering drugs by the adult(s) who is bed sharing.

6. Safe sleep environments (ABM, 2006; AAP 2005)
   a. Place babies in the supine position for sleep.
   b. Use a firm, flat surface and avoid waterbeds, couches, sofas, pillows, soft materials, or loose bedding.
   c. Use only a thin blanket to cover the infant.
   d. Ensure that the head will not be covered. In a cold room, the infant could be kept in an infant sleeper to maintain warmth.
   e. Avoid the use of quilts, duvets, comforters, pillows, and stuffed animals in the infant's sleep environment.
   f. Never put an infant down to sleep on a pillow or adjacent to a pillow.
   g. Never leave an infant alone on an adult bed.
   h. Ensure that there are no spaces between the mattress and headboard, walls, and other surfaces, which may entrap the infant and lead to suffocation. Placement of a firm mattress directly on the floor away from walls may be a safe alternative.

X. Support Systems for Mothers

A. Mothers who have a strong support system for breastfeeding have better outcomes (Ekstrom, Widstrom, & Nissen, 2003; Rose et al., 2004; Sikorski, 2003).

1. There is a correlation between low parental confidence and a high perception of insufficiency (McCarter-Spaulding & Kerarney 2001).

2. Enhancing a mother's self-efficacy and increasing her confidence in her ability to breastfeed will help her persevere if she encounters difficulties (Blythe et al., 2002).

3. A mother's self-esteem will increase with a positive breastfeeding experience (Locklin & Naber, 1993).

4. Interventions need to shift from education to enhancing the mother's confidence regarding breastfeeding (Ertim et al., 2001).

B. Mother-to-mother support groups are a valuable resource.

1. They reinforce women's traditional patterns of seeking and receiving advice from relatives and friends.

2. They educate women about options and help them make informed choices.

3. Open communication and cooperation with the medical community and breastfeeding professionals empower mothers to make informed decisions.

4. They provide anticipatory guidance to help mothers learn what to expect, avoid potential problems, and resolve issues before they become obstacles.

C. Opposition to breastfeeding often manifests itself as subtle undermining of the mother's efforts.

1. Questions and comments that prompt mothers to explain and defend their decision to breastfeed can undermine a mother's confidence and cause her to doubt her decision or her capability to breastfeed.
   a. A mother who is confident about her decision to breastfeed is less likely to yield to the opinions or rude remarks of a stranger.
   b. Objections from people close to the mother are more difficult to cope with.
   c. Developing friendships and relationships with people who are supportive of breastfeeding or who are breastfeeding mothers themselves may help her become more confident with breastfeeding (Dykes et al., 2003).

2. Employers who have had previous experience with breastfeeding employees often react more positively (Dunn et al., 2004).
   a. A mother can avoid the stress and tension of an unsupportive work environment by speaking frankly with her employer about any special needs she will have.
   b. Negative attitudes result more from lack of understanding and experience than outright opposition (Bridges et al., 1997).
   c. Unreasonable and unfair treatment by an employer should be reported to the human resources department, local labor relations board, or in the United States, the Equal Employment Opportunity Commission.

3. Physician lack of support is difficult for a mother. A checklist may help parents determine if their physician truly supports breastfeeding (Newman & Pitman, 2000).

4. In many cultures, the baby's grandmother has a pivotal role in a mother's breastfeeding experience (Ekstrom et al., 2003).
   a. Some grandparents perceive breastfeeding as contributing to lack of sleep and a crying baby.
   b. Many health and breastfeeding organizations have information geared directly to grandparents (TDH, 2002).

5. Opposition from the baby's father is especially difficult.
    a. A father's opposition will weigh greatly on the decision to initiate or continue breastfeeding (Chang & Chan, 2003; Kong & Lee, 2004; Rose et al., 2004).
    b. As a man's role changes from mate to father, it may be difficult for him to regard the woman's breasts as something other than sexual.
    c. Opposition may stem from concern for the well-being of the mother and baby; educating the father can address misconceptions.
    d. Networking with families of older nursing babies and children will enable the father to meet other breastfeeding families and find it more acceptable.
    e. Avoid placing yourself in the middle of a conflict between a mother and an unsupportive partner. If you suspect domestic violence, provide hotline numbers and local community resources.

References

Academy of Breastfeeding Medicine (ABM). Academy of Breastfeeding Medicine Protocol on Co-Sleeping. Available at: http://www.bfmed.org/ace-files/protocol/cosleeping.pdf. Accessed October 11, 2006.

Academy of Breastfeeding Medicine (ABM). Academy of Breastfeeding Medicine Protocol on Contraception during Breastfeeding. Available at: http://www.bfmed.org/ace-files/protocol/finalcontraceptionprotocolsent2.pdf. Accessed January 13, 2006.

Ainsworth MDS, Blehar MC, Waters E, Wall S. *Patterns of Attachment—Psychological Study of the Strange Situation.* Hillsdale, NJ: Lawrence Erlbaum Associates; 1978.

American Academy of Pediatrics Task Force on Sudden Infant Death Syndrome. The Changing Concept of Sudden Infant Death Syndrome: Diagnostic Coding Shifts, Controversies Regarding Sleeping Environment, and New Variables to Consider in Reducing Risk. *Pediatrics.* November 2005b;116(5):1245–1255.

Aney M. Babywise linked to dehydration, failure to thrive. *AAP News.* 1998;14(4):21.

Arnestad AM, Andersen A, Vege Å, Rognum TO. Changes in the epidemiological pattern of sudden infant death syndrome in southeast Norway, 1984–1998: implications for future prevention and research. *Arch Dis Child.* 2001;85:108–115.

Ball HL. Breastfeeding, bed-sharing and infant sleep. *Birth.* 2003;30:181–188.

BarYam NB, Darby L. Fathers and breastfeeding: a review of the literature. *J Hum Lact.* 1997;13:45–50.

Beck C. A checklist to identify women at risk for developing postpartum depression. *J Obstet Gynecol Neonatal Nurs.* 1998;27:39–46.

Bjarnadottir R, Gottfredsdottir H, Siqurdardottir K, et al. Comparative study of the effects of a progestogen-only pill containing desogestrel and an intrauterine contraceptive device in lactating women. *BJOG.* 2001;108:1174–1180.

Blair PS, Fleming PJ, Smith IJ, et al. Babies sleeping with parents: case-control study of factors influencing the risk of the sudden infant death syndrome. BMJ. 1999; 319:1457–1462.

Blythe R et al. Effect of maternal confidence on breastfeeding duration: An application of breastfeeding self-efficacy theory. *Birth.* 2002;29(4):278-284.

Bocar DL, Moore K. Acquiring the parental role: a theoretical perspective. In: *Lactation Consultant Series.* Franklin Park, IL: La Leche League International; 1987.

Bowlby J. *Attachment and Loss: Attachment.* New York: Basic Books; 1969.

Bridges C et al. Employer attitudes toward breastfeeding in the workplace. *J Hum Lact.* 1997;13:215-219.

Briere J, Runtz M. The long-term effects of sexual abuse: a review and synthesis. *New Dir Ment Health Serv.* 1991;51:3-13.

Centers for Disease Control (CDC). Births: Final data for 2002. *National Vital Statistics Report.* 52(10);2003.

Chang JH, Chan WT. Analysis of factors associated with initiation and duration of breast-feeding: A study in Taitung Taiwan. *Acta Paediatr Taiwan.* 2003;44(1):29-34.

Cooper P et al. Psychosocial factors associated with the early termination of breastfeeding. *J Psychosom Res.* 1993;37:171-176.

Danli S, Qingxiang S, Guowei S. A multicentered clinical trial of the long-acting injectable contraceptive Depo Provera in Chinese women. *Contraception.* 2000; 62:15-18.

Delight E, Goodall J, Jones PW. What do parents expect antenatally and do babies teach them? *Arch Dis Child.* 1991;66:1309-1314.

Dewan N, Wood L, Maxwell S, et al. Breast-feeding knowledge and attitudes of teenage mothers in Liverpool. *J Hum Nutr Diet.* 2002;15:33-37.

Diaz S, Cardenas H, Brandeis A, et al. Early difference in the endocrine profile of long and short lactational amenorrhea. *J Clin Endocrinol Metab.* 1991;72:196-201.

Diaz S, Cardenas H, Brandeis A, et al. Relative contributions of anovulation and luteal phase defect to the reduced pregnancy rate of breastfeeding women. *Fertil Steril.* 1992;58:498-503.

Dunn B et al. Breastfeeding practices in Colorado businesses. *J Hum Lact.* 2004;20(2): 170-177.

Dunson TR, McLaurin VL, Grubb GS, Rosman AW. A multicenter clinical trial of a progestin-only oral contraceptive in lactating women. *Contraception.* 1993; 47:23-35.

Dykes F, Moran VH, Burt S, Edwards J. Adolescent mothers and breastfeeding: Experiences and support needs: an exploratory study. *J Hum Lact.* 2003;19:391-401.

Ekstrom A, Widstrom AM, Nissen E. Breastfeeding support from partners and grandmothers: perceptions of Swedish women. *Birth.* 2003;30:261-266.

Erikson EH. *Childhood and Society.* New York: W.W. Norton; 1950.

Ertim I et al. The timing and predictors of the early termination of breastfeeding. *Pediatrics.* 2001;107(3):543-548.

Finkelhor D. The international epidemiology of child sexual abuse. *Child Abuse Negl.* 1994;18:409-417.

Fleming A, Corter C, Stallings J, Steiner M. Testosterone and prolactin are associated with emotional responses to infant cries in new fathers. *Horm Behav.* 2002; 42:399–413.

Fleming PJ, Blair PS, Bacon C, et al. Environment of infants during sleep and risk of the sudden infant death syndrome: results of 1993–5 case-control study for confidential inquiry into stillbirths and deaths in infancy. *BMJ.* 1996;313:191–195.

Freed G, Fraley JK, Schanler RJ. Attitudes of expectant fathers regarding breastfeeding. *Pediatrics.* 1992;90:224–227.

Gale S, Harlow B. Postpartum mood disorders: a review of clinical and epidemiological factors. Review. *J Psychosom Obstet Gynaecol.* 2003;24:257–266.

Gamble D, Morse J. Fathers of breastfed infants: postponing and types of involvement. *J Obstet Gynecol Neonatal Nurs.* 1992;22:358–365.

Gellen J. The feasibility of suppressing ovarian activity following the end of amenorrhea by increasing the frequency of suckling. *Int J Gynecol Obstet.* 1992; 39:321–325.

Gold M. *The Good News About Depression: Cures and Treatments in the New Age of Psychiatry,* rev ed. New York: Bantam; 1995.

Goto K, Miririan M, Adams M, et al. More awakenings and heart rate variability during sleep in preterm infants. *Pediatrics.* 1999;10:603–609.

Graham M. Parental sensitivity to infant cues: similarities and differences between mothers and fathers. *J Pediatr Nurs.* 1993;8:376–384.

Gray R, Apelo R, Campbell O, et al. The return of ovarian function during lactation: Results of studies from the US and the Philippines. In: Gray R, Leridon H, Spira A, eds. *Biomedical and Demographic Determinants of Reproduction.* Oxford: Colorado Press; 1993:428–445.

Greenwood K, Littlejohn P. Breastfeeding intentions and outcomes of adolescent mothers in the Starting Out program. *Breastfeed Rev.* 2002;10:19–23.

Hauck FR, Herman SM, Donovan M, et al. Sleep environment and the risk of Sudden Infant Death Syndrome in an urban population: the Chicago Infant Mortality Study. *Pediatrics.* 2003;111:1207–1214.

Jenni O, Fuhrer H, Iglowstein I, et al. A longitudinal study of bed sharing and sleep problems among Swiss children in the first 10 years of life. *Pediatrics.* 2005;115 (Suppl):233–240.

Jordan P, Wall V. Breastfeeding and fathers: illuminating the darker side. *Birth.* 1990;17:210–213.

Kelsey J. Hormonal contraception and lactation. *J Hum Lact.* 1996;12:315–318.

Kemp JS, Unger B, Wilkins D, et al. Unsafe sleep practices and an analysis of bedsharing among infants dying suddenly and unexpectedly: results of a four-year, population-based, death-scene investigation study of sudden infant death syndrome and related deaths. *Pediatrics.* 2000;106:341–349.

Kendall-Tackett K. Breastfeeding and the sexual abuse survivor. *J Hum Lact.* 1998; 14:125–133.

Kendall-Tackett K. *The Hidden Feelings of Motherhood: Coping with Stress, Depression and Burnout.* Oakland, CA: New Harbinger Publisher; 2001.

Kennedy KI, Kotelchuck M, Visness CM, et al. Users' understanding of the lactational amenorrhea method and the occurrence of pregnancy. *J Hum Lact.* 1998;14:209–218.

Kippley S. Breastfeeding survey results similar to 1971 study. *CCL News.* 1986;13:10 and *CCL News.* 1987;13:5.

Kippley S, Kippley JF. The relation between breastfeeding and amenorrhea. *J Obstet Gynecol Neonatal Nursing.* 1972;1:15–21.

Klaus MH, Kennell JH. *Parent-Infant Bonding.* 2nd ed. St. Louis: C.V. Mosby; 1982.

Koetsawang S. The effects of contraceptive methods on the quality and quantity of breast milk. *Int J Gynaecol Obstet.* 1987;25(Suppl):115–127.

Kong S, Lee D. Factors influencing decision to breastfeed. *J Adv Nurs.* 2004;46(4): 369–379.

Labbok MH, Hight Laukaran V, Peterson AE, et al. Multicentre study of the lactational amenorrhea method (LAM). I. Efficacy, duration and implications for clinical application. *Contraception.* 1997;55:327–336.

Leffler D. U.S. high school age girls may be receptive to breastfeeding promotion. *J Hum Lact.* 2000;16:36–40.

Lizarraga J et al. Psychosocial and economic factors associated with infant feeding intentions of adolescent mothers. *J Adolesc Health.* 1992;13:676–681.

Locklin M, Naber S. Does breastfeeding empower women? Insights from a select group of educated, low-income, minority women. *Birth.* 1993;20:30–35.

March of Dimes/National Foundation. *Facts You Should Know About Teen Pregnancy.* White Plains, NY: March of Dimes; 2002.

McCarter-Spaulding D, Kerarney M. Parenting self-efficacy and perception of insufficient breast milk. *JOGNN.* 2001;30(5):515–522.

McCoy RC, Corwin MJ, Willinger M, et al. Frequency of bed sharing and its relationship to breastfeeding. *J Dev Behav Pediatr.* 2004;25:141–149.

McKenna JJ. An anthropological perspective on the sudden infant death syndrome (SIDS): the role of parental breathing cues and speech breathing adaptations. *Med Anthropol.* 1986;10:9–92.

McKenna JJ, McDade T. Why babies should never sleep alone: a review of the co-sleeping controversy in relation to SIDS, bedsharing and breast feeding. *Paediatr Respir Rev.* 2005;6:134–152.

McKenna JJ, Thoman EB, Anders TF, et al. Infant-parent co-sleeping in an evolutionary perspective: implications for understanding infant sleep development and the sudden infant death syndrome. *Sleep.* 1993;16:263–282.

McNeilly A. Lactational amenorrhea. *Endocrinol Metab Clin North Am.* 1993;22:59–73.

McNeilly A, Tay CC, Glasier A. Physiological mechanisms underlying lactational amenorrhea. *Ann NY Acad Sci.* 1994;709:145–155.

Misri S. Shouldn't I be happy? Emotional problems of pregnant and postpartum women. New York: Free Press; 2002.

Moody L. Case studies of moms who had problems using Babywise or Preparation for Parenting, 2002. Available at: www.angelfire.com/md2/moodyfamily/casestudies.html.

Nakamura S, Wond M, Danello MA. Review of the hazards associated with children placed in adult beds. *Arch Pediatr Adolesc Med.* 1999;153:1019–1023.

National Center for Health Statistics (NCHS). Births to teenagers in the United States, 1940–2000. *Natl Vital Stat Rep;* September 25, 2001. Available at http://www.cdc.gov/nchs/data/nvsr/nvsr49/nvsr49_10.pdf. Accessed December 4, 2006.

Newman J, Pitman T. *The Ultimate Breastfeeding Book of Answers.* Roseville, CA: Prima Pub; 2000.

Oates M. Perinatal psychiatric disorders: A leading cause of maternal morbidity and mortality. *Br Med Bull.* 2003;67(1):219–229.

Rose V et al. Factors influencing infant feeding method in an urban community. *J Natl Med Assoc.* 2004;96(3):325–331.

Rubin R. Attainment of the maternal role: Part 1, Processes. *Nurs Res.* 1967a; 16:237–245.

Rubin R. Attainment of the maternal role. Part II, Models and referents. *Nurs Res.* 1967b; 16:342–346.

Sears W, Gotsch G. *Becoming a Father.* 2nd ed. Schaumburg, IL: La Leche League International; 2003.

Sikorski J, Renfrew MJ, Pindoria S, Wade A. Support for breastfeeding mothers: a systematic review. *Paediatr Perinat Epidemiol.* 2003;17:407–417.

Sivin I, Diaz S, Croxatto HB, et al. Contraceptives for lactating women: A comparative trial of a progesterone-releasing vaginal ring and the copper T 380A IUD. *Contraception.* 1997;55:225–232.

Speroff L. Postpartum contraception: issues and choices. *Dialogues in Contraception.* 1992–1993;3:1–3, 67.

Tay C, Glasier AF, McNeilly AS. Twenty-four hour patterns of prolactin secretion during lactation and the relationship to suckling and the resumption of fertility in breast-feeding women. *Hum Reprod.* 1996;11:950–955.

Taylor J, Cabral H. Are women with an unintended pregnancy less likely to breastfeed? *J Fam Pract.* 2002;51(5):431–436.

Texas Department of Health (TDH), Bureau of Nutrition Services. Just for Grandparents. 2002; #13-06-11288.

Vestermark V, Hoqdall CK, Plenov G, Birch M. Postpartum amenorrhoea and breastfeeding in a Danish sample. *J Biosoc Sci.* 1994;26:1–7.

Webb C. Is the Babywise method right for you? what you should know about Babywise and Growing Kids God's Way. Tulsa Kids; July 2003.

Williams M. Epigee Birth Control Guide. Available at: www.epigee.org. Updated August 1, 2003.

Williams N. Counseling challenges: Helping mothers handle conflicting information. *Leaven.* 1998;34(2):19–20.

Williams N. Dancing with differences: Helping mothers handle conflicting information, including scheduled feeding and sleep training. La Leche League Int'l 1999 Conference, Orlando, FL; July 5, 1999.

Willinger M, Ko CE, Hoffman HJ, et al. Trends in infant bed sharing in the United States, 1993–2000. *Arch Pediatr Adolesc Med.* 2003;157:43–49.

Internet Resources for Postpartum Depression Information

British Columbia Reproductive Mental Health Program—Guidelines for healthcare professionals. Available at: http://www.rcp.gov.bc.ca/guidelines.htm. Accessed November 15, 2006.

Emedicine Consumer Health. Available at: http://www.emedicinehealth.com/postpartum_depression/article_em.htm. Accessed November 15, 2006.

March of Dimes. Discusses complications including baby blues and postpartum depression. Available at: http://www.marchofdimes.com/pnhec. Accessed November 15, 2006.

Mayo Clinic. Online site to empower people to manage their health by providing useful and up-to-date information and tools. Available at: http://www.mayoclinic.com/health/postpartum-depression/DS00546. Accessed November 15, 2006.

MedlinePlus. Postpartum Depression. Brings together authoritative information from National Library of Medicine (NLM), the National Institutes of Health (NIH), and other government agencies and health-related organizations. Available at: http://www.nlm.nih.gov/medlineplus/postpartumdepression.html. Accessed November 15, 2006.

Medscape Women's Health. Part of WebMD. Do your own research on various subjects pertaining to women's health. Available at: http://www.medscape.com/womenshealth-home?src=pdown. Accessed November 15, 2006.

Online PPD Support Group. Devoted to mothers and families affected by postpartum depression. Offers information, advice, and support through a mailing list, chat room, and forum. Available at: http://www.ppdsupportpage.com. Accessed November 15, 2006.

Pacific Postpartum Support Society. Non-profit society dedicated to supporting the needs of distressed postpartum mothers and their families. Available at: http://www.postpartum.org. Accessed November 15, 2006.

Postpartum Adjustment Support Services of Canada (PASS-Can). Source for pregnancy and parenting information, interaction, resources and products in multiple forms of media. Available at: http://iparentingcanada.com. Accessed November 15, 2006.

Postpartum Depression Links. Extensive list of links to various subjects relating to PPD. Available at: http://www.psycom.net/depression.central.post-partum.html. Accessed November 15, 2006.

Postpartum Support International. Social support network, information center, and research guide concerning PPD. Offers information on research, conferences, early detection, and resources for new parents and professionals. Available at: http://www.postpartum.net. Accessed November 15, 2006.

Pregnancy and Parenting. Message board hosted by ivillage. Offers tips, support, and advice on trying to conceive, pregnancy, parenting, toddlers, school-age children, and teens. Available at: http://parenting.ivillage.com/messageboards. Accessed November 15, 2006.

The Postpartum Stress Centre. Specializes in the diagnosis and treatment of prenatal and postpartum depression and anxiety disorders; offers general counseling services, too. Available at: http://www.postpartumstress.com/index.html. Accessed November 15, 2006.

WellMother.com. Online resource for women and their families. Website owned by Shaila Misri, MD, FRCP(C) that offers support and resources on a number of issues related to the emotional challenges of women, specifically: menstruation, PMS, pregnancy, pregnancy loss, postpartum challenges, and menopause. Available at: http://www.wellmother.com. Accessed November 15, 2006.

MATERNAL MENTAL HEALTH AND BREASTFEEDING

Kathleen Kendall-Tackett, PhD, IBCLC

OBJECTIVES

- Recognize the symptoms of depression and other mood disorders in new mothers.
- Describe the causes of postpartum depression.
- Provide information to mothers on treatment options for depression that are compatible with breastfeeding.
- Describe how maternal mood disorders that occur in the first postpartum year can impact breastfeeding.

Introduction

A mother's emotional state can have a dramatic influence on her well-being in the first postpartum year. Depression, posttraumatic stress disorder (PTSD), and other conditions can cause mothers to quit breastfeeding and have a negative impact on their relationships with their babies (Kendall-Tackett, 2005). Even when mothers are depressed, however, breastfeeding protects babies from the harmful effects of their mothers' depression (Jones, McFall, & Diego, 2004). And when breastfeeding is going well, it is mildly protective of maternal mood (Groër, 2005; Kendall-Tackett, 2005).

I. Postpartum Depression

A. Overview.

1. Postpartum depression is relatively common, affecting 10% to 20% of new mothers worldwide (Kendall-Tackett, 2005).

2. Some populations, however, such as low-income ethnic minority mothers, may have rates as high as 40% to 50% (McKee et al., 2001). But in cultures where there are rituals that support new mothers, rates of postpartum depression and other conditions are quite low (Stern & Kruckman, 1983).

3. Symptoms of depression include moods of sadness, anhedonia (inability to experience pleasure in normally pleasurable activities), sleep difficulties unrelated to infant care, fatigue, inability to concentrate, hopelessness, and thoughts of death. For a diagnosis of depression these symptoms must be present for at least two weeks.

4. Depression also may manifest as somatic complaints or severe fatigue. In many cultures, these symptoms are more acceptable than depression. Another indication of possible depression is increased use of health care services for the mother or her baby.

5. "Baby blues" are often mild and self-limiting. But many believe that the blues are an early manifestation of depression and therefore should not be ignored (see Chapter 4).

6. Most treatment options for depression are compatible with breastfeeding.

B. Causes of depression in new mothers.

1. The factors that underlay depression in mothers vary from woman to woman.

2. Causes of depression in new mothers fall into five categories.
   a. Physiological causes.
      i. Fatigue and sleep difficulties can both cause and be the consequence of depression. Depression causes sleep problems, leading to fatigue, which in turn causes more depression. Medications can be helpful in addressing sleep difficulties, as can cognitive therapy and helping the mother cope with disrupted sleep (e.g., more support during the day so she can get some rest).
      ii. Pain and depression have many similarities and may share a common etiology. Postpartum pain can trigger depression and should be dealt with promptly.
      iii. Immune system activation, particularly elevations of the pro-inflammatory cytokines interleukin-1β (IL-1β), IL-6, and tumor necrosis factor-α also increase the risk of depression. Cytokines increase inflammation. Because they are anti-inflammatory, Omega-3 fatty acids are thought to be effective in the prevention and treatment of depression. Conventional (O'Brien, Scott, & Dinan, 2006) and herbal (including St. John's Wort) antidepressants also appear to have an anti-inflammatory action (Bratman & Girman, 2003), which may be a reason for their efficacy.
      iv. At this point, there is very little evidence supporting a hormonal etiology of postpartum depression (Kendall-Tackett, 2005).
   b. Negative birth experiences.
      i. Negative birth experiences are relatively common. In one study, 40% of a representative U.S. sample of mothers described giving birth in predominantly negative terms (Genevie & Margolies, 1987).

    ii. Objective aspects of birth (e.g., cesarean vs. vaginal) only account for some reactions. Mothers who have cesarean births are at somewhat increased risk of having a negative reaction, but that is not always true. Subjective aspects of birth, such as those that are listed below, are more likely to lead to a woman's negative assessment of giving birth.
- Did she believe that giving birth was dangerous to herself or her baby?
- Did she feel in control of either the medical situation or herself during labor?
- Did she feel supported during labor and birth?

    iii. Birth experiences can cause psychological trauma. One review study found that 1.5% to 6% of women met the full criteria of PTSD following birth (Beck, 2004). In comparison, 7.5% of residents of lower Manhattan in New York City met the full criteria for PTSD following the 9/11 terrorist attacks (Galea et al., 2003).

    iv. Even when women do not meet full criteria, they may manifest symptoms of PTSD. One study found that 30% of mothers had symptoms of PTSD after giving birth (Soet, Brack, & DiIorio, 2003). These symptoms include intrusive thoughts about the birth while they are awake or when they try to sleep, emotional numbing, and dissociation (see Section II).

    v. Mothers are more vulnerable to PTSD if they have had prior episodes of depression or PTSD, are abuse survivors (which increases the risk of both PTSD and depression), had prior episodes of loss (including childbearing loss), or were depressed during pregnancy.

c. Infant characteristics.

    i. Infants with a "difficult" temperament can trigger depression in mothers. These babies are often highly sensitive to their surroundings, don't fall into regular schedules or routines, cry a lot in the first few months, have an intense need to be with their mothers, and often do not sleep well at night.

    ii. These babies can undermine a woman's sense of competence and self-efficacy, especially if this is her first baby. In one study, low self-efficacy was related to the effect of temperament on maternal depression. In other words, the infant's difficult temperament caused the mothers' depression by making them feel incompetent (Cutrona & Troutman, 1986).

    iii. Infant illness, preterm birth, and disability also can cause depression in mothers, particularly if the babies are at high risk. However, this reaction is often delayed and may not manifest itself until the babies are out of danger, or even several months after they are discharged.

    iv. Kangaroo Care and social support for parents both have been effective techniques to help mothers cope with the demands of their preterm or disabled infants (Capuzzi, 1989; Feldman et al., 2002). Perinatal home visiting has mixed results and seems effective only for mothers who perceive that there is a need for it (Affleck et al., 1989).

d. Psychological characteristics.

    i. *Attributional style* refers to how people explain events in their lives. Are they optimists or pessimists? Pessimists attribute negative events to some intrinsic flaw in themselves, see negative situations as unchangeable, and think that negative events influence every aspect of their lives. These beliefs increase the risk of depression and are specifically addressed in cognitive-behavioral therapy.

    ii. *Previous psychiatric history* includes the psychiatric history of the mother and her first-degree relatives. A mother who has had prior episodes of depression or PTSD is at increased risk. This includes depression during pregnancy, which some studies have found is even more common than depression after birth. However, this elevated risk does not mean depression is inevitable. With proper support for the mother, depression can be avoided.

    iii. *Self-esteem, self-efficacy,* and *expectations* refer to how mothers feel about themselves as mothers. Do they feel competent? Are their expectations of themselves and their babies realistic? Feeling incompetent and having unrealistic expectations increases the risk of depression.

e. Social factors.

    i. *Abusive* or *dysfunctional family of origin.* Childhood sexual abuse, in particular, dramatically increases the lifetime risk of depression. But all forms of child maltreatment increase risk.

    ii. *Loss.* This situation might include loss of a parent during childhood (particularly loss of a mother), childbearing loss, and loss of a partner through death or divorce.

    iii. *Lack of social support.* Social support includes emotional and instrumental support that can be provided by a woman's partner, friends, relatives, and professionals. Partner support is a key source. But for women without partner support, support from others can prevent depression. U.S. culture is generally poor at providing support for new mothers. Individual practitioners can encourage mothers to seek this type of support for themselves by offering referrals to mothering organizations and by giving them "permission" to ask for help.

    iv. *Socioeconomic status.* Despite the popular myth, postpartum depression is not more common in white middle-class women. Lower-income women are not only more vulnerable (unless they have good support), but when they become depressed, fewer resources are available to help them recover.

    v. *Stressful life events.* Mothers who have endured recent stressful events, even positive ones (e.g., moving to a new home), may find themselves depressed.

3. Each of these risk factors alone can cause depression. However, many mothers have multiple risk factors that combined can dramatically increase the risk of depression.

4. By helping mothers identify the sources of their depression, intervention can be targeted more specifically.

C. Breastfeeding and depression.

1. Depressed mothers are more likely to quit breastfeeding (Kendall-Tackett, 2005).

2. Mothers who were not breastfeeding were significantly more likely to be depressed in two studies (Astbury et al., 1994; Taj & Sikander, 2003). Overall, breastfeeding appears to be mildly protective of maternal mood (Kendall-Tackett, 2005).

3. However, breastfeeding difficulties can increase the risk of depression. Some of the risk factors include nipple pain, overall breastfeeding problem severity, and worrying about breastfeeding.

4. When the breastfeeding issues were resolved, the maternal mood states returned to normal (Amir et al. 1996).

D. Assessment of postpartum depression.

1. Assessment inventories.
   a. *Edinburgh Postnatal Depression Scale.* The most commonly used postpartum depression screening tool in the world. It is copyright free and available at http://www.GraniteScientific.com.
   c. Beck's *Postpartum Depression Screening Scale.* A more in-depth scale available at Western Psychological Services (http://www.wpspublish.com).

2. Red flag symptoms that require immediate medical attention for the mother.
   - She has not slept in two or three days.
   - She is losing weight rapidly.
   - She cannot get out of bed.
   - She is ignoring basic grooming.
   - She seems hopeless.
   - She says her children would be better off without her.
   - She is actively abusing substances.
   - She makes strange or bizarre statements (e.g., plans to give her children away to strangers).

E. Treatment options.
   A variety of treatment options are available that are effective for mild, moderate, and severe depression. Most of these options are compatible with breastfeeding, and several can be safely combined.

1. Vitamin and mineral supplements.
   a. People who are depressed are often low in vitamins B_6 and B_{12} as well as folic acid and choline (Bratman & Girman, 2003).

b. Some of the most promising supplements are the Omega-3 fatty acids. Studies have found docosahexaenoic acid (DHA) to be effective for the prevention of depression, and eicosapentaenoic acid (EPA) (with or without DHA) as a possible adjunct to medications used to treat depression. DHA and EPA can come from food (e.g., cold water fish such as salmon and mackerel), but mothers are often deficient in them because contaminants may make it unsafe to consume seafood during pregnancy and lactation. Mothers can also obtain DHA and EPA from fish oil, or vegetarian DHA supplements or DHA-fortified foods (Freeman et al., 2006; Hibbeln, 2002; Peet & Stokes, 2005).

c. Omega-3 found in flax seed and other plant sources is α-linolenic acid (ALA), the parent essential fatty acid to EPA and DHA. However, the body's conversion of ALA to EPA/DHA is inefficient. ALA does not have efficacy in the prevention or treatment of depression (Bratman & Girman, 2003; Kendall-Tackett, 2005).

d. One study of mothers found that those who had high levels of DHA during pregnancy had babies with more mature sleep patterns in the first few days of life than babies of mothers who were low in DHA. Quality of infant sleep could have an indirect effect on their mothers' mental health, with babies who have more mature sleep patterns allowing their mothers to get more rest (Cheruku et al., 2002).

2. Exercise.
   a. Exercise has proven as effective as sertraline, an antidepressant drug, in randomized trials for the treatment of even major depression. Patients assigned to the exercise condition are also less likely to relapse once treatment ends (Babyak et al., 2000).
   b. Exercising two to three times a week for about 20 minutes a session is enough to get an antidepressant effect.
   c. Exercise can be combined with other treatment modalities.

3. Therapy.
   a. Two forms of therapy have proven efficacious for the treatment of even severe depression: cognitive-behavioral therapy and interpersonal therapy (O'Hara et al., 2000; Rupke, Blecke, & Renfrow, 2006).
   b. Both of these types of therapy have proven as effective as medications in randomized clinical trials.

4. Herbal medications.
   a. St. John's wort (*Hypericum perforatum*) is an effective treatment for mild-to-moderate depression and for major depression (van Gurp et al., 2002).
   b. It is currently considered safe for breastfeeding mothers (Hale, 2006). Mothers should tell their health care providers that they are taking it because it can interact with several classes of prescription medications (e.g., oral contraceptives, cyclosporins, and antidepressants).

c. Kava, another herb that is sometimes paired with St, John's wort for treatment of anxiety, is a sedative and currently contraindicated for breastfeeding mothers (Hale, 2006).

5. Antidepressant medications.

a. Most antidepressants are compatible with breastfeeding. Medications with inert metabolites (e.g., sertraline and paroxetine) are preferred for breastfeeding mothers because they result in lower exposure of the baby to the medication.

b. Only one class of antidepressants—monoamine oxidase inhibitors—is always contraindicated for breastfeeding mothers (e.g., Nardil, Parnate) (Thomas Hale, PhD, personal communication, 2006).

II. Other Conditions

Several conditions can either occur alone or co-occur with postpartum depression.

A. Posttraumatic stress disorder.

1. Women may experience PTSD as a result of a prior trauma-producing event (e.g., childhood abuse, rape or assault, car accident, natural disaster) or as a result of the birth itself.

2. A key aspect of what makes a traumatic event harmful is whether the mother believed that either her or a loved-one's life was in danger. In terms of the mother's reaction, her perception is what counts. For birth, it does not matter if the mother's perception of risk is not medically "true." If she believes that she or her baby might have died, then she is likely to have a reaction.

3. To meet full criteria for PTSD, women must have symptoms in three domains: intrusion, avoidance, and hyperarousal. Even when someone does not meet the full criteria, however, they may still have troublesome symptoms. For example, emotional numbness after a traumatic birth may make it difficult initially for a mother to bond with her baby. Intrusive thoughts, nightmares, and chronic hyperarousal may compromise the quality of a mother's sleep, further impairing her mental health.

B. Bipolar disorder.

1. Bipolar disorder can manifest for the first time in the postpartum period.

2. Postpartum bipolar disorder is tricky to diagnose because it almost always manifests as major depression. When the depression is treated, often with the selective serotonin reuptake inhibitor (SSRI) class of antidepressants, these medications can trigger a manic episode.

3. Postpartum bipolar disorder can occur with or without psychosis and tends to run in families.

C. Eating disorders.

1. Eating disorders can occur during pregnancy and during the postpartum period.

2. Active eating disorders during pregnancy increase the rate of postpartum depression.

D. Obsessive-compulsive disorder (OCD).

1. OCD is characterized by recurrent, unwelcome thoughts, ideas, and doubts that give way to obsessions. The exact incidence of postpartum OCD is not known, but a high percentage of women with postpartum OCD also have postpartum depression (Kendall-Tackett, 2005).

2. OCD can manifest itself as repetitive thoughts of infant harm. Generally speaking, these thoughts do not lead to an increased risk that the mother will harm her baby. In fact, she will often go to extreme measures to keep anything from happening to her baby (Abramowicz et al., 2002).

3. OCD and co-occurring depression are treated with SSRIs.

E. Maternal stress.

1. From a physiological standpoint, stress and depression are similar in that both have high levels of the stress hormone cortisol.

2. Elevated cortisol levels can impact breastfeeding. One study found that for women with higher levels of cortisol, often after a stressful birth, lactogenesis II was delayed by several days (Grajeda & Perez-Escamilla, 2002).

3. Groër and colleagues (2005) found that mothers who were stressed, fatigued, or had negative moods had lower levels of prolactin in their milk and blood than mothers who were not tired and stressed.

III. Adverse Childhood Experiences (ACE)

A. Definition and incidence.

1. ACE includes childhood physical and sexual abuse, emotional abuse, neglect, witnessing domestic violence between parents or a parent and his/her partner, parental mental illness, substance abuse, or criminal activity.

2. These types of experiences are common. In one large, middle-class U.S. sample, 51% had experienced at least one type of ACE (Felitti et al., 2001). Samples with higher risk populations tend to have even higher rates.

3. These types of experiences can impact mothers postpartum, most notably by increasing the risk of depression and PTSD. This risk is especially elevated in mothers who are sexual abuse survivors.

4. Women who have these types of experiences may have higher rates of intention to breastfeed and breastfeeding initiation rates. However, they may encounter problems and cease breastfeeding prematurely (Kendall-Tackett, 2004).

5. Practitioners may need to work with mothers who are abuse survivors to modify breastfeeding so that it is more comfortable. Depending on the mother's experience, some strategies that may help include: using distraction while breastfeeding; avoiding nighttime feedings; reducing the amount of skin-to-skin contact; and pumping milk and using a bottle. Be flexible and help the mother find a way that works best for her.

References

Abramowitz JS, Schwartz SA, Moore KM, Luenzmann KR. Obsessive-compulsive symptoms in pregnancy and the puerperium: a review of the literature. *J Anx Disord.* 2002;426:1–18.

Affleck G, Tennen H, Rowe J, et al. Effects of formal support on mothers' adaptation to the hospital-to-home transition of high-risk infants: the benefits and costs of helping. *Child Develop.* 1989;60:488–501.

Amir LH, Dennerstein L, Garland SM, et al. Psychological aspects of nipple pain in lactating women. *J Psychosom Obstet Gynecol.* 1996;17:53–58.

Astbury J, Brown S, Lumley J, Small R. Birth events, birth experiences, and social differences in postnatal depression. *Aust J Public Health.* 1994;18:176–184.

Babyak M, Blumenthal JA, Herman S, et al. Exercise treatment for major depression: maintenance of therapeutic benefit at 10 months. *Psychosom Med.* 2000;62:633–638.

Beck CT. Posttraumatic stress disorder due to childbirth. *Nurs Res.* 2004;53:28–35.

Bratman S, Girman AM. *Handbook of Herbs and Supplements and Their Therapeutic Uses.* St. Louis: C.V. Mosby; 2003.

Capuzzi, C. Maternal attachment to handicapped infants and the relationship to social support. *Res Nurs Health.* 1989;12:161–167.

Cheruku SR, Montgomery-Downs HE, Farkas SL, et al. Higher maternal plasma docosahexaenoic acid during pregnancy is associated with more mature neonatal sleep-state patterning. *Am J Clin Nutr.* 2002;76:608–613.

Cutrona CE, Troutman BR. Social support, infant temperament, and parenting self-efficacy: a mediational model of postpartum depression. *Child Develop.* 1986;57:1507–1518.

Feldman R, Eidelman AI, Sirota L, Weller A. Comparison of skin-to-skin (kangaroo) and traditional care: parenting outcomes and preterm infant development. *Pediatrics.* 2002;110:16–26.

Felitti VJ, Anda RF, Nordenberg D, et al. Relationship of childhood abuse and household dysfunction to many of the leading causes of death in adults. In: Franey K, Geffner R, and Falconer R, eds. *The Cost of Child Maltreatment: Who Pays? We All Do.* San Diego, CA: Family Violence and Sexual Assault Institute; 2001:53–69.

Freeman MP, Hibbeln JR, Wisner KL, et al. Randomized dose-ranging pilot trial of omega-3 fatty acids for postpartum depression. *Acta Psychia Scand.* 2006;113:31–35.

Galea S, Vlahov D, Resnick H, et al. Trends of probable post-traumatic stress disorder in New York City after the September 11 terrorist attacks. *Am J Epidemiol.* 2003; 158:514–524.

Genevie L, Margolies E. *The Motherhood Report: How Women Feel About Being Mothers.* New York: Macmillan; 1987.

Grajeda R, Perez-Escamilla R. Stress during labor and delivery is associated with delayed onset of lactation among urban Guatemalan women. *J Nutr.* 2002; 132:3055–3060.

Groër M. Differences between exclusive breastfeeders, formula-feeders, and controls: a study of stress, mood, and endocrine variables. *Biol Res Nurs.* 2005;7:106–117.

Groër M, Davis M, Casey K, et al. Neuroendocrine and immune relationships in postpartum fatigue. *MCN Am J Matern Child Nurs.* 2005; 30:133–138.

Hale T. *Medications and Mothers' Milk.* 12th ed. Amarillo, TX: Hale Publishing; 2006.

Hibbeln JR. Seafood consumption, the DHA content of mothers' milk and prevalence rates of postpartum depression: a cross-national, ecological analysis. *J Affect Dis.* 2002;69:15–29.

Jones NA, McFall BA, Diego MA. Patterns of brain electrical activity in infants of depressed mothers who breastfeed and bottle feed: the mediating role of infant temperament. *Biol Psychol.* 2004;67:103–124.

Kendall-Tackett KA. *Breastfeeding and the Sexual Abuse Survivor.* Lactation Consultant Series 2, Unit 9. Schaumburg, IL: La Leche League International; 2004.

Kendall-Tackett KA. *Depression in New Mothers.* Binghamton, NY: Haworth; 2005.

McKee MD, Cunningham M, Jankowski KR, Zayas L. Health-related functional status in pregnancy: relationship to depression and social support in a multi-ethnic population. *Obstet Gynecol.* 2001;97:988–993.

O'Brien SM, Scott LV, Dinan TG. Antidepressant therapy and C-reactive protein levels. *Br J Psychiatry.* 2006;188:449–452.

O'Hara MW, Stuart S, Gorman LL, Wenzel A. Efficacy of interpersonal psychotherapy for postpartum depression. *Arch Gen Psych.* 2000;57:1039–1045.

Peet M, Stokes C. Omega-3 fatty acids in the treatment of psychiatric disorders. *Drugs.* 2005;65:1051–1059.

Rupke SJ, Blecke D, Renfrow M. Cognitive therapy for depression. *Am Fam Physician.* 2006;73:83–86.

Soet JE, Brack GA, DiIorio C. Prevalence and predictors of women's experience of psychological trauma during childbirth. *Birth.* 2003;30:36–46.

Stern G, Kruckman L. Multi-disciplinary perspectives on postpartum depression: An anthropological critique. *Soc Sci Med.* 1983;17:1027–1041.

Taj R, Sikander KS. Effects of maternal depression on breastfeeding. *J Pakistani Med Assoc.* 2003;53:8–11.

van Gurp G, Meterissian GB, Haiek LN, et al. St. John's wort or sertraline?: Randomized controlled trial in primary care. *Can Fam Physician.* 2002;48:905–912.

Internet Resources

Information on depression, abuse and neglect, breastfeeding, and other women's issues is presented in articles, conference presentations, and other educational materials written by Kathleen Kendall-Tackett, PhD, IBCLC; use and reprints are free with acknowledgment of source. Available at: http://www.GraniteScientific.com. Accessed November 16, 2006.

Includes "7 Natural Laws of Breastfeeding" and excerpts of *Breastfeeding Made Simple*, Mohrbacher, N., Kendall-Tackett, K., Oakland, CA: New Harbinger Publications; 2005. Available at: http://www.BreastfeedingMadeSimple.com. Accessed November 16, 2006.

Resources and information for those who may be experiencing prenatal or postnatal mood or anxiety disorders. Sponsored by Postpartum Support International. Available at: http://www.Postpartum.net. Accessed November 16, 2006.

Information for families about mental health and pregnancy. Depression after Delivery has now combined with Postpartum Support International, but archived articles are still available on this site. Available at: http://www.DepressionafterDelivery.com. Accessed November 16, 2006.

Suggested Readings

Hassmen P, Koivula N, Uutela A. Physical exercise and psychological well-being: a population study in Finland. *Prevent Med.* 2000;30:17–25.

Kendall-Tackett KA. *Hidden Feelings of Motherhood.* 2nd ed. Amarillo, TX: Hale Publishing; 2005.

Mohrbacher N, Kendall-Tackett KA. *Breastfeeding Made Simple.* Oakland, CA: New Harbinger Publications; 2005.

Breastfeeding and Working Women

Cathy Carothers, BLA, IBCLC, and Barbara Wilson-Clay, BSEd, IBCLC

OBJECTIVES

- Identify ways employment impacts breastfeeding initiation and duration.
- List benefits to employers who provide lactation support for employees.
- List benefits to mothers and babies when breastfeeding is continued after the mother returns to work.
- Identify common barriers to sustaining lactation among women returning to work.
- Identify common barriers of employers in establishing worksite lactation support.
- Identify strategies for assisting employers with establishing lactation support programs for employees.
- Describe basic workplace requirements to support the lactating employee.
- State factors to consider in choosing appropriate breast pumps.
- Describe the safe storage of breast milk.
- Identify key information that should be discussed with childcare providers.
- List occupational hazards in the workplace in relation to breastfeeding.

Introduction

The majority of mothers today with young children work outside the home. While separation can pose challenges for breastfeeding mothers, women have developed many successful strategies to maintain their breastfeeding relationships. These creative options include maternal leave of absence for up to one year following birth, flexible scheduling, home-based employment, onsite child care, bringing the infant to the mother for feedings, expressing milk in the workplace for missed feedings, and reverse cycle feeding. The lactation consultant helps the employed mother to reach her goals for breastfeeding through anticipatory guidance so that mothers can plan a course of action to support their working and mothering goals. This counseling occurs during the prenatal period and continues in the early postpartum days and after the mother returns to work.

To properly assist the mother, the lactation consultant must understand the physiology of lactation to help the mother establish and maintain an adequate milk supply. The lactation consultant also must be familiar with alternate methods of milk expression, including both hand expression and the use of breast pumps. He or she must be able to counsel on the use of alternate feeding devices, safe storage and handling of human milk, and coping methods for dealing with the challenges of combining employment with breastfeeding. In addition, the lactation consultant should understand the key components of a worksite lactation program that can enable women to meet their breastfeeding goals and be able to address employer barriers to providing onsite support for breastfeeding employees.

I. Impact of Employment on Breastfeeding Initiation and Duration

A. Employment among women and mothers is the rule rather than the exception.

B. Sixty-one percent of women in the United States and 76% of women in Sweden with children under the age of six work outside the home (OECD, 2002).

C. Seventy percent of women with children under the age of 3 worked full-time, with one-third of these women returning to work within three months and two-thirds returning to work within six months (USBC, 2002).

D. Eighty-four percent of working women return to the work force within six months.

E. Low-income women and African-American women in the United States are more likely to return to work earlier than higher income earners and are more likely to be employed in jobs that present numerous challenges to the continuation of breastfeeding (Lindberg, 1996).

F. Some studies show that intention to work can affect breastfeeding initiation. In particular, women planning to work part-time are more likely to initiate breastfeeding than women planning to work full-time (Fein & Roe, 1998; Scott et al., 2001).

G. Duration of breastfeeding is significantly affected when a mother returns to work (Biagioli, 2003).

H. The number of hours worked impacts duration. The more hours a week she works, the shorter the duration (Table 6-1) (Fein & Roe, 1998).

I. U.S. welfare reform requirements have significantly impacted breastfeeding rates (Haider, Jacknowitz, & Schoeni, 2003).

1. Mothers affected by the reform are more likely to return to work sooner than they planned and face difficulties maintaining lactation.

Table 6-1 Breastfeeding duration relative to hours worked per week

Hours Worked Per Week	Not Working	< 20 hours	20–34 hours	> 35 hours
Average Duration of Breastfeeding	25.1 weeks	24.4 weeks	22.5 weeks	16.5 weeks

    2. Estimates are that if welfare reform had not been enacted, national breastfeeding rates six months after birth would have been 5.5% higher than they were in 2000 (Haider et al., 2003).

  J. Many women do not view employment and breastfeeding to be compatible.

    1. Compared to unemployed women, full-time employed women are less likely to continue breastfeeding to six months.

    2. Types of occupations impact breastfeeding duration. Women classified as professional, administrative, or managerial are more inclined to breastfeed longer than women employed in low wage jobs or jobs requiring lower skills (Galtry, 1997; Hanson et al., 2003).

  K. The duration of maternal leave significantly affects breastfeeding duration (Roe et al., 1999).

    1. For each week of maternity leave taken, breastfeeding duration increases by approximately one-half of a week (Roe et al., 1999).

    2. Returning to work within 12 weeks postpartum is related to the greatest decrease in breastfeeding duration (Galtry, 2003; Gielen et al., 1991; Taveras, 2003).

  L. Intention and actual breastfeeding practices can improve duration rates of breastfeeding. Women who breastfeed exclusively during the first postpartum month and intend to fully or partially breastfeed are more likely to breastfeed longer than six months after returning to work (Piper & Parks, 1996).

II. Supporting Breastfeeding is a "Win–Win" for Employers, Mothers, and Babies

  A. For mothers, continuing to breastfeed results in:

    1. Optimal outcomes for her baby's health, growth, and development.

    2. Significant reduction in numerous acute infections and chronic diseases in infants (AAP, 2005).

    3. Continued emotional bonding with baby.

    4. Fewer missed days of work because her baby is healthier (Cohen, Mrtek, & Mrtek, 1995).

5. Lower health care costs (Ball & Wright, 1999).

6. Less energy, time, and cost to purchase, store, and prepare infant formula.

7. Benefits of oxytocin released during pumping sessions with increased feelings of relaxation and sense of well-being.

8. Strong sense of "reconnection" when mother and child are reunited following separation at work (Bocar, 1997; Neifert, 1998).

B. For employers, breastfeeding results in:

1. Lower absenteeism rates due to baby-related illnesses, and shorter absences when they do miss work compared with women who do not breastfeed (Cohen et al., 1995). For an employee earning $15/hour, each one day of absence costs the company $160 (Faught, 1994).

2. Lower health care costs for the employer (Ball & Wright, 1999).

C. Value of worksite lactation support programs.

1. Lower rates of maternal absenteeism (Cohen et al., 1995).

2. Reduced turnover rates and improved employee loyalty to the company (Galtry, 1997; Lyness et al., 1999; Ortiz, McGilligan, & Kelly, 2004).

3. Lower health care costs (Cohen et al., 1995).

4. Higher job satisfaction (Galtry, 1997).

5. Longer duration of breastfeeding (Bar-Yam, 1998a; Cohen and Mrtek, 1994; Whaley et al., 2002)

III. Components of a Successful Lactation Support Program (US DHHS, 2003)

A. Space to express milk.

1. A place to express milk comfortably and in privacy assists with milk ejection and enables mothers to have a more productive pumping experience.

2. Options for private breastfeeding areas include:
   a. Converting small unused spaces such as large closets, offices, or other small rooms.
   b. Creating space within a women's lounge.
   c. Installing walls, partitions, or dividers in corners or areas of rooms.
   d. Creating multi-user stations within a single room divided by partitions or curtains.

3. Requirements for the room: central area that is easy to access, private with ability to be locked; nearby access to running water; electrical outlet; comfortable chair; well-lit; ventilated; and heated/air conditioned.

4. Nice to include: breast pump with table or counter, telephone, parenting literature, soft lighting, storage space, footstool, and breastfeeding artwork.

5. Use of a quality bilateral electric breast pump can facilitate quick milk expression (Corbett-Dick & Bezek, 1997). Options include:
   a. Employer provides a hospital-grade multi-user pump and attachment kits.
   b. Employer provides a hospital-grade multi-user pump and the employee purchases the attachment kit.
   c. Employer provides or subsidizes a portable electric breast pump for employees.
   d. The mother provides her own equipment.

6. A place to store milk is necessary. Options include:
   a. Employer provides small refrigerators in milk expression rooms.
   b. Employee brings cooler packs for milk storage.
   c. Public refrigerators in the work area (though not preferred by women and could pose an issue regarding safety of the milk).

B. Time to express milk (Wyatt, 2002).

1. Established lunch and morning/afternoon breaks are usually sufficient for milk expression during a standard work day (Slusser et al., 2004).

2. Milk expression needs vary according to the baby's age.
   a. A mother of a baby less than 4-months-old may need three 20-minute milk expression breaks during a standard eight-hour work period.
   b. A mother of a 6-month-old may need to express milk only two times/day because her baby is likely to be starting solid foods.
   c. Mothers of babies older than 12 months may need to express milk only once or twice during the work period.

C. Education.

1. Standard information about the company lactation program in employee benefits materials, wellness or work life program initiatives, company newsletter, and posters/flyers posted in the workplace.

2. Identify pregnant employees and provide information. Options include information packets, and prenatal lunch-time classes and support groups led by a lactation consultant.

3. Back-to-work consults for new mothers with a lactation consultant to tailor a milk expression schedule to fit her job situation.

4. Resource center with books, videos, and materials on ways to maintain lactation after returning to work.

5. Promotion of the program to supervisors and colleagues through flyers, newsletters, e-mail listservs, and staff meeting presentations.

D. Support (Whaley, 2003; Wyatt, 2002).

1. Support from the employer is highly valued among breastfeeding women.

2. Access to other breastfeeding employees enhances confidence and helps mothers reach their maternal goals for breastfeeding.

3. Consultations with a lactation consultant help the woman address concerns with establishing breastfeeding and maintaining milk supply once she is separated from her baby.

IV. Identified Barriers to Sustaining Lactation After Returning to Work (US DHHS, 2003)

A. Barriers of women.

1. Real or perceived low milk supply (Arlotti et al., 1998; Lewallen et al., 2006; McLeod, Pullon, & Cookson, 2002; Zinn, 2000).

2. Lack of accommodations in the workplace to express milk (Corbett-Dick & Bezek, 1997).

3. Lack of time to pump with resultant diminishing milk supply (Arthur, Saenz, & Replogle, 2003).

4. Fatigue, stress, and exhaustion (Frank, 1998; Nichols & Roux, 2004; Wambach, 1998).

5. Feeling overwhelmed with demands of fulfilling job requirements and meeting the needs of their child (Hochschild & Machong, 2003).

6. Childcare concerns and reliance upon family for help with children (Best Start, 1996; Corbett-Dick & Bezek, 1997).

7. Concerns over employers' and colleagues' support (Corbett-Dick & Bezek, 1997; Frank, 1998).

B. Identified barriers to providing support among employers.

1. Lack of awareness of the numbers of women breastfeeding, or the ways breastfeeding can decrease employee absenteeism and lower health care costs to the company (Bridges, Frank & Curtin, 1997; Libbus & Bullock, 2002).

2. Belief that breastfeeding employees will be too fatigued and therefore more unproductive on the job (Brown, Poag, & Kasprzycki, 2001).

3. Belief that breastfeeding or pumping in the workplace will interfere with an employee's productivity (Libbus & Bullock, 2002).

4. Lack of space to accommodate a lactation room and lack of time for employees to pump (Brown et al., 2001).

5. Liability concerns (Brown et al., 2001).

6. Belief that breastfeeding is a personal decision and not the employer's responsibility (Dunn et al., 2004).

7. Concerns that co-workers will complain or have to cover for an employee who takes time to pump during the work period (Brown et al., 2001).

8. Lack of knowledge in how to set up a lactation support program (Brown et al., 2001).

V. Counseling Strategies for Mothers

A. During the prenatal period, ways the lactation consultant can help mothers:

1. Help women understand reasons to initiate and continue breastfeeding after returning to work.

2. Provide practical strategies, encouragement, and support for breastfeeding (Meek, 2001).

3. Help women understand reasons to express milk while separated from the baby, including:
   a. Protecting the baby from illnesses and allergies.
   b. Providing greater comfort for the mother.
   c. Preventing painful engorgement, mastitis, and leaking.
   d. Maintaining milk supply

4. Offer support and solutions to help her reach *her* goals for infant feeding. For instance, some mothers will choose not to express milk at work or are unable to due to worksite constraints, and will need strategies for being more comfortable when they are separated from their babies.

5. Identify breastfeeding classes in the community to help her have good information to initiate and maintain breastfeeding.

6. Develop a plan for combining employment with breastfeeding, including:
   a. Timing her return to work with optimal maternity leave possible (at least 12 weeks or longer is optimal).
   b. Exploring work options that will enable her to spend as much time as possible with her baby. These can include: job sharing (Vanek & Vanek, 2001); part-time employment (Hills-Bonczyk et al., 1993; Ryan, Wenjun, & Acosta, 2002); gradual phase-back (part-time before full-time); or working at home/telecommuting (Table 6-2).

7. Dialogue with her supervisor about milk expression options, including time needed, milk expression locations, and milk storage.

8. Develop realistic milk expression schedules.

9. Discuss strategies for addressing potential interruptions in the work period that may affect lactation.

10. Explore options for milk expression, including: hand expression, breast pumping, having baby brought to the mother during breaks, or going to the childcare center to feed the baby during one or more breaks during the work period.

11. Assist in selection of appropriate breast pump equipment. See Chapter 30: Milk Expression, Storage, and Handling.

12. Ethical issues related to breast pumps.

Table 6-2 Descriptions of flexible work programs and their benefits for new mothers and employers.

Benefit	Definition	Advantages for New Mothers	Advantages for Employers
Earned time	Sick leave, vacation time and personal days are grouped into one set of paid days off. Workers take these days at their own discretion.	Mothers do not have to justify time off to their supervisors. Often, earned time accrues over several years, giving new mothers substantial paid leave after childbirth.	Promotes loyalty because workers feel trusted and valued. Workers often willing to work extra time as need arises because their needs were met when they arose.
Part-time	Workers work less than 35–40 hours/week. Benefits are usually prorated to hours worked.	Gives new mothers more time at home. Often includes flexibility of which hours are worked.	Retains workers with valuable experience and training. Saves recruiting and training new workers.
Job sharing	Two workers each work part-time and share the responsibilities and benefits of one job.	Gives mothers more time at home while keeping the same job.	Retains workers with valuable experience and training. Saves recruiting and training new workers.
Phase back	Workers return from leave to full-time work load gradually over several weeks or months.	Longer return to work adjustment period for mother and baby. More time with infant, when breastfeeding is being established.	Retains workers with experience. Promotes loyalty and dedication of workers.
Flex-time	Workers arrange to work hours to suit their schedules, i.e., 7 AM–3 PM, or 10 AM–6 PM	Can work with spouse's schedule to require less paid child care. Can arrange hours around best times of day to be with baby. Shorter commutes in less traffic.	Workplace covered for more hours/day. Workers better able to focus when schedules suit their needs.
Compressed work week	Workers work more hours on fewer days, i.e., 7 AM–7 PM, 3 days/week.	Allows new mothers full days at home with their babies.	Workers better able to focus when schedules suit their needs. Retains workers with experience and training.
Telecommuting	Workers work all or part of their jobs from home.	Can work around baby's schedule. Less commuting time. Less work clothing and travel expenses.	Retains workers with experience and training. Saves office and parking space.
On-site or near-site day care	Day care provided on or near site, often sponsored by the company.	Can visit baby for nursing etc. during the work day. Commuting time is with baby.	Promotes loyalty among workers. Workers better able to focus when baby is accessible.

Source: Reprinted by permission: Bar-Yam N. Workplace lactation support, part 1: A return to work breastfeeding assessment tool. *J Hum Lact.* 1998;14:249–254.

   a. The lactation consultant is obligated to "remain free of conflict of interest while fulfilling the objectives and maintaining the integrity of the lactation consultant profession" and to "provide information about appropriate products in a manner that is neither false nor misleading" (Galtry, 1997).
   b. If the lactation consultant provides equipment, she must be aware of the product liability issues.
      i. This awareness includes issues related to the safety of reusing or sharing breast pumps designed and labeled by the manufacturer as "single user items" (Gielen et al., 1991).
      ii. The lactation consultant is expected to remain current in terms of research regarding the safety and efficacy of equipment related to supporting lactation.
      iii. The lactation consultant must assist in "trouble shooting" equipment.
         1. To identify worn out valves as an issue that negatively affects strength of suction.
         2. To identify a need to increase pump flange size.
         3. To educate mothers on ways to prevent mold growth in tubing.
   13. Explore childcare options with providers who support her decision to breastfeed. Encourage the mother to explore providers close to her workplace to facilitate feeding baby either during the work period or immediately before and after work.
B. Before the mother returns to work, the lactation consultant can help her (Table 6-3).
   1. Successfully establish breastfeeding in the hospital and during her early weeks at home. This includes:
      a. Developing an abundant milk supply (the most frequent reason for weaning is real or perceived insufficient milk supply [Bourgoin et al., 1997]).
      b. Frequent breastfeeds/removal of milk during the early stage of breastfeeding (lactogenesis II) increases development of prolactin receptors that affect long-term milk supply (Cox, Owens, & Hartmann, 1996).
   2. Address coping strategies, including getting help with household chores, dealing with fatigue and stress, eating healthy meals, establishing good breastfeeding patterns, and gaining help from family members to protect her health and energy.
   3. Provide anticipatory guidance to assist in prevention of engorgement, mastitis, and maintaining milk supply once she is separated from her baby.
   4. Provide the mother with realistic expectations for early pumping attempts.
      a. It is normal not to express much milk at first (around ½ oz or 15 ml. is common with the first few pumping sessions after 3–4 days postpartum).
      b. Her body will learn to respond to the stimulation of hand expression or breast pumping in order to trigger milk ejection.

Table 6-3   Return-to-work breastfeeding assessment worksheet.

	Yes	No	Notes

Type of Job

1. What is the client's job?
2. Does she have her own office?
3. Does she keep her own calendar/control her own time?
4. Does the client's job involve travel out of town or out of her office?
5. Are most of her colleagues men or women?*

Space

Bathrooms are not acceptable breastfeeding/pumping spaces!

1. Is there designated private breastfeeding/pumping space (Nursing Mothers' Room/NMR) in the workplace?
2. Does the space have a sink, a chair, and electrical outlets?
3. Are pumps available there?
4. Where is the space in relation to the client's workspace?
5. How long does it take to get from the workspace to the NMR?
6. Where will the client store her milk?
7. If there is no designated space, where will the mother pump?
8. Can she use the same space every day?
9. Are there electrical outlets there?
10. Where is the nearest sink?

Time

Pumping should not come at the expense of the mother's lunch!

1. How old will the baby be upon return to work?
2. How often will the client be pumping/breastfeeding when she first returns to work?
3. When will the client pump?
4. What type of pump will she use? Is there a double pump?
5. How many parts on the pump must be cleaned out with each use?
6. Can breaks be taken reliably at the same time every day?
7. If there is on-site or near-site day care, can the mother go to the baby to nurse?

Support

1. What at work knows that the client plans to breastfeed/pump at work?
2. Does the supervisor need to be informed or consulted?
3. If so, what are his/her feedings about the client's plan?
4. Are there other new mothers at work (at the same workplace or colleagues at other workplaces) who are nursing or planning to nurse at work?
5. Are there mothers at work who have done so in the past?

	Yes	No	Notes

6. What are her partner's feelings about the mother's plan to nurse and work?

7. Do day care providers know how to handle breast milk?

8. How do they feel about it?

9. Will on-site or near-site providers call the mother to nurse, if she requests it?

Gatekeepers

1. If there is no lactation support program, who can help the client find time and space to pump/breastfeed?

2. Who is responsible for signing up spare offices/conference rooms?

3. Who keeps the calendar, answers the phone, greets visitors?

Supervisor

1. Must the supervisor be consulted regarding making time and/or space available to pump/breastfeed?

2. What is the relationship between the client and her supervisor?

3. Has the client addressed this issue with her supervisor?

4. If so, what was the response?

5. If not, what are her concerns about doing so?

Breastfeeding-Friendly Benefits

1. Are there any policies in the workplace regarding nursing mothers?

2. Are there any policies regarding flexibility for new mothers returning to work?

3. Does the client have access to any of the following programs?

   a. earned time   e. flex-time

   b. part-time   f. compressed work week

   c. job sharing   g. telecommuting

   d. phase back   h. on-site or near-site day care

4. If so, has the client thought about taking advantage of one or more of them!

5. What is the procedure for doing so?

6. If not, with whom would the client speak to try to arrange one or more of these programs/

   a. supervisor   d. Employee Relations Officer

   b. Human Resources Officer   e. Other (specify)

   c. Benefits Officer

Note: Space for answers is not displayed to scale.

*In some workplaces, men are more understanding and supportive than women and sometimes it is the reverse, but it is good information to have.

Source: Reprinted by permission: Bar-Yam N. Workplace lactation support, part 1: A return-to-work breastfeeding assessment tool. *J Hum Lact.* 1998;14:249–254.

c. Pumping sessions of 12 to 15 minutes are generally sufficient to obtain milk for practice feeds and to begin storing milk in the freezer.

d. Label milk with baby's name and date of expression, and freeze for later use when she returns to work.

5. Help the mother determine the amount of breastmilk her baby will need while the two are apart.

a. The amount of milk her baby needs will depend on many factors, including whether she is exclusively breastfeeding, age of her baby, and the number of hours she is separated from her baby.

b. Typically, as babies grow, they may take less milk as they begin to eat solid foods.

6. Begin expressing milk around two to four weeks postpartum and storing it for later use when she returns to work (Bocar, 1997; Wyatt, 2002;). The earlier the mother returns to work, the more frequently she will need to express milk when she is away from her baby.

7. Strategies to facilitate milk expression are covered in Chapter 30: Milk Expression, Storage, and Handling.

8. Provide general guidelines on safe storage of human milk (see Chapter 30). Note that milk storage guidelines are generally more liberal for healthy infants than storage for hospitalized infants.)

9. Provide strategies for introducing expressed milk to the baby.

a. Pumped milk can be offered by an alternative method of the mother's choice to help the baby become accustomed to being fed as he or she will be fed by the childcare provider.

b. Offering the baby a full feed is not necessary to accustom the baby to an alternative feed.

c. Small volumes can serve to familiarize baby with alternative feeding methods and might be less stressful.

d. Offer expressed milk when baby is not overly hungry; it is difficult for babies to learn new tasks when they are uncomfortable.

e. Feedings can be best offered by someone other than the mother.

f. Waiting too long to introduce a bottle can cause problems with bottle refusal (Fein & Roe, 1998).

g. Many mothers choose to use a cup for giving expressed milk to baby.

10. Develop realistic expectations about her first days back on the job.

a. Suggest that she return to work on a part-time basis or a partial work week schedule to shorten the first week away from the baby.

11. Identify community sources for support to boost her confidence in her ability to combine breastfeeding and employment.

C. After the mother returns to work, the lactation consultant can help provide information.

   1. Addressing lactation challenges brought on by separation from her baby (such as engorgement, leaking, and concerns about milk supply).

   2. Practical strategies for milk expression and storage tailored to the unique work and childcare situation she faces.

      a. Some mothers prefer the "5–15–5" rule, with two very short pump-for-comfort sessions in the midmorning and mid-afternoon, and a longer break at lunch to express milk.

   3. Addressing childcare provider's concerns about safety of handling human milk.

      a. Milk is not currently classified by the Occupational Safety and Health Administration as requiring "universal precautions" while handling (Kearny and Cronenwett, 1991; see Appendix C).

      b. If concerns about handling milk are expressed, mothers can pre-package milk by using solid, labeled containers (no soft plastic bags that could tear and leak).

      c. Empty, used bottles are put in a bag for the mother to clean so that the worker never handles the milk, only the bottles.

   4. General information for childcare providers.

      a. Infants in childcare have higher rates of diarrhea and upper respiratory infections; breastfeeding helps lower the rate of illnesses (Cohen et al., 1995).

      b. Wash hands after diaper changes and before feeding.

      c. Check storage date on label and use milk that most closely matches baby's age.

      d. Thaw milk in the refrigerator or gently warm in hot water.

      e. Avoid thawing milk at room temperature because this enables bacteria to multiply.

      f. Avoid quick heating of milk on the stove or microwave, because this increases the risk of uneven distribution of the heat that can injure the baby (Katcher & Lanese, 1985).

      g. Discard leftover milk that was thawed or warmed and used by the baby at the feeding.

      h. Gently shake the milk to mix the layers.

      i. Give the baby no other food without parental authorization.

      j. Expect the baby's appetite to change from feeding to feeding.

      k. Try to avoid feeding baby large quantities of milk in the hour before the mother arrives.

      l. Hold the baby for all feeds; do not prop the bottle.

      m. Milk can be offered in a bottle, cup, spoon, by dropper, or chilled to the consistency of ice milk and spooned to the older baby (older than 4 months).

      n. Allow the baby to be in charge of the feed rather than the caregiver controlling the feeds or forcing the infant to eat.

5. Dealing with baby's changing feeding patterns.
   a. Many babies sleep long hours when mother is gone as a way of coping with the long separation. This "reverse cycle breastfeeding" means baby wants to be held and nursed when mother is with the baby.
   b. Mothers can view this time as a way to rest and cuddle with baby.
   c. Mothers can ask the childcare provider to follow baby's feeding cues rather than waking her baby to feed.
6. Addressing feelings of sadness at the separation from her infant.

VI. Assisting Employers with Providing Lactation Support

A. The lactation consultant is a valuable resource for employers by helping them explore solutions for supporting breastfeeding employees.
B. Provide information and professional materials for employers that explain the business case for breastfeeding, and simple steps for establishing a lactation support program.
C. Offer to serve on a company task force to explore strategies for supporting breastfeeding employees.
D. Provide individual technical assistance to employers who want to establish a worksite lactation program. In some cases, the lactation consultant might be employed by the company to establish a corporate lactation program or to offer assistance to employees.
E. Provide resources for breastfeeding employees at the worksite, and be available for one-on-one assistance to address breastfeeding concerns.
F. Encourage recognition programs in the community to recognize worksites that provide support to breastfeeding employees. Examples: Texas "Mother-Friendly Worksite" designation (recognizing all worksites that achieve established criteria for providing a supportive environment) or individual awards to outstanding employers.

VII. The Lactation Consultant's Role as a Community Advocate for Working Mothers

A. The lactation consultant is in a pivotal role within the community for encouraging policies and programs to support working mothers with breastfeeding.
B. Advocate for legislation that supports breastfeeding mothers. This can include legislation requiring or encouraging employers to provide a supportive environment (examples: California, Connecticut, Georgia, Hawaii, Illinois, Minnesota, Oklahoma, Rhode Island, Tennessee, Texas and Washington in the United States) as well as legislation requiring childcare providers to provide accommodations for breastfeeding mothers (example: Mississippi).

C. Offer to speak at community business and service organization meetings, or at employer organizations that meet regularly.

D. Set up displays at job fairs or health fairs in the community to provide information on the importance of combining breastfeeding and employment.

E. Provide prenatal education about breastfeeding at lunch-time seminars with pregnant workers at selected worksites.

F. Offer to facilitate a working mother's support group meeting at worksites in the community that meets during lunch or in the evenings.

G. Provide companies with information about supporting breastfeeding, and available resources in the community.

H. Begin a coalition, or ask the existing community breastfeeding coalition to conduct outreach with local worksites.

I. Meet with local legislative representatives to discuss breastfeeding policy issues in your area.

J. Alert the media about advancements in breastfeeding support in community worksites. Publicity helps women view continued breastfeeding as the social norm, provides positive public relations to employers, and encourages other worksites to follow their lead.

VIII. Occupational Hazards and the Breastfeeding Woman

A. It is undeniably true that the presence of environmental contaminants has exposed human populations to elevated levels of toxins, some of which appear in human milk. This fact argues more for the reduction of such exposure than against breastfeeding. The long-term effects of toxic exposure via breast milk are not yet known. Analysis of human milk after accidental exposure to PCBs, DDE, and heptachlor has not demonstrated that the infants were harmed by breastfeeding, although level of exposure might be a mitigating factor (Kurinij et al., 1989).

B. It is prudent for pregnant and lactating women to avoid unnecessary exposure to hazardous chemicals, fumes, and materials.

C. Occupational exposures typically involve trace metals, solvents, and halogenated hydrocarbons (Lindburg, 1996).

D. Exposure to passive cigarette smoke should be avoided.

E. Water-based toxins are more rapidly excreted.

F. Artists and ceramic workers must consider lead exposure; clothing should be changed before handling the baby; hand-washing and breathing filters should be used.

G. Household herbicides, pesticides, and cleaning solvents should not be directly handled or inhaled.

H. Protective clothing, masks, goggles, and air filters are prudent strategies for lactating women who work around toxic materials.

I. Health care workers should practice universal precautions (see Appendix C), especially given the potential for exposure to human immunodeficiency virus and hepatitis C.

J. Accidental exposures to toxins or potential infection should be reported to the mother's health care provider; milk or blood can be tested.

References

American Academy of Pediatrics Policy Statement on Breastfeeding and the Use of Human Milk. *Pediatrics.* 2005;115:496–506. Available at http://www.aap.org/advocacy/releases/feb05breastfeeding.htm. Accessed December 7, 2006.

Arlotti J, Cottrell B, Lee S, Curtin J. Breastfeeding among low-income women with and without peer support. *J Community Health Nurs.* 1998;5:163–178.

Arthur C, Saenz RB, Replogle WH. The employment-related breastfeeding decisions of physician mothers. *J Miss State Med Assoc.* 2003;44:383–387.

Ball T, Wright A. Health care costs of formula-feeding in the first year of life. *Pediatrics.* 1999;103:871–876.

Bar-Yam N. Workplace lactation support, part 1: A return-to-work breastfeeding assessment tool. *J Hum Lact.* 1998a;14:249–254a.

Best Start Social Marketing. Research brief: USDA WIC National Breastfeeding Loving Support Campaign, 1996; Tampa, FL: Best Start Social Marketing.

Biagioli F. Returning to work while breastfeeding. *Am Fam Physician.* 2003: 68:2201–2208.

Bocar D. Combining breastfeeding and employment: increasing success. *J Perinat Neonat Nurs.* 1997;11:23–43.

Bourgoin G, Lahaie N, Rheaume B, et al. *Can J Public Health.* 1997;88:238–241.

Bridges CB, Frank DI, Curtin J. Employer attitudes toward breastfeeding in the workplace. *J Hum Lact.* 1997;13:215–219.

Brown C, Poag S, Kasprzycki C. Exploring large employers' and small employers' knowledge, attitudes, and practices on breastfeeding support in the workplace. *J Hum Lact.* 2001;17:39–46.

Cohen R, Mrtek MB. The impact of two corporate lactation programs on the incidence and duration of breastfeeding by employed mothers. *Am J Health Promot.* 1994; 8:436–441.

Cohen R, Mrtek M, Mrtek RG. Comparison of maternal absenteeism and infant illness rates among breast-feeding and formula-feeding women in two corporations. *Am J Health Promot.* 1995;10:148–153.

Corbett-Dick P, Bezek SK. Breastfeeding promotion for the employed mother. *J Pediatr Health Care.* 1997;11:12–19.

Cox, DB, Owens RA, Hartmann PE. Blood and milk prolactin and the rate of milk synthesis in women. *Exp Physiol.* 1996;81:1007–1020.

Dunn BF, Zavela KJ, Cline AD, Cost PA. Breastfeeding practices in Colorado businesses. *J Hum Lact.* 2004;20(2):217–218.

Faught, L. Lactation programs benefit the family and the cooperation. *J Compensation & Benefits.* 1994; September/October: 44–47.

Fein SB, Roe B. The effect of work status on initiation and duration of breastfeeding. *Am J Pub Health.* 1998;88:1042–1046.

Frank E. Breastfeeding and maternal employment: two rights don't make a wrong. *Lancet.* 1998;352:1083–1085.

Galtry J. Lactation and the labor market: breastfeeding, labor market changes, and public policy in the United States. *Health Care Women Int.* 1997;18:467–480.

Galtry J. The impact on breastfeeding of labour market policy and practice in Ireland, Sweden, and the USA. *Soc Sci Med.* 2003;57:167–177.

Gielen, AC, Faden RR, O'Campo P, et al. Maternal employment during the early postpartum period: effects on initiation and continuation of breastfeeding. *Pediatrics.* 1991;87:298–305.

Haider SJ, Jacknowitz A, Schoeni RF. Welfare work requirements and child well-being: evidence from the effects on breastfeeding. *Demography.* 2003;40:479–497.

Hanson, M, Hellerstedt WL, Desvarieux M, Duval SJ. Correlates of breast-feeding in a rural population. *Am J Health Behav.* 2003;27:432–444.

Hills-Bonczyk SG, Avery MD, Savik K, et al. Women's experiences with combining breastfeeding and employment. *J Nurse Midwifery.* 1993;38:257–266.

Hochschild A, Machung A. *The Second Shift.* New York: Penguin Books; 2003.

Katcher A, Lanese M. Breastfeeding by employed mothers: a reasonable accommodation in the workplace. *Pediatrics.* 1985;75:644–647.

Kearny M, Cronenwett L. Breastfeeding and employment. *J Obstet Gynecol Neonatal Nurs.* 1991;20:471–280.

Kurinij N, Shiono P, Ezrine S, Rhoades G. Does maternal employment affect breastfeeding? *Am J Public Health.* 1989;79:1247–1250.

Lewallen LP, Dick MJ, Flowers J, et al. Breastfeeding support and early cessation. *J Obstet Gynecol Neonatal Nurs.* 2006;35:166–172.

Libbus M, Bullock L. Breastfeeding and employment: an assessment of employer attitudes. *J Hum Lact.* 2002;18:247–251.

Lindberg LD. Trends in the relationship between breastfeeding and postpartum employment in the United States. *Soc Biol.* 1996;43:191–202.

Lyness K, Thompson C, Francesco A, Judiesch M. Work and pregnancy: Individual and organizational factors influencing organizational commitment, timing of maternity leave, and return to work. *Sex Roles.* 1999;41:485–508.

McLeod D, Pullon S, Cookson T. Factors influencing continuation of breastfeeding in a cohort of women. *J Hum Lact.* 2002;18:335–343.

Meek JY. Breastfeeding in the workplace. *Pediatr Clin North Am.* 2001;48:461–474.

Neifert M. *Dr. Mom's Guide to Breastfeeding.* New York: Penguin Putnam; 1998.

Nichols MR, Roux GM. Maternal perspectives on postpartum return to the workplace. *J Obstet Gynecol Neonatal Nurs.* 2004;33:463–471.

Organization for Economic Cooperation and Development. OECD employment outlook 2002. Chapter 2. In: *Women at Work: Who Are They and How Are They Faring?* Available at: http://www.oecd.org/dataoecd/28/58/18960381.pdf. Accessed November 17, 2006.

Ortiz J, McGilligan K, Kelly P. Duration of breast milk expression among working mothers enrolled in an employer-sponsored lactation program. *Pediatr Nurs.* 2004; 30:111–119.

Piper B, Parks PL. Predicting the duration of lactation: evidence from a national survey. *Birth.* 1996;23:7–12.

Roe B, Whittington LA, Fein SB, Teisl ME. Is there competition between breastfeeding and maternal employment? *Demography.* 1999;36:157–171.

Ryan AS, Wenjun Z, Acosta A. Breastfeeding continues to increase into the new millennium. *Pediatrics.* 2002;110:1103–1109.

Scott J, Landers M, Huges R, Binns C. Factors associated with breastfeeding at discharge and duration of breastfeeding. *J Paediatr Child Health.* 2001;37:254–261.

Slusser WM, Lange L, Eickson V, et al. Breast milk expression in the workplace: a look at frequency and time. *J Hum Lact.* 2004;20:164–169.

Taveras E. Clinician support and psychosocial risk factors associated with breastfeeding discontinuation. *Pediatrics.* 2003;112(1 Pt 1):108–115.

United States Breastfeeding Committee (USBC). Workplace breastfeeding support [issue paper]. Raleigh, NC: 2002. Available at: http://www.usbreastfeeding.org. Accessed November 17, 2006.

U.S. Department of Health and Human Services, Health Resources and Services Administration, Maternal and Child Health Bureau. 2003. Research Brief: Using Loving Support to Develop Breastfeeding-Friendly Worksites Support Kit. Rockville, MD.

Vanek EP, Vanek JA. Job sharing as an employment alternative in group medical practice. *Med Group Manage J.* 2001:48:20–24.

Wambach K. Maternal fatigue in breastfeeding primiparae during the first nine weeks postpartum. *J Hum Lact.* 1998;14:219–229.

Whaley S, Meehan K, Lange L, et al. Predictors of breastfeeding duration for employees of the Special Supplemental Nutrition Program for Women, Infants, and Children (WIC). *Am Diet Assoc.* 2002;102:1290–1293.

Wyatt SN. Challenges of the working breastfeeding mother: workplace solution. *AAOHN J.* 2002;50:61–66.

Zinn B. Supporting the employed breastfeeding mother. *J Midwifery Women's Health.* 2000;145;216–226.

Suggested Readings

Auerbach K. Assisting the employed breastfeeding mother. *J Nurse Midwifery.* 1990; 35:26–34.

Bar-Yam N. Workplace lactation support, part II: Working with the workplace. *J Hum Lact.* 1998b;14:321–325b.

Lauwers J, Swisher A. When breastfeeding is interrupted. Chapter 24. In: Lauwers J, Swisher A, eds. *Counseling the Nursing Mother.* Sudbury, MA: Jones and Bartlett Publishers; 2005:485–495.

Nichols L. Then comes the baby in the baby carriage: the economic resource use of new mothers. *Abstracts International.* 2001;61:2925-A.

Petersen DJ, Boller HR. Employers' duty to accommodate breast-feeding, working mothers. *Employee Relations Law Journal.* 2004;30:80-88.

Walker M. Physical, Medical, emotional, and environmental challenges to the breastfeeding mother. Chapter 9. In: Walker M, ed. *Breastfeeding Management for the Clinician.* Sudbury, MA: Jones and Bartlett Publishers; 2005.

Wambach K, Rojjanasrirat W. Maternal employment and breastfeeding. Chapter 17. In: Riordan J, ed. *Breastfeeding and Human Lactation.* Sudbury, MA: Jones and Bartlett Publishers; 2005.

CARING FOR VULNERABLE POPULATIONS

Cynthia Turner-Maffei, MA, IBCLC

OBJECTIVES

- Describe cultural competency vis-à-vis breastfeeding.
- Identify two strategies that have been successful in promoting breastfeeding in vulnerable populations.
- Demonstrate awareness of the rationale for special concerns regarding breastfeeding and vulnerable populations.

Introduction

Lactation consultants strive to promote, support, and protect breastfeeding among all families. The benefits of breastfeeding are particularly advantageous for families living in vulnerable situations. Special emphasis must be placed on meeting the needs of those who are less able to access breastfeeding help because of financial, language, geographic, and cultural barriers. Lactation consultants should endeavor to develop cultural competency in order to address these barriers. Lactation consultants should be aware of the need to assist families in disaster situations, whether related to natural events, wars, or other events.

I. Issues of Vulnerable Populations Regarding Breastfeeding

A. Low-income families.

1. In some nations, low-income mothers breastfeed at the highest rates; in other nations, the reverse is true.

2. Perceived value of breastfeeding versus formula.

   a. Formula is beyond the economic reach of low-income families in many developing nations.

   b. Often, formula has a greater perceived value than breast milk. The ability to purchase formula is a status symbol in some communities.

    c. Gifts of formula from health care providers and health systems have been associated with a decline in exclusive breastfeeding (Donnelly et al., 2000), an increase in cessation of breastfeeding within the first 2 weeks, and early introduction of solid foods (Howard et al., 2000).

3. In some nations, those who receive a lower wage do not receive the degree of workplace accommodation of nursing or milk expression breaks that is attained by higher wage-earning cohorts.

4. Accessibility of breastfeeding help.
    a. Low-income populations often have limited access to health care services, including breastfeeding help.
    b. Where lactation care is available largely on a fee-for-service basis, breastfeeding help may be beyond the financial means of many families.

5. Minority families.
    a. Traditions, beliefs, and values surrounding breastfeeding vary widely among the world's cultures.
    b. Statements of authority figures can be received positively or negatively by members of minority cultures.
      i. Some cultures value authority figures; others seek authority within.
      ii. Authority-based breastfeeding promotion programs have the potential to be counterproductive if not carefully designed. Rejection of medical advice might be perceived as an act of autonomy by some individuals (Carter, 1995).

6. The racial and ethnic prejudices prevalent within the majority culture can influence the choices of individuals of minority cultures.

7. Access to health care services, including breastfeeding care, may be limited within minority communities due to financial, language, geographic, and cultural barriers.

B. Immigrant families.

1. Immigrant families often assume very different breastfeeding patterns in their new nation (Homer, Sheehan, & Cooke, 2002).

2. Some have theorized that these changes in breastfeeding patterns might reflect women's assimilation of the infant feeding norms of their new nation (Balcazar, Trier, & Cobas, 1995; Romero-Gwynn & Carias, 1989). In many developed countries, breastfeeding is relatively invisible, practiced largely in private homes, while bottle-feeding is the visible cultural norm. One study found that while recent immigrants to the United States were more likely to breastfeed than U.S.-born women, their likelihood of breastfeeding declined 4% with every year lived in the United States (Gibson-Davis & Brooks-Gunn, 2006).

3. Other factors that may influence breastfeeding include:
    a. Degree of visibility of breastfeeding as the cultural norm.

b. Degree of cultural acceptability of breastfeeding.

c. Availability and affordability of breastmilk substitutes.

d. Presence or absence of support provided by larger family networks.

e. Difficulty of integrating breastfeeding with employment outside the home. Ease of integrating breastfeeding and employment ranges widely. Women working in low-wage positions may have more difficulty getting approval for breaks for breastfeeding or milk expression.

4. Disasters and emergencies.

a. Families have an urgent need for infant feeding support during man-made and natural disaster situations ranging from tsunamis and floods to wars and refugee crises. The resultant trauma, lack of access to safe water and food, insufficient medical care, violence, and displacement can have a long-lasting, unspoken effect on all aspects of daily life, including infant feeding.

b. Breastfeeding makes an unparalleled contribution to the health of children living in emergency situations. Research from Guinea-Bissau demonstrates that weaned children suffered a six-fold higher mortality than those who continued to breastfeed during the first three months of war (Jakobsen et al., 2003).

c. The visibility and accessibility of donated formula and powdered milk, along with general lack of awareness of women's abilities to continue to lactate and to re-lactate in emergency situations can be a deterrent to continued breastfeeding.

d. Lactation consultants are encouraged to work with local disaster relief groups to increase knowledge of the importance of supporting ongoing breastfeeding and to ensure that relief workers have adequate knowledge and skill to do so.

e. Lactation consultants should familiarize themselves with resources such as *Infant Feeding in Emergencies* (Emergency Nutrition Network, 2004) and *Infant Feeding in Emergencies: A Guide for Mothers* (World Health Organization, 1997), as well as the position statements of the International Lactation Consultant Association (ILCA) and other organizations regarding this topic (ILCA, 2005).

C. Cultural competency.

1. Cultural competency is a key skill for lactation consultants. Cultural competence has been defined as: "The level of knowledge-based skills required to provide effective clinical care to patients from a particular ethnic or racial group" (U.S. Department of Health & Human Services, 2006).

2. The first step toward developing cultural competency is for each provider to undertake self-assessment. Care is enhanced when each care provider identifies and endeavors to remain conscious of his or her own cultural values and biases (Gabriel, Gabriel, & Lawrence, 1986).

3. Care providers and their clients might have divergent beliefs about issues such as the etiology of problems, appropriate care plans, and so on.
   a. Exploring the client's viewpoint is key in arriving at mutually acceptable care plans.
   b. Cultural beliefs and practices such as avoiding feeding babies colostrum have an impact on breastfeeding (Gunnlaugsson & Einarsdottir, 1993; Hizel et al., 2006). The practice of feeding an infant other foods (including formula) during the first days of life might lead health care workers to assume incorrectly that a mother has chosen not to breastfeed.
      i. Respectful questions can be asked so the lactation consultant can begin to determine if a mother's cultural traditions are helpful, harmless, or harmful to the breastfeeding relationship (Riordan, 2005, p. 715).
      ii. The identity of the most influential person in a woman's feeding decision varies among cultures. Some identified individuals are the mother's relatives (particularly the mother's mother), peers, partners, and health care providers (Bryant, 1982; Freed, Jones, & Schanler, 1992; Martens, 1997; Narayanan et al., 2005; Sciacca et al., 1995; Susin, Giugliani, & Kummer, 2005; Wiemann, DuBois, & Berenson, 1998).
      iii. Several sources have identified general medical beliefs and values of different cultures. Such information can provide a framework for initial exploration with clients (Taylor, 1985; Waxler-Morrison, Anderson, & Richardson, 1990; Winikoff, Castle & Laukaran, 1988).
      iv. While it is possible to generalize about the experience of many groups of people, it is impossible to predict the meaning of an experience for any individual. Truly culturally competent care makes no assumptions about the experience, practices, or viewpoints of others.
      v. New educational media and strategies should be designed, tested, and evaluated based on input from members of the target community.
D. Strategies for individual encounters.
   1. Establish an environment of trust and respect.
      a. Ask respectful, open-ended questions.
      b. Inquire about and practice sensitivity to differing customs regarding eye contact, body language, touching the mother and the baby.
E. Seek to understand the unique perspective of each woman.
   1. Invite each woman to express her knowledge and concerns.
      a. A series of questions designed for this purpose (Kleinman, 1980) can be helpful in elaborating a woman's understanding and cultural knowledge of the situation.
      b. Without such knowledge, the care provider might unwittingly provide information that violates a client's belief structure.
   2. Acknowledge any expressed concerns.

3. Offer understanding and carefully targeted educational messages (Bryant et al., 1992).

4. Invite the client's feedback regarding suggested action plans.

    a. One author suggests, "If I tell you something and your mother has told you something different, please let me know and we'll see how we can work together" (Taylor, 1985).

    b. For example, the goal of treatment of the postpartum woman in the humoral health practices of many of the world's cultures is to keep the woman warm, eating, drinking, and surrounding herself with substances classified as "hot," and to avoid those that are associated with cold. This woman may perceive her lactation consultant's suggestion to apply ice to her engorged breasts as contradictory to her cultural practices.

5. Making provisions for an interpreter is necessary. Children should not be depended upon to convey medical information between mothers and health care providers. Provide written materials in the mother's native language at an easy reading level.

F. Include partners and family members in encounters as much as possible.

1. Develop careful follow-up plans.

    a. Integrate breastfeeding follow-up with other services (pediatric follow-up) to the extent possible.

    b. Identify whether the woman is expected to contact the consultant or vice-versa.

    c. Many clients move frequently and do not have regular access to a telephone. Establish backup communication plans.

G. Know that women who have familial or financial problems might require special attention and extra counseling sessions so that they can be helped to identify how to achieve and sustain exclusive breastfeeding (Haider, 1997).

1. Develop and invite her to participate in a peer counseling program.

    a. Peer counseling programs have been identified among the most effective strategies for breastfeeding promotion and preservation (Agrasada et al., 2005; Gross et al., 1998; Leite et al., 2005; Long et al., 1995; Martens, 2002).

    b. "[P]eers are more persuasive spokespersons than health professionals or celebrities because they offset the lack of role models and doubts many women have about the ability of low-income women to lactate successfully" (Bryant et al., 1992).

    c. Women who have had successful breastfeeding experiences and who are members of the target community are recruited and trained to counsel and support pregnant and parenting mothers.

    d. Peer counseling programs are often low-cost methods of providing breastfeeding help.

II. Improving Support for Vulnerable Populations in the Health Care System

A. Integrate breastfeeding support into comprehensive medical care.

    1. Several researchers have shown that providing continuous lactation care within the framework of comprehensive prenatal, postpartum, and pediatric care is most effective in increasing incidence (Brent et al., 1995; Kistin et al., 1990; Li et al., 2004), duration (Jones, 1986; Labarere et al., 2005), and exclusivity (Labarere et al., 2005; Lutter et al., 1997) of breastfeeding.

    2. Encourage breastfeeding training for all health care providers.

    3. Increase awareness of community breastfeeding support systems and services among health care providers.

B. Develop cultural competency programs within health care systems and among health care providers.

    1. Identify individuals within the target community who are willing to serve as "cultural brokers" (Fadiman, 1997) to provide cultural interpretation when needed for lactation consultants and other members of the health care team.

    2. Encourage cultural assessment to identify the major values, health beliefs, and practices of target populations (Tripp-Reimer, Brink, & Saunders, 1984).

    3. Encourage systems and providers to study the impact of health care practices (for example, distribution of formula samples) on breastfeeding outcomes.

    4. Explore barriers to breastfeeding through interviews with community members and use this information to design new programs and strategies (Riordan & Gill-Hopple, 2001).

C. Offer education regarding the identification of breastfeeding as the safest infant feeding method in all situations, including emergencies.

Summary

Through self-assessment, cultural awareness, respectful counseling, and developed skill, lactation consultants can help vulnerable families have satisfying breastfeeding experiences. Just as breastfeeding is an empowering and satisfying experience for many women and their families, working with families who are in vulnerable situations provides many opportunities for professional growth and fulfillment for lactation consultants.

References

Agrasada GV, Gustafsson J, Kylberg E, et al. 2005. Postnatal peer counseling on exclusive breastfeeding of low-birthweight infants: a randomized, controlled trial. *Acta Paediatr.* 2005;94:1109–1115.

Balcazar H, Trier CM, Cobas JA. What predicts breastfeeding intention in Mexican-American and Non-Hispanic white women? Evidence from a national survey. *Birth*. 1995;22:74–80.

Brent NB, Redd B, Dworetz A, et al. Breastfeeding in a low-income population. *Arch Pediatr Adolesc Med*. 1995:149:798–803.

Bryant CA. Impact of kin, friend and neighbor networks on infant feeding practices. *Soc Sci Med*. 1982;17:57–65.

Bryant CA, Coreil J, D'Angelo S, et al. A new strategy for promoting breastfeeding among economically disadvantaged women and adolescents. *NAACOG's Clin Iss Perinat Women's Health Iss: Breastfeeding*. 1992;3:723–730.

Carter P. *Feminism, Breasts and Breastfeeding*. New York: St. Martin's Press; 1995.

Donnelly A, Snowden HM, Renfrew MJ, et al. Commercial hospital discharge packs for breastfeeding women. *Cochrane Database Syst Rev*. 2000;(2):CD002075.

Emergency Nutrition Network. *Infant Feeding in Emergencies*. Oxford, UK: ENN; 2004.

Fadiman A. *The Spirit Catches You and You Fall Down: A Hmong Child, Her American Doctors, and the Collision of Two Cultures*. New York: Noonday Press; 1997.

Freed GL, Jones TM, Schanler RJ. 1992. Prenatal determination of demographic and attitudinal factors regarding feeding practice in an indigent population. *Am J Perinatol*. 1992;9:420–424.

Gabriel A, Gabriel KR, Lawrence RA. Cultural values and biomedical knowledge: choices in infant feeding. *Soc Sci Med*. 1986;23(5):501–509.

Gibson-Davis CM, Brooks-Gunn J. Couples' immigration status and ethnicity as determinants of breastfeeding. *Am J Public Health*. 2006;96:641–646.

Gross SM, Caulfield LE, Bentley ME, et al. Counseling and motivational videotapes increase duration of breast-feeding in African-American WIC participants who initiate breastfeeding. *J Am Diet Assoc*. 1998;98:43–148.

Gunnlaugsson G, Einarsdottir J. Colostrum and ideas about bad milk: A case study from Guinea-Bissau. *Soc Sci Med*. 1993;326:283–288.

Haider R. Reasons for failure of breast-feeding counselling: Mothers' perspective in Bangladesh. *Bull of WHO*. 1997;75:191–196.

Hizel S, Ceyhun G, Tanzer F, et al. Traditional beliefs as forgotten influencing factors on breast-feeding performance in Turkey. *Saudi Med J*. 2006;27:511–518.

Homer CS, Sheehan A, Cooke M. Initial infant feeding decisions and duration of breastfeeding in women from English, Arabic and Chinese-speaking backgrounds in Australia. *Breastfeed Rev*. 2002;10:27–31.

Howard C, Howard F, Lawrence R, et al. Office prenatal formula advertising and its effect on breastfeeding patterns. *Obstet Gynecol*. 2000;95:296–303.

International Lactation Consultant Association. Position on infant feeding in emergencies. 2005. Available at: http://www.ilca.org/pubs/InfantFeeding-EmergPP.pdf. Accessed December 6, 2006.

Jakobsen M, Sodemann M, Nylen G, et al. Breastfeeding status as a predictor of mortality among refugee children in an emergency situation in Guinea-Bissau. *Trop Med Int Health.* 2003;8:992–996.

Jones D. Effect of a lactation nurse on the success of breastfeeding: a randomized controlled trial. *J Epidemiol Comm Health.* 1986;40:45–49.

Kistin N, Benton D, Rao S, et al. Breastfeeding rates among black urban low-income women: effect of prenatal education. *Pediatrics.* 1990;86:741–746.

Kleinman A. *Patients and Healers in the Context of Culture.* Berkeley, CA: University of California Press; 1980.

Labarere J, Gelbert-Baudino N, Ayral AS, et al. Efficacy of breastfeeding support provided by trained clinicians during an early, routine, preventive visit: a prospective, randomized, open trial of 226 mother-infant pairs. *Pediatrics.* 2005; 115(2):e13946.

Leite AJ, Puccini RF, Atalah AN, et al. Effectiveness of home-based peer counselling to promote breastfeeding in the northeast of Brazil: a randomized clinical trial. *Acta Paediatr.* 2005;94:741–746.

Li L, Zhang M, Scott JA, et al. 2004. Factors associated with the initiation and duration of breastfeeding by Chinese mothers in Perth, Western Australia. *J Hum Lact.* 2004; 20:188–195.

Long DG, Funk-Archuleta MA, Geiger CJ, et al. 1995. Peer counselor program increases breastfeeding rates in Utah Native American WIC Population. *J Hum Lact.* 1995; 11:279–284.

Lutter CK, PerezEscamilla R, Segall A, et al. The effectiveness of a hospital-based program to promote exclusive breast-feeding among low-income women in Brazil. *Am J Public Health.* 1997;87:659–663.

Martens PJ. Prenatal infant feeding intent and perceived social support for breastfeeding in Manitoba First Nations communities: a role for health care providers. *Int J Circumpolar Health.* 1997;56:104–120.

Martens PJ. Increasing breastfeeding initiation and duration at a community level: an evaluation of Sagkeeng First Nation's community health nurse and peer counsellor programs. *J Hum Lact.* 2002;18:236–246.

Narayanan I, Dutta AK, Philips E, Ansari Z. Attitudes, practices, and socio-cultural factors related to breastfeeding: pointers for intervention programmes. In: Atkinson SA et al., eds. *Breastfeeding, Nutrition, Infection and Infant Growth in Developed and Emerging Countries.* St. John's, Canada: ARTS Biomedical Publishers and Distributors; 2005.

Riordan J, Gill-Hopple K. Breastfeeding care in multicultural populations. *J Obstet Gynecol Neonatal Nurs.* 2001;30:216–223.

Riordan J. *Breastfeeding and Human Lactation, Third Edition.* Sudbury, MA: Jones and Bartlett Publishers; 2005.

Romero-Gwynn E, Carias L. Breast-feeding intentions and practices among Hispanic mothers in Southern California. *Pediatrics.* 1989;84:626–632.

Sciacca JP, Phipps BL, Dube DA, Ratliff MI. Influences on breast-feeding by lower-income women: an incentive-based, partner-supported educational program. *J Am Diet Assoc.* 1995;95:323–328.

Susin LR, Giugliani ER, Kummer SC. [Influence of grandmothers on breastfeeding practices.] *Rev Saude Publica.* 2005;39:141–147. (Portuguese).

Taylor MM. *Transcultural Aspects of Breastfeeding–USA.* Lactation Consultant Series, Unit 2. Wayne, NJ: Avery Publishing Group; 1985.

Tripp-Reimer T, Brink PJ, Saunders JM. Cultural assessment: content and process. *Nurs Outlook.* 1984;32:78–82.

U.S. Department of Health & Human Services. Health Careers Opportunity Program Definitions. Washington, DC: DHHS; 2006. Available at http://bhpr.hrsa.gov/diversity/definitions.htm#Cultural%20Competence. Accessed November 27, 2006.

Waxler-Morrison N, Anderson J, Richardson E. *Cross-Cultural Caring: A Handbook for Health Professionals.* Vancouver, BC: University of British Columbia; 1990.

Wiemann CM, DuBois JC, Berenson AB. Racial/ethnic differences in the decision to breastfeed among adolescent mothers. *Pediatrics.* 1998;101:e11.

Winikoff B, Castle MA, Laukaran VH, eds. *Feeding Infants in Four Societies: Causes and Consequences of Mothers' Choices.* New York: Greenwood Press; 1988.

World Health Organization, Regional Office for Europe. Infant feeding in emergencies: A guide for mothers. Copenhagen, Author, 1997. Available at: http://www.euro.who.int/document/e56303.pdf. Accessed November 27, 2006.

Professional Development

Education and Change

Karin Cadwell, PhD, FAAN, RN, IBCLC

OBJECTIVE

- List resources for professional education and change in lactation.

Introduction

Almost all national and international statements regarding lactation call for changes to improve education for health care providers and lactation management based on evidence. Changing current practice is a slow process that needs a well thought-out plan. This chapter proposes the use of evidence-based practice as the foundation to make changes.

I. Blueprint for Policy Makers to Promote, Protect, and Support Breastfeeding (UNICEF, 1999) (See Chapter 2: International Initiatives to Promote, Protect, and Support Breastfeeding)

A. Establish national breastfeeding committees.

B. Promote the Baby-Friendly Hospital Initiative™ (BFHI).

C. Implement and enforce the International Code on Marketing Breast-milk Substitutes.

D. Establish maternity protection.

E. Train medical personnel and health care workers.

F. Support exclusive and sustained breastfeeding throughout the community.

G. Provide resources for support groups.

H. Promote breastfeeding campaigns.

I. Integrate breastfeeding messages into child health activities.

J. Improve women's social and economic status.

II. The Evidence-Based Practice Paradigm is an Emerging Model for Objective Examination of the Validity of Policy and is an Underpinning of Change

A. The paradigm offers tools to address the tension between folklore and medicine by authority and between observed experience and authority.

B. Evidence-based practice might level the field by providing a forum for interdisciplinary discussion.

C. A hierarchy of evidence has been accepted in medical research literature (Guyatt et al., 1995).

   1. Systematic reviews and meta-analyses.

   2. Randomized controlled trials.

   3. Cohort studies.

   4. Case-control studies.

   5. Cross-sectional surveys.

   6. Case reports.

D. Planning for change.

   1. Form a multidisciplinary practice committee.

   2. Develop a philosophy of care.

   3. Gather information.

     a. Explore the basis for current practice.

     b. Standards and guidelines from professional organizations.

     c. Review standards from regulatory agencies.

     d. Examine hospital policies and procedures.

     e. Search the published literature.

     f. Grade the literature by using the following framework:

       i. Rituals versus rationales: Define current practices as rituals (for example, "We have always done it this way.") or rationales (based on scientific principles, standards of care, and evidence).

       ii. Evaluate using current protocols.

       iii. Develop best practices for the breastfeeding family.

E. Evaluate current practice.

   1. No published standards or guidelines for care, but research support (for example, cup feeding for preterm infants),

   2. No published standards or guidelines for care and poor research support (for example, cabbage leaves for engorgement).

   3. Published standards and guidelines for care and literature support (for example, unrestricted breastfeeding times and frequency).

F. Benefits of evidence-based care.

    1. Practices are defensible during budget cuts and restrictions.

    2. Promotion of multidisciplinary collaboration.

    3. Assurance of patient safety.

    4. Reduction of liability.

G. Successful implementation of research into practice is a function of the interplay of three core elements:

    1. Level and nature of the evidence.

    2. Context or environment into which the research is to be placed.

    3. Method or way in which the process is facilitated (Rycroft-Malone, 2004).

H. Evidence-based examinations of breastfeeding policies and practices have been published.

    1. International Lactation Consultant Association. *Clinical Guidelines for the Establishment of Exclusive Breastfeeding* (2005). Available at www.ilca.org.

    2. World Health Organization (WHO), Division of Child Health and Development. *Evidence for the Ten Steps to Successful Breastfeeding* (1998).

    3. The Healthy Children Project. *Toward Evidence-Based Breastfeeding Practice.* (2000).

    4. The Academy of Breastfeeding Medicine has as a central goal the development of evidence-based clinical protocols for managing common medical problems that may impact breastfeeding success. These protocols can be found at www.bfmed.org.

III. Three Levels of Objectives for Lactation Management Education (Naylor et al., 1994)

A. Level I: Awareness.

    1. Target group: medical students (pre-service education).

    2. Example objective: discuss, in general terms, findings from the basic and social sciences of lactation.
       a. Describe the general benefits of breastfeeding for the infant.

B. Level II: Generalist.

    1. Target group: pediatricians, obstetric-gynecology physicians and residents, family medicine residents, and advanced practice nurses.

    2. Example objective: Apply the findings from the basic and social sciences to breastfeeding and lactation issues.
       a. Describe the unique properties of human milk for human infants.
       b. Describe the advantages of preterm milk for the preterm infant.

C. Level III: Specialist.

    1. Target group: advanced/independent study, fellowships.

    2. Example objective: Critique the findings from the basic and social sciences and evaluate their applicability to clinical management issues.
        a. Discuss in detail the components of human milk and their functions.
        b. Describe in detail the suitability of preterm human milk for the preterm infant.

IV. Education Specific to the Field of Breastfeeding and Human Lactation Has Been Developed by WHO and the United Nations Children's Fund

A. Promoting Breastfeeding in Health Facilities: A short course for administrators and policy makers.

    1. Goal: to sensitize administrators and directors of health facilities to the importance of breastfeeding and the BFHI.

    2. Target group: health facility directors and administrators.

    3. Length: A 10- to 12-hour course.

B. Breastfeeding Management and Promotion Course.

    1. Goal: to change maternity care to be breastfeeding-friendly.

    2. Target group: all staff of a maternity facility.

    3. Length: 20-hour course (includes 3 hours of clinical practice).

C. Breastfeeding Counseling Training Course.

    1. Goal: To develop clinical and counseling skills in breastfeeding.

    2. Target group: key health workers in all parts of the health system.

    3. Length: 40-hour course plus 8 hours of clinical practice.

D. Training Guide in Lactation Management.

    1. Goal: to prepare a cadre who can become trainers or BFHI assessors.

    2. Target group: trainers, policy makers, doctors, and senior community workers.

    3. Length: 80-hour course plus 6 hours of clinical practice.

V. Components of Professional Knowledge According to Schein (1972)

A. An underlying discipline or basic science component upon which the practice rests or from which it is developed.

B. An applied science or "engineering" component from which many of the day-to-day diagnostic procedures and problem solutions are derived.

C. A skills and attitudinal component that concerns the actual performance of services to the client using the underlying basic and applied knowledge.

References

Guyatt GH, Sackett DL, Sinclair JC, et al. User's guides to the medical literature. IX. A method for grading health care recommendations. *JAMA.* 1995;274:1800–1804.

Healthy Children 2000 Project, Inc. Sandwich, MA: Healthy Children's Center for Breastfeeding. Available at: http://www.healthychildren.cc. Accessed November 28, 2006.

International Lactation Consultant Association. Revised as, *Clinical Guidelines for the Establishment of Exclusive Breastfeeding;* Raleigh, NC: ILCA; 2005. Available at: http: www.ilca.org.

Naylor AJ, Creer AE, Woodward-Lopez G, Dixon S. Lactation management education for physicians. *Semin Perinatol.* 1994;18:525–531.

Rycroft-Malone J, Harvey G, Seers K, et al. An exploration of the factors that influence the implementation of evidence into practice. *J Clin Nurs.* 2004;13:913–924.

Schein E. *Professional Education.* New York: McGraw Books; 1972:43.

United Nations Children's Fund (UNICEF). *Breastfeeding: Foundation for a Healthy Future.* New York: UNICEF; 1999.

World Health Organization (WHO). *Evidence for the Ten Steps to Successful Breastfeeding.* Geneva: WHO; 1998.

Suggested Readings

AWHONN: Achieving Consistent Quality Care. Washington, DC: Association of Women's Health, Obstetric and Neonatal Nurses; 1998.

Breastfeeding Support Consultants. Creating Change . . . in the face of Resistance. Chalfont, PA: BSC; 1995.

Cadwell AL, Turner-Maffei C. *Toward evidence-based breastfeeding practice.* Sandwich, MA: Health Education Associates, Inc.; 1999.

Cadwell K. Using the quality improvement process to affect breastfeeding protocols in United States hospitals. *J Hum Lact.* 1997;13:5–9.

Canadian Task Force on the Periodic Health Examination. The periodic health examination. *Can Med Assoc J.* 1979;121:1193–1254.

DeGeorges KM. Evidence! Show me the evidence! Untangling the web of evidence-based health care. *AWHONN Lifelines.* 1999;3:47–48.

Dickerson K, Manheimer E. The Cochrane collaboration: evaluation of health care and services using systematic reviews of the results of randomized controlled trials. *Clin Obstet Gynecol.* 1998;41:315–331.

Dolan MS. Interpretation of the literature. *Clin Obstet Gynecol.* 1998;41:307–314.

Enkin M, Keirse MJNC, Renfrew M, Neilson J. *A Guide to Effective Care in Pregnancy and Childbirth.* 2nd ed. Oxford, UK: Oxford University Press; 1995.

Family and Reproductive Health, Division of Child Health and Development. *Evidence for the Ten Steps to Successful Breastfeeding.* Geneva: World Health Organization; 1998.

Heinig MJ. Evidence-based practice: art versus science? *J Hum Lact.* 1999;15:183–184.

Greenhalgh T. *How to Read a Paper: The Basics of Evidence Based Medicine.* 3rd ed. London: BMJ Publishing Group; 2006.

Leff EW, Schriefer J, Hagan JF, DeMarco PA. Improving breastfeeding support: a community health improvement project. *J Qual Improv.* 1995;21:521–529.

McKibbon KA. Evidence-based practice. *Bull Med Library Assoc.* 1998;86:396–401.

Sikorsk J, Renfrew MJ. Support for breastfeeding mothers. *Birth.* 1999;26:131.

Simpson KR, Knox GE. Strategies for developing an evidence-based approach to perinatal care. MCN *Am J Matern Child Nurs.* 1999;24:122–131.

Sinclair JC, et al. Introduction to neonatal systematic reviews. *Pediatrics.* 1997; 100:892–895.

United States Preventive Services Task Force. Breastfeeding Counseling, Washington, DC: US Department of Health and Human Services; 2003.

Walker M. *Breastfeeding Management for the Clinician: Using the Evidence.* Sudbury, MA: Jones and Bartlett Publishers; 2006.

Wood MJ. Nursing practice research and evidence-based practice. *Clin Nurs Res.* 2006; 15:83–85.

World Health Organization (WHO). *Global Strategy on Infant and Young Child Feeding.* Geneva: WHO; 2003.

World Health Organization and Wellstart International. Promoting breastfeeding in health facilities: A short course for administrators and policy makers. WHO/NUTR/96.3. Geneva: WHO; 1996.

INTERPRETATION OF STATISTICS AND QUANTITATIVE RESEARCH

Patricia J. Martens, CertEd, MSc, IBCLC, PhD

OBJECTIVES

- Describe basic statistical concepts and how these relate to an understanding of quantitative research and its application to clinical practice.
- Describe basic epidemiologic concepts and how these relate to an understanding of research and its clinical application.
- Describe basic data collection tools and how to critique them.
- Describe a framework for critiquing quantitative research.

Introduction

This chapter focuses on understanding the basics of quantitative research, which is research based on numerical data collection and analysis. Many studies use only a numerical approach, such as a study on the average breast milk intake of full-term babies at different points in time, or a study on initiation and duration rates of breast-feeding. Quantitative research is considered "generalizable" in the sense that it is expected to give you an idea of what a typical result is, how variable you would expect the result to be, and what you would estimate the population value to be based on the results of a sample of people from that population. Some people refer to quantitative research as "wide and thin" (in contrast to qualitative research being "narrow and deep"), meaning that you get a broad idea of a numerical value for a large population from the findings of your research, or an idea of which treatment works "better" from a number-viewpoint, but you also may miss the subtleties of the qualitative information about why you see what you do, or the rich context of the findings. Many people advocate for a mixed methods approach that combines the strengths of both quantitative and qualitative research into a single study.

Part 1: Basic Statistical Concepts

I. Four Types of Quantitative Data (This Makes a Difference as to the Type of Statistical Test to Use)

A. Two types of categorical data.

1. *Nominal:* distinctive named categories, but having no implied order.
   a. Example: eye color.
2. *Ordinal:* distinctive categories, but having an implied order.
   a. Example: satisfaction rating scale with categories of very unsatisfied, unsatisfied, neutral, satisfied, very satisfied (Likert scale).

B. Two types of continuous data.

1. *Interval:* data that are continuous, where the interval between numbers has real meaning but the numbers do not have a "true zero," that is, if you double the number, the true quantity doesn't double.
   a. Example: Celsius temperature, where each degree of temperature has a constant interval. From 15° to 16°C is the same interval change as from 30° to 31°C but from 15° to 30°C really doesn't double the amount of heat.
2. *Ratio:* data that are continuous and also have a "true zero" so that the ratio is meaningful.
   a. Example: Pulse rate of 120 beats per minute is really double a pulse rate of 60 beats per minute.

II. Measuring the "Typical" (That is, Measures of Central Tendency) Mean, Median, and Mode, and When to Use Each One. All of These Measures Are Ways to Give a Picture of the Typical Result in Your Data Set.

A. Mean: arithmetic average.

1. Sum of all of the data, divided by N (where N is the total number of data points).
   a. Example: five babies have birth weights of 2500, 3000, 3500, 3500, and 4500 g, so the mean is the sum divided by the number of data points, or 17,000 g/5 = 3400 g.
2. Used for continuous data (ratio, interval).

B. Median.

1. Halfway point of the dataset, where half of the data points are located above and half below the middle point.
2. Used for continuous and ordinal data.
3. Especially useful for *skewed* data (defined in IV.B.3.).

C. Mode.

    1. Most frequently occurring number of the dataset.

    2. Used for continuous, ordinal, and nominal data.

D. Example: For a dataset of birth weights (in grams) for five newborns at 2500, 3000, 3500, 3500, and 4500 g, the *mean* is 17,000 g/5=3400 g; the *median* is the halfway point (3rd value) = 3500 g; and the *mode* is the most frequently occurring value = 3500 g.

III. Measuring the Variability for Continuous Data (Range, Variance, and Standard Deviation and How to Interpret These Measures

A. Range.

    1. Difference between the highest and lowest values.

    2. Easy to calculate, but only uses most extreme values to describe the dataset.

B. Variance.

    1. Calculated by taking every data point's distance from the mean, squaring that difference, adding these together, and dividing the sum by $(n - 1)$, that is, one less than the sample size.

    2. Uses all data points, but the variance is in *squared units*, and as such is not easy to understand practically.

C. Standard deviation (SD).

    1. The square root of the variance (see above).

    2. Useful to describe normally distributed continuous datasets, because 95% of the data should be within ± 2 SD (read as "plus or minus 2 standard deviations) from the mean (next section explains SD).

D. Example: For a dataset of birth weights (in grams) for five newborns at 2500, 3000, 3500, 3500, and 4500 g, the *range* is 4500–2500 or 2000 g, the *variance* is 550,000 grams squared (g^2), and the SD is 742 g.

IV. The Importance of a *Normal Distribution* for Continuous Data

A. Characteristics of a normally distributed continuous dataset.

    1. Shows a specific pattern; the most frequently occurring number (mode) will be the halfway point (median), which will also be the arithmetic average (mean). The further away the datum is from the mean, the rarer it is to see a data point.

    2. A total of 68% of the data fall within ± 1 SD from the mean, and 95% of the data fall within ± 2 SD from the mean.

B. Using a histogram to graph continuous data.

1. Group data into equal intervals (often 8 to 14 intervals) and count how many data points fit into each interval. Then graph these data.

2. Normally distributed data show a histogram shape that is high in the middle, very symmetrical, and the mean, median, and mode values are similar.

3. Skewed data show a histogram shape that has a long "tail" either to the left (negatively skewed, lots of low numbers) or to the right (positively skewed, lots of high numbers). The mean, median, and mode values are not the same, and often the median is a better measure than the mean to get a sense of the "typical" value.

4. Bimodal data show a histogram with two "peaks," meaning that there may be two very different groups within the dataset.

C. Example: Figure 9-1 is a sample dataset of newborn birth weights ($N = 812$ newborns), with the mean = 3624 g, SD = 464 g, median = 3605 g, and mode = 3595 g. It exhibits a pattern close to a perfect normal distribution.

1. The largest number of babies ($n = \sim 275$ babies) fit into the grouping from around 3450 to 3800 g, and very few babies (≤ 20) fit into each of the groupings from approximately 2300 to 2600 g, and from 4600 to 5000 g. (Note: there is an overlay of a perfect normal distribution shape.)

2. The mean, median, and mode values are similar, and appear in the middle of the histogram where it peaks.

3. There is no "*skewness*," that is, no tail at the low or high end.

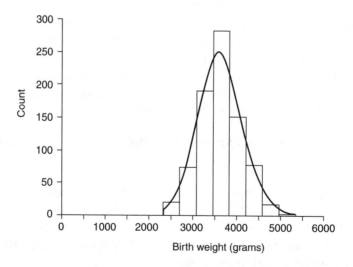

Figure 9-1   Histogram of newborn birth weights, showing frequencies of birth weight categories overlaid by a perfect normal distribution curve

4. In a perfect normal distribution, 68% of the data would be within ±1 SD of the mean (that is, 3624 ± 464 g, or from 3160 to 4088 g), and 95% within ±2 SD of the mean (from 2696 to 4552 g). In this dataset, 73% of the data are within ±1 SD, and 95% are within ±2 SD, close to the perfect normal distribution.

5. In the perfect normal distribution, you would have 2.5% of the data higher, and 2.5% of the data lower than ±2 SD, for a total of 5% of data outside of *normal*. In this sample, 2.5% of the data are higher, and 2.8% lower than ± 2 SD from the mean.

D. Interpreting continuous data for clinical practice.

1. From a sample study (Gagnon et al., 2005), the data can be interpreted as follows.

   a. Fact: The length of hospital stay of Canadian newborns in this study was given as a mean of 29.9 hours, with an SD of 5.4 hours. Interpretation: the typical length of hospital stay was around 29.9 hours, but 95% of the newborns stayed between 29.9 ± 2 (5.4) or 19.1 to 40.7 hours (almost 1 day to almost 2 days). Clue for lactation consultants: would this generalize to your setting and clientele?

   b. Fact: median age at first supplementation was 8.4 hours, range of 1.6 to 43.9 hours. Interpretation: 50% of newborns were supplemented before 8.4 hours, and 50% after 8.4 hours. Clue for lactation consultants: Although the range is interesting (i.e., the lowest and the highest values), these are the extreme values and may not represent the "typical." The median/mean is much more useful. The authors' use of a median rather than a mean implies "skewed" data instead of normally distributed data (in this case, a "tail" of high values). Note: If the mean ± 2 SD yields a negative value (impossible to have a negative length of stay), then it is skewed data and should be reported as the median.

V. Standard Error and 95% Confidence Intervals of the Mean

A. Standard error (SE) of the mean.

1. From your smaller sample of the population, SE helps you to estimate a range within where you would expect the true population mean to be found, based on your study sample.

2. SE is calculated from the SD and the sample size N. SE = SD divided by the square root of N.

3. Expect to find the true population mean somewhere around ± 2 SE of the mean in your sample.

4. The larger the sample size (N), the smaller the SE, and the narrower the interval in which you can approximate the true population mean (payoff for using large sample sizes in a study, so you have a narrower estimate of the true population mean).

B. 95% Confidence interval (CI) of the mean.

1. The interval represented by the mean ± 2 SE is called the 95% CI or 95% confidence limit of the mean.

2. We are 95% sure that the true population mean lies within this interval (statistics always has uncertainty attached to its estimates).

C. Example of the normally distributed dataset of newborn birth weights for $N = 812$ newborns, where the mean = 3624 g, SD = 464 g, and SE = 16 g.

1. From this study, we are 95% certain that the true population mean of full-term newborns' birth weight lies somewhere between 3592 and 3656 g. These are the calculations:
   a. SE = SD divided by the square root of N, or 464/square root of 812 = 16 g.
   b. 95% CI of the mean is 3624 ± 2 (SE) or 3624 ± 2 (16); that is, from 3592 to 3656 g.

D. Interpreting SE and 95% CI of the mean in clinical practice.

1. Use caution when reading publications showing the mean ± a number. Determine if this number is the SD, 2 SD, SE or 95% CI. Interpretation varies: SD describes the entire dataset, with ± 1 SD encompassing 68% and ± 2 SD encompassing 95% of the data points; SE describes the estimate of the population mean, with the mean ± 2 SE (also called the 95% CI) giving the interval in which to expect the true population mean 95% of the time.

VI. Reading Graphs

There are several ways to display data, but the most common are error bar charts, box plots, and pie charts.

A. Error bar charts.

1. These show the mean (arithmetic average) and a line to indicate the variation.

2. Determine what the line represents, because this differs among various publications and could represent either: ± 1 SD, ± 2 SD, ± 1 SE, or ± 2 SE.

3. Example: Figure 9-2 shows mean birth weights of full-term newborns by gestational age ($N = 809$), with the lines showing ± 2 SE (that is, 95% CI) indicating the estimate of the population mean for each gestational age.
   a. Wider intervals imply smaller sample size on which to base the population mean of 37 weeks gestation ($n = 32$) and 42 weeks ($n = 14$); compared to 40 weeks ($n = 300$). The larger the sample size, the narrower the SE and the narrower the estimate of the true population mean.

B. Box plots.

1. The median is a line within the rectangle. The lower (Q1) and upper (Q3) edges of the rectangle are the 25th and 75th percentiles, respectively. Thus, Q1 and below is 25% of the data points, the median and below is 50%, and Q3 and below is 75% of the data points.

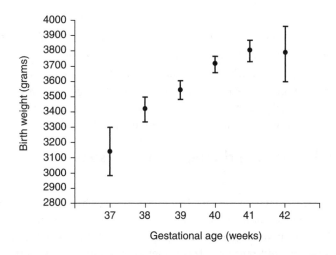

Figure 9-2   Error bar plot of birth weight by gestational age, showing 95% confidence intervals of the mean birth weight for each age

2. The "T"-shaped lines extending from each end are called *whiskers*. Different textbooks suggest different ways to draw these, such as at the 10th and 90th percentiles, or at the most extreme low and high values, or 1.5 times the distance between Q1 and Q3 (as shown in Figure 9-3) where data points outside these whiskers are considered *outliers*.

3. Example: In Figure 9-3, the median is 3600 g and the box is at 3300 and 3900 g, so 25% of babies have birth weights below 3300, 50% below 3600, and 75% below 3900 g.

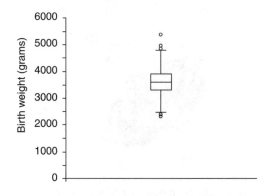

Figure 9-3   Box plot showing the birth weights of full-term newborns

C. Pie charts.

1. A pie chart displays what percentage of the data fits into each category, with the entire circle representing 100% of the data.

2. Example: Compare Figures 9-4 and 9-5. Figure 9-4 gives the reader the information about the relative percentage of each category. Figure 9-5 gives the identical information in the form of a bar chart, but the reader may get a better idea of the relative percentages from the pie chart format.

VII. Statistical Testing and Inferential Statistics

A. Terminology.

1. *Inferential statistics:* Generalizes beyond the research sample and makes statements (infers) about the population, with realistic uncertainty about the conclusions. Your study has a target population of interest from which a sample is drawn that should represent this target population. Your results should then generalize (infer) to the target population from which you took your sample.

2. *Dependent and independent variables:* the dependent variable (also known as the *outcome variable*) is the measure in which you are interested as the outcome of your research question. The independent variable(s), also known as the *explanatory variable(s)*, are those measures that are used in explaining the outcome measure.
a. Example: In a study to examine factors influencing the duration of breastfeeding, breastfeeding duration is the outcome variable, and explanatory variables could include maternal age, parity, and/or type of postpartum counseling.

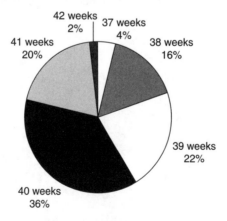

Figure 9-4   Pie chart showing the frequency of gestational age categories in a study of full-term newborns

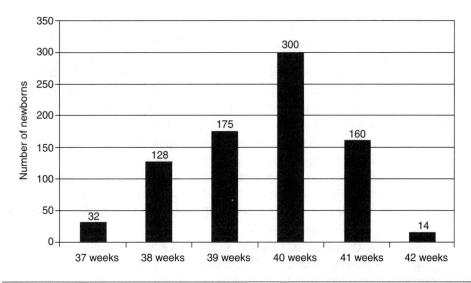

Figure 9-5   Bar chart showing frequency of gestational age categories in a study of full-term newborns

3. *Null hypothesis and alternate hypothesis:* The "default setting" of statistics is that there is no relationship between the explanatory and outcome variables; this is called the null hypothesis. A researcher needs to find enough proof to reject the null hypothesis (that is, show that there is no relationship or difference) and accept the alternate hypothesis (that there is a relationship or difference).
   a. Example: The *null hypothesis* states that there is *no* relationship between how long a baby is breastfed and whether or not the woman received postpartum support. The *alternate hypothesis* states that there is a relationship between breastfeeding duration and postpartum support.

4. *P-value* and the meaning of $P < .05$: Statistical testing depends upon the ideas of probability.
   a. The *P*-value states the probability of seeing your research result based on chance alone, that is, assuming that the null hypothesis is correct and your result is simply part of a normal distribution of results where no relationship exists.
   b. $P < .05$ (read, *P* less than point zero five) states that if the null hypothesis were correct, you would only see a result like this less than 5% of the time (.05 means .05 out of 1, or 5 out of 100, or 5%).
   c. If the *P*-value of a statistical test is less than 5%, you reject the null hypothesis and conclude the alternate hypothesis (that is, there is a relationship that is *statistically significant*).

      d. Examples of *P*-values less than 5%, $P < .05$, $P < .01$, and $P < .001$ (less than 5%, 1% and .1%, respectively), conclude that there is a statistically significant finding.

      e. Examples of *P*-values greater than 5%, $P < .34$, $P < .08$, and $P < .20$ (34%, 8%, and 20%, respectively), are *not statistically significant* (NS), and conclude the null hypothesis (that there is no difference or no relationship).

5. *Type 1 error:* Conclusion that there is a statistically significant difference even though the null hypothesis was correct at the population level (could be thought of as the "over-enthusiast" error; see Table 9-1).

      a. The *P*-value indicates the level of type 1 error, with $P < .05$ meaning that 5% of the time you could see this difference by chance alone (5% of the time, or 1 in 20 times, you could wrongly conclude a difference even though the null hypothesis was correct).

6. *Type 2 error:* Concludes that there is no difference (that is, concluding that the null hypothesis is correct) even though there really is a difference at the population level (could be thought of as the "skeptic" error; see Table 9-1). (Also refer to Martens, 1995).

      a. A Type 2 error may occur when the sample size (*N*) of a study is small.

      b. For studies that conclude no significant difference, ensure that the power of the study is sufficient to find a difference if it truly exists (see *power* below).

7. *Power of a study:* How likely you are to find a real difference if it exists, given your sample size.

      a. Good studies are designed with a power of at least 80%.

      b. Statistical calculations prior to the study can ensure adequate power, so there is less chance of committing a type 2 error.

Table 9-1 Type I and Type II Errors

		Reality at the population level	
		Null hypothesis is true (no difference)	*Alternate hypothesis is true (real difference)*
Results based on your research project	*Conclude "no difference" (accept the null hypothesis)*	Correct conclusion	Type II error
	Conclude difference exists (reject the null hypothesis and accept the alternate hypothesis)	Type I error	Correct conclusion

8. *Statistical significance versus clinical significance:* A study can show statistically significant results, but because of very large sample sizes there actually may only be a small difference, so decide on whether this much difference is *clinically significant,* that is, whether it has any clinical impact.

    a. Example: In a research study involving many subjects, a new drug (costing twice as much as a standard drug already in use) increases milk production by a small but statistically significant amount of 1 milliliter per 24 hours (1 mL/24 h). This statistic is probably not clinically significant to justify the extra cost. Alternatively, if this drug increased a woman's milk supply by a substantial amount (50 mL/24 h, for example), then it may be clinically as well as statistically significant.

B. Statistical tests.

    1. Statistical tests indicate if there is enough proof to reject the null hypothesis and conclude the alternate hypothesis.

        a. If $P < .05$, then reject the null hypothesis and accept the alternate hypothesis (that a statistically significant relationship or difference exists).

    2. The type of statistical test chosen depends upon the type of data you are analyzing. Table 9-2 describes several commonly used statistical tests.

        a. *Parametric tests* assume that the data are normally distributed, whereas *non-parametric* tests do not assume this.

    3. Statistical tests can show associations between variables, but this does not necessarily mean causation (that one caused the other; see research design section for more on causation).

Part 2: Basic Epidemiologic Concepts

I. Basic Epidemiologic Terms to Determine Risk

A. Ways to compare "exposed" and "unexposed" as to the risk of a certain "disease." See Table 9-3 for examples.

    1. *Relative risk (RR)* compares the probability of getting the disease in the exposed group versus the unexposed group.

        a. Example (Table 9-3): The RR of being supplemented if the baby has a high birth weight equals the probability of getting the disease in the exposed versus the unexposed groups = (67/142 divided by 204/558) = (0.472/0.366) = 1.29.

    2. *Odds ratio (OR)* compares the odds of getting a disease in the exposed group versus the unexposed group. An *odds* is a fraction of the number of times that an event happened divided by the number of times it did not.

        a. Example (see Table 9-3): OR = odds of getting the disease in the exposed versus the unexposed groups = (67/75 divided by 204/354) = 1.55.

Table 9-2   Common Statistical Tests

Statistical Test	Type of Data	Test Statistic	Example	What You Would Conclude
t-test (Student's t-test)	Compares the means of two different groups. Outcome variable: continuous data. Explanatory variable: categorical data (two "groups").	t	Is there a difference in the mean birth weight of male and female full-term newborns? Males: 3692 g (95% CI 3648–3736); Females: 3557 g (95% CI 3512–3602); $t = 4.18$, df, 809 two-tailed, $P < .001$	Yes, since $P < .05$ (P is actually much less, at .001). Male newborns have a higher average birth weight compared to females.
Paired t-test	Compares two different measures of the *same* person. Outcome variable: continuous data. Explanatory variable: categorical data (one "group" measured twice).	t	Is the hospital discharge weight of a full-term newborn less than the birth weight? Mean birth weight 3629 g. Mean discharge weight 3443 g. Mean difference: -186 g (95% CI -179 to -194 g), paired t-test: $t = -48.5$, df 771, one-tailed, $P < .00001$	Yes, since $P < .05$. There is a weight loss of full-term newborns that is probably somewhere between 179 and 194 g. Note that this is called a "one-tailed" test because it has a directional hypothesis ("less") rather than just a difference (is there any difference?). A one-tailed test has more power.
Analysis of variance (ANOVA)	Compares the means of more than two different groups (are the group means different, or	F	Is there a difference in birth weight for those full-term newborns who are exclusively breastfed,	No, because $P > .05$ (the P-value is greater than .05 or 5%). $P = 0.49$. The notation "NS" is often used for "not

Table 9-2   Common Statistical Tests—continued

Statistical Test	Type of Data	Test Statistic	Example	What You Would Conclude
	similar?) Outcome variable: continuous data. Explanatory variable: categorical data (several "groups"). Note: if you find $P < .05$, a subsequent statistical test (such as a Duncan or Tukey multiple test) must be done to find out which of the groups differ from each other.		exclusively formula-fed, or partially breastfed while in hospital? Means of groups: Formula-fed 3588 g, Partial 3648 g Exclusively breastfed 3618 g ANOVA test: F = 0.71, df 2, 810; P = 0.49, NS	statistically significant." So, we would conclude that there is no evidence to show that differences in birth weight are predictors of type of feeding in hospital.

Non-parametric equivalents of the above tests are used when the outcome measure is ordinal data, or when there is a breech in the assumptions of continuous data (such as non-normally distributed continuous data), and compare medians rather than means:

t-test: Mann Whitney U test

paired t-test: Wilcoxon test

ANOVA: Kruskal-Wallis test

Statistical Test	Type of Data	Test Statistic	Example	What You Would Conclude
Chi-square test	Compares proportions (are the proportions in two or more groups different?) Categorical data.	χ^2	Are primiparous women more likely to experience a caesarean section birth than multiparous women? N = 807 women (287 primiparas, 520 multiparas). χ^2 = 16.1, df 1, $P <$ .0001.	Yes, since $P < .05$. Primiparas (20.9%) were twice as likely as multiparas (10.6%) to experience caesarean section birth.

continues

Table 9-2 Common Statistical Tests—continued

Statistical Test	Type of Data	Test Statistic	Example	What You Would Conclude
Alternatives to Chi-square test: Fisher's exact test: for small counts McNemar test: paired data (that is, two categorical measures of the same person)				
Correlation (Pearson's correlation)	Looks at the relationship between two continuous variables (you measure two different things about the same person, over many people), and asks the question, "is it a linear relationship? Correlations take values between -1 (strong negative relationship, with one getting larger as the other gets smaller) and $+1$ (strong positive relationship, with one getting larger as the other gets larger), with "0" meaning no relationship. The amount of variation explained by this relationship is equal to the square of the correlation coefficient r.	r	Is there a correlation between healthy, full-term newborn birth weight and the percent weight loss in hospital? $r = 0.128$, df 773; $P < .0004$	Yes. The correlation is positive (that is, the higher the birth weight, the higher the weight loss). However, this relationship does not explain much of the variation ($r^2 = .016$, or 1.6% of the total variation).

Table 9-2 Common Statistical Tests—continued

Statistical Test	Type of Data	Test Statistic	Example	What you would conclude
Non-parametric equivalent of the Pearson's correlation: Spearman's correlation, used for continuous data that is non-normal, or ordinal data.				
Multiple regression	Looks at the unique contribution of several explanatory variables on a continuous outcome measure. Explanatory variables can be continuous or categorical.		What are the predictors of birth weight of full-term newborns? Birth weight (grams) = $-2065 + 142$ (gestational age in weeks) -114 (female) $+ 142$ (multiparous) $+ 129$ (caesarean section birth) Model: F = 38.5; df 4, 798; $P <$ .0001, $r^2 = 0.16$. Each explanatory variable was significant ($P < .05$).	This model explains 16% of the variation in birth weight ($r^2 = 0.16$), and shows the unique contribution of each explanatory variable. You can calculate the mean birth weight of a newborn from the equation (such as, for a male baby born at 40 weeks to a multiparous mother vaginally: Birth weight = $-2065 + 142$ (40) -114 (0) $+ 142$ (1) $+ 129$ (0) = 3757 g.
Logistic regression	Looks at the unique contribution of several explanatory variables on a categorical outcome variable (yes/no). Explanatory variables can be		What factors are associated with a breastfed baby being exclusively breastfed (this is a yes/no measure) while in a hospital? Explanatory variables include: parity, sex of	Parity and the sex of the newborn are not statistically significant factors associated with exclusive breastfeeding. Statistically significant factors ($P < .05$): Both caesarean section

continues

Table 9-2   Common Statistical Tests—continued

Statistical Test	Type of Data	Test Statistic	Example	What You Would Conclude
	continuous or categorical. Odds ratios (OR) show the unique contribution of each explanatory variable on the outcome.		newborn, high birth weight (> 4000 g) or not, type of delivery (caesarean section or not), and use of a spinal epidural during delivery. $N = 696$, model $P < .001$, $r^2 = 0.05$; parity ($P = .71$, NS); sex ($P = .20$, NS); type of delivery ($P < .0005$, OR $= .42$); epidural ($P < .02$, OR $= .63$); normal birth weight ($P < .02$, OR $= 1.6$)	delivery and having an epidural are statistically significant factors in reducing the chance of being exclusively breastfed (the OR is less than 1); being of normal birth weight significantly increases the chance of being exclusively breastfed.

Table 9-3   Is the Risk of Being Supplemented Associated with a Full-Term Breastfed Newborn's Birth Weight?*

	Breastfed Newborns in Hospital: Exclusive or Supplemented		
	Supplemented ("Diseased")	Exclusively Breastfed ("Not Diseased")	n
High birth weight ("exposed")	67 (47.2%)	75	142
Normal birth weight ("not exposed")	204 (36.6%)	354	558
	271	429	700

*Chi-square $= 5.38$, 1 df, $P < .025$ (because the P-value is less than 0.05, it means there is a "statistically significant" association between high birth weight and supplementation).

3. For both RR and OR: 1 means that there is the same risk, greater than 1 (> 1) means a bigger risk, and less than 1 (< 1) means a smaller risk.

4. RR and OR are very close numerically only if the prevalence of disease is small, that is, less than 10% ($< 10\%$; Zhang, 1998).

5. Certain types of statistical analyses (such as logistic regression) and study designs (such as case-control studies) produce OR values rather than RR.

6. Various other measures are used in epidemiologic studies (such as risk difference, attributable risk [exposed], and population-attributable risk; see Table 9-4).

7. Number needed to treat (NNT).
   a. Usually used to describe a positive intervention, such as a pharmaceutical or program intervention. Calculated by 1/RD, where RD is the *risk difference* (Table 9-4).
   b. How many people would you need to treat to see the effect?
   c. Example: In a longitudinal study on infant feeding and later type 2 diabetes, it was found that 10% of adults who had been exclusively breastfed, and 17% of adults who had been exclusively formula-fed, had adult type 2 diabetes. The RD is 17% $-$ 10% = 7% (or .07 as a fraction of 1 rather than a percent). So, the NNT = (1/.07) = 14, meaning that 14 babies must be exclusively breastfed in order to prevent one case of adult type 2 diabetes.

II. Basic Research Designs

A. Study designs can be described through a series of questions (Figure 9-6).
   1. Is the study descriptive or analytical?
   2. If analytical, is there artificial manipulation (*experimentation*), or not?
   3. Artificial manipulation (*experimental studies*), that is, intervention is under the control of the researcher.
      a. Are people or sites randomly assigned to receive or not receive the intervention? (*randomized controlled trial*). For example: Women experiencing sore nipples postpartum are randomly assigned two types of nipple cream and followed to see which produces the fastest healing.
      b. Are people or sites selected to be as similar as possible prior to the intervention, but not randomly assigned (*quasi-experimental comparison group*)? For example: Two hospital sites that are very similar to each other are chosen, and one site begins a new rooming-in policy intervention while the other does not. In-hospital exclusive breastfeeding rates are measured at both sites over the next several months to see if the policy had an effect.

Table 9-4   Epidemiologic Concepts, Meanings, and Examples

Measure	Other Names	What It Means	Example from Table 3	Interpreting the Example
Relative Risk (RR)	Risk ratio Rate ratio	Compares two groups. What is the risk for disease in the exposed group compared to the unexposed group?	Of breastfed full-term newborns ($N = 700$), 47.2% of high birth weight babies were supplemented, but only 36.6% of other newborns. RR = 1.29 OR = 1.55	A high birth weight newborn was 1.29 times (29%) more likely to be supplemented compared to a normal birth weight newborn. Note that the OR similarly shows that there is a greater chance or "odds" of (OR = 1.55), but not as intuitive as RR. OR and RR are very close only if the outcome is rare.
Risk difference (RD)	Rate difference Absolute risk reduction		Of breastfed full-term newborns ($N = 700$), 47.2% of high birth weight babies were supplemented, but only 36.6% of other newborns. RD = .472–.366 = .106 (or 10.6% difference)	10.6% more babies were supplemented in the high birth weight group. This gives an idea of how large the true difference is (Note: you can have a large RR, but a very small risk difference. For example, if only 1% of high birth weight babies and .78% of the others were supplemented, the RR would still be 1.29, but the

Table 9-4 Epidemiologic Concepts, Meanings, and Examples–continued

Measure	Other Names	What It Means	Example from Table 3	Interpreting the Example
				risk difference is a very small amount (1% − .78% = .22%)
Attributable risk (exposed)	Attributable fraction exposed (or proportion exposed, or risk percent exposed)	Among those "exposed" to the risk factor, what proportion of "disease" resulted because of being exposed?	Attributable risk (exposed) = (RR −1)/RR = (1.29 −1)/1.29 = 0.225 or 22.5%	Among those having the risk factor of high birth weight, .225 (or 22.5%) of them were supplemented because of this risk factor. In other words, some of these babies would have been supplemented just because supplementation also occurred in the non-risk (non-high birth weight) babies. Thus, 22.5% of the high birth weight babies were supplemented due to being high birth weight.
Population attributable risk	Etiologic fraction, Population attributable fraction, Population attributable proportion,	Among the entire (whole) population, what proportion of the disease cases resulted because of being exposed?	Population attributable risk P (RR −1)/[P(RR − 1) + 1] = .203 (1.29 −1)/[.203 (1.29−1) + 1] = .056 or 5.6%	Of all the supplemented newborns, 5.6% of them were supplemented because they were "exposed"

continues

Table 9-4   Epidemiologic Concepts, Meanings, and Examples—continued

Measure	Other Names	What it means	Example from Table 3	Interpreting the Example
	Population attributable risk percent		Note: to calculate population attributable risk, you need to know the overall proportion of high birth weight (P) in your population. In Table 9-3, P, which is 142 of the 700 babies, or 20.3%.	(because they were of high birth weight).

4. No artificial manipulation (observational studies).
   a. Is information collected concurrently (*cross-sectional study*), or over time (*longitudinal study*)?
   b. If cross-sectional, you cannot say that one factor "causes" the other, only that they are "associated." For example: Using national survey data, you find that low income is associated with low breastfeeding rates of babies. This is an association, but one does not necessarily cause the other.
   c. If longitudinal, then:
      i. *Cohort study:* Do you follow people forward from "exposure" to "disease" to see the effects of exposure or non-exposure on future risk of disease?

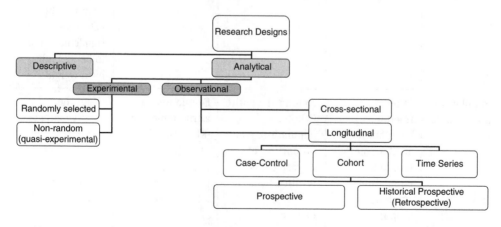

Figure 9-6   Research design schema

Do you start now and go forward in time (prospective), or do you have a "cohort" somewhere in the past and you follow them forward (historical prospective)? For example: Interviewing women in their third trimester about their social supports and confidence levels ("exposures"), and following them through time to see if they breastfeed or not ("disease").

ii. *Case-control study:* Do you go backward from "disease" to "exposure", that is, compare those people with and without the disease as to their past exposure to certain risk factors being studied? For example: Selecting groups of adults with and without diabetes ("disease"), and taking a history of their past "exposure" such as breastfeeding status, eating patterns, and past exercise to see if exposure patterns differ between the two groups.

iii. *Time series study* (with or without a comparison site): Do you measure rates of a population over time, to see if any trends are occurring (and if these can be related to naturally occurring interventions in the community; called *natural experiments*). For example: Community breastfeeding rates are tracked year-by-year over 15 years, and qualitative data about occurrences in policy or programs in the community are layered on these trends to see what influenced the trends.

B. Each study design has its strengths and limitations in terms of validity. There are also various threats to validity (Campbell, Stanley & Gage, 1963).

1. *Internal validity:* Refers to the strength of evidence for causation. For example, does X really cause Y?

   a. Examples of threats to internal validity are (see Martens 2002a, b): non-blinding (the people in the experiment know which treatment group they are in); selection bias (the groups differed before the intervention even occurred); maturation (did something change naturally over time, despite the intervention?).

   b. Randomized controlled trials (RCTs) are considered to have high internal validity, but not all interventions can be randomized ethically (you can't randomize babies to be breastfed or not!).

   c. Evaluation criteria for the type of evidence: the *Clinical Guidelines for the Establishment of Exclusive Breastfeeding* (ILCA, 2005) considers internal validity of a research study by classifying the strength of the evidence according to a hierarchy similar to Figure 9-7.

2. *External validity:* Refers to whether the results of the study are generalizable to settings beyond the study itself.

   a. Does the study reflect the "real world" or are the restrictions to enrollment, the setting, or the conditions of the intervention quite different than your clinical setting or the ordinary care a person would receive?

   b. Although RCTs are high in internal validity, they may be less than ideal for generalizability because of their highly restrictive enrollment and artificial

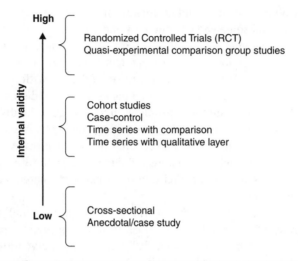

Figure 9-7   Hierarchy of internal validity (causality) for research designs

setting. Thus, quasi-experimental or observational studies may better generalize into other "real world" settings.

Part 3: Basic Research Tools and Instruments

I. Instrument Measures

A. Measures can be derived from various sources, such as chart audits or direct measures using *instruments*. These instruments can take the form of measurement instruments such as weigh scales, or tools such as surveys.

II. For Any Instrument You Need to Assess Its Reliability and Validity

A. Reliability: How reproducible are the results?

1. Example: Weighing a baby on a scale several times should give you the same (or similar) results if the scale is *reliable*.

B. Validity: How close to the truth are the results?

1. Example: How close is a scale to the true weight? A scale can be giving a similar weight over several weighings (reliable), but could be consistently weighing too high or too low (therefore, not valid). Only by calibrating the scale to a valid standard and then doing serial weighings would the data be valid.

C. Non-validity: You can "hit the mark" (that is, be close to the truth; validity) or you can get repeatable results (that is, close to each other; reliability) without being valid (Figure 9-8). If you have non-repeatability (non-reliability), then you cannot have validity.

III. Survey Instruments

A. Need to be tested for reliability.

1. Test–retest (that is, do people get similar results when doing the test a second time after a period when nothing has changed?); inter-rater reliability (if there is more than one surveyor, do they code in a similar way?); intra-rater reliability (is one surveyor coding consistently over time?).

2. Statistical tests used to indicate reliability include Cronbach alpha (from 0 to 1, with closer to 1 meaning better reliability), Cohen kappa (where two observers rate the same event to see if there is close agreement; ≥ 0.7 is considered good agreement).

B. Need to be tested for validity.

1. Construct validity. Does the tool measure all aspects of the concept it is designed to measure? You need to do a literature search to see what concepts should be included when designing a tool.

2. Content validity, face validity. Does the content of the survey make sense to the experts in the field and the current literature? A peer review from experts in the field is useful.

3. Concurrent validity. Does this tool perform similarly to another validated tool that is supposed to measure a similar construct? Example: Does a new tool to measure the effectiveness of breastfeeding in the early postpartum period give similar results to a tool already tested in the literature?

4. Predictive validity. Does this tool measure something that is statistically predictive of some logical variable in the future? Example: You hypothesize that

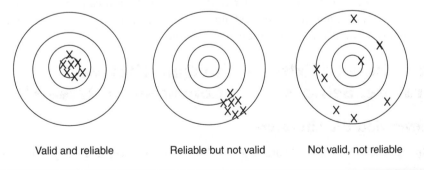

Valid and reliable   Reliable but not valid   Not valid, not reliable

Figure 9-8 A diagram illustrating validity and reliability in terms of "hitting the mark" of a target

a tool measuring the intent to breastfeed should statistically predict the real infant feeding choice at birth. If it does, then the tool has predictive validity.

C. Checklist for using survey instruments.

1. Always pilot test a survey with people similar to those who will be in the study.

2. Look for surveys that have been used before, that have been tested for validity and reliability.

3. Avoid common problems in survey questions.

   a. Avoid double negatives. Bad example: Do you not breastfeed in situations that are not private? Better wording: Do you breastfeed in public situations?.

   b. Avoid asking more than one item in a question. Bad example: Answer "yes" or "no": Do you like cheese or pickles? Problem: The surveyor doesn't know if the person liked cheese only, pickles only, or both if they answered "yes." Better wording is to ask separate questions.

   c. Avoid overlapping categories. Bad question: Is your baby 2–4 months old, or 4–6 months old? Problem: Which question should be checked off if the baby is 4 months old? Better wording: Is your baby 2–4 months old or 5–6 months old?

   d. Avoid leading or biased questions.

   e. Avoid questions that are not applicable to all respondents, unless you allow people to skip questions.

D. A survey is a tool to collect data for many different research designs (longitudinal, cross-sectional, RCTs, and so on) and not a study design itself.

IV. Importance of Definitions (*Operationalizing the Construct*)

A. It is important to understand the way in which a construct was operationalized, that is, how an idea or concept was actually defined for measurement.

1. Example: In a study of health outcomes, "breastfed" babies are compared to "non-breastfed" babies. To understand the study and critically analyze the results, it is important to understand how these constructs ("breastfed" and "non-breastfed") were operationalized (defined).

Part 4: How to Critique the Quantitative Literature: Being a Good Consumer of Research

I. Reviewing the Literature

A. Internet search engines. Search various Web-based sources using key words or phrases.

    1. *PubMed* (United States National Library of Medicine and the National Institutes of Health) is a free search engine of health-related published articles (http://www.ncbi.nlm.nih.gov/entrez/query.fcgi?CMD=search&DB=PubMed).

B. Published conference abstracts. Called "grey" literature because they have not undergone rigorous peer review nor are they published in a peer-reviewed journal, the abstracts may provide anecdotal evidence, preliminary or unconfirmed study results of interest, and suggestions for further research.

C. Tips for searching the literature.

    1. Be careful of the single study. One study alone is probably not sufficient evidence on which to base practice. The concept of $P < .05$ implies that 5% of the time (or 1 time out of 20), you could make a type 1 error and jump to the alternate hypothesis in error. Several repeated studies that all find similar results give a much stronger case on which to base practice.

    2. Look for *systematic reviews*, which are summaries of the literature done through critical appraisals of study design and methodology for all the literature on a specific topic.

        a. The Cochrane Library contains systematic reviews of RCTs on relevant medical topics that are compiled by worldwide experts.

        b. A good example: *Clinical Guidelines for the Establishment of Exclusive Breastfeeding* (ILCA, 2005), which rates the evidence for each management strategy.

    3. Look for *meta-analyses*, which statistically combine the results from several studies as if they were all part of one big study. This increases the sample size and reduces the possibility of type 2 errors in the many smaller studies.

        a. For example: A 2005 meta-analysis of the relationship between breastfeeding and a decreased risk of overweight combined 11 studies to yield an odds ratio of .96 (95% CI, .94–.98) for each month of breastfeeding (Harder et al., 2005).

II. Critiquing Quantitative Research Articles

A. When critiquing research articles, or designing research yourself, you need to ensure that certain criteria are met. Table 9-5 is a summary checklist.

B. If you are submitting a research proposal to the International Lactation Consultant Association (ILCA) Research Committee, a similar checklist will be used to critique the proposal (with additional checks of the budget, the proposed timeline, and the potential for the study to further the understanding of breastfeeding issues). Information for applying is available on the ILCA website, Research section (available at: http://www.ilca.org/research/ index.php; accessed November 27, 2006).

Table 9-5   Checklist for Evaluating Quantitative Studies

Section	Comments
1. Problem statement and hypothesis	Is the problem clearly stated? Are the research questions, objectives, and hypotheses clearly stated? Are the population, variables, and any relationships identified? Is the problem researchable?
2. Purpose/significance	Is there an identified and supported need for the study?
3. Abstract	Never rely solely on an abstract when analyzing a study, because you may be missing important details. Only use abstracts as a screening tool for finding which studies relate to your topic of interest. Does the abstract summarize important findings in a clear manner? Does it reflect the true findings of the actual full study?
4. Literature review and background	Is there an adequate review of the literature that outlines previous findings related to the present problem? Does it present a well-rounded review? Does the review logically guide the reader to the present study? Are there sufficient background facts? Does the literature review contain systematic reviews and meta-analyses if available?
5. Conceptual framework or theory	Is there a conceptual framework or a theory that links together the study variables, and makes sense as to the problem and hypotheses being studied?
6. Methodology	
A. Design	Is the design clearly explained, and appropriate for the problem? What are the strengths and limitations of this type of study design? What is the degree of internal/external validity?
B. Variables	What are the independent (explanatory) and dependent (outcome) variables, and how have these been defined and measured? Do these variables adequately operationalize the constructs?

Table 9-5 Checklist for Evaluating Quantitative Studies—continued

Section	Comments
C. Population and Sampling	Are the type of sampling, the selection process, and the exclusion/inclusion criteria given? Is the "representativeness" of the sample (in terms of representing a certain target population) described? Does this sample generalize to your particular clinical population?
D. Sample size	Is the sample size justified? Is there adequate power to detect an expected difference (80% or more power)?
E. Procedures and tools	Are the data collection methods appropriate for the design and setting? If instruments and tools are used, are they described adequately, including validity and reliability of the tools?
F. Ethical considerations	Did participants have a consent process? Was this research protocol reviewed by a credible ethical review committee? Are the procedures ethical? Did the researcher ensure privacy and confidentiality of the research subjects?
7. Data analysis	
A. Statistical analysis	Are the statistical tests appropriate for the design, sample size, and type of data collected? If there are skewed data, is the median result given? Are the P-values given, so you can determine the statistical significance, and the possibility of type 2 error?
B. Loss to follow-up	Is there a careful explanation of who was "lost to follow-up" in the study, and why they did not complete the study? Would this bias the study results (that is, were those who completed the study different from those who did not)?
8. Results	Has the research question been answered in a clear manner? Is the result clinically significant, or only statistically significant? If the conclusion is "no difference," was there adequate sample size (that is, did the study have sufficient power)?

continues

Table 9-5   Checklist for Evaluating Quantitative Studies—continued

Section	Comments
9. Discussion and interpretation	Do the discussion and interpretation follow from the results given, or do they go beyond the results of the study? Are the conclusions true to the study results? Are limitations of the study discussed?
10. Generalizability	What is the real world interpretation of the study? Does it generalize to your clientele? Is the result clinically significant and not just statistically significant? Does the additional burden justify any additional cost? Is there a calculation of the RR, RD, PAR, NNT? If not, could you do these calculations to determine if it has real world significance?
11. Sponsorship	Who sponsored or funded the study? Could this lead to potential bias? If so, examine the definitions used, the sample sizes used, and the conclusions given. If a potential bias exists, make sure that this research appears in a peer-reviewed medical journal, and not just in the "grey literature."

References

Campbell, DT, Stanley, JC, Gag L. *Experimental and Quasi-Experimental Designs for Research*. Chicago: McNally, 1963.

Gagnon AJ, Leduc G, Waghorn K, Platt RW. In-hospital formula supplementation of healthy breastfeeding newborns. *J Hum Lact*. 2005;21:397–405.

Harder T, Bergmann R, Kallischnigg G, Plagemann A. Duration of breastfeeding and risk of overweight: a meta-analysis. *Am J Epidemiol*. 2005;162:397–403.

ILCA. Overfield ML, Ryan CA, Spangler A, Tully MR (eds). *Clinical Guidelines for the Establishment of Exclusive Breastfeeding*. 2nd ed. Raleigh, NC: International Lactation Consultant Association; 2005. Available at: http://www.ilca.org/education/2005clinicalguidelines.php. Accessed November 29, 2006.

Martens PJ. A mini-lesson in statistics: what causes treatment groups to be deemed 'not statistically different'? *J Hum Lact*. 1995;11:117–121.

Martens PJ. Will your breastfeeding intervention make a difference? What the lactation consultant needs to know about program evaluation. *J Hum Lact.* 2002a;18:379–381.

Martens PJ. "First, do no harm": evaluating research for clinical practice. *Current Issues in Clinical Lactation.* 2002b:37–47.

Zhang J. What's the relative risk? A method of correcting the odds ratio in cohort studies of common outcomes. *JAMA.* 1998;280:1690–1691.

Suggested Readings

Barnett V. *Sample Survey: Principles & Methods.* 3rd ed. New York: Oxford University Press; 2002.

Bhopal R. *Concepts of Epidemiology: An Integrated Introduction to the Ideas, Theories, Principles and Methods of Epidemiology.* New York: Oxford University Press; 2002.

Harmon-Jones C. Reading and evaluating breastfeeding research. *Leaven.* 2005; 41:99–103.

Last JM, Spasoff RA, Harris SS, Thuriaux MC, eds. A *Dictionary of Epidemiology.* 4th ed. Edited for the International Epidemiological Association. New York: Oxford University Press; 2001.

Norman GR, Streiner DL. *PDQ (PrettyDarnedQuick) Statistics.* 3rd ed. Hamilton, Canada: B.C. Decker; 2003.

Streiner DL, Norman GR. *PDQ (PrettyDarnedQuick) Epidemiology.* 2nd ed. Hamilton, Canada: B.C. Decker; 1998.

Young TK. *Population Health: Concepts and Methods.* 2nd ed. New York: Oxford University Press; 2005.

INTERPRETATION OF RESEARCH: QUALITATIVE METHODOLOGY

Sara L. Gill, PhD, RN, IBCLC

OBJECTIVES

- Define qualitative research.
- Describe qualitative methodologies.
- Describe the major phases of a qualitative research project.
- Discuss issues of scientific rigor in qualitative studies.

Introduction

The term *qualitative research* is a very general term that includes a range of methods and designs. The intent of qualitative research is to describe and explain phenomena within a holistic framework. All qualitative methods approach research questions holistically with the focus on the human experience and the ways in which people create meaning in their lives. Qualitative methodologies provide a means of exploring the depth, richness, and complexity of phenomena. Research subjects in qualitative studies are referred to as respondents, participants, or informants. In ethnography, *key informants* provide the researcher with information about the culture. Key informants have special knowledge about the phenomena under study. They often help the researcher locate information or individuals (informants) to interview.

I. Assumptions of Qualitative Research

A. Multiple constructed realities.

1. Reality, based on perception, is different for each person.

2. The qualitative researcher must consider multiple perspectives in an attempt to fully understand a phenomenon.

B. Subject–object interaction.

   1. Researcher and participant interact to influence each other.

C. Subject has tacit knowledge.

D. Simultaneous mutual shaping.

   1. There is no attempt to determine causality but a belief that it is impossible to differentiate cause from effect.

E. Value-bound inquiry.

   1. Influenced by the researcher in the choice of method that guides the investigation.

II. Qualitative Research Traditions

Each type of qualitative method is guided by a particular philosophy. This philosophy guides the research questions asked, the observations made, and the data interpretation.

A. Anthropology.

   1. Domain: culture.

   2. Research tradition: ethnography, ethnoscience.

   3. Example:

      a. Black Non-Hispanic mothers' perceptions about the promotion of infant-feeding methods by nurses and physicians (Cricco-Lizza, 2006).

      b. In this ethnographic study, 11 key informants described their perceptions about the promotion of infant-feeding methods by physicians and nurses.

B. Philosophy.

   1. Domain: lived experience.

   2. Research tradition: phenomenology, hermeneutics.

   3. Example:

      a. Getting to know you: mothers' experiences of kangaroo care (Roller, 2005).

      b. Mothers' experiences of providing kangaroo care to their preterm babies was the focus of this phenomenologic study.

C. Sociology.

   1. Domain: social settings.

   2. Research tradition: grounded theory.

   3. Example:

      a. Constructing compatibility: managing breastfeeding and weaning from the mother's perspective (Hauck & Irurita, 2002).

      b. The purpose of this grounded theory study was to describe the process of managing the latter stages of breastfeeding and weaning.

D. Sociolinguistics.

    1. Domain: communication.

    2. Research tradition: narrative analysis, discourse analysis.

    3. Example:

        a. Adolescent mothers four years later: narratives of the self and visions of the future (SmithBattle & Wynn Leonard, 1998).

        b. Using narrative analysis, researchers examined adolescent mothers' narratives of self and their visions of the future.

E. History.

    1. Domain: past events, behavior.

    2. Research tradition: historical.

    3. Example:

        a. Historical analysis of siderail use in American hospitals (Brush & Capezuti, 2001).

        b. The purpose of this historical research study was to explore siderail use in American hospitals in the 20th century.

III. Characteristics of Qualitative Research

A. Natural setting for conducting the investigation.

B. Researcher is the "instrument."

    1. The researcher gathers data through interviews and observations rather than using survey tools, measurement instruments, or observation checklists, etc. (pen and paper measures).

C. Uses tacit knowledge to understand the world of the informants.

D. Often (but not exclusively) uses qualitative data and methods.

    1. Deals with narrative (words).

    2. Interpretative.

E. Purposive sampling.

    1. Participants are selected for the study based on their knowledge about the phenomena of interest.

F. Inductive data analysis: putting pieces together to make a whole.

G. Emergent research design: the research design emerges during the course of the study.

H. Tentative application.

    1. Generalizability is not a goal of qualitative research, so qualitative researchers do not make broad applications of the study findings.

I. Focus-determined boundaries.

    1. The qualitative researcher sets boundaries to the inquiry based on the research question, perceptions of the participants, setting, and values. The findings have no meaning in abstractions.

IV. Most Commonly Used Interpretative Methodologies

Method is selected according to the nature of the problem and what is known about the phenomenon to be studied.

    A. Basic qualitative description.

        1. Generic form of qualitative research.

        2. Offers a topical/thematic summary/survey of events.

        3. Least interpreted of qualitative descriptions.

        4. Example:

            a. What is the problem with breastfeeding? A qualitative analysis of infant feeding perceptions (Stewart-Knox, Gardiner, & Wright, 2003).

            b. These researchers used qualitative content analysis to identify themes related to infant feeding decisions.

    B. Phenomenology.

        1. Focus is on the discovery of meaning of people's lived experience.

        2. Goal is to describe fully the lived experience and the perceptions to which it gives rise.

        3. Source of data is in-depth conversations.

        4. Steps in the process include bracketing, intuiting, analyzing, describing.

            a. Bracketing: Researcher awareness of their preconceived thoughts and opinions about the phenomena of interest.

            b. Intuiting: Researcher is open to the meaning of the phenomena from the participants' perspectives.

            c. Analyzing: Researcher identifies the structure of the phenomena under study.

            d. Describing: Researcher represents a particular perspective/interpretation of the phenomena.

    C. Ethnography.

        1. Goal is to describe and interpret cultural behavior.

        2. Culture is inferred from the group's words, actions, and artifacts.

        3. Assumption is that cultures guide the way people structure their experience.

        4. Seeks an *emic* (insider) perspective of the culture.

        5. Sources of data: observations, in-depth interviews, records, charts, and physical evidence.

D. Grounded theory.

    1. Best identifies and analyzes complex processes.

    2. Generates theory from data. Theory is grounded in and connected to the data.

    3. Goal is to generate comprehensive explanations of phenomena that are grounded in reality.

    4. Data collection, data analysis, and sampling occur simultaneously.

    5. Sources of data: in-depth interviews (occasionally observations).

    6. Steps include constant comparison, categories, core category, and basic social process.

V. Phases in Qualitative Design

Qualitative methodologies use a flexible rather than linear approach.

A. Orientation and overview.

    1. Identify a problem.
        a. Broad topic or focus topic.
        b. No hypotheses.

    2. Literature review.

    3. Address ethical issues.
        a. More of a concern than in quantitative methodologies because of the close relationship between the researcher and participants.

    4. Gaining entry (access to setting and/or participants in which the researcher is interested).

B. Focused exploration.

    1. Conducting the study.

    2. Data analysis after data "saturation".
        a. Data collection continues until no new information is obtained during interviews or participant observation (the point of saturation). At this point, there is redundancy in the information.

C. Confirmation and closure.

    1. Exiting the setting.

    2. Ensuring trustworthiness.
        a. Trustworthiness is similar to reliability and validity in quantitative research. When a study is trustworthy, the reader is reassured that the findings accurately reflect the viewpoints and experiences of the participants.

    3. Dissemination.

VI. Sampling

A. Purposive. Seek participants who have knowledge about the phenomena and can share that information.

B. Interview/observe people who have experience.

    1. At informant's convenience because of time commitments.

C. Data saturation used to decide when to stop sampling.

D. Entry to setting must be negotiated with key members of the setting.

VII. Types of Data

A. Interviews.

    1. Semi-structured using open-ended questions.

    2. Examine one or two topics in detail.

    3. Follows participant's lead in asking further questions; the researcher avoids asking leading questions.

    4. Sensitive to language.

    5. Checks to make sure the researcher understands what the participant is saying.

    6. As interviews progress, researcher may add additional questions.

    7. Types of questions.
        a. Behaviors or experiences.
        b. Opinions or beliefs.
        c. Feelings.
        d. Knowledge.
        e. Sensory.
        f. Background or demographics.

B. Participant observation.

    1. Purpose.
        a. A means of describing through observations the ways in which people construct their reality.
        b. A means of describing through observations the activities and interactions of a setting.
        c. Data are recorded as field notes.

    2. Steps in participant observation.
        a. Gaining entry (permission to conduct the study).
        b. Initial contact.
           i. Researcher introduction.
           ii. Explanation of study purpose.

   3. Develop trust and a cooperative relationship with the participants.
      a. Be unobtrusive.
      b. Be honest.
      c. Be unassuming.
   4. Observe (Goetz & LeCompte, 1984).
      a. Who is present in the setting?
      b. What is happening in the setting?
      c. When does this activity occur?
      d. Where is this activity happening?
      e. Why is the activity happening?
      f. How is the activity organized?
C. Document review.
   1. May include a review of written records such as diaries, letters, newspapers, meeting minutes, and legal documents.
D. Artifacts.
   1. May include an analysis of items made or used by the culture such as feeding vessels or feeding utensils.

VIII. Data Analysis

A. Start data analysis when researcher begins to collect data.
B. Iterative process.
   1. Data analysis guides further data collection.
C. Product is rich, thick description (a very thorough description of the setting, interactions, and features of the phenomena).
D. Computer software programs (Nudist, Atlas.ti, and others) are available for organization and management of qualitative data.

IX. Trustworthiness

The researcher must persuade the readers that findings accurately reflect the experiences and viewpoints of the participants. Rigor or trustworthiness in qualitative research ensures that data collection and analysis are truthful. Trustworthiness in qualitative research is similar to reliability and validity in quantitative research.

A. Credibility.
   1. Techniques are employed that make it more likely that credible findings and interpretations will be produced.
   2. Prolonged engagement in the setting that is long enough to learn the culture, develop trust, and minimize misinformation.

3. Persistent observation to identify characteristics and elements in the situation most relevant to the problem.

4. Triangulation involves the use of corroborating evidence to draw conclusions about the phenomena. Triangulation allows for a multidimensional perspective of the phenomena of interest. Triangulation can enhance the credibility of a study. *Triangulation* refers to the use of multiple and different:
   a. Data sources.
   b. Data collection methods.
   c. Investigators.
   d. Theories.

5. *Peer debriefing* occurs when the researcher exposes himself or herself to a disinterested peer to keep the inquirer honest, test working hypotheses, and to test the next step in the methodological design.

6. *Negative case analysis.* Looking for disconfirming data (data that challenge the researcher's understanding of the phenomena) in both past and future observations/interviews. Analyzing disconfirming data will provide new understanding about the emerging conceptualization.

7. *Member checks.* Data and beginning interpretations are confirmed by study participants.

B. Dependability.

1. The stability of qualitative data over time and conditions. An inquiry audit, a scrutiny of the data collection and analysis by an external reviewer, is used to ensure dependability.

C. Confirmability.

1. Refers to the objectivity of the data. Inquiry audits are used to ensure confirmability. The researcher must develop an audit trail, materials consistently and conscientiously recorded and organized throughout the researcher process documenting both data collection and analysis strategies, which allows an independent auditor to come to conclusions about the data.

D. Transferability.

1. Refers to the extent to which the findings can be transferred to other settings.

2. It is the responsibility of the researcher to provide thick description that makes transferability judgments possible on the part of the potential appliers.

X. Ethical Concerns

A. The same ethical principles for quantitative methods apply to qualitative methods. Given the nature of qualitative methods, implementation of these principles throughout the research process may be different.

B. Concern around issues of harm, consent, deception, privacy, and confidentiality of data.

C. Prior to data collection, Institutional Review Board approval must be obtained as well as permission from the data collection site.

D. Consent is ongoing in qualitative studies.

E. Anonymity must be preserved.

1. More than changing persons' names.

2. Remove as many identifiers as possible.

3. Report demographic characteristics as group data.

4. Change the name of institutions, cities, suburbs, etc.

F. Participants have the right:

1. To be fully informed of the study's purpose.

2. To be aware of the time required and amount of involvement for participation.

3. To confidentiality and anonymity.

4. To ask questions of the investigator.

5. To refuse to participate without negative ramifications.

6. To refuse to answer any questions.

7. To withdraw from the study at any time.

8. To know what to expect during the research process.

9. To know what information is being obtained about them.

10. To know who will have access to the information.

11. To know how the information will be used.

G. Questions to ask of a qualitative study (Mays & Pope, 1995).

1. Did the researcher explicitly describe the methods used?

2. Was the context clearly described?

3. Was the sampling strategy clearly described and appropriate for the method used?

4. How was the fieldwork undertaken? Was it described in detail?

5. Did the researcher maintain an audit trail? Was it inspected by others?

6. Were the procedures for data analysis clearly described? Did they relate to the original research questions? How were themes and concepts identified from the data?

7. Was the analysis repeated by more than one researcher?

8. Did the investigator give evidence of seeking out observations that might have contradicted or modified the analysis (that is, negative or discomfirming cases)?

9. Was sufficient evidence presented in the written account to show the relationship between the interpretation (themes, categories, etc.) and the evidence (quotations)?

References

Brush BL, Capezuti E. Historical analysis of siderail use in American hospitals. *J Nurs Scholarship*. 2001;33:381–385.

Cricco-Lizza, R. Black Non-Hispanic mothers' perceptions about the promotion of infant-feeding methods by nurses and physicians. *J Obstet Gynecol Neonat Nurs*. 2006;35:173–180.

Hauck YL, Irurita VF. Constructing compatibility: managing breast-feeding and weaning from the mother's perspective. *Qual Health Res*. 2002;12:897–914.

Mays N, Pope C. Qualitative research: rigour and qualitative research. *BMJ*. 1995; 311:109–112.

Roller CG. Getting to know you: mothers' experiences of kangaroo care. *J Obstet Gynecol Neonat Nurs*. 2005;34:210–217.

SmithBattle L, Wynn Leonard V. Adolescent mothers four years later: narratives of the self and visions of the future. *Adv Nurs Sci*. 1998;20:36–49.

Stewart-Knox B, Gardiner K, Wright M. What is the problem with breast-feeding? A qualitative analysis of infant feeding perceptions. *J Hum Nutr Diet*. 2003; 16:265–273.

Suggested Readings

Beck CT. Qualitative research: the evaluation of its credibility, fittingness, and auditability. *West J Nurs Res*. 1993;15:263–266.

Beck CT. Initiation into qualitative data analysis. *J Nurs Edu*. 2003;42:231–234.

Burns N, Groves SK. *The Practice of Nursing Research*. 5th ed. St. Louis: Elsevier Saunders; 2005.

Creswell JW. *Qualitative Inquiry and Research Design: Choosing Among Five Traditions*. Thousand Oaks, CA: Sage Publications; 1998.

Denzin NK, Lincoln YS, eds. *Handbook of Qualitative Research*. Thousand Oaks, CA: Sage Publications; 1994.

Goetz JP, LeCompte MD. *Ethnography and Qualitative Design in Educational Research*. Orlando, FL: Academic Press; 1984.

Lincoln YS, Guba EG. *Naturalistic Inquiry*. Newbury Park, CA: Sage Publications; 1985.

Morse JM. Myth #93: reliability and validity are not relevant to qualitative inquiry. *Qual Health Res*. 1999;9:717–718.

Polit DF, Beck CT. *Nursing Research: Principles and Methods*. 7th ed. Philadelphia: Lippincott; 2004.

Sandelowski M. Whatever happened to qualitative description? *Res Nurs Health.* 2000;
23:334–340.

Savage J. Participant observation: standing in the shoes of others? *Qual Health Res.*
2000;10:324–339.

Spradley J. *The Ethnographic Interview.* New York: Holt, Rinehart and Winston; 1979.

Spradley JP. *Participant Observation.* New York: Holt, Rinehart and Wilson; 1980.

Strauss A, Corbin J. *Basics of Qualitative Research: Grounded Theory Procedures and
Techniques.* Newbury Park, CA: Sage Publications; 1990.

Van Manen M. *Researching Lived Experience.* New York: State University of New York
Press; 1990.

A Legal Primer for Lactation Consultants

Priscilla G. Bornmann, JD

OBJECTIVES

- List ways in which the lactation consultant patient/client relationship can be created.
- Describe legal actions most likely to be brought against lactation consultants.
- Define "informed consent" and discuss how it relates to the lactation consultant.
- Describe the use of technology as it relates to lactation consultant practice.
- Discuss at least three techniques a lactation consultant should use when testifying at a deposition or trial.

Introduction

This chapter is designed to provide accurate general information regarding legal matters that the lactation consultant might encounter in practice. Although the information relates specifically to the United States, the intent and general concepts in this chapter would most likely have parallels in other countries. The International Lactation Consultant Association (ILCA) website (www.ilca.org) contains forms prepared in a format that is readily convertible to personal use. Readers should feel free to reproduce or retype these forms for their personal use or for the use of their offices. However, they should not be used without reading the outline material that relates to them, nor should they be used without the user's absolute certainty that they have not been changed to fit the user's specific circumstances (including any requirements specific to the relevant jurisdiction). These forms are not to be resold. If legal advice or other expert assistance is required, the services of a competent professional should be sought. To obtain copyright permissions, please contact the copyright holder, P.G. Bornmann and Jones and Bartlett Publishers, Inc. Copyright © 2006 by Priscilla G. Bornmann, J.D. All rights reserved McKinley & Bornmann, P.L.C. 100 North Pitt Street, Suite 201, Tel: (703) 299-8713. E-mail: pgbornmann@cavtel.net.

I. The Lactation Consultant/Patient/Client Professional Relationship

A. Creation of the lactation consultant/patient/client relationship.

1. There is generally no duty to render care or attention unless the lactation consultant agrees to do so. However, if the lactation consultant "accepts" a patient/client, duties are created that are contractual in nature.[1] Those duties that are created exist whether or not the lactation consultant is being paid for services.[2]

   a. Duty to render the appropriate level of care (unless authorized to withdraw).

   b. Duty to refer, if unable to render appropriate care.

   c. Duty not to abandon patient/client.

2. The contract creating the patient/client relationship may be created either by:

   a. *Express agreement*, defined as an actual agreement, the terms of which are stated either orally or in writing. For example: lactation consultant agrees to counsel participants in a health plan.

   b. *Implied agreement*, a contract inferred in law as a matter of reason and justice from the acts or conduct of the parties or the circumstances surrounding the transaction. For example: This could result from a telephone conversation in which patient/client asks to make an appointment for a specific condition (not merely to "see" a lactation consultant).[3]

3. Occurrences that may create a lactation consultant/patient/client relationship.

   a. Periodic visits, but for different reasons: each appointment is a new contract.

   b. Ongoing visits for a *chronic* condition requiring patient/client to appear for follow-up: one contract.

   c. Making an appointment.

      i. This usually constitutes an agreement to meet to determine *whether* to enter a patient/client relationship.

      ii. However, in some cases a patient/client relationship is created by the act of making an appointment.
      Example: Virginia case: A blind woman and her 4-year-old guide dog went to a doctor's office. The doctor demanded that the guide dog be removed, refused to treat the woman, and did not assist her in finding

---

[1]*MacNamara v. Emmons*, 36 Cal. App. 2d., 199, 204-205, 97 P.2d 503, 507 (1939).

[2]Failure to pay an account may constitute grounds for a lactation consultant to terminate a client relationship, so long as the lactation consultant does not attempt to do so at a critical time, the lactation consultant provides notice to the client, and the lactation consultant gives the client an opportunity to obtain proper care elsewhere.

[3]But see, *Tsoukas v. Lapid*, 191 Ill. 2d 561, 738 N.E.2d 936 (Ill. 2000), in which the court held that a health maintenance organization (HMO) patient's telephone calls to a physician listed in an HMO directory did not establish a physician–patient relationship between the parties.

other medical attention. The court noted the appointment had been made "for the treatment of a vaginal infection," and thus created a relationship and duties . . . was more than a mere appointment to see a physician.[4] Two questions would be relevant to a lactation consultant: (1) Did the patient/client entrust her treatment to the lactation consultant? and (2) Did the lactation consultant accept the case?[5]

    iii. Practice Tip: Think before turning away someone who arrives pursuant to an appointment. If the person needs immediate counseling or care, give it. If not, the lactation consultant may make alternate arrangements or refer to another competent practitioner.

  d. Examination probably creates a relationship.[6]

Practice Tip: If you discover a problem beyond your competency, don't just walk away. Advise patient/client of your concerns and about the need to obtain follow-up care, and refer to a competent practitioner.

  e. Phone calls may create a relationship. Their content determines whether this is so. To avoid creating a relationship by telephone:[7]

    i. The person receiving the call should identify her/himself and obtain the name of the individual to whom she is speaking.

    ii. The person receiving the call may listen to the caller's complaints.

    iii. If an appointment is made, it should be made clear that the appointment is being made for evaluation in order to determine whether the lactation consultant can accept the new patient/client.

    iv. If no appointment is made, the person receiving the call should inform the caller of her options. For example, she may go to the local emergency room, phone an appropriate physician, or phone another lactation consultant.

    v. If the lactation consultant gives comments in the nature of advice, a lactation consultant/patient/client relationship has been created.

---

[4]*Lyons v. Grether*, 218 Va. 630, 239 S.E.2d 103 (1977).

[5]*Parkell v. Fitzporter*, 301 Mo. 217, 256 S.W. 239 (1923); *Hanson v. Pock*, 57 Mont. 51, 187 P. 282 (1920); *Peterson v. Phelps*, 23 Minn. 319, 143 N.W. 793 (1913).

[6]*Green v. Walker*, 910 F.2d 291 (5th Cir. 1990); see also, *Harris v. Kreuzer*, 2006 W.L. 68765 (Va. Jan. 13, 2006) VLW#006-6-013 23 pages. (Physician's consent to examine patient formed a limited relationship for purpose of the examination imposing on the physician a duty, limited solely to the exercise of due care consistent with the applicable standard of care so as not to cause harm to the patient in the actual conduct of the examination.)

[7]*Hamil v. Bashline*, 224 Pa. Super. 407, 307 A.2d 57 (1973); b*ut see, Fabien v. Matzko*, 235 Pa. Super 267, 344 A.2d 569 (1975) and *Childs v. Weis*, 440 S.W.2d 104 (Tex. Civ. App. 1969); but *see, Tsoukas v. Lapid*, 191 Ill. 2d 561, 738 N.E.2d 936 (Ill. 2000) in which the court held that an HMO patient's telephone calls to a physician listed in an HMO directory did not establish a physician–patient relationship between the parties.

4. Occurrences that usually do not create a lactation consultant/patient/client relationship.
   a. Request by a physician that the lactation consultant see a patient/client or review the patient/client's record. (However, if doctor is "relying" on the lactation consultant and the lactation consultant knows this, a relationship may be implied (see the patient/client soon).
   b. Lactation consultant's hospital affiliation. Generally no relationship exists as to persons who once were in the hospital, but are no longer inpatients. However, this rule may not apply if the call is to a hospital "hot line." In an emergency, it would be best to see and/or refer.

B. Duration and termination of the lactation consultant/patient/client relationship.
   1. Duration. Usually no duration is specified, so the law fills in by requiring the lactation consultant to continue care until:
      a. The need for lactation consultant services no longer exists OR
      b. The patient/client withdraws from care OR
      c. The lactation consultant withdraws in a manner that does not constitute "abandonment" of the patient/client.
   2. Termination. The relationship exists until:
      a. The need for lactation consultant services no longer exists *OR*
      b. The lactation consultant and patient/client mutually agree to discontinue relationship *OR*
      c. Patient/client discharges lactation consultant either expressly or by seeking lactation consultant services from another provider *OR*
      d. lactation consultant unilaterally withdraws from relationship by:
         i. Giving patient/client appropriate notice of intent to withdraw.
            (a) Talk by phone or in person:
            (b) Send certified letter, return receipt requested, stating: (1) status of patient/client; (2) need for follow-up care; (3) intention to withdraw by definite stated date (date must give time for patient/client to seek alternative care); (4) that client may seek lactation consultant for emergencies until date stated and (5) state that subsequent physician or lactation consultant can obtain a copy of all records with written permission from patient/client. Note: a patient/client's failure to pay will not justify the lactation consultant's unilateral withdrawal without giving sufficient opportunity to obtain alternative care.
         ii. Referring to a competent replacement or to a specialist when patient/client's problem is outside lactation consultant competence.[8]
   3. Situations that may constitute abandonment.
      a. Lactation consultant called to consult (this is a limited contract). To avoid problems, take three steps.

---

[8]*Brandt v. Grubin*, 131 N.J. Super 182, 329 A.2d 82, 89 (1974).

      i. Tell patient/client verbally and write in chart: "I have been called by Dr. ____ to evaluate____."

     ii. Perform service needed.

    iii. Tell patient/client verbally and write in chart: "I am signing off this case and will no longer follow this patient/client. However, I (or business name) will remain available if I am notified that additional consultations or assistance is required."

  b. Failure to attend the patient/client when required under a general contract for treatment.

  c. Substitution of lactation consultants. The patient/client is not abandoned if the replacement is competent. To avoid problems:

      i. Notify replacement of case details verbally and in writing.

     ii. If possible, give notice to patient/client of intent to substitute.

    iii. Advise new patient/client of group's rotation procedure.

  d. Patient/client's failure to keep follow-up appointment or to follow medical advice. Under such circumstances a lactation consultant has a duty to:

      i. Be sure patient/client understands nature of condition *AND*

     ii. Be sure patient/client is informed of risks of failing to seek medical attention *AND*

    iii. Provide the patient/client with an opportunity to visit the lactation consultant for counseling or care.

  e. *Practice Tip*: Call the patient/client with information in d (i–iii) above. Follow up with a letter to patient/client sent by certified mail, return receipt requested, which contains the same information.

II. Consent, Informed Consent, and the Lactation Consultant in the United States

These comments on consent and the doctrine of informed consent, as it has been applied in the United States, are not specific to breastfeeding issues because no cases related to breastfeeding have been reported. However, it is hoped that an overview of general principles may help lactation consultants better understand this common law doctrine, which is gaining acceptance in a wide variety of medical settings.[9]

  A. Consent principles.

    The distinction between *consent* and *informed consent* is legally significant. Consent occurs when the patient/client, or one authorized on her behalf, agrees to a course of treatment or the performance of a medical procedure. It requires only

---

[9]*Ketchup v Howard*, 247 Ga. App. 54, 00 FCDR 206, 2000 WL 1747538 (Ga. Ct. App., Nov. 29, 2000) [held that medical professionals, including dentists, must obtain informed consent from patients by advising them about procedures' known risks and available treatment alternatives]; *Matthis v. Mastromonaco*, 733 A.2d 456 (1999) [held that the informed consent doctrine applies to noninvasive procedures as well as invasive ones].

that the patient/client, or her representative, understand the nature of the proposed treatment.[10] If the lactation consultant fails to obtain consent and proceeds to touch the patient/client, the lactation consultant may be guilty of a battery (of touching the patient/client without consent), and liable for an award of nominal damages, even though no real injury results.

B. Informed consent.

Even if a patient/client's consent is given, a lactation consultant could be found liable to a patient/client for not obtaining *informed* consent. What information is needed as the basis for informed consent? The courts have generally held that a patient/client's informed consent is given only if the following areas have been discussed:

1. The nature of the patient/client's problem or illness.

2. The nature of the proposed therapy or treatment.

3. Reasonable alternative therapies or treatments.

4. The chance of success with the proposed therapy or treatment.

5. Substantial risks inherent in the therapy or treatment.

6. Any risks[11] related to failing to undergo therapy or treatment.

Note: Although a written consent form will be considered as evidence that the patient/client's informed consent was obtained, it is not usually conclusive.[12] A suit for lack of informed consent is generally based on negligence.[13] The

---

[10]Note, however, the client's consent, or even insistence on a certain treatment plan or procedure will not relieve a health care provider from the obligation to treat patients within the accepted standard of care. *Metzler v. New York State Board for Professional Medical Conduct,* 610 N.Y.S.2d 334 (AD 3 Dept 1994) [homeopathic treatment].

[11]It is well settled that only material risks need to be disclosed. There is no duty to disclose all conceivable risks *(Gouse v. Cassell,* 532 Pa. 197, 615 A.2d 33 [1992]), risks that are not reasonably foreseeable *(Hondroulis v. Schumacher,* 546, So. 2d 466 [La. 1989]), or those risks that are minimal (*Penwick v. Christensen,* 912 S.W.2d 275 [Tex. App. Houston, 14th Dist, 1995] *writ denied* [June 28, 1996]; *rehearing of writ of error filed* [July 12, 1996] *rehearing of writ of error overruled* [Aug 1, 1996]). However, establishing whether a particular risk is more than merely "conceivable," or "reasonably foreseeable," or greater than "minimal" is an imprecise exercise that has spawned much litigation.

[12]*Siegel v. Mt. Sinai Hospital,* 62 Ohio App. 2d 12, 403 N.E.2d 202 (1978).

[13]The case law of the state of Pennsylvania is an exception to this rule. In Pennsylvania, if informed consent was not given, this is treated as the legal equivalent of no consent having been given, and the action is then an action for battery (not negligence). *Gouse v. Cassel,* 532 Pa. 197, 615 A.2d 331, 334 (1992); *Sagala v. Tavares,* 533 A.2d 165(Pa. Super. 1987); *Boyer v. Smith,* 345 Pa. Super Ct. 66, 497 A.2d 646 (1985); *Salis v. United States,* 522 F. Supp 989 (MD Pa. 1981); *Gray v. Grunnagle,* 423 Pa. 144, 233 A.2d 633 (1966). Consider also *People v. Messinger,* No. 9467694FH (Mich, Ingham County Cir. Ct. Feb. 2, 1995) [jury acquitted a father charged with involuntary manslaughter on grounds that his decision to disconnect premature infant son's respirator was the result of informed decision to withdraw life sustaining treatment in the child's "best interests"]; *Dewes v. Indian Health Service,* 504 F. Supp 203 (D S.D. 1980).

patient/client must prove not only that the lactation consultant breached a duty to give or obtain such consent, but also that this caused injury or damage. This usually requires that the patient/client prove she would have elected a different treatment or course of therapy had she been properly informed.[14]

Standard consent forms alone ordinarily do not provide sufficient information about the disclosures made to the patient/client to establish that the patient/client's consent was an adequately informed one.[15] On the other hand, a consent form will be given effect as a defense if all the evidence supports a conclusion that the patient/client was informed about the treatment to which he or she consented.[16]

Theoretically, a patient/client, or her representative, could waive the obligation to obtain informed consent if the patient/client or her representative insisted that she not be informed of the nature of the treatment or the accompanying risks.[17] However, the actual occurrence of such a waiver is difficult to foresee in a breastfeeding context.

For lactation consultants in a busy practice, adequate legal protection may be obtained in relation to courses of treatment often recommended by writing up an information sheet, and frequently updating the same. The lactation consultant should ask the mother (or both parents, if they are available) to sign and date two identical forms, below a typed statement saying that she or they acknowledge(s) receipt of the information. One copy of the form should remain in the lactation consultant's files, and the other should be given to the mother or both parents. When determining the information to include in such a form, consider the following recommendations:

[14]*Canterbury v. Spence*, 464 F.2d 772, 780 (D.C. Cir.), *cert. denied*, 409 U.S. 1064 (1972); *St. Gemme v. Tomlin*, 118 Ill. App. 3d 766, 74 Ill. Dec. 264, 455 N.E.2d 294 (1983). The 1992 Code of Medical Ethics prepared by the Council on Ethical and Judicial Affairs of the American Medical Association states that a patient's right of self-decision can be effectively exercised only if the patient possesses enough information to make an intelligent choice, that the patient should make the ultimate decision on accepting treatment, and that a physician's ethical obligation is to present the medical facts accurately to the patient and assist that patient in making choices from the therapeutic alternatives consistent with good medical practice. *Also see, Koegan v. Holy Family Hospital*, 95 Wash.2d 306, 622 P.2d 1246 (1980).

[15]*Pegram v. Sisco*, 406 F. Supp 776 (WD Ark. 1976) *aff'd* 547 F.2d 1172 (8th Cir. l976); *LePelley v. Grefenson*, 101 Idaho 422, 614 P.2d 962 (1980); *Karl J. Pizzalotto MD Ltd v. Wilson*, 437 So. 2d 859 (La. 1983) remd 444 So. 2d 143 (La. App. 1983); *LaCaze v. Collier*, 434 So. 2d 1039 (1983); *Roberson v. Menorah Medical Center*, 588 S.W.2d 134 (Mo. App. 1979); *Gray v. Grunnagle*, 423 Pa. 144, 233 A.2d 633 (1966); *Cross v. Trapp*, 294 S.E.2d 446 (W.Va. 1982).

[16]See *Rogers v. Brown*, 416 So. 2d 624 (La. App. 1982). In this case, the client's consent was established on the basis of a consent form where the physician and nurse testified that risks of treatment were fully explained to the client and the form was completed, signed, and given to the client.

[17]*Putensen v. Clay Adams, Inc.*, 12 Cal. App. 3d 1064, 91 Cal. Rptr. 319 (1970).

a. Consult with other lactation consultants to determine what risks and alternative modes they explain to their patient/clients.
b. Consult current medical literature to determine the frequency and severity of risks and the availability of reasonable alternative modes of treatment.
c. Supplement the above with those additional risks that are serious or life-threatening even though infrequently encountered.
d. Add to the form additional information that you believe the average prudent patient/client(s) would want to have explained to allow her/them to give informed consent.

The existence of a duty to obtain informed consent is not dependent on prior legal recognition of this doctrine in the forum. The absence of any law recognizing informed consent liability at the time of the defendant's alleged breach will not preclude imposing informed consent liability if making more extensive disclosures would have been recognized as good and acceptable medical practice at the time.[18] The duty to obtain informed consent is based on the right of patient/clients to control what will be done with their own bodies.[19]

Some states in the United States limit use of the informed consent doctrine to cases involving surgical or operative medical procedures.[20] A few other states have held that their informed consent statutes do not apply to "routine medical procedures."[21] In such jurisdictions, it is doubtful that the doctrine of informed consent would be relevant to most breastfeeding situations. However, there is recent case law that holds that the doctrine of informed consent applies to noninvasive, as well as invasive, medical procedures.[22]

Currently, the *primary treating physician* has the duty to obtain the patient/client's informed consent for treatment, but not always those personnel who merely consult with,[23] refer to,[24] or assist[25] the attending

---

[18]*Halley v. Birbiglia*, 3901 Mass. 540, 458 N.E.2d 710 (1983).

[19]*Canterbury v. Spence*, 150 App. D.C. 263, 464 F.2d 772 (D.C. Cir. 1972) *cert. denied* 409 U.S. 1064 (1972); *Sard v. Hardy*, 281 Md. 432, 379 A.2d 1014 (1977); *Smith v. Shannon*, 100 Wash.2d, 666 P.2d 351 (1983). However, in many jurisdictions, this duty arises out of the fiduciary nature of the physician–patient relationship and may not apply to lactation consultants. *Nelson v. Gaunt,* 125 Cal. App. 3d 623, 178 Cal. Rptr. (1981).

[20]*Boyer v. Smith*, 345 Pa. Super. Ct. 66, 497 A.2d 646 (1985)[holding that the defendant had no duty to obtain a patient's informed consent to the administration of a therapeutic drug].

[21]*Novak v. Texada, Miller, Masterson & Davis Clinic*, 514 So. 2d 524 (La. App. 1987) *cert. denied* 515 So. 2d 807 (La. (1987) [administration of a flu shot held to be a "routine" medical procedure to which Louisiana's informed consent statute did not apply]; *Daniels v. State*, 532 ASo. 2d 218 (La. App. 1988) [treating a closed wrist fracture found to be a routine medical procedure to which Louisiana's informed consent statute did not apply].

[22]*Matthis v. Mastromonaco,* 160 N.J. 26, 733 A.2d 456 (N.J. 1999).

[23]*Halley v. Birbiglia*, 390 Mass. 540, 458 N.E.2d 240 (1982).

[24]*Stovall v Harms*, 214 Kan. 835, 522 P.2d 353 (1974); *Llera v. Wisner*, 171 Mont. 254, 557 P.2d 805 (1976); *Johnson v. Whitehurst*, 652 S.W.2d 441 (Tex. App. 1983).

[25]*Harnish v. Children's Hospital Medical Center*, 387 Mass. 152, 439 N.E.2d 240 (1982).

physician.[26] Depending upon the jurisdiction, a hospital or clinic may be able to escape liability for failing to obtain the patient/client's informed consent before performing a procedure or conducting a course of treatment prescribed by the patient/client's physician.[27] However, in some jurisdictions it is possible to impose *respondeat superior* liability on the hospital at which the patient/client received medical treatment without her or his informed consent, if it can be shown that the physician who breached the duty to obtain informed consent was a hospital employee. Under certain circumstances, if the employee is the agent for a hospital, both the employee and the hospital may be held responsible.[28]

C. Who should consent?

1. The duty to obtain consent is owed to the patient/client. However, if the patient/client is a minor or under a disability, the patient/client may not be legally competent to give consent. In such cases, the lactation consultant should obtain the consent from the patient/client's parent or guardian. Moreover, in breastfeeding cases, who is the patient/client: the mother alone or the mother and the baby? Although there is no existing case law, because breastfeeding has physical ramifications for both mother and baby, it appears that both have "patient/client" status.

D. Who can give consent for an infant?

1. *The general rule* in the United States is that competent adults are capable of giving valid consent. Prior to the age of majority, which usually is designated by state statute, an individual is considered incapable of consenting to medical

[26]*Beard v. Brunswick Hospital Center,* 632 N.Y.S.2d 805 (App. Div. 2d Dept, 1995)[a physician who assisted a surgeon, but who was not the primary surgeon, found not liable]; *Foflygen v. Zemel,* 420 Pa. Super. 18, 615 A.2d 1380 (Pa. 1993) [a physician taking a patient's medical history in conjunction with the patient's admission to the hospital for medical treatment, and a nurse assisting the treating physician during the procedure held not liable]; *Barnes v. Gorman,* 605 So. 2d 805 (Miss. 1992) [consent obtained by a licensed practical nurse may not be adequate], but see, *Perez v. Park Madison Professional Lab* (lst Dept., 1995) 212 App. Div. 2d 271, 630 N.Y.S.2d 37, *partial summary judgment granted, cause dismd.* (N.Y. App. Div. lst Dept) 1995 N.Y. App. Div. LEXIS 7844 *and app. dismd. without op.* 87 N.Y.2d 896, 640 N.Y.S.2d 880, 663 N.E.2d 922; (*Sangiulo v. Leventhal,* 132 Misc2d 680, 505 N.Y.S.2d 507 (1986) [a "substitute physician" administering part of a course of treatment started by a physician for whom he was covering found not liable].

[27]*Davis v. Hoffman, M.D.,* 972 F. Supp 308, 1997 WL 416261 (ED Pa., 1997) [hospital not responsible for independent contractor's failure to obtain patient's informed consent]; *Geise v. Stice,* 567 N.W.2d 156, 252 Neb. 913 (Neb 1997) [hospital had no duty to obtain informed consent since physician was not an employee of the hospital]; *Gross v. Oklahoma Blood Institute,* 856 P.2d 998 (Okla. App. 1990), *but see, Keel v. St. Elizabeth Medical Center,* 842 S.W.2d 860 (Ky. 1990).

[28]*Koegan v. Holy Family Hospital,* 95 Wash.2d 306, 622 P.2d 1246 (1980); *Shenefield v. Greenwich Hospital Ass'n,* 10 Conn. App 239, 522 A.2d 829 (1987) [Physician as agent for hospital.]. *But see* the following cases holding hospitals not liable for the failures of staff physicians to obtain informed consent: *Harnish v. Children's Hospital Medical Center,* 387 Mass. 152, 439 N.E.2d 240 (1982); *Roberson v. Menorah Medical Center,* 588 S.W.2d 134 (Mo. App. 1979); *Cross v. Trapp,* 294 S.E.2d 446 (W. Va. 1982).

care or treatment. Thus, it is necessary to obtain the consent of an infant's parent or guardian to consent on the infant's behalf.[29] A parent with legal custodial rights over a child has the authority to consent to medical care and treatment for that child. So, if parents are divorced or legally separated (that is, a separation agreement has been signed), the parent granted legal authority for the care, custody, and control of the child has the right to consent to treatment, to the exclusion of the other parent.

2. *If the parent herself is a minor*, the legal waters are muddied and her ability to consent to treatment for her child is less clear. Best practice would suggest that the lactation consultant receive the consent of the other parent (if that parent is not a minor) or from the minor's parents (grandparents) or guardian, unless the minor parent is considered to be "emancipated" or a "mature minor."

3. *Emancipation* has been defined as "the relinquishment by the parent of control and authority over the minor child, conferring on him (child) the right to his earnings and terminating the parents' legal duty to support the child."[30] Emancipation generally occurs when a minor lives away from her parents, supports herself, and conducts her own affairs. Some states have statutes defining particular circumstances that qualify a child as emancipated.[31] Other states, to avoid encouraging runaways, require that this relationship be consensual between the child and the parent. In the absence of such a statute, the following have been considered to confer emancipated or "mature minor"[32] status on a minor:
   a. Military duty.[33]
   b. Marriage.[34]
   c. Living apart from the child's family independently of their support and services.[35]

Emancipated minors are granted the same legal status as if already at the age of full majority. They are able to provide consent for their own medical care, and so may be able to consent to such care for their children as well. However, if

---

[29]In some jurisdictions, children over a certain age may consent to particular treatments for themselves, such as for infectious disease, family planning, out-patient substance abuse rehabilitation, and out-patient mental health treatment.

[30]*Wallace v. Cox*, 136 Tenn. 69, 188 S.W. 611, 612 (1916).

[31]E.g., see §16.1-331, *et seq.*, 3, Code of Virginia, which provides that a petition for emancipation may be filed for any minor who has reached her sixteenth birthday.

[32]*Belcher v. Charleston Area Medical Center*, 188 W. Va. 105, 422 S.E.2d 827 (1992).

[33]*Swenson v. Swenson*, 241 Mo. App. 21, 227 S.W.2d 103 (1950).

[34]*Bach v. Long Island Jewish Hospital*, 49 Misc.2d 207, 267 N.Y.S.2d 289 (1966).

[35]*Smith v Seigly*, 72 Wash.2d 16, 431 P.2d 719 (1967).

the emancipated minor parent has a spouse of legal age, the lactation consultant is advised to obtain the consent of the spouse for the treatment of the infant whenever possible.

4. *If the lactation consultant believes the parent is incompetent*, another problem situation is presented, even if there has been no adjudication of the parent's incompetence. Under such circumstances, it would be best if the lactation consultant could also obtain the permission of the parent's parent (grandparent) or guardian under such conditions.

III. Legal Actions Most Likely to Be Brought Against Lactation Consultants

A. Battery
   1. Description. A technical battery occurs if a lactation consultant, in the course of treatment, exceeds the consent given by the patient/client. Although no wrongful intent is present, and in fact there may be a sincere purpose to aid the patient/client, recovery is permitted (unless there is an emergency).
   2. Elements (in most states).
      a. Duty. To respect the rights of other persons to freedom from harmful or offensive bodily contact.
      b. Intent. Lactation consultant intended to physically contact patient/client.
      c. Breach. Unconsented to, harmful, or offensive contact with one person by another.
      d. Causation. Causation of injury presumed (no need to prove causation).
      e. Damage. Injury (to dignity) presumed (no need to prove injury only amount of damages).
   3. Example: Giving a bottle to a baby whose parents have directed to be exclusively breastfed and be given no water and no artificial nipples (Figure 11-1).
B. Professional negligence (includes failure to diagnose, initiate treatment, refer or consult, provide attention or care, or obtain informed consent).
   1. Description. Professional negligence occurs if, when rendering professional services, a lactation consultant fails to exercise that degree of skill and learning commonly applied under all the circumstances in the community by the average prudent reputable member of the profession, with the result of injury, loss, or damage to the recipient of those services or to those entitled to rely upon them.
   2. Elements (in most states).
      a. Duty. To use due care on rendering lactation consultant services.

Parents' Names
Parents' Address
Date

By Certified Mail, Return Receipt Requested to:

HOSPITAL and address
PEDIATRICIAN and address
OBSTETRICIAN and address

Dear _____:

I expect to deliver my child at _____ (name of hospital) on or about
_____ (date). I have made the decision to breastfeed. Consequently, I direct that
my newborn not be given water, formula, artificial nipples (this prohibition includes teats,
dummies, and pacifiers) or any substance other than human milk except in the case of an
unavoidable medical emergency under circumstances where consent cannot be given either by
myself or my husband, _____ (husband's full name).

In the event of an emergency for which supplemental feeding is necessary, donor human
milk should be used. Given this advance notice, there is virtually no reason why my newborn
should be given formula, because there is time for donor milk to be ordered.

IN LETTER TO OBSTETRICIAN, ADD THE FOLLOWING: Please place this
letter in my medical record.

IN LETTER TO PEDIATRICIAN, ADD THE FOLLOWING: Please place a copy
of this letter in a place where you will see it immediately upon my baby's birth.

IN LETTER TO HOSPITAL, ADD THE FOLLOWING: I am enclosing two copies
of this letter. Please place a copy of this letter in both my medical record and that of my
infant.

Sincerely,

Figure 11-1   Sample letter from parent informing hospital that infant is to be breast-fed only and directing not to give water and not to use nipples

b. Breach. Act/omission causing lactation consultant to fail to provide standard of care as would be provided by the "ordinary, prudent lactation consultant" under similar circumstances.

c. Causation. Direct or proximate causation of injury must be proved.

d. Damage. Dollar value of resulting injury.

3. Example: *Baptist Memorial Hospital-Union County v. Johnson,* No 98-IA-00175-SCT (Supreme Court of Mississippi 2000).

Parents brought negligence action against hospital for mistakenly placing their infant with an unidentified female patient/client, who breastfed the infant. In response to parents' request for discovery of the patient/client's identity and medical records, the hospital affirmatively asserted the patient/client's medical privilege of confidentiality. At the hearing on parents' motion to compel, the judge compelled discovery of the patient/client's identity and production of her medical records, and also entered an interlocutory order asking for determination of scope of statutory patient/client–physician privilege. On appeal, the state Supreme Court held that: (1) the hospital must disclose identity of unidentified female patient/client, who mistakenly breastfed the infant, as a witness to hospital's alleged conduct, and (2) the hospital must produce woman's medical records to trial court for in-camera review, subject to issuance of protective orders to determine whether infant's health was at risk.

C. Infliction of emotional distress.

1. Description. A cause of action by which a person may seek redress for extreme emotional disturbance suffered due to the negligent or intentional conduct of another person.

2. Elements (these vary widely by state, but read much like the following).

a. Duty. To refrain from harmful conduct.

b. Breach. The lactation consultant acts in an extreme and outrageous manner exceeding the bounds of decency observed by a civilized society.

c. Intent. The lactation consultant knew or should have known his or her conduct was likely to cause plaintiff severe emotional distress.

d. Causation. The lactation consultant's actions directly and proximately caused the plaintiff to suffer actual and severe emotional distress (more than embarrassment or humiliation).

e. Damage. Dollar value of resulting severe mental distress.

3. Examples:

a. *Garcia v. Lawrence Hospital,* 5 A.D.3d 227, 773 N.Y.S.2d 59 (N.Y. 2004). Background: Patient/client alleged that the hospital was negligent in bringing her day-old baby to her for breastfeeding after she was medically sedated, and then leaving them alone together unsupervised after the sedative allegedly caused patient/client to fall asleep on top of the baby, smothering him to death. The Court granted patient/client's motion for leave to amend her complaint so as to include a cause of action for emotional injury, and hospital appealed.

Held: Patient/client had cause of action for emotional injury under a zone-of-danger theory. Although patient/client did not observe the injury she inflicted and was never personally exposed to unreasonable risk of bodily harm, there was an especial likelihood of genuine and serious mental distress, arising from special circumstances.

b. *Volm v. Legacy Health Systems, Inc.*, 237 F. Supp. 2d 1166 (United States District Court, D. Oregon 2002).

Background: Lactation consultant sued health care corporation that had banned consultant from all of its hospital and clinic facilities, and individual doctors and nurses, alleging violations of Sherman Act, Oregon Antitrust Act, Oregon Unlawful Trade Practices Act, and intentional interference with economic relations, implied duty of good faith, defamation, and intentional infliction of emotional distress under Oregon law.

Held: Individual physicians' and nurses' alleged conduct in setting out to destroy lactation consultant's career, intentionally encouraging hostile atmosphere toward her, holding repeated meetings in which they blamed consultant for all problems existing at hospital, and leveling allegations of wrongdoing without providing her information necessary to address them, was not sufficient to constitute extraordinary transgression of bounds of socially tolerable conduct, as required to support claim for intentional infliction of emotional distress under Oregon law.

c. *Champagne v. Mid-Maine Medical Center*, 711 A.2d 842 (Me. 1998).

Background: Mother, whose newborn baby was mistakenly breastfed by another patient/client in maternity ward at hospital, sued hospital and nursing student to recover for invasion of privacy, battery, intentional infliction of emotional distress, and negligent infliction of emotional distress. The Court found that the mother was not the indirect victim of alleged negligence, as would warrant recovery for negligent infliction of emotional distress, because the mother did not witness baby being nursed by the wrong mother and did not learn about the incident until about one hour afterward. More specifically, the Court held that: (1) the mother was not direct or indirect victim of alleged negligence, as required to recover for negligent infliction of emotional distress; (2) the mother failed to show causal relationship between the alleged failure to inform her of the risks created by the breastfeeding incident and the emotional distress she claimed; and (3) the incident could not be characterized as so extreme and outrageous as to exceed all possible bounds of decency in a civilized community.

D. Breach of warranty.

    1. Description. A statement of fact respecting the quality or outcome or particular result to be achieved by agreeing to receive certain medical services or treatments, made by the medical service provider to induce the patient/client to consent to those services and/or treatments, and relied upon by the patient/client, which is not fulfilled.

    2. Elements (in most states).

        a. Duty. Lactation consultant promises or "guarantees" a result.

        b. Intent. No proof of fraudulent intent or untruthfulness required.

        c. Breach. Promised result not achieved.

        d. Causation. Direct or proximate causation of damage must be proved.

        e. Damage. Dollar value of the difference between the value of the expected outcome and the value of the actual outcome.

    3. Example:

        a. *Hawkins v. McGee*, 84 N.H. 114, 146 A. 641 (1929).

        Background: Hawkins consulted McGee, a surgeon, about scar tissue that was the result of a severe burn caused by contact with an electric wire, which Hawkins had experienced about nine years prior. The surgeon suggested the removal of the scar tissue from the palm of the plaintiff's right hand and replacing it with a skin graft taken from the plaintiff's chest. Evidence was produced to the effect that before the operation was performed, Hawkins and his father went to McGee's office and that McGee, in answer to the question, "How long will the boy be in the hospital?" replied, "Three or four days, not over four; then the boy can go home and it will be just a few days when he will go back to work with a good hand." The court found these statements could only be construed as expression of opinions or predictions, even though those estimates were exceeded. However, the evidence also showed that Dr. McGee said before the operation was decided upon, "I will guarantee to make the hand a hundred per cent perfect hand or a hundred per cent good hand." Because after the operation, the boy grew hair from the palm of his hand, the result was not "perfect" or "one hundred per cent good." Thus, the court found that Dr. McGee had given a warranty as to the result of the operation, which had been breached and that damages were due McGee.

E. Unauthorized practice of medicine (governed by state statute).

    1. Description. Practicing medicine (as defined in the medical practice act for the applicable state) without the authority (license) to do so. State legislatures, through licensing laws, determine what is and what is not the practice of medicine. However, legislatures often authorize several professions to practice in the same, related, or similar fields and as a result these have overlapping

practice areas. Thus, courts as well as legislatures have recognized that licensing laws do not create monopolies for professions[36] and not all practice areas are exclusive.[37]

2. Overlapping scopes of practice. Because scopes of practices overlap, the only question is whether a lactation consultant's activity is within the scope of lactation consultant practice. If not, and it is reserved by statutes to one of the other professions, then it is illegal for a lactation consultant to engage in it. However, if it is within the scope of lactation consultant practice, then it is not important whether other professions are also permitted to engage in it. Many lactation consultants are also registered nurses or other licensed health care professionals whose statutorily defined scope(s) of practice includes some lactation care activities. For those lactation consultants who do not hold some other health care license, the territory is not so well defined.[38]

3. The *practice of medicine* generally includes the right to diagnose, treat, and prescribe. Some states' statutes specifically exempt any person licensed or certified to practice a limited field of the healing arts under their laws, if those persons strictly confine themselves to the field for which they are licensed or certified and do not assume the title of physician or surgeon, and don't hold themselves out as qualified to prescribe drugs in any form or to perform operative surgery.[39]

4. *Diagnosis* is generally defined as the identification of a disease based on its signs and symptoms. However, many states make a distinction between a "medical diagnosis" (the identification of a disease and its cause based on its

---

[36]*In Re Carpenter's Estate*, 196 Mich. 561 (1917).

[37]*Sermchief v. Gonzales*, 600 S.W.2d 683 (Mo. 1983) ("Having found that the nurses' acts were authorized by [the Nursing Practice Act], it follows that such acts do not constitute the unlawful practice of medicine); *Professional Health Care Ina v. Bigsby*, 709 P.2d 86, 88 (Colo., 1985) (acts of a nurse practitioner who was indirectly supervised by a physician and who followed protocols and directions that he established "constituted only the practice of professional nursing and could not be construed to be the illegal practice of medicine"); *Prentice Medical Corporation v. Todd*, 145 Ill. App.3d 692, 495 N.E.2d 1044, 99 Ill. Dec. 303 (Ill. App. Ct., 1986) (nurse who practiced under standing orders and cooperated with supervising physicians was not holding herself out as practicing medicine, despite the fact that she referred to her "practice"); *Hofson v. Orenreich*, 168 A.D.2d 243, 562 N.Y.S. 2d 479 (New York 1990) (New York Supreme Court determined that a jury was justified in finding that a nurse who incised and drained three acne cysts and removed blackheads was not engaged in the unauthorized practice of medicine).

[38]But see, International Lactation Consultant Association, "Standards of Practice for International Board Certified Lactation Consultants " available at www.ilco.org (go to "Resources" and then to "Downloadable Publications") and International Board of Lactation Consultant Examiners, "IBLCE Competency Statements" and "Clinical Competencies for IBLCE Practice" available at www.iblce.org (click on "Professional Standards").

[39]Examples include § 71-1.103(16) of the Laws of Nebraska and Delaware Code title 24 §1702(9).

signs and symptoms) and a "nursing diagnosis"[40] (the identification of and discrimination between physical and psychosocial signs and symptoms essential to the effective execution and management of the nursing regimen). The main difference between these two types of diagnosis is that the nursing diagnosis does not make a final conclusion about the identity and cause of the underlying disease.

F. Failure to report child neglect/abuse (governed by state statute).

1. Reporting is required. In most states, health care workers and others who have direct contact with children and who observe something suggesting possible child abuse or neglect[41] are required by law to report suspected child abuse. This report should be made according to the state laws where the lactation consultant works, as described by the procedures in place in the lactation consultant's work setting. The justification for overriding patient/client confidentiality is the state's interest in protecting public health.

Although similar in many respects, the specific requirements of each state's laws are different and the avenues for reporting may be different for lactation consultants in different settings, but the lactation consultant's responsibility remains the same. The protocol for notifying authorities should be taken seriously and followed to the letter. In the event no protocols are in position for the lactation consultant's workplace, the lactation consultant should first follow through by reporting to the patient/client's physician and local authorities and secondly follow-up by taking steps to make certain a protocol is put in place (an employment lawyer can help with this). When reporting, the lactation consultant should take care to report objective observations (and not accuse) to protect against any risk of becoming the subject of a retaliatory charge of slander.

2. Failure to report. If a lactation consultant fails to report as required, he or she risks being charged with a criminal offense, which most states classify as a misdemeanor.

---

[40]See the discussion of Pennsylvania law in Kabla, Edward J., "Legalities of a telephone nurse triage system," *Physicians News Digest* at http://www.physiciansnews.com/law/998kabala.html. ("Registered nurses are typically authorized to make assessment of persons who are ill and to render a nursing diagnosis in their capacity as professionals. For example: a nursing diagnosis could be a situation where the nurse finds or fails to find symptoms described by a physician in standing orders or protocols. The nurse would identify symptoms for the purpose of administering courses of treatment prescribed by the physicians. The nursing regimen is always designed to function in consultation with the treating physicians or other physicians licensed in Pennsylvania. Further, the protocols used in the nursing regimen would have been developed by a facility or practice with specific knowledge as to the capability of their nursing staff and the accessibility of the physicians.")

[41]Some states, like Iowa, recognize that what most people think of as an issue of "neglect" is covered under the child abuse category of "denial of Critical Care."

3. Sources of information. Lactation consultants can check for their state's rules by going to the Administration for Children and Families Web site (http://www.acf.dhhs.gov), which maintains a database of state requirements (http://nccanch.acf.hhs.gov/pubs/reslist/rl_dsp.cfm?rs_id=5&trate_chno= 11-11172). If the lactation consultant's state is not listed or the suspected abuse took place outside the state in which the lactation consultant practices, it is possible to use the Childhelp USA National Abuse Hotline at 800-4-A-CHILD (800-422-4453) to obtain relevant information.

4. Immunity from suit if reported in good faith. Most states' statutes confer immunity from civil and criminal suits that might otherwise be brought against those persons who report in good faith.

5. False reports may result in a criminal conviction. Persons who knowingly or intentionally make a false report may be convicted for a felony.

G. Violation of unfair and deceptive trade practice statutes (State "Little FTC Acts" or Consumer Protection Acts).

1. Description. U.S. Supreme Court decisions in the 1970s established that the "learned professions" have commercial aspects and thus are not immune from antitrust law.[42] These were the forerunners of state court rulings holding that the entrepreneurial and business aspects of medical practices are not exempt from little Federal Trade Commission (FTC) act coverage.

State or "little" FTC acts prohibit "unfair" or "deceptive" acts or practices in trade or commerce. Such causes of action are often included in health care suits because they are attractive to plaintiffs, because many of these acts provide for the recovery of attorney fees and/or treble damages for willful, knowing, or bad faith violations.

Note that brochures and Web sites that provide medically related information to consumers often also serve as advertisements. In addition, Web sites may provide hyperlinks to other sites. These raise a host of concerns, including the ethical and legal obligations governing marketing and referral practices, which could become the subject of little FTC act litigation.

2. Examples:
a. *Quimby v. Fine*, 724 P.2d 403 (Wash. App. 1986).
Although lack of informed consent claims are usually brought as negligence cases, some states have recognized this conduct as a violation of consumer protection law(s), particularly if the lack of informed consent "relates to the entrepreneurial aspects of the medical practice"—such as setting prices, billing, collection, obtaining, retaining and dismissing patient/clients."

---

[42]*Goldfarb v. Virginia State Bar*, 421 U.S. 773 (1975); *National Society of Professional Engineers v. U.S.*, 435 U.S. 679 (1978).

      b. *Mother & Unborn Baby Care of N. Texas v. State*, 749 S.W.2d 533, 542 (Tex. App. 1988).
      A facility run by anti-abortion activists was found to have violated the Texas act in holding itself out, in the yellow pages and statements to prospective patient/clients, as an abortion clinic and then trying to dissuade patient/clients from having abortions.

      c. *Gadsden v. Newman*, 807 F. Supp. 1412, 1420 (C.D. Ill. 1992).
      Plaintiff alleged that defendant psychiatrist had an undisclosed contract with a hospital that included financial incentives, self-referrals, and increased billings.

      d. *Vassolo v. Baxter Healthcare Corp.*, 696 N.E.2d 909, 915, 924 (Mass. 1998).
      Patient/client brought a claim against a breast implant manufacturer based on that manufacturer's failure to disclose the risks of its product to her health care provider.

H. Copyright infringement.

  1. Description. Unauthorized use of copyrighted material. See 17 U.S.C. §501.

  2. Examples:
    a. Making multiple copies of a journal article for numerous hospital staff members to keep at their desks for reference.
    b. Using a cartoon as a slide to illustrate a presentation for which you receive an honorarium, without first obtaining the artist's permission to use it in this way.

I. Trademark/service mark/certification mark infringement.

  1. Description. The unauthorized use or colorable imitation of the mark already appropriated by another, on goods or services of a similar class. See U.S.C. § 1051, et seq.

  2. Trademarks apply to products. A trademark is any word, phrase, slogan, or design that is used by a person or entity to define its products and distinguish them from the products of others.[43]

  3. Service marks apply to services. A service mark is the same as a trademark except that it identifies and distinguishes services rather than products.[44] Registered service marks that are familiar to lactation consultants include the words "International Board of Lactation Consultant Examiners" and the IBLCE's logo.

---

[43]15 U.S.C. § 1127.

[44]*Reddy Communications v. Environmental Action Foundation*, 477 F. Supp. 936, 943 (D.D.C. 1979) ("Service marks might just as well have been called trade marks for services, leaving conventional trade marks to be referred to as trade marks for goods, but the different term is probably more convenient . . . .").

4. Certification marks apply to products or services. Unlike trademarks or service marks, a certification mark[45] is not used by the owner of the mark, but instead is applied by other persons to their goods or services, with authorization from the owner of the mark.

The certifier/owner of a certification mark does not produce the goods or perform the services in connection with which the mark is used, and thus does not control their nature or quality. What the certifier/owner of the certification mark does control is the use of the mark by others on their goods or in connection with their services, by taking steps to ensure that the mark is applied only to goods or services that contain the requisite characteristics or meet the specified requirement which the certifier/owner has established or adopted for the certification.

Examples of registered certification marks which are familiar to lactation consultants include the acronyms "IBCLC" and "RLC" and the phrases "International Board Certified Lactation Consultant" and "Registered Lactation Consultant."

5. Infringement. Identical standards govern the determination whether a trademark, service mark, or certification mark has been infringed.
   a. Example of infringement: A lactation consultant uses the initials "IBCLC" when he/she did not successfully complete the IBLCE examination, or when the lactation consultant has failed to timely recertify as required to maintain certification. This would be actionable as an infringement of the "IBCLC" service mark, which is owned and has been registered by the IBLCE.

IV. Use of Technology in Lactation Consultant Practice

The rapid proliferation of technological advances continues to influence the way lactation consultants practice. Devices and concepts such as fax machines, video conferencing, e-mail, the Internet, cellular phones, networked computer systems, and satellite communications shape the way lactation consultants serve their patients/clients on a day-to-day basis. Certainly, technology provides the means for more efficient and effective methods of performing services, but these same advances that can improve a lactation consultant's ability to serve patients/clients may also present a number of ethical pitfalls for the unwary practitioner.

   A. Facsimiles (faxes) and client confidentiality.

   Due to an inadvertent mistake, you or another staff member fax a medical record to the wrong number. The mistake is discovered later that afternoon after you

---

[45]A certification mark "certifies" the "regional or other origin, material, mode of manufacture, quality, accuracy, or other characteristics of such person's goods or services or that the work or labor on the goods or services was performed by members of a union or other organization." 15 U.S.C. § 1127.

receive a call from the pediatrician inquiring as to why he/she has not yet received the faxed records. After making a check, you discover that the fax was sent to the wrong location.

1. Has there been a breach of patient/client confidentiality?

2. What steps should or must you take to recover the medical record from the recipient and to minimize any potential damage to your patient's/client's confidentiality?

3. Have you personally committed an ethical violation?

4. Would the issues be any different if the message had been sent to the wrong e-mail address instead?

B. Cell phones and client confidentiality.

Has it occurred to you that it is possible to breach a patient's/client's confidentiality when you talk to her? This can happen if someone is eavesdropping on your conversation. In today's world, the biggest eavesdropping risk is posed not by the person lurking behind the door, but by a third party's interception of a cellular phone call. Does a lactation consultant who uses a cell phone to discuss patient/client matters breach the ethical obligation to protect patient/client confidentiality?[46] The answer to this question is anything but clear. In fact, the most accurate answer is, "It depends . . ."

There is no lactation consultant ethical history upon which to base an answer.[47] However, parallel cases in other professional contexts indicate that whether a lactation consultant's use of a cellular phone to communicate with patients/clients violates a duty of confidentiality "depends" on whether there is a reasonable expectation of privacy in the communication. Determining if a lactation consultant has a "reasonable expectation of privacy" in a means of communication is a two-part inquiry: First, one must determine whether the lactation consultant has a subjective belief that the chosen mode of communication is private. Second, the belief must be objectively reasonable.[48]

There are two types of cellular phones—analog and digital—and the expected level of privacy in using each differs greatly. Conversations over analog phones are particularly susceptible to interception by third parties. On the other hand, digital cellular phones work differently and are believed to provide greater security against interception, although they are not completely secure. Moreover, even if a

---

[46]Tenet #6, Code of Ethics for International Board Certified Lactation Consultants (Dec. 1, 2004).

[47]The IBLCE's Ethics and Discipline Committee issues opinions only on matters that have come before it and this issue has not been the subject of a complaint.

[48]See generally, *Katz v. United States*, 389 U.S. 347 (1967).

digital phone is used, this does not necessarily mean the call is being transmitted through a digital network.[49]

As cellular phones become more prevalent and demands on lactation consultants have become even greater, it is likely that increasing numbers of lactation consultants will use cell phones to communicate with their patients/clients. Keep in mind the following guidelines before using cell phones to discuss any confidential information.

- Tell your patients/clients when you are using a cell phone, informing them of the risks of doing this, and providing them with the opportunity to consent.

- Consider purchasing a scrambler to prevent the interception of analog cellular calls if you frequently use a cell phone to call clients about confidential matters.

- Check to see whether ILCA or the IBLCE have issued ethical guidelines or whether the legislatures or courts in your jurisdiction have rules on the reasonable expectation of privacy in cellular communications.

- Check with your professional liability insurance carrier to see if it has issued any guidance on the issue.

- When possible, use a land-line phone instead of a cell phone.

- If in doubt, do not use a cell phone.

C. Internet issues.

Problems can arise when a lactation consultant participates on electronic bulletin boards, on-line services, or the Internet. Because this is a new area, the ethical rules and codes of conduct that apply to this part of a lactation consultant's practice are just beginning to evolve, so there is little precedent.[50] These tips may help lactation consultants avoid liability for false or misleading advertising, breach of confidentiality, malpractice, or the unauthorized practice of medicine as a result of their electronic communications. Because Internet sources are not equally reliable, it is imperative that you consider the purpose for which this information could possibly be used before presenting it to a patient/client who might rely on its accuracy.

1. False or misleading advertising.
   a. Web sites. Potentially, a Web site is a great place to advertise to a wide audience. Just remember that all of the rules that generally govern advertising will apply to anything you say to a prospective client or patient

---

[49]The caller and/or recipient may be in an area in which digital service is not available, or may be on an analog or cordless phone. Most digital phones have the capability of switching back and forth from digital to analog to address this very problem.

[50]States whose laws expressly address advertising through "electronic media" obviously govern advertising on the Internet.

(by way of any medium, not just electronic communications). Generally, advertising must be truthful and incapable of misleading even an unsophisticated consumer.

  b. E-mail solicitations. No parameters for these have been established, but there seems no reason to distinguish them from other mass mailing strategies or targeted mailing tactics.

2. Breach of confidentiality.

  a. Interception. E-mail and Internet communications may be subject to interception. Therefore, be especially wary of posting any message that could be construed to be "medical advice." The safest course is to limit on-line communication to information, rather than advice, whether partaking in bulletin board discourse or drafting a Web page. To minimize the possibility that your comments will be construed as medical advice, you may decide to place a written disclaimer either at the beginning or the end of the text.[51]

  b. Consider including a message at the top or bottom of your transmissions similar to the following:

  CONFIDENTIALITY NOTE: This message is intended only for the addressee(s) named herein and may contain information that is privileged and confidential under applicable law. For these reasons, this communication may not be forwarded without the prior written permission of the original author. If the reader of this message is not the intended recipient, you are hereby notified that the disclosure, copying, distribution, or the taking of any action in reliance on the contents of this information is strictly prohibited. If you have received this communication in error, please call collect to _____, so we may arrange to retrieve this transmission at no cost to you.

  Although taking this precaution "can't hurt," it is not always a successful measure. Around the country, courts have issued varying opinions regarding the effectiveness of such a message in diminishing the sender's liability for the unintended recipient's use of information received by mistake.

  c. Misdirection and mis-forwarding. Unlike faxes or "snail mail" (i.e., regular mail services), the risk of misdirected e-mail is higher simply because one can write and send an e-mail much faster than a letter or fax. Also, the intended recipient(s) can easily forward these communications to other unintended recipients. A partial solution to this dilemma is the "envelope within the envelope" approach. When using this approach, the entire text of

---

[51]You should be aware, however, that some legal commentators claim that a disclaimer alone may not be sufficient, and could even be used as evidence that you "knew" the communication was not confidential.

the primary e-mail is the message on unintended transmission. Then the sensitive information is added to the e-mail as an attachment.

3. Professional negligence.
   a. E-mail. Another area of concern is the lack of professionalism that often accompanies the use of e-mail. Often people who routinely review outgoing first-class mail for spelling, grammar, style, and neatness fail to review their outgoing e-mail. It is also important to be careful with the substance of what your e-mail says. Many courts have held that employees have no protectable privacy interest in the messages sent from their employer's computers, so it is reasonable to expect that your messages may be reviewed. In addition, e-mails result in a written record that is not completely deleted from the computer or network when you hit the "delete" button. The rule is simple: unless you are comfortable having the text of your e-mail discussed on television news, don't send it over the office system.
   b. Bulletin boards. A bulletin board is no different from a cocktail party in cyberspace. You can end up in a lactation consultant–patient or lactation consultant–client relationship without intending that to happen. Whether you have formed such a relationship with someone will be judged by the client's or patient's subjective belief that such a relationship exists, provided that belief is "reasonable." There are two basic issues: (1) maintaining competence; and (2) avoiding negligence. Think about whether you would feel comfortable giving advice to someone who called you and gave you the same skeletal facts that you receive in an e-mail. If you would want more information, be sure to ask for it or don't answer the questions. If you need to do research, do it, or don't answer the questions. If you need to observe the mother and/or baby, say so, and don't answer the question. The safest tactic is to completely avoid giving "medical advice" (refer to the information given under "confidentiality" above).

4. Unauthorized practice of medicine.
   Do you know where the client is located? You may not. If your message includes a "diagnosis" or a "prescription," or any other action that falls within the state's or country's unauthorized practice statutes (as judged on the basis of 20/20 hindsight) and if the client or patient lives in a state or country that vigorously enforces those laws, you could be risking a legal action.

D. Summary

Although technology continues to change rapidly and almost on a day-to-day basis, the ethical and legal principles that govern lactation consultant practice do not. Competence, confidentiality, diligence, honesty, and service to the public are time-honored concepts that form the foundation for all lactation consultant practice.

V. ABCs of Testifying at a Deposition or a Trial

Lactation consultants occasionally become involved in litigation. If you are deposed, or called to testify at trial, try to determine whether you are being called as a "fact witness" or an "expert witness." The roles are equally important, but slightly different.

A. Fact witness.

    1. *Fact witnesses* have first-hand knowledge relevant to the issues in a case. They may testify either because they have volunteered to do so, or because they have been required to testify by receiving a subpoena. If you have worked directly with the mother–infant dyad, you would be qualified to serve as a fact witness. Generally, fact witnesses must limit their testimony to facts, although courts may "let in" opinions that may be helpful to the understanding of their testimony. Although fact witnesses are not usually paid for their testimony, they are entitled to reimbursement of their expenses. (Note: A fact witness in one case may serve as an expert witness in another. Many fact witnesses have the background necessary to qualify as an expert witness.)

B. Expert witness.

    1. *Expert witnesses* testify because they have knowledge, skill, experience, training, education, or expertise that may prove helpful to the judge or jury. Expert witnesses testify voluntarily, by agreement with one of the attorneys or the court. It is best if lactation consultants testifying as expert witnesses have no prior contact with the litigants. The role of an expert witness is to review the records, know the case, suggest authorities and references that support the case, etc. Meetings may be held with counsel to discuss areas of contemplated interrogation and possible cross-examination, the selection of exhibits, and the documents to be introduced. Expert witnesses are entitled to payment for their services and to reimbursement of their expenses.

C. Behavior during a deposition or trial.

The following pointers are general instructions on how to act at a deposition or at trial. You should not follow them strictly but use them as guidelines. Everyone makes mistakes; however, these suggestions should help you to avoid them.

    1. Tell the truth.

        a. Honesty. In a lawsuit, as in all other matters, honesty is the best policy. A lie may lose the case. Telling the truth, however, demands more than refraining from telling a deliberate falsehood. Telling the truth requires that witnesses testify accurately about what they know. Everything you say must be right, must be correct, and must be accurate.

        b. Accuracy. To be accurate in all of your answers, you must be aware that technically you cannot possibly tell what you did yesterday, what you saw yesterday, or what you heard yesterday. Technically, you can only testify to what you remember seeing yesterday, or what you remember hearing yesterday.

    c. Memory. Memory is not perfect. You can talk about what you saw, what you heard, and what you did as though memory were a fact, but you are really only remembering something. That's an important distinction. Obviously, there are some things that you do remember, and you remember them clearly, and there can be no question about them. But there will probably be many things about which you may be uncertain. In those instances, you can testify only about what you remember.

2. Do not act as the advocate for any party.

    a. Objectivity. Attempt to testify objectively and only about that which you are knowledgeable. This means that you will probably answer all kinds of questions about breastfeeding. But in most cases, do not give an opinion about any other topic because it will only serve to diminish your credibility. For example: in a custody case, do you really *know* what is truly best for the child? Unless you are brought in as a character witness for a friend (and not as a lactation consultant), avoid taking either parent's "side."

3. Educate "your" attorney.

    a. Give the attorney your resumé so he or she has the information necessary to qualify you as an expert witness. Be prepared to explain your credentials, which include formal schooling, employment history, and other relevant experience. If you are an IBCLC, give the attorney an IBLCE brochure and make sure the lawyer understands the credential. If it is foreseeable that your testimony may be countered by that of some other health care provider, explain in detail how little formal background in breastfeeding most professional schools include in their curriculums. If you are an IBCLC, encourage the attorney to call your regional IBLCE office and talk with someone there about the reasons for a voluntary certification instead of a licensing procedure and the constitutional requirement for the alternative pathway. Then do the same yourself, so you can testify without hesitation.

4. Ask "your" attorney about the mother and baby.

    a. Background of the case. In many cases, you will not know the people involved, so it is important that you ask about the background of the breastfeeding dyad. For example, does the mother smoke? (If so, then be prepared to rebut any inferences to the effect that her breast milk may be harmful to the child.) Does she drink alcohol? Take illegal drugs? Have there been any neglect or abuse issues? You know what's relevant. The attorney may not.

5. Supply "your" attorney with copies of the references upon which you will rely.

    a. Authoritative reference materials. If you know the issues that are likely to arise during the trial, assemble copies of the most authoritative articles and other materials, and give them to the attorney to read. If possible, supply the attorney with a set of questions to ask.

6. Be prepared to quote a fee.
   a. Determining your fee. The attorney will not be able to tell you precisely how long the proceeding will take. So be prepared to quote an hourly fee and to charge 50% of that hourly fee for your travel time. This charge for testifying should be about the same as what you would charge for a private consultation of the same duration.

7. Ask "your" attorney whether you should bring some general references when you testify.
   a. What to bring to a deposition or trial. Many times no references are necessary. But if having up-to-date respected lactation texts with you (such as, Lawrence & Lawrence, 2005; or Riordan, 2005) will calm your nerves, why not bring it along? Impress on the attorney that these are generally accepted as authoritative, in case they could be used in cross-examination.

8. Be prepared for the hypothetical question.
   a. Practice scenarios. Either or both attorneys may describe a scenario based on a particular set of facts and then ask you to comment on it in your "professional opinion" or to a "reasonable degree of medical certainty." Be aware that usually when this is done, they are asking about some issue very central to the case. Think about the question before answering. Then answer with clarity. If additional facts would make a difference, say so at the outset. Unless the question is very simple, avoid giving a bare "yes" or "no" answer.

9. Educate the people in the courtroom or conference room.
   a. Generally, you truly will be *the expert* on human lactation at any trial or deposition. The only time that there will be someone there who knows as much as you will be if another lactation consultant is called to testify. Try to remember how little the average person in our society knows about breastfeeding, and to remember to define basic terms and to simply describe basic processes (for example, the effect of stimulation on milk supply). When possible, give a little background about the basic anthropological/social/medical theory on which your answer is built. Judges and lawyers are usually fascinated by a lactation consultant's testimony.

10. Admit what you do not know.
    a. The issue here is credibility. You cannot be effective if you aren't prepared to do this.

11. Straighten out confusion.
    a. Be clear. If you should get confused about a point, straighten the matter out while the testimony is being taken. (If you are testifying at a deposition, you will have an opportunity to read the testimony over afterward and make

any necessary corrections, but it is better to make your corrections at the time of the deposition.)

b. Example: The opposing lawyer may ask you a question that will remind you of a related question that you have already answered. The new questions may remind you that when you answered the previous one, you made a mistake. The worst tactic you can take is to try and cover up that mistake by giving an incorrect answer. The best one is to correct the mistake then and there. Say, "Excuse me, I just remembered back there you asked me X and I said Y. I was mistaken. I should have told you Z."

12. Do not guess.

a. Give exacting answers. If you do not remember something, admit it. If you do not know something, admit it. You may feel embarrassed. You may feel that you should be able to remember, but unless you really do remember, do not guess. There is nothing to gain by guessing. If you guess rightly, you have not won anything. If you guess wrongly, you have lost. You cannot answer accurately if you do not hear or understand a question, so be sure that you hear and understand it before you try to answer it. If you do not hear it, ask to have it repeated. If you do not understand it, ask to have it explained. It is important that you understand each question the way the lawyer intends you to understand it. It is likewise important that anyone else who hears or reads your answer understand it the same way that you mean it. Language is inexact. It is much easier to be general than to be specific. Therefore, the defense attorney's questions may have several meanings, and your answers may have several meanings. Be sure that your answers are as exact as they can be, so that no one can misinterpret them.

13. Give accurate estimates.

a. Beware of questions involving time and dates. If you estimate, make sure everyone understands you are estimating.

14. Clarify multiple meanings.

a. You will be asked questions that have multiple meanings. You will have to answer them, so if there is any doubt in your mind as to whether a question has a multiple meaning, either make certain that you understand what the questioner means (by asking the person, "Do you mean . . .?) or make sure that what you mean is clear.

15. Answer background questions as accurately as possible.

a. Sample questions. The lawyers will ask you for background information, which may include your address, when and where you were born, where you went to school, and what jobs you have held. You may not be able to remember all such details, but do your best. If you do not remember, tell the questioner that you do not remember or give the best possible estimate. For example, "Well I'm not sure, but it seems to me it may have been back in 1995 or 1996, about then."

16. Beware of a question that assumes fact.
    a. Questions. You might be asked a question that assumes a fact that isn't true or assumes that you have testified to a fact when you haven't. You have heard the question, "Have you stopped beating your wife yet?" You can't answer it "yes" or "no" without getting into trouble because it assumes a fact that isn't true.
    b. Example: The questioner may ask, "When did you first see the baby?" and you may say, "Well, I'm not sure, on July 5th or 6th. I don't know, somewhere along in there." Later, the questioner will ask, "Well, after you first saw the baby on July 5th, what happened?" This assumes you had testified that you first saw the baby on July 5th when in fact you testified you weren't sure when you first saw the baby.

17. Watch out for alternative questions.
    a. Questions. Another type of question to watch out for is a question in the alternative, such as, "Well, now is it one or is it two? Which is it?" The danger is that you may know it isn't one, but you don't know whether it's two or not. Your mind may reason that if it's either one or two, and you know it's not one, then it must be two. So you answer, "It's two," when you really don't know.
    b. Other options. The fallacy in this type reasoning is easy to see. "What color is this pencil? Is it red or is it blue?" You can see that it is obviously yellow. So just because questions are put to you in the alternative doesn't mean that the given alternatives are the only options.

18. Be alert to paraphrases.
    a. Assert your truth and accuracy. The opposing attorney may paraphrase part of your testimony. He or she may say, "Well, now, let me see if I understand you correctly; if I am mistaken, you correct me," and then state what he or she understands your testimony to be. If any word or phrase is used that you do not think is correct, call it to the lawyer's attention.
    b. Qualify statements. Even if the paraphrase sounds perfect to you, do not give an unqualified "yes," because you may be saying "yes" to something you really didn't intend. A word may have meaning that you didn't understand or appreciate. The most you can say is, "Yes, that sounds about right," or "As far as I can tell, that's about right." Otherwise, you are putting your stamp of approval on every word used. You are letting the attorney tell your story in his or her words, some of which you may not have fully understood.

19. Take your time.
    a. Consider. Give the question as much thought as is required to understand it and form your answer and then give the answer. Never give a snap answer, but bear in mind that if you take a long time to answer each question, a judge or jury may think you are making up your answers.

b. Interruptions. Do not answer while the questioner is still talking. If you are talking and the questioner is talking, you should stop. One of two things is happening:

   i. You are answering before the questioner has finished the question, in which case you should stop because you can't listen to the question and understand it while you are answering it.

   ii. The questioner is interrupting you before you have completed your answer to the first question, in which case you should also stop.

   iii. Solution. When you stop because you have been interrupted, pay no attention to the question being asked, but keep in mind what you were about to reply to the first question. If you don't, chances are you will forget it. When the questioner finishes talking, say, "Pardon me, I wasn't through with my last answer." Then give your answer and ask, "Now, what was your next question?"

20. Answer concisely.

   a. Be crisp. Answer a question concisely and then wait for the next question. Say what you need to say, but don't go off on a tangent.

   b. Be non-confrontational. You should not be evasive or argumentative, nor should you nit-pick about language. Don't hide anything. You are only to answer the question, but the question must be asked before you give an answer.

   c. Don't invite more questions. You can do this by the inflection of your voice. For example, the questioner may ask what shoe you put on first this morning. If you answer, "Well, I don't remember what shoe I put on first this morning," with the accent on "this" you are inviting another question.

21. Be aware of your speech and appearance.

   a. Professional presentation. Talk loudly enough so everybody can hear you. Don't chew gum, and keep your hands away from your mouth so that you can speak distinctly. Speak up so the court reporter can hear you. You must give an audible "yes" or "no" answer. The reporter cannot hear nods of the head. "Yes" or "no" sounds better than "uh-huh" or "yeah." Dress conservatively and be well-groomed.

22. Look the judge (and jurors, if any) in the eye.

   a. Direct eye contact. Do not be afraid to look the judge and jurors in the eye while you are testifying. They are naturally sympathetic to a witness and want to hear what is said. Look at them most of the time and speak frankly and openly as you would to a friend or neighbor.

23. Do not look at "your" lawyer for approval.

   a. Don't look for help when you are on the stand. You are on your own. If you look at your lawyer when a question is asked on cross-examination or look for approval after answering a question, the jury will notice and will get a bad impression. You must appear confident about your answers.

24. Do not be defensive.
    a. Don't argue with opposing lawyers. They have a right to question you, so do not become defensive or give evasive answers. You are not there to convince them how right you are or how wrong the other side is. You are not there to do anything except answer every question as accurately, courteously, and concisely as possible.

25. Do not lose your temper.
    a. You should appear to be completely disinterested. Do not lose your temper no matter how hard you are pressed.

26. Be courteous.
    a. One of the best ways to make a good impression is to be courteous. Be sure to address the judge as "Your Honor."

27. Avoid joking.
    a. Be serious. Avoid wisecracking and joking. A lawsuit is a serious matter.
    b. No levity. This is particularly true for depositions. Remarks that everyone present understands as a joke can haunt you after they are transcribed. This is because voice inflection, facial expression, and body posture made the difference. But there it is in black and white, "I could have killed her!"

28. Do not be reluctant to admit to discussions with "your" attorney.
    a. Be honest. If you are asked whether you have talked to "your" lawyer, admit it freely. The same thing goes for when you are asked if you are being paid. It can be particularly effective to say, "Although I am earning a fee, that will not affect the content of my answers."

29. Beware of the "have you told me everything" question.
    a. Summary. At the end, the other attorney may decide to ask you, "Have you told me everything about how this happened?" Chances are you have not because you were not asked questions about everything. You are only required to answer what was asked, so don't "close the book" by saying, "Yes, this is all." Instead, what you can say is, "Yes, as far as I can recall, that's about all. I have tried to answer your questions. I believe I have answered them the best I know how."

30. Relax.
    a. If you relax and talk as you would to neighbors or friends, you will make a more credible impression.

31. Reread these instructions the night before you testify so that you will have them firmly in your mind. They will help you.

VI. Reported Cases of Interest to Lactation Consultants

A. *Baptist Memorial Hospital v. Johnson*, 754 So. 2d 165 (Miss. 2000).
B. *Champagne v. Mid-Maine Medical Center*, 711 A.2d 842 (Me. 1998).
C. *Garcia v. Lawrence Hospital*, 5 A.D.3d 227, 773 N.Y.S.2d 59 (N.Y. 2004).
D. *Volm v. Legacy Health Systems, Inc.*, 237 F. Supp. 2d 1166 (U.S.D.C. D. Or. 2002).

References

Lawrence RA, Lawrence RM. *Breastfeeding: A Guide for the Medical Profession*. 6th ed. St. Louis: C.V. Mosby; 2005.
Riordan J. *Breastfeeding and Human Lactation*. 3rd ed. Sudbury, MA: Jones and Bartlett Publishers; 2005.

Suggested Readings

Bornmann, P. *Legal Considerations and the Lactation Consultant—USA*. Unit 3. The Lactation Consultant Series. Wayne, NJ: Avery Publishing Group; 1986.
Harper FW, James F Jr, Gray OS. *The Law of Torts*. 2nd ed. Boston: Little Brown; 1986.
International Board of Lactation Consultant Examiners. *Code of Ethics for International Board Certified Lactation Consultants* (December 1, 2004). Available at: http://www.iblce.org/ethics.htm. Accessed December 1, 2006.
International Board of Lactation Consultant Examiners. *Clinical Competencies for IBCLC Practice*. Available at: http://www.iblce.org/cllinical%20competencies.htm. Accessed December 1, 2006.
International Board of Lactation Consultant Examiners. *IBLCE Competency Statements*. Available at: http://www.iblce.org/competency%20statements.htm. Accessed December 1, 2006.
International Lactation Consultant Association. *Standards of Practice for International Board Certified Lactation Consultants*. Raleigh, NC: ILCA; 2005. Available at: http://www.ilca.org/pubs/Standards-of-Practice-web.pdf.
Jameton, A. *Nursing Practice: The Ethical Issues*. Upper Saddle River, NY: Prentice Hall; 1984.
Pallash B. Advocating effectively. *Association Management* (subscription service), Vol. 54, No. 1, January 2002.
Smith LJ. Expert witness: what to emphasize. *Journal of Human Lactation*. 1991; 7:3:141.
Suhler A., Bornmann P, Scott J. The lactation consultant as expert witness. *Journal of Human Lactation*. 1991;7(3):129–140.
Taraska J. *Legal Guide for Physicians*. New York: Matthew Bender (as supplemented through 2002).
Wold C. *Managing Your Medical Practice*. New York: Matthew Bender (as supplemented through 2002).

Science of Lactation

Breastfeeding Anatomy and Physiology

MATERNAL BREASTFEEDING ANATOMY

Marsha Walker, RN, IBCLC
Revised by Judith Lauwers, BA, IBCLC

> *"Such a spectacular survival strategy that we call ourselves after
> the mammary gland, mammals . . . animals that suckle their young."*
>
> **Gabrielle Palmer, author and activist**

OBJECTIVES

- Describe the process of breast development.
- Locate the major structures of the breast.
- Describe the function of the major structures of the breast.
- Discuss variations of breast anatomical structures.

Introduction

The medical term for the breast is the *mammary gland*, which comes from the Latin word *mamma*, meaning "the breast." The mammary gland is the only organ that is not fully developed at birth. It undergoes four major phases of growth and development: in utero, during the first two years of life, at puberty, and finally during pregnancy and lactation. The breast provides both nutrition and nurturing. The lactation consultant requires a basic understanding of the structures and functions of the breast in order to provide proper breastfeeding management guidelines and to troubleshoot problems.

I. Breast Development

A. Embryo and neonate.

    1. Week 3 to 4: Breast development begins with a primitive milk streak running bilaterally from the axilla to the groin.

2. Week 4 to 5: Milk streak becomes mammary milk ridge, or milk line. Paired breasts develop from this line of glandular tissue.

3. Week 7 to 8: Thickening and inward growth into the chest wall continue.

4. Week 12 to 16: Specialized cells differentiate into smooth muscle of nipple and areola.

5. Week 15 to 25: Epithelial strips are formed, which represent future secretory alveoli.
   a. Lactiferous ducts and their branches form and open into a shallow epithelial depression known as the mammary pit.
   b. The mammary pit becomes elevated, forming the nipple and areola.
   c. An inverted nipple results when the pit fails to elevate.

6. After 32 weeks: A lumen (canal) forms in each part of the branching system.

7. Near term: 15 to 25 mammary ducts form the fetal mammary gland.

8. Neonate.
   a. Galactorrhea (also called *witch's milk*): Secretion of colostral-like fluid from neonate mammary tissue due to influence of maternal hormones (Collaborative Group, 2002; Lee et al., 2003; Madlon-Kay, 1986).
   b. Recommend not to express neonatal colostrum, as this may lead to mastitis in the newborn (Collaborative Group, 2002; Lee et al., 2003).

B. Puberty and pregnancy.

   1. Breasts keep pace with general physical growth.

   2. Growth of the breast parenchyma begins and continues.
      a. Ductal and lobular growth.
      b. Surrounding fat pad.
      c. Ducts, lobes, and alveoli.

   3. Onset of menses at 10 to 12 years of age.
      a. Primary and secondary ducts grow and divide.
      b. Terminal end buds form, which later become alveoli (small sacs where milk is secreted) in the mature female breast.
      c. Proliferation and active growth of ductal tissue takes place during each menstrual cycle.

   4. Complete development of mammary function occurs with pregnancy.

C. Anomalies in breast development.

   1. Some illnesses, chemotherapy, therapeutic radiation to the chest, chest surgery, or injuries to the chest might affect development.

   2. Programmed apoptosis (cell death) has been suggested as one theory for lower breast cancer rates in women who have breastfed (Collaborative Group, 2002; Lee et al., 2003; Tryggvadottir et al., 2001).

II. General Anatomy of a Mature Breast

A. Exterior breast (Figure 12-1).

1. Located in the superficial fascia (fibrous tissue beneath the skin) between the second rib and the sixth intercostal space.

2. Tail of Spence: Mammary glandular tissue that projects into the axillary region.
   a. Distinguished from supernumerary tissue because it connects to the duct system.
   b. Potential area of milk pooling and mastitis (Lee et al., 2003).

3. Skin surface contains the nipple, areola, and Montgomery glands.

4. Size is not related to functional capacity.
   a. Fat composition of the breast gives it its size and shape.
   b. Size may indicate milk storage potential (Daly & Hartmann, 1995; Hartmann et al., 1996).

B. Nipple areola complex.

1. Nipple.
   a. Conical elevation located in the center of the areola.
   b. Nipple features.
      i. Four to 18 milk duct openings (Ramsay et al., 2005a; Walker, 2006).
      ii. Smooth muscle fibers that function as a closure mechanism to keep milk from continuously leaking.

Figure 12-1   Quadrants of the left breast and axillary Tail of Spence

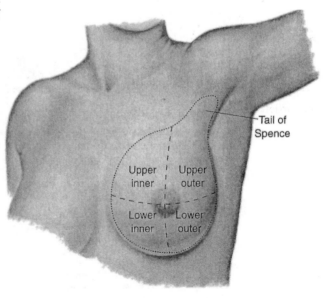

    iii. Sebaceous and apocrine sweat glands.
    iv. Dense innervation of sensory nerve endings.
  c. Nipple erection
    i. Muscle arrangement of longitudinal inner muscles and outer circular and radial muscles make the nipple erect when contracted.
    ii. Erect nipple is supported by fibro-elastic tissue and local venostasis that decrease the surface area of the areola.
    iii. Erect nipple changes shape to a smaller, firmer, and more prominent projection to aid the infant in latching.
2. Areola.
  a. Circular, dark pigmented area that surrounds the nipple.
    i. Elastic like the nipple.
    ii. Constructed of smooth muscle and collagenous, elastic, connective tissue fibers in radial and circular arrangement.
    iii. Usually darkens and enlarges during pregnancy.
  b. Montgomery's tubercles are located around the areola.
    i. Contain ductular openings of sebaceous and lactiferous glands and sweat glands.
    ii. Enlarge during pregnancy and resemble small, raised pimples.
    iii. Secrete small amount of milk and a substance that lubricates and protects the nipples.
C. Parenchyma: Functional parts of the breast (Figures 12-2 and 12-3).

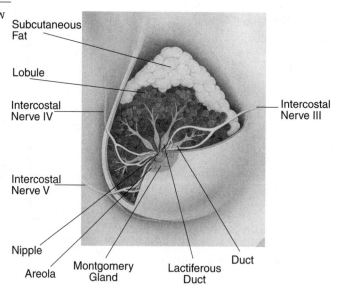

Figure 12-2 Frontal view of lactating breast. *Source:* Riordan, J. *Breastfeeding and Human Lactation, 3rd ed.* Jones and Bartlett Publishers, 2005.

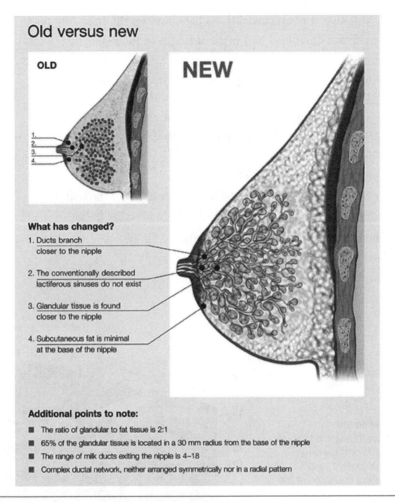

Figure 12-3   Side view of lactating breast
Source: Medela A.G., Switzerland, 2006. Printed with permission.

1. Alveolar gland with branching, ductular alveoli.
   a. Composed of secretory acinar units in which the ducts terminate.
   b. Clusters of alveoli cells are each surrounded by a contractile unit of myoepithelial cells that are responsible for ejecting milk into the ductules.

2. An intricate system of ductules from 15 to 25 lobes converge into larger lactiferous ducts behind the nipple.
   a. Ducts widen temporarily in response to milk ejection reflex and narrow when the feed is complete (Ramsay et al., 2004, 2005b).

b. Milk that is not removed flows backward up the collecting ducts.

3. Lactiferous ducts lead to 4 to 18 openings in the nipple.

D. Stroma: Supporting tissues of the breast.

1. Connective tissue, fat tissue, blood vessels, nerves, and lymphatics.

2. Cooper's ligaments.
   a. Suspensory ligaments running vertically through the breast.
   b. Attach the deep layer of subcutaneous tissue to the dermis layer of the skin.

E. Vascular anatomy (Figure 12-4).

1. The breast is highly vascular.

2. Internal mammary artery supplies 60% of blood to the breast.

3. Lateral thoracic artery supplies 30% of blood to the breast.

4 Blood vessels within the breast enlarge.

5. Surges of estrogen stimulate growth of the ducts.

6. Surges of progesterone cause glandular tissue to expand.

Key
1. Subclavian artery
2. Superior thoracic artery
3. Internal thoracic artery
4. Major pectoralis muscle
5. Perforating branches of the internal mammary artery
6. Arterial plexus around areola
7. Intercoastal arteries
8. Pectoral branches of the lateral thoracic artery
9. Circumflex scapular artery
10. Minor pectoralis muscle
11. Subscapular artery
12. Lateral thoracic artery
13. Pectoral branch of the thoracoacromial artery
14. Axillary artery
15. Deltoid branch of the thoracoacromial artery

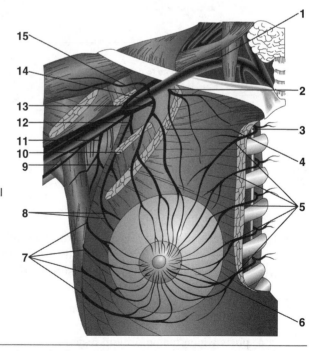

Figure 12-4   Arterial blood supply to the breast

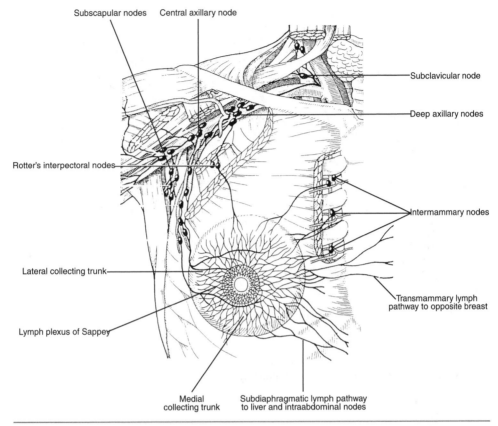

Figure 12-5   Lymph drainage of breast

F. Lymphatic system (Figure 12-5).

   1. Collects excess fluids from tissue spaces, bacteria, and cast-off cell parts.

   2. Drains mainly to the axillary lymph nodes.

G. Innervation (Figure 12-6).

   1. Breast innervation derives mainly from branches of the fourth, fifth, and sixth intercostal nerves.

   2. Nerve supply to the innermost areas of the breast is sparse.

   3. The fourth intercostal nerve penetrates the posterior aspect of the breast.

      a. It supplies the greatest amount of sensation to the areola, at the four o'clock position on the left breast and at the eight o'clock position on the right breast.

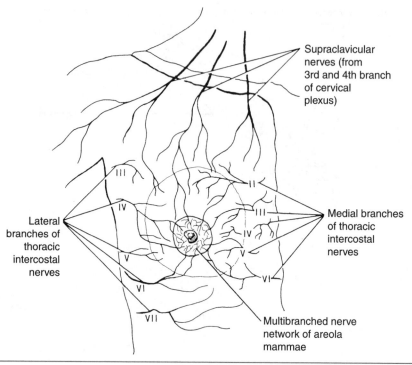

Figure 12-6   Innervation of the mammary gland

b. It becomes more superficial as it reaches the areola, where it divides into five branches.

c. The lowermost branch penetrates the areola at the five o'clock position on the left breast and at the seven o'clock position on the right breast.

d. Trauma to this nerve might result in some loss of sensation in the breast.

e. If the lowermost branch is severed, loss of sensation to the nipple and areola might result.

f. Aberrant sensory or autonomic nerve distributions in the nipple/areola complex.

   i. Could affect the milk ejection reflex and secretion of prolactin and oxytocin.

   ii. Trauma or severing of this nerve could result from breast augmentation or reduction surgery.

III. Variations

A. Breasts vary in size, shape, color, and placement on the chest wall (Table 12-1; Figure 12-7).

Table 12-1   Breast Types Classified by Physical Characteristics

Type 1	Round breasts, normal lower, medial, and lateral quadrants
Type 2	Hypoplasia of the lower medial quadrant
Type 3	Hypoplasia of the lower medial and lateral quadrants
Type 4	Severe constrictions, minimal breast base

   1. Nonpregnant woman: Mature breast weighs about 200 g.

   2. Pregnancy near term: Breast weighs between 400 and 600 g.

   3. Lactation: Breast can weigh 600 to 800 g.

B. Breast malformations

   1. Hypermastia: Presence of an accessory mammary gland.

     a. Accessory or supernumerary nipple develops along the milk line (Velanovich, 1995).

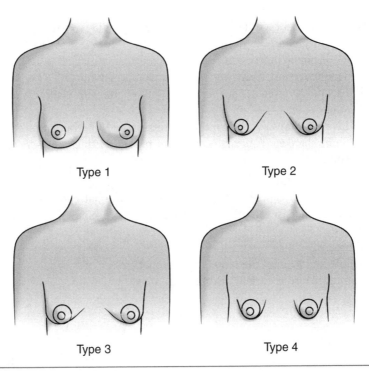

Type 1   Type 2

Type 3   Type 4

Figure 12-7   Breast classifications

b. Often prominent during pregnancy and lactation.

c. May be associated with renal or other organ-system anomalies (Berman & Davis, 1994).

d. Accessory glandular tissue can lactate and undergo malignant changes (Collaborative Group, 2002; Lee et al., 2003).

2. Hyperthelia: Nipple without accompanying mammary tissue.

3. Hypertrophy: Abnormally large breast.

4. Hypomastia: Abnormally small breast.

5. Hyperplasia: Overdevelopment of the breast—hyperplastic breast.

6. Hypoplasia: Underdevelopment of the breast—hypoplastic breast.

   a. Tubular or tuberous shape because of lack of glandular tissue.

   b. Breasts may have large areolas.

   c. Breasts are frequently asymmetric and widely spaced.

   d. May present increased risk for insufficient milk (Huggins, Petok, & Mireles, 2000).

   e. Unilateral hypoplasia of the breast combined with hypoplasia of the thorax, and pectoral muscles—Poland's syndrome.

C. Nipple variations (Figure 12-8).

1. Tied, retracted, or inverted nipple.

   a. Poor nipple protractility is common in primigravid women.

   b. Protractility improves during pregnancy.

   c. Types of nipple protrusion.

      i. True inversion: Stays inverted with compression, rare.

      ii. Pseudo-inverted: Appears inverted but everts with compression and/or stimulation.

      iii. Everted: Stays everted with compression and/or stimulation.

      iv. Short shanked: Appears everted but retracts with compression and/or stimulation.

2. Other nipple variations.

   a. Bulbous: Large nipple that may be difficult for a baby to grasp.

   b. Dimpled: Increases the risk for maceration as the nipple lies enveloped by the areola.

   c. Bifurcated.

   d. Double and/or multiple nipples close together.

   e. Skin tag: More prevalent during pregnancy.

Type of Nipple	Before Stimulation	After Stimulation

Common nipple

The majority of mothers have what is referred to as a *common nipple*. It protrudes slightly when at rest and becomes erect and more graspable when stimulated. A baby has no trouble finding and grasping this nipple in order to pull in a large amount of breast tissue and stretch it to the roof of his mouth.

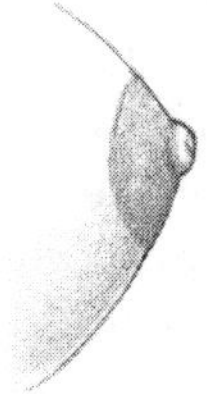

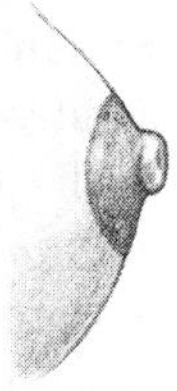

Flat and/or Short Shanked nipple

The *flat nipple* may be soft and pliable and have the ability to ridge, therefore it molds to the infants mouth without problem. The *flat nipple may have a short shank* that makes it less easy to ridge and for the baby to find and grasp. In response to stimulation, this nipple may remain unchanged or may retract with compression. Slight movement inward or outward may be present, but not enough to aid the baby in finding and initially grasping the breast on center. This nipple may benefit from the use of a syringe to increase protractility.

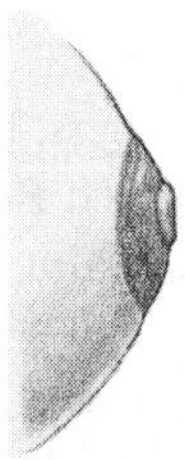

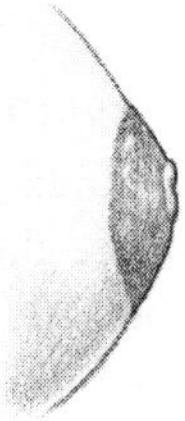

Pseudo-inverted nipple

An *pseudo-inverted* nipple may appear inverted but becomes erect after compression and/or stimulation. This nipple needs no correction and presents no problems with grasp ability.

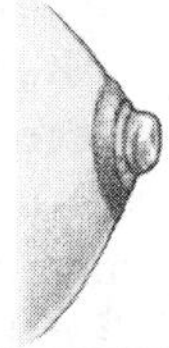

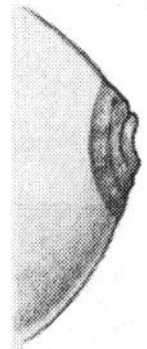

Retracted nipple

The *retracted nipple* is the most common type of inverted nipple. Initially, this nipple appears to be graspable. However, on stimulation, it retracts, making attachment difficult. This nipple responds well to techniques that increase nipple protrusion.

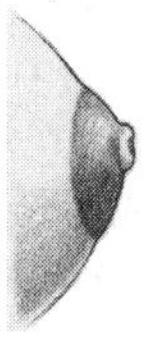

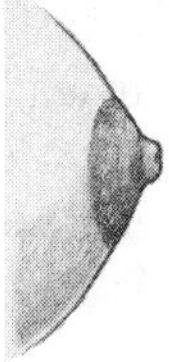

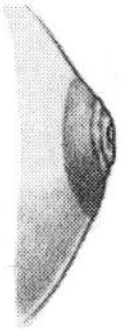

Inverted nipple

The truly *inverted nipple* is retracted both at rest and when stimulated. Such a nipple is very uncommon and more difficult for the baby to grasp. All techniques used to enhance protractility of breast tissue can be used to improve attachment. Even if the nipple remains retracted, the baby should be able to latch on if the mother helps form her breast into the mouth

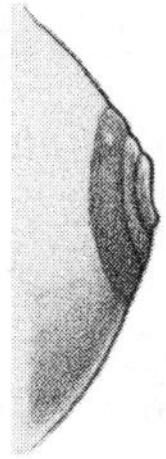

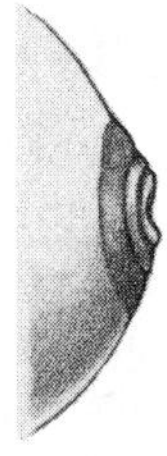

Figure 12-8   Five basic types of nipples
Source: Reprinted from Lauwers, J., and Swisher, A. *Counseling the Nursing Mother,* 4th ed. Jones and Bartlett Publishers, 2005.

References

Berman MA, Davis GD. Lactation from axillary breast tissue in the absence of a supernumerary nipple: a case report. *J Reprod Med*. 1994;39:657–659.

Collaborative Group on Hormonal Factors in Breast Cancer. Breast cancer and breastfeeding: collaborative reanalysis of individual data from 47 epidemiological studies in 30 countries. *Lancet*. 2002;360:187–195.

Daly S, Hartmann P. Infant demand and milk supply. Part 1: infant demand and milk production in lactating women. *J Hum Lact*. 1995;11:21–26.

Hartmann, PE, Owens RA, Cox DB, Kent JC. Breast development and control of milk synthesis. *Food Nutr Bull*. 1996;17:292–304.

Huggins KE, Petok ES, Mireles O. Markers of lactation insufficiency: a study of 34 mothers. In: *Current Issues in Clinical Lactation-2000*. Sudbury, MA: Jones and Bartlett Publishers; 2000:25–35.

Lee SY, Kim MT, Kim SW, et al. Effect of lifetime lactation on breast cancer risk: a Korean women's cohort study. *Int J Cancer*. 2003;105:390–393.

Madlon-Kay DJ. "Witch's milk." Galactorrhea in the newborn. *Am J Dis Child*. 1986; 140:250–253.

Ramsay DT, Kent JC, Owens RA, Hartmann PE. Ultrasound imaging of milk ejection in the breast of lactating women. *Pediatrics*. 2004;113:361–367.

Ramsay JC, Kent C, Hartmann RA, Hartmann PE. Anatomy of the lactating human breast redefined with ultrasound imaging. *J Anat*. 2005a;206:525.

Ramsay DT, Mitoulas LR, Kent JC, et al. The use of ultrasound to characterize milk ejection in women using an electric breast pump. *J Hum Lact*. 2005b;21:421–428.

Tryggvadottir L, Tulinius H, Eyfjord JE, Sigurvinsson T. Breastfeeding and reduced risk of breast cancer in an Icelandic cohort study. *Am J Epidemiol*. 2001;154:37–42.

Velanovich, V. Ectopic breast tissue, supernumerary breasts, and supernumerary nipples. *South Med J*. 1995;88:903–906.

Walker M. *Breastfeeding Management for the Clinician: Using the Evidence*. Sudbury, MA: Jones and Bartlett Publishers; 2006:55, 388.

Suggested Readings

Auerbach KG, Riordan J. *Clinical Lactation: A Visual Guide*. Sudbury, MA: Jones and Bartlett Publishers; 2000.

Harris JR, Lippman ME, Morrow M, Osborne CK. *Diseases of the Breast*. Baltimore: Lippincott Williams & Wilkins; 2004.

Imaginis. The Breast Cancer Resource. Breast anatomy and physiology. Available at: http://imaginis.com/breasthealth/breast_anatomy.asp. Accessed December 6, 2006.

Lauwers J, Swisher A. *Counseling the Nursing Mother*. 3rd ed. Sudbury, MA: Jones and Bartlett Publishers; 2005.

Lawrence RA, Lawrence RM. *Breastfeeding: A Guide for the Medical Profession.* 6th ed. St. Louis: C.V. Mosby; 2005.

Love S, Lindsey K. *Dr. Susan Love's Breast Book.* 3rd ed. HarperCollins Publishers; 2000.

Mohrbacher N, Stock J. *The Breastfeeding Answer Book.* Schaumburg, IL: La Leche League International; 2003.

Osborne MP. Breast development and anatomy. In: Harris JR, Henderson IC, Hellman S, Kinney DW, eds. *Diseases of the Breast.* Philadelphia: Lippincott; 2000:1–14.

Poland's syndrome. Available at: http://www.polands-syndrome.com. Accessed December 6, 2006.

Riordan J. *Breastfeeding and Human Lactation.* 3rd ed. Sudbury, MA: Jones and Bartlett Publishers; 2005.

Wilson-Clay B, Hoover K. *The Breastfeeding Atlas.* 3rd ed. Austin, TX: LactNews Press; 2005.

INFANT ANATOMY FOR FEEDING

Chele Marmet, BS, MA, IBCLC, and Ellen Shell, IBCLC
Revised by Catherine Watson Genna, BS, IBCLC

OBJECTIVES

- Locate and name the cranial and facial bones, sutures, fontanelles, joints, and processes on the infant skull.
- Name and describe the function of the 12 pairs of cranial nerves.
- Locate, name, and describe the function and innervation of the muscles of sucking and mastication.
- Locate, name, and describe the anatomical features of an infant's oral cavity.
- Identify the reference, atypical, and abnormal infant head and oral cavity.
- Describe the oral reflexes related to breastfeeding.

Introduction

Familiarity with the anatomy of the infant's head is important as a basis for understanding the normal structure and function in infant feeding and as a reference for analyzing and correcting breastfeeding problems. The term *reference* is a nonjudgmental word used to describe the most common example or the greatest representation of a population, rather than the term *norm*. It is necessary to distinguish between normal variations and abnormalities, both of which might cause breastfeeding problems. The lactation consultant requires an understanding of how infant anatomical structures and motions combine to enable the infant to take in nutrients and to determine his or her requisite milk supply. The newborn's oral anatomy is his or her primary way of relating to the world (Bosma, 1972; Brazelton, 1995). Appropriate and accurate anatomical assessment aids the lactation consultant in assessing the normal and recognizing deviations that are amenable to intervention.

I. Basic Concepts of Anatomic Terminology

A. Reference: used to describe the most common example.

B. Body planes: used to facilitate uniformity in descriptions of the body (Kapit & Elson, 1993).

1. Midsagittal: the plane vertically dividing the body through the midline into right and left halves.

2. Sagittal: any plane that is parallel to the midsagittal line, vertically dividing the body into right and left portions.

3. Coronal (frontal): any plane dividing the body into anterior (ventral) and posterior (dorsal) portions at right angles to the sagittal plane.

4. Transverse: (cross, horizontal) plane dividing the body into superior (upper) and inferior (lower) portions.

C. Directions and positions.

1. Cranial, superior, rostral: uppermost or above.

2. Caudal, inferior: lowermost or below.

3. Anterior, ventral: toward the front.

4. Posterior, dorsal: toward the back.

5. Medial: nearest the midline of the body.

6. Lateral: toward the side.

7. Proximal: nearest the point of attachment or origin.

8. Distal: away from the point of attachment or origin.

9. Superficial: on the surface.

10. Deep: below the surface.

11. Ipsilateral: pertaining to the same side.

12. Contralateral: pertaining to the opposite side.

D. Terms.

1. Alveolus: a small cavity.

2. Process: projections on a bone.

3. Meatus: a passage or channel, especially the external opening of a canal.

4. Foramen: a natural hole or passage, especially one into or through a bone.

5. Lumen: the cavity or channel within a tube or tubular organ.

6. Sinus: a recess, cavity, or hollow space.

7. Protuberance: a projecting part, process, or swelling.

8. Fontanel: junctions of cranial bones covered by a tough membrane.

E. Body positions.

    1. Prone: lying face down.

    2. Supine: lying on the back.

F. Joints.

    1. Temporomandibular: opens and closes the jaw; lateral displacement of the mandible.

    2. Suture: a joint that does not move; the bones are united by a thin layer of fibrous tissue.

G. Muscles.

    1. Involuntary: contraction not induced by will.

    2. Voluntary: movement using willful control.

    3. Visceral/smooth: found in digestive and respiratory tracts.

    4. Cardiac/striated: involuntary muscle possessing a striated appearance of voluntary muscles but with less separation between the cells, allowing coordination of contraction.

    5. Skeletal/striated: voluntary, striated; gross and fine motor movements.

    6. Origin: the more fixed attachment of a muscle that serves as a basis of action.

    7. Insertion: the movable attachment where the effects of movement are produced.

H. Systems: groups of organs that form the general structural plan of the body.

    1. Skeletal: bones, cartilage, and membranous structures that protect and support the soft parts of the body and that supply levers for movement.

    2. Muscular: facilitates movement.

    3. Cardiovascular: pumps and distributes blood.

    4. Lymphatic: drains tissue spaces, provides for intercellular waste disposal, and carries absorbed fat in the blood.

    5. Nervous: controlling system for cognition, movement, and autonomic functions.

    6. Endocrine: chemical regulator of body functions.

    7. Integument: skin (hair, nails, sebaceous, and sweat glands); insulation, temperature, and water regulation.

    8. Respiratory: brings oxygen to and eliminates carbon dioxide from the blood.

    9. Digestive: converts food into substances that the body can absorb and utilize.

    10. Urinary: forms and eliminates urine and maintains homeostasis.

11. Immune: protection from and reaction to disease and infection.

12. Reproductive: perpetuation of the species.

II. Skeletal System of the Infant's Head, Face, and Neck

A. Bones (Diamond, Scheibel, & Elson, 1991; Grant, 1956).

1. Occipital: forms the back and base of the cranium; contains the foramen magnum through which the spinal cord passes.

2. Frontal: forms the forehead, roof of the nasal cavity, and orbits (bony sockets containing the eyes).

3. Parietal: sides and roof of the cranium.

4. Temporal: sides and base of the cranium; houses the middle and inner ear structures.

5. Ethmoid: between the nasal bones and sphenoid; forms part of the anterior cranial floor, medial walls of the orbits, and part of the nasal septum.

6. Nasal: upper bridge of the nose.

7. Vomer: posterior nasal cavity; forms a portion of the nasal septum.

8. Lacrimal: anterior, medial wall of the orbit.

9. Zygomatic arch: prominence of the cheeks and part of the lateral wall and floor of the orbits.

10. Palatine: posterior nasal cavity between the maxillae and sphenoid.

11. Maxilla: upper jaw.

12. Mandible: lower jaw.

13. Inferior nasal concha: lateral wall of the nasal cavity.

14. Hyoid bone: horseshoe-shaped bone suspended from the styloid process of the temporal bone.

B. Passages.

1. Choanae: posterior nasal apertures, paired passages from the nasal cavity to the nasopharynx. Breastfeeding widens the choanae, unless tongue tie is present (Palmer, 1998).

C. Sutures: found only in the skull.

1. Coronal: line of articulation between the frontal bone and the two parietal bones.

2. Sagittal: line of articulation between the two parietal bones in the midline.

3. Lambdoidal: anterior articulation between the occipital and parietal bones.

D. Fontanels: the membranous intervals between the angles of the cranial bones in infants.

1. Anterior fontanel: a diamond-shaped interval where the frontal angles of the parietal bones meet the two separate halves of the frontal bones.

2. Posterior fontanel: a triangular interval at the union of the lambdoid and sagittal sutures.

3. Sphenoidal fontanel: irregularly shaped interval on either side of the skull.

4. Mastoid fontanel: interval on either side of the skull.

III. Innervation of the Mouth and Suckling Motion (Netter, 2006)

A. Cranial nerves.

1. CN I olfactory: smell.

2. CN II optic: sight.

3. CN III oculomotor: innervates external muscles for several movements of the eye.

4. CN IV trochlear: innervates muscles that move the eye up and down.

5. CN V trigeminal: three branches; muscles of mastication.

6. CN VI abducens: moves the eye up temporarily.

7. CN VII facial: muscles for facial expression.

8. CN VIII vestibulocochlear: hearing and equilibrium.

9. CN IX glossopharyngeal: taste.

10. CN X vagus: larynx, pharynx.

11. CN XI spinal accessory: muscles of the neck and shoulder.

12. CN XII hypoglossal: muscles of the tongue.

B. Cranial nerves related to suckling (Table 13-1).

1. Cranial nerves related to swallowing; 26 muscles and six cranial nerves must coordinate for swallowing (Table 13-2).

Table 13-1 Cranial Nerves Related to Suckling

Structure	Cranial Nerve/Sensory	Cranial Nerve/Motor
Mouth	CN V (shape/texture)	CN VII
Tongue	CNVII, IX (taste)	CN XII
Jaw	CN V (position of TMJ)	CN

Source: Adapted from Wolf LS, Glass RP. *Feeding and Swallowing Disorders in Infancy: Assessment and Management.* Tucson, AZ: Therapy Skill Builders; 1992.

Table 13-2 Cranial Nerves Related to Swallowing

Structure	Cranial Nerve/Sensory	Cranial Nerve/Motor
Palate	CN V, IX	CN V, VII, IX, X
Tongue	CN IX	CN V, VII, XII
Pharynx	CN V, X	CN IX, X
Larynx	CN X	CN IX, X

Source: Adapted from Wolf LS, Glass RP. *Feeding and Swallowing Disorders in Infancy: Assessment and Management.* Tucson, AZ: Therapy Skill Builders; 1992.

IV. Muscles Related to Suckling

A. Muscles used in mastication and suckling (Figure 13-1; Figure 13-2).

   1. Temporalis: raises the mandible; closes the mouth; draws the mandible backward.

   2. Masseter: closes the jaw (Gomes et al., 2006).

   3. Medial pterygoid: raises the mandible; closes the mouth.

   4. Lateral pterygoid: brings the jaw forward.

   5. Buccinator: compresses the cheek and retracts the angle (Gomes et al., 2006).

   6. Orbicularis oris: closes the lips.

   7. Mentalis: elevates center of lower lip (Jacinto-Goncalves et al., 2004).

Figure 13-1   Muscles and nerves used in suckling and swallowing, sagittal section. *Source:* Adapted from M. Biancuzzo, *Breastfeeding the Newborn: Clinical Strategies for Nurses.* St. Louis: Mosby, Inc.

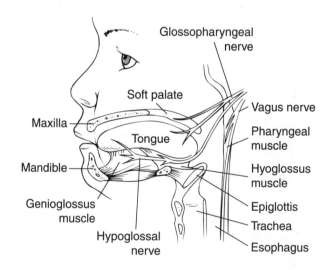

Figure 13-2 Lateral view.
Source: Adapted from
M. Biancuzzo, *Breastfeeding
the Newborn: Clinical
Strategies for Nurses.* St.
Louis: Mosby, Inc.

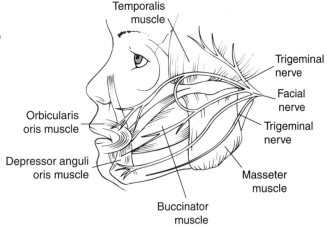

B. Muscles that move the tongue (Takemoto, 2001).

1. Genioglossus: depresses and extends/protrudes tongue forward.

2. Styloglossus: draws the tongue upward and backward.

3. Stylohyoid: draws the hyoid and tongue upward.

4. Digastric: raises the hyoid or opens the mouth.

5. Mylohyoid: elevates the hyoid; supports the mouth floor.

6. Hyoglossus: depresses the tongue.

7. Geniohyoid: elevates and draws the hyoid forward.

8. Intrinsic musculature of tongue: shapes the tongue.
   a. Superior longitudinal: elevates tip and sides of tongue, makes tongue concave.
   b. Inferior longitudinal: curls tongue tip downward, makes tongue convex.
   c. Transverse lingual: narrows and increases thickness of tongue.
   d. Lateral lingual: broadens and lengthens tongue.

C. Muscles that move in the throat.

1. Sternohyoid: depresses the hyoid and larynx.

2. Omohyoid: depresses the hyoid.

3. Sternothyroid: depresses the thyroid cartilage.

4. Thyrohyoid: raises and changes the form of the larynx.

V. Anatomy of the Head, Mouth, and Pharynx of the Newborn as It Relates to Feeding (Morris & Klein, 2000)

A. Oral cavity (mouth).

1. Bounded by the roof, floor, lips, and cheeks.

2. Roof consists of the palatine process of the maxilla and the palatine bone (hard palate).

3. Transitions posteriorly into the soft palate and uvula.

4. Floor consists of the mandible spanned by the mylohyoid, geniohyoid, and front of the digastric muscle.

5. The orbicularis oris surrounds the lips.

6. Cheeks are defined by the buccinator and masseter muscles; sucking pads that consist of fatty tissue are encased in the cheek to provide stability for the cheek during sucking, lateral borders for the tongue.

7. Mandible is small and retracted.

8. The tongue fills the entire oral cavity and touches the roof and floor of the mouth as well as the lateral gum lines and cheeks.

9. Lingual frenulum: a fold of mucous membrane extending from the floor of the mouth to the midline of the under surface of the tongue, should regress during mid-gestation (Hogan, Westcott, & Griffiths, 2005; Dollberg et al., 2006).

10. Labial frenae: the membranes that attach the lips to the gum ridges, inferiorly and superiorly (Oldfield, 1955).

B. Pharynx: a soft muscular tube at the back of the throat.

1. Oropharynx: composed of the area between the elevated soft palate and the epiglottis.

2. Nasopharynx: section of the pharynx between the nasal choanae and the elevated soft palate; the eustachian tubes originate in the nasopharynx.

3. Hypopharynx: extends from the base of the epiglottis to the cricopharyngeal sphincter.

C. Larynx: gateway to the trachea composed of cartilage suspended by muscles and ligaments to the hyoid bone and cervical vertebrae.

1. Contains the epiglottis, which folds down to cover the airway during swallowing.

2. Contains the vocal folds or cords, which also close during swallowing in order to protect the airway.

D. Trachea: a semirigid tube that branches into the primary bronchi leading to each lung; the posterior aspect is a membranous wall that abuts the soft tissue of the esophagus.

E. Esophagus: a thin, muscular tube that extends to the stomach and distends as food is propelled through it by peristaltic motion.

VI. Palate

A. Function

1. The hard palate assists with positioning and stability of the nipple within the mouth.

2. The soft palate works with the tongue to create the posterior seal of the oral cavity.

3. The soft palate elevates during the swallow, contacting the pharyngeal walls and closing off the nasal cavity, directing the bolus toward the hypopharynx.

B. Reference palate.

1. The hard palate should be intact and smoothly contoured.

a. In utero and after birth, the shape of the hard palate is contoured by the continual pressure of the tongue as it rests against the palate with the mouth closed.

2. Submucous clefts of the soft palate cannot be visualized.

a. Might see a translucent zone in the middle of the soft palate.

b. Bifid uvula.

c. Absent or notched posterior nasal spine.

d. Paranasal bulge (transverse bony ridge alongside the nose) (Stahl, 1998).

Figure 13-3   Midsagittal section of cranial and oral anatomy of an adult while swallowing

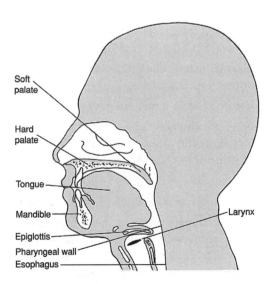

Figure 13-4 Midsagittal section of cranial and oral anatomy of an infant while swallowing

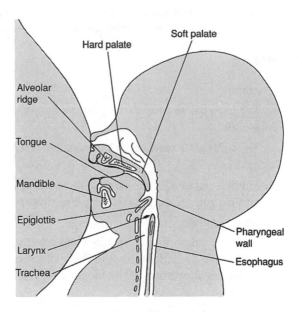

C. Variations and abnormalities of the palate. Note that tongue movements shape the palate (Palmer, 1998).

1. High palate: the palate or a portion of the palate is very high, altering the shallow saucer shape.

2. Wide palate or flat palate: reduced arch.

3. Narrow palate: reduced horizontal spread of palate.

4. Short and long palates: shorter or longer than the typical one inch from the alveolar ridge (gum ridge) to the point where the soft palate folds.

5. Channel palate: midline groove usually from the prolonged presence of orotracheal tubes.

6. V-shaped arch: a high, narrow palate that is narrower anteriorly.

7. Bony prominences: uncommon; more common is an Epstein pearl (accumulation of epithelial cells; also called a retention cyst) located at the juncture of the hard and soft palates.

8. Sloped palate: sudden declines in the normal curve.

9. Bubble palate: concavities of the hard palate confined with a rim.

10. Cleft: a complete opening in the hard or soft palate resulting from the failure of the primary palate and/or palatal shelves to meet and fuse during the seventh to eighth week of gestation (Danner & Wilson-Clay, 1986; Miller & Miller, 1986; Mohrbacher, 1994).

VII. Mandible Placement

A. Reference.

1. Upper and lower jaw loosely opposed.

2. Both gum ridges in direct opposition.

B. Deviations.

1. Recessed jaw: the lower gum ridge is posterior to the upper gum ridge.

2. Micrognathia: an excessively small or posteriorly positioned mandible; internally, the tongue is also posteriorly positioned in relation to the oral cavity.

VIII. Tongue

A. Reference.

1. Brings the nipple into the mouth, shaping it and stabilizing its position.

2. May provide a compression force to move milk toward the nipple (Ardran et al., 1958). When the mandible drops, negative pressure in the mouth causes milk to flow from the nipple (Ramsay & Hartmann, 2005).

3. Forms a central groove to stabilize the teat and channel fluid toward the pharynx.

4. Assists in forming a bolus in preparation for the swallow.

5. The tongue is soft with a rounded tip.

6. Lies on the bottom of the mouth with a slight central groove.

B. Variations and anomalies.

1. Tongue tip elevation: the tip of the tongue is in opposition to the upper gum ridge or the palate behind the alveolar ridge.

2. Humped: in an anterior-posterior direction.

3. Bunched: compressed in a lateral direction.

4. Retracted: held posteriorly in the mouth behind the inferior alveolar ridge.

5. Protruded: the tip rests forward, well past the lips.

6. Tongue-tie or ankyloglossia - a short or tight lingual frenulum (Coryllos et al., 2004; Amir, James, & Beatty, 2005; Messner et al., 2000; Jain, 1996; Griffiths, 2004; Riche et al., 2005).

IX. Oral Reflexes

A. Adaptive.

1. Rooting response: touching or stroking the baby's lips or cheek causes turning of the head toward the stimulus and opens the mouth (gape response).

2. Sucking reflex: a light touch of the nipple or a finger to the lips or tongue initiates the complex movements of the suckle.

3. Swallowing: elicited by a bolus of fluid impacting the sensory receptors of the soft palate and back of the mouth; has both reflexive and voluntary properties (Figures 13-4 and 13-5) triggered at the valeculae in newborns.

4. Protrusion reflex- baby's tongue moves down and forward in anticipation of grasping and drawing the breast into the mouth.

B. Protective.

1. Gag reflex: protects the baby from ingesting items that are too large for the esophagus; is elicited in the newborn at the mid-tongue area.

2. Cough reflex: mechanism that protects the airway from the aspiration of liquids.

References

Amir, LH, James JP, Beatty J. Review of tongue tie release at a tertiary maternity hospital. *J Paediatr Child Health.* 2005;41:243–245.

Ardran, GM et al. A cineradiographic study of breast feeding. *Br J Radiol.* March 1958; 31 (363):156-162.

Bosma JF, ed. *Oral Sensation and Perception: The Mouth of the Infant.* Springfield, IL: Charles C Thomas; 1972.

Brazelton TB. Neonatal behavioral assessment scale. In: *Clinics in Developmental Medicine,* No. 88. Philadelphia: Lippincott; 1995.

Coryllos E et al: Congenital Tongue-Tie and Its Impact on Breastfeeding. AAP Breastfeeding Section: Breastfeeding, Best for Baby and Mother; 2004.

Danner S, Wilson-Clay B. Breastfeeding the infant with cleft lip/palate. Lactation Consultant Series. Auerbach KG, ed. Schaumburg, IL: La Leche League International, Unit 10; 1986.

Diamond MD, Scheibel AB, Elson LM. *The Human Brain Coloring Book.* New York: Harper Collins; 1991.

Dollberg S et al. Immediate nipple pain relief after frenotomy in breast-fed infants with ankyloglossia: a randomized, prospective study. *J Pediatr Surg.* September 2006; 41(9):1598-1600.

Gomes, CF et al. Surface electromyography of facial muscles during natural and artificial feeding of infants. *J Pediatr (Rio J).* April 2006; 82(2):103-109.

Grant JCB. *An Atlas of Anatomy.* Baltimore: Williams & Wilkins; 1956.

Griffiths, DM. Do tongue ties affect breastfeeding? *J Hum Lact.* 2004;20:409–414.

Hogan M, Westcott C, Griffiths M. Randomized, controlled trial of division of tongue-tie in infants with feeding problems. *J Paediatr Child Health.* 2005;41:246–250.

Jacinto-Goncalves, Gaviao MB, Berzin F, et al. Electromyographic activity of perioral muscle in breastfed and bottlefed infants. *J Clin Pediatr Dent.* 2004;29:57–62.

Jain E. Tongue-Tie: Impact on Breastfeeding. Complete Management Including Frenotomy (video). Calgary, Alberta, Canada: Lakeview Breastfeeding Clinic; 1996.

Kapit W, Elson L. *The Anatomy Coloring Book*. New York: Addison Wesley; 1993.

Messner AH, Lalakea ML, Aby J, et al. Ankyloglossia: incidence and associated feeding difficulties. *Arch Otol Head Neck Surg*. 2000;126:36–39.

Miller JG, Miller JH. The controversial issue of breastfeeding for infants with cleft palate. St Innisfail, Alberta, Canada: Med Medical Research and Publishing; 1996.

Mohrbacher N. Nursing a baby with a cleft lip or palate. *Leaven*. 1994; Mar/Apr:19–23.

Morris S, Klein M. *Pre-feeding Skills*. 2nd ed. Tucson, AZ: Therapy Skill Builders; 2000.

Netter F. *Atlas of Human Anatomy*. Elsevier Health Sciences; 2006.

Oldfield MC. Congenitally short frenula of the upper lip and tongue. *Lancet*. 1955; 1:528–530.

Palmer B. The influence of breastfeeding on development of the oral cavity: a commentary. *J Hum Lact*. 1998;14:93–98.

Ramsay DT, Hartmann P. Milk removal from the breast. *Breastfeed Rev*. March 2005;13(1):5-7.

Riche LA, Baker NJ, Madlon-Kay DJ, DeFor TA: Newborn tongue-tie: prevalence and effect on breast-feeding. *J Am Board Fam Pract*. 2005;18:1–7.

Stahl S. Classic and occult submucous cleft palates: a histopathologic analysis. *Cleft Palate Craniofac J*. 1998;35:351–358.

Takemoto, H. Morphological Analyses of the Human Tongue Musculature for Three-Dimensional Modeling. *J Speech Lang Hear Res*. February 2001;44(1):95–107.

Suggested Readings

Bly L. The Components of Normal Movement During the First Year of Life and Abnormal Motor Development (monograph). Neuro-Developmental Treatment Association, Inc. Oak Park, IL: NDTA; 1983.

Gray H. *Gray's Anatomy*. New York: Barnes and Noble Books; 2005.

Ingram TTS. Clinical significance of the infantile feeding reflexes. *Physiol Behavior*. 1962;26:327–329.

Marmet C, Shell E. Training neonates to suck correctly. *MCN Am J Matern Child Nurs*. 1984;9:401–407.

Milani-Comparetti A. The neurophysiologic and clinical implications of studies on fetal motor behavior. *Semin Perinatol*. 1981;5:183–189.

PHYSIOLOGY OF THE BREAST DURING PREGNANCY AND LACTATION

Marsha Walker, RN, IBCLC
Revised by Gini Baker, RN, MPH, IBCLC

OBJECTIVES

- Discuss the hormonal control of mammary growth during pregnancy.
- Describe the processes of lactogenesis I, II, and III.
- List the hormones of lactation and their function.
- Describe the neuro-endocrine control of milk ejection.
- Discuss the feedback inhibitor of lactation.
- Define autocrine (local) control of milk synthesis.
- Explain the process of milk synthesis.

Introduction

The breast is a remarkable endocrine organ that experiences growth, differentiation, and lactation in response to a complex interplay of hormones and stimulation. *Mammogenesis,* which is the development of the mammary gland and related structures within the breast, occurs throughout fetal, adolescent, and adult life. It is a time of cellular division and proliferation. The stages of breast changes during pregnancy and into breastfeeding are: (1) *mammogenesis,* where there is cellular division and proliferation; (2) *lactogenesis I,* which is beginning secretory cellular activity and accumulation of colostrum from about 10 to 12 weeks gestation; (3) *lactogenesis II,* after placental delivery the establishing of fuller milk supplies; and (4) *lactogenesis III,* the stage of mature milk production and supply (also known as galactopoesis) (Uvnas-Moberg & Eriksson, 1996).

The hormonal environment of pregnancy finishes preparing the breasts to assume the role of nourishing the infant following birth. After delivery, a profound change occurs in the hormonal milieu, enabling an elaborate system of neuro-endocrine feedback to produce and deliver milk of a changing composition to meet the needs and stores of the infant as he or she grows and develops. The breasts are capable of full lactation from about 16 weeks of pregnancy onward. Milk does not "come in" because it is already present before delivery, during lactogenesis I in the form of *colostrum.*

Milk production is under endocrine or hormonal control before delivery of the placenta, and changes to autocrine control during lactogenesis II. Abundant production is suppressed by inhibiting hormones until placental delivery, when the change in hormonal checks and balances followed by the stimulus of infant suckling signals the breasts to produce copious amounts of milk. The lactation consultant benefits from a familiarity with this cascade of events and its influence on lactation.

I. Mammogenesis: Breast Development

A. The breasts during pregnancy.
1. Final preparation for lactation.
   a. Early in the first trimester, mammary epithelial cells proliferate, ductal sprouting and branching are initiated, and lobular formation occurs.
   b. Ducts proliferate into the fatty pad, and the ductal end buds differentiate into alveoli.
   c. Increases occur in mammary blood flow, interstitial water, and electrolyte concentrations.
   d. Mammary blood vessels increase their luminal diameters and form new capillaries around the lobules.
   e. During the last trimester, secretory cells fill with fat droplets and the alveoli are distended with colostrum.
   f. Mammary cells become competent to secrete milk proteins at midpregnancy but are kept in check by high circulating levels of steroids, particularly progesterone.
   g. Most milk products secreted during pregnancy find their way back into the plasma via the leaky junctions (spaces between the mammary alveolar cells).
2. Breasts during pregnancy: hormonal control.
   a. Milk supply is hormonally driven: endocrine control system.
   b. Placental lactogen, prolactin, and chorionic gonadotrophin: accelerated growth.
   c. 17 beta-estradiol is required for mammary growth and epithelial proliferation during pregnancy.
   d. Glucocorticoids enhance formation of the lobules during pregnancy.
   e. Estrogen.

       i. Increases during pregnancy.

      ii. Stimulates ductular sprouting.

  f. Prolactin.

       i. Necessary for complete growth of the gland (Uvnas-Moberg et al., 1990).

      ii. Secreted by the anterior pituitary gland.

     iii. Stimulates prolactin receptor sites for the initiation of milk secretion located on the alveolar cell surfaces.

     iv. Lactogenesis II occurs earlier if the woman has breastfed before, possibly due to increased number of prolactin receptor sites (Zuppa et al., 1988).

      v. Levels rise during sleep and throughout pregnancy (Cregan, Mitoulas, & Hartmann, 2002).

     vi. In non-nursing mothers, prolactin drops to pre-pregnant levels at two weeks postpartum.

    vii. Prolactin is prevented from exerting its effect on milk secretion by the elevated levels of progesterone.

   viii. Prolactin-inhibiting factor is secreted by the hypothalamus in order to negatively control prolactin's effects.

  g. Progesterone.

       i. Increases during pregnancy.

      ii. Progesterone stimulates lobuloalveolar growth while suppressing secretory activity.

     iii. Lobular formation occurs in response to progesterone.

     iv. Sensitizes mammary cells to the effects of insulin and growth factors.

      v. May be involved in the final preparation of the gland for copious milk production (lactogenesis II).

II. Lactogenesis I

A. Beginning of secretory cellular activity and milk production.

B. Occurs around 16 to 18 weeks prenatally.

C. Breast is first capable of synthesizing unique milk components; human placental lactogen is thought to be responsible.

D. Thyroid hormones increase the responsiveness of mammary cells to prolactin and can improve lactation performance.

E. Three main hormones are necessary for lactation to begin: prolactin, insulin, and hydrocortisone.

F. Supportive metabolic hormones include insulin, cortisol, thyroid-parathyroid hormone, and growth hormone.

G. The antepartum secretion, or colostrum, shows a gradually increasing presence of lactose, casein, and alpha-lactalbumin.

H. Colostrum (milk) is available to the infant at delivery (milk does not have to "come in").

III. Lactogenesis II

A. Lactogenesis II is the onset of copious milk secretion.

1. Between 30 and 72 hours following delivery of the placenta.

2. Women do not typically begin feeling increased breast fullness until 50 to 73 hours (2–3 days) after birth (Riordan, 2005).

3. Initially under endocrine control and now under autocrine control (DeCoopman, 1993; Wilde et al., 1995a, 1995b).

B. Placental expulsion following delivery precipitates an abrupt decline in levels of human placental lactogen, estrogen, and progesterone.

1. Decline in progesterone levels is thought to be the initiating event for Lactogenesis II, because progesterone is a prolactin inhibitor.

2. This decline in progesterone acts in the presence of lactogenic hormones, such as prolactin and glucocorticoids for full lactogenic activity.

3. A sharp rise in citrate and alpha-lactalbumin occurs at the onset of lactogenesis II.

C. May be delayed by outside factors.

1. Maternal fluid loads in labor (Cotterman, 2004; Lauwers & Swisher, 2005).

2. Maternal health status (Kaplan & Schenken, 1990; Whitworth, 1988).

3. Women who have type 1 diabetes mellitus; there might be a temporary imbalance in the amount of insulin required for glucose homeostasis and insulin required for the initiation of lactation.

4. Retained placental fragments.

D. Prolactin.

1. Plasma prolactin levels increase sharply after placenta delivery and rise and fall with the frequency, intensity, and duration of nipple stimulation. Prolactin levels fall about 50% in the first week postpartum. Breast milk prolactin levels have been detected in mature milk up to 40 weeks postpartum (Riordan, 2005).

2. Frequent feeding in early lactation stimulates development of prolactin receptor sites in the mammary gland. The theory is that the controlling factor in breast milk production is the number of prolactin receptor sites and not the amount of prolactin in circulating blood (Riordan, 2005).

3. While prolactin is necessary for milk secretion, its levels are not directly related to the volume of milk produced; that is, prolactin becomes permissive in its function.

4. Prolactin release occurs only in response to direct stimulation of the nipple/areola, that is, autocrine control, in lactogenesis III.

IV. Lactogenesis III

A. Previously called *galactopoesis*: maintenance of lactation.

B. Milk contains a small whey protein called *feedback inhibitor of lactation* (*FIL*).

   1. Role of FIL appears to be to slow milk synthesis when the breast is full.

   2. Rate of milk synthesis slows when milk accumulates in the breast; more FIL is present.

   3. Rate of milk synthesis speeds up when milk is removed from the breast and less FIL is present.

   4. Ability to continue making milk is now dependent on autocrine control (milk removal), which is dependent upon the hypothalamus.

   5. More frequent milk removal theoretically will produce more milk.

C. Foremilk and hindmilk.

   1. All milk starts out as concentrated milk, sometimes referred to as *hindmilk*.

   2. When milk remains in the breast, it draws in water and lactose and becomes more dilute *foremilk*.

D. Calorie content of mature milk (Kent et al., 2006; Daly et al., 1992; Daly & Hartmann, 1995a, b; Cregan & Hartmann, 1999; Cregan et al., 2002; Mitoulas et al., 2002; Ramsay et al., 2005; Ramsay & Hartmann 2005; Walker, 2006).

   1. Colostrum mean energy value is 67 kcal/dL or 18.76 kcal/oz.

   2. Mature milk mean energy value is 75 kcal/dL or 21 kcal/oz.

   3. Caloric content varies widely throughout each feeding and the day due to changing fat content.

   4. The amount of fat in human milk changes during each feeding depending on the time since the last feeding.

   5. Fat content in human milk is influenced by several factors including maternal metabolism, maternal weight, maternal diet, and frequency of feeds.

V. Involution

A. Occurs when the milk-producing system in the breast is no longer being used.

B. Complete involution varies among women and may occur approximately 40 days after complete cessation of breastfeeding.

C. Is dependent upon type of weaning process, whether abrupt or gradual.

D. Anecdotally, women report that the longer they are actively producing milk, the longer it takes for the production to go away completely.

E. How many children a woman has breastfed in the past can affect the number of prolactin receptor sites.

F. Affected by maternal medical influences such as body type, obesity, maternal diet, rate of metabolism, and maternal medications.

VI. General Information

A. Milk production.

1. Volume of milk removed from the breast at a feeding/expression.

2. Is correlated to the needs of the baby.

B. Milk synthesis (accumulation of milk within the breast).

1. Rate of milk synthesis: Rate at which newly synthesized milk is accumulating within the breast.

2. Local or autocrine control regulates the short-term milk synthesis of the breasts.

3. Milk synthesis responds to the varying amount of residual milk remaining in the breast after a feeding (FIL factor).

4. Degree to which milk is removed signals the amount of milk to be made for the next feeding.

5. The greater the degree of milk removal at a feeding, the greater the rate of milk synthesis after that feed (DeCarvalho et al., 1983).

6. Milk synthesis is controlled independently in each breast.

7. Storage capacity of breasts varies greatly among women.

8. Measured storage capacity of a breast increases with breast size.

9. Small breasts are capable of secreting as much milk over a 24-hour period as large breasts.

C. Milk synthesis process.

1. Cells lining both the alveoli and the smaller ductules appear capable of secreting milk.

2. Degree of fullness in breast and rate of short-term synthesis are inversely related (Daly et al, 1992, 1993, 1996; Walker, 2006).

3. Wide variability in rate of milk synthesis ranging from 17 to 33 mL/h (Arthur et al, 1989a, 1989b).

4. The milk is stored in the alveoli and in small ducts adjacent to the cells that secrete it, compressing and flattening the cells.

5. Five pathways are involved in milk synthesis (Arthur PG et al., 1989; Arthur, Smith, & Hartmann, 1989; Daly et al., 1996).

a. Pathway I: protein secretion.

i. Most important proteins synthesized by the mammary cell are casein, lactoferrin, alpha-lactalbumin, and lysozyme.

    ii. Protein synthesis begins in the nucleus with the transcription of specific mRNAs that code for milk proteins and pass into the cytoplasm, where they serve as templates.

    iii. Proteins pass to the Golgi apparatus, where phosphate and sugar groups are added.

    iv. Calcium enters this compartment and aggregates the casein molecules into micelles containing large amounts of calcium and phosphate.

    v. Secretory vesicles migrate to the apical membrane, fuse with it, and release their contents.

  b. Pathway II: lactose secretion.

    i. Alpha-lactalbumin forms a complex with the enzyme galactosyl-transferase, catalyzing the synthesis of lactose from glucose and UDP-galactose.

    ii. Lactose concentration is 200 mM, or about 7% by weight.

    iii. Another 30 mM of sugar is added to the milk as glycosyl groups on milk proteins; these are oligosaccharides that vary according to the mother's ABO blood type and are involved in disease protection.

  c. Pathway III: milk fat synthesis (Daly et al., 1993; De Carvalho et al., 1993).

    i. Substrate for milk fat synthesis comes from two sources.

    ii. Mammary alveolar cells synthesize the shorter chain fatty acids (10–16 carbons) from glucose.

    iii. Fatty acids derived from plasma sources are synthesized in adipose tissue and are the longer chain fatty acids (16–20 carbons).

  d. Pathway IV: monovalent ion secretion into milk.

    i. Low ion concentrations of sodium, potassium, and chloride are maintained by mechanisms in the apical membrane.

  e. Pathway V: plasma protein secretion into milk.

    i. A plasma membrane receptor binds immunoglobulin A (IgA) from the plasma to the mammary alveolar cell. IgA is released from the apical membrane into the milk.

    ii. Other hormones (such as prolactin, insulin, growth factors, and so on) have receptors on mammary cells and most likely find their way into milk through pathway V.

D. Milk release (also referred to as *milk ejection reflex* or *let down reflex*) (De Coopman 1993).

  1. Neuroendocrine involvement in milk ejection.

    a. Occurs with:

      i. Direct stimulation to sensory neurons in the areola.

      ii. Impulses from the cerebral cortex, ears, and eyes can also elicit the release of oxytocin through exteroceptive stimuli (such as hearing a baby cry) (Uvnas-Moberg et al., 1990).

      b. Some women feel the milk ejection reflex as increased pressure or tingling within the breast or as shooting pains, whereas some women never feel the milk ejection reflex.

      c. Response to oxytocin release from the posterior pituitary.

          i. Mothers, especially multiparous women, with each breastfeeding will also feel uterine cramping for the first few days after birth.

         ii. Mothers might also report increased thirst, a warm or flushed feeling, increased heat from the breasts, or a feeling of sleepiness or calmness.

      d. Milk ejection signs can be seen when the baby begins gulping milk (when the rapid pattern of two sucks per second decreases to one suck or so per second with swallowing).

      e. Milk ejection reflex serves to increase the intraductal mammary pressure and to maintain it at levels that are sufficient to overcome the resistance to the outflow of milk from the breast.

2. Oxytocin.

      a. A simultaneous and closed secretion of oxytocin occurs into brain regions of the lactating mother (Febo, Numan, & Ferris, 2005; Jonas et al., 2006; Winberg, 2005; Uvnas-Moberg & Petersson, 2004; Mezzacappa et al., 2001).

          i. Has a calming affect.

         ii. Lowers maternal blood pressure.

        iii. Decreases cortisol levels, decreases anxiety and aggressive behavior.

        iv. Permeates the areas of the brain associated with mothering and bonding behaviors.

      b. Causes a contraction of the myoepithelial cells surrounding the alveoli, forcing milk into the collecting ducts of the breast.

      c. Nipple stimulation causes oxytocin release of brief 3 to 4 second bursts into the bloodstream every 5 to 15 minutes (Neville, 2001).

      d. Variable and intermittent bursts of oxytocin are also seen from pre-nursing stimuli and mechanical stimulation from a breast pump (Boutte et al., 1985; Fewtrell et al., 2001; Zoppou, Barry, & Mercer, 1997).

      e. Oxytocin causes shortening of the ducts without constricting them, thus increasing milk pressure (Neville, 2001).

References

Arthur PG, Jones TJ, Spruce J, Hartmann PE. Measuring short-term rates of milk synthesis in breast-feeding mothers. *Q J Exp Physiol.* 1989;74:419–428.

Arthur PD, Smith M, Hartmann PE. Milk lactose, citrate, and glucose as markers of lactogenesis in normal and diabetic women. *J Pediatr Gastroenterol Nutr.* 1989; 9:488–496.

Boutte CA, Garza C, Fraley JK, et al. Comparison of hand- and electric-operated breast pumps. *Hum Nutr Appl Nutr.* 1985;39:426–430.

Cotterman K. Reverse pressure softening: a simple tool to prepare areola for easier latching during engorgement. *J Hum Lact.* 2004;20:227–237.

Cox DB, Owens RA, Hartmann PE. Blood and milk prolactin and the rate of milk synthesis in women. *Exp Physiol.* 1996;81:1007–1020.

Cox, DB, Owens RA, Hartmann PE. *Studies on human lactation: the development of the computerized breast measurement system* (1998). Available at http://mammary.nih. gov/reviews/lactation/Hartmann001/index.html. Accessed December 7, 2006.

Cregan MD, Hartmann PE. Computerized breast measurement from conception to weaning: clinical implications. *J Hum Lact.* 1999;15:89–96.

Cregan MD, Mitoulas LR, Hartmann PE. Milk prolactin, feed volume and duration between feeds in women breastfeeding their full-term infants over a 24 h period. *Exp Physiol.* 2002;87:207–214.

Daly SEJ, Di Rosso A, Owens RA, Hartmann PE. Degree of breast emptying explains changes in the fat content, but not fatty acid composition, of human milk. *Exp Physiol.* 1993;78:741–755.

Daly SEJ, Hartmann PE. Infant demand and milk supply. Part 1: infant demand and milk supply in lactating women. *J Hum Lact.* 1995a;11:21–31.

Daly S, Hartmann PE. Infant demand and milk supply. Part 2: the short-term control of milk synthesis in lactating women. *J Hum Lact.* 1995b;11:27–37.

Daly SEJ, Kent JC, Owens RA, Hartmann PE. Frequency and degree of milk removal and the short-term control of human milk synthesis. *Exp Physiol.* 1996;81:861–875.

Daly SEJ, Kent JC, Owens RA, et al. The determination of short-term volume changes and the rate of synthesis of human milk using computerized breast measurement. *Exp Physiol.* 1992;77:79–87.

Daly SEJ, Owens RA, Hartmann PE. The short-term synthesis and infant-regulated removal of milk in lactating women. *Exp Physiol.* 1993;78:209–220.

DeCarvalho MD, Robertson S, Friedman A, Klaus M. Effect of frequent breast-feeding on early milk production and infant weight gain. *Pediatrics.* 1983;72:307–311.

De Coopman J. Breastfeeding after pituitary resection: support for a theory of autocrine control of milk supply? *J Hum Lact.* 1993;9:35–40.

Febo M, Numan M, Ferris CF. Functional magnetic resonance imaging shows oxytocin activates brain regions associated with mother-pup bonding during suckling. *J Neurosci.* 2005;25:11637–11644.

Fewtrell M, Lucas P, Collier S, Lucas A. Randomized study comparing the efficacy of a novel manual breast pump with a mini-electric breast pump in mothers of term infants. *J Hum Lact.* 2001;17:126–131.

Jonas W, Wiklund I, Nissen E, et al. Newborn skin temperature two days postpartum during breastfeeding related to different labour ward practices. *Early Hum Dev.* 2006; July 28 [Epub ahead of print].

Kaplan CR, Schenken RS. Endocrinology of the breast (Chapt 3). In: Mitchell GW, Bassett LW, eds. *The Female Breast and Its Disorders.* Baltimore: Williams & Wilkins; 1990:22–44.

Kent JC, Mitoulas LR, Cregan MD, Ramsay DT, Doherty DA, Hartmann PE. Volume and frequency of breastfeedings and fat content of breast milk throughout the day. *Pediatrics*. 2006;117:e387–e395.

Lauwers J, Swisher A. *Counseling the Nursing Mother: A Lactation Consultant's Guide*. Sudbury, MA: Jones and Bartlett Publishers; 2005:414.

Mezzacappa ES, Kelsey RM, Myers MM, Katkin ES. Breast-feeding and maternal cardiovascular function. *Psychophysiology*. 2001;38:988–997.

Mitoulas LR, Kent JC, Cox DB, et al. Variation in fat, lactose and protein in human milk over 24 h and throughout the first year of lactation. *Br J Nutr*. 2002;88:29–37.

Neville MC. Anatomy and physiology of lactation. *Pediatr Clin North Am*. 2001;48:13.

Ramsay DT, Hartmann PE. Milk removal from the breast. *Breastfeed Rev*. 2005;13:5–7.

Ramsay DT, Mitoulas LR, Kent JC, et al. The use of ultrasound to characterize milk ejection in women using an electric breast pump. *J Hum Lact*. 2005;21:421–428.

Riordan J. *Breastfeeding and Human Lactation*. 2nd ed. Sudbury, MA: Jones and Bartlett Publishers; 2005.

Uvnas-Moberg K, Eriksson M. Breastfeeding: physiological, endocrine and behavioral adaptations caused by oxytocin and local neurogenic activity in the nipple and mammary gland. *Acta Paediatr*. 1996;85:525–530.

Uvnas-Moberg K, Petersson M. Oxytocin—biochemical link for human relations. Mediator of antistress, well-being, social interaction, growth, healing. *Lakartidningen*. 2004;101:2634–2639. (in Swedish).

Uvnas-Moberg K, Widstrom A-M, Werner S, et al. Oxytocin and prolactin levels in breast-feeding women. *Acta Obstet Gynecol Scand*. 1990;69:301–306.

Walker M. *Breastfeeding Management for the Clinician*. Sudbury, MA: Jones and Bartlett; 2006.

Whitworth N. Lactation in humans. *Psychoneuroendocrinology*. 1988;13:171–188.

Wilde CJ, Addey CVP, Boddy LM, Peaker M, Autocrine regulation of milk secretion by a protein in milk. *Biochem J*. 1995a;305:51–58.

Wilde CJ, Prentice A, Peaker M. Breastfeeding: matching supply with demand in human lactation. *Proc Nutr Soc*. 1995b;54:401–406.

Winberg J. Mother and newborn baby: mutual regulation of physiology and behavior— a selective review. *Dev Psychobiol*. 2005;47:217–229.

Zoppou C, Barry SI, Mercer GN. Dynamics of human milk extraction: a comparative study of breast feeding and breast pumping. *Bull Math Biol*. 1997;59:953–973.

Zuppa AA, Tornesello A, Papacci P, et al. Relationship between maternal parity, basal prolactin levels and neonatal breast milk intake. *Biol Neonate*. 1988;53:144–147.

Physiology of Infant Suckling

Amy Spangler, MN, RN, IBCLC

OBJECTIVES

- Define the terms sucking and suckling.
- Define nutritive and nonnutritive modes of suckling.
- Describe oral motor and feeding development.
- Describe the suckling cycle.
- List factors that can influence or contribute to suckling abnormalities.

Introduction

The dynamic and intricate coordination between sucking, swallowing, and breathing superimposed on a background of the infant's behavioral state make infant feeding a complicated, multidimensional task (Wolf & Glass, 1992). During pregnancy, the developing fetus receives nutrients through the placental circulation and waste products are excreted through the maternal circulation. At birth, dramatic changes occur, after which the newborn must ingest food by mouth, digest and absorb nutrients, and excrete metabolic wastes. All of these activities occur in a setting of rapid growth, high nutritional needs, and body systems that are not yet fully developed. The lactation consultant benefits from an understanding of oral motor development, the mechanics of suckling, and the mechanisms that control suckling behavior.

I. Oral Anatomy

Muscular activity and changing pressure gradients combine to move air and food from the nasal and oral cavity to the stomach (Kennedy & Kent, 1988). To facilitate the safe transport of air and food through the same and adjacent structures, a system of valves that includes the lips, soft palate, tongue, epiglottis, and cricopharyngeal sphincter channels food and air in the proper direction at the proper time (Morris, 1982). The resting position of the valves favors respiration, with most of the valves changing position to allow swallowing.

A. Birth to six months of age.

1. Oral cavity is short from top to bottom and bounded by the roof, floor, lips, and cheeks.

2. Hard palate is short, wide, and slightly arched with a corrugated surface (rugae).

3. Soft palate and epiglottis are closely approximated.

4. Sucking fat pads in the cheeks are present.

5. Tongue fills the oral cavity. Tongue tip protrudes past the alveolar ridge, maintaining contact with the lower lip.

6. Frenulum anchors the tongue to the floor of the mouth.

7. Jaw is recessed with the lower gum line slightly behind the upper gum line.

B. Six months to one year of age.

1. Oral cavity elongates vertically and becomes more spacious.

2. Soft palate and epiglottis are no longer in close proximity. Larynx must elevate further to allow epiglottis to seal completely during swallowing.

3. Tongue moves back into the mouth, and the tip is behind the alveolar ridge. Lateral tongue movements facilitate manipulation of food.

4. Sucking fat pads and other adipose tissue in the cheeks diminish. This allows for greater movement of the lips and cheeks.

5. Teeth erupt.

II. Oral Reflex Development (Wolf & Glass, 1992)

Oral reflexes develop very early in utero. Swallowing plays a crucial role in infant survival and develops at an early age (Bosma, 1985; Pritchard, 1966). The fetus:

- Exhibits swallowing at 12 to 14 weeks gestation (Bosma, 1985; Ianniruberto & Tajani, 1981).

- Exhibits sucking as early as 15 to 18 weeks (Ianniruberto & Tajani, 1981) along with the gag reflex (Ianniruberto & Tajani, 1981; Tucker, 1985).

In the extrauterine environment, sucking activity has been observed:

- At 27 to 28 weeks but the pattern is disorganized and random.

- By 32 weeks a burst–pause pattern is clearly emerging but still lacks coordination.

- At 34 to 35 weeks sucking and related components for effective feeding are present (Brake et al., 1988; Casaer et al., 1982; Hack, Estabrook, & Robertson, 1985; Wolf & Glass, 1992).

There are two categories of oral reflexes:

- Adaptive (rooting and sucking).

- Protective (gag and cough).

When a reflex loses its functional significance, it diminishes or disappears. Reflexes that are essential to survival persist, such as gag and swallowing.

- Swallowing plays a role in the regulation of amniotic fluid volume during pregnancy.
- Near term, the normal fetus swallows approximately one-half of the total volume of amniotic fluid each day (Diamant, 1985).
- An imbalance in the regulation of amniotic fluid is an early indicator of anatomical defects in the fetus (Fisher, Painter, & Milmoe, 1981).

A. Gag reflex.

   1. Stimulus: posterior tongue/pharynx.

   2. Appears: 18 weeks gestation.

   3. Disappears: Peaks at 40 weeks gestation; diminishes by 6 months but persists.

B. Phasic bite reflex.

   1. Stimulus: Gums.

   2. Appears: 28 weeks gestation.

   3. Disappears: 9 to 12 months.

C. Rooting reflex.

   1. Stimulus: mouth corner/lips/cheek.

   2. Appears: 32 weeks gestation.

   3. Disappears: peaks at 40 weeks gestation; disappears by 3 to 6 months.

D. Sucking reflex.

   1. Stimulus: mouth/tongue.

   2. Appears: 15 to 18 weeks gestation.

   3. Disappears: 6 to 12 months.

E. Swallowing reflex.

   1. Stimulus: pharynx.

   2. Appears: 12 to 14 weeks gestation.

   3. Disappears: persists.

F. Tongue protrusion reflex.

   1. Stimulus: Tongue/lips.

   2. Appears: 28 weeks gestation.

   3. Disappears: 6 months.

III. Science of Suckling

Suckling and sucking are often used interchangeably to describe mouth movements with or without the ingestion of food by the infant.

- Some authors make a clear distinction between suckling and sucking (Arvedson & Brodsky, 1993; Lawrence, 2005; Wolf & Glass, 1992).
- During the first weeks after birth, the physiologic flexion acquired as a result of the limited space inside the uterus contributes to successful oral feeding (Arvedson & Brodsky, 1993).
- Arvedson and Brodsky (1993) describe two distinct suck phases, suckling and sucking.

A. Suckling.
  1. The first pattern to develop.
  2. Involves a backward and forward movement of the tongue.
  3. The tongue moves forward for half of the suckle pattern, with the backward phase being the most pronounced.
  4. Tongue protrusion does not extend beyond the border of the lips (Arvedson & Brodsky, 1993).
  5. The sides of the tongue move upward to form a central groove, helping in formation of the liquid bolus and in movement of the bolus posteriorly.

B. Sucking.
  1. Second phase, which develops between 6 and 9 months of age, when the tongue has more room for movement because of the downward and forward growth of the oral cavity.
  2. During sucking, the tongue raises and lowers, and the jaw makes smaller vertical excursions.
  3. Arvedson and Brodsky (1993) describe the developmental sequence from suckling to sucking as one of several developmental steps demonstrating readiness for thicker liquids and soft foods.

Lawrence (2005) differentiates between suckling and sucking as follows:

- Suckling is the means by which nourishment is taken at the breast, that is, breastfeeding.
- Sucking is the drawing into the mouth by means of a partial vacuum, that is, bottle-feeding.

Wolf and Glass (1992) use sucking to describe the rhythmic movements of the infant's mouth and tongue either:

- On a bottle or breast to obtain nourishment or
- On a pacifier, finger, or other object to modulate state or explore the environment (Arvedson & Brodsky, 1993; Lawrence, 2005).

C. All mammals are characterized by their ability to lactate.
  1. Suckling patterns are unique to each mammal species.

2. When healthy, full-term infants are placed on their mother's abdomen immediately after birth, they can seek and move to the breast, latch-on, and suckle within the first hour (Righard & Alade, 1990).

   a. This raises the question of the impact of separation of a mother and infant on breastfeeding initiation and duration, and the extent to which the interruption produces lasting harm (Righard & Alade, 1990).

D. The principal mechanism of milk removal common to all mammals is the contractile response of the mammary myoepithelium under the hormonal influence of oxytocin from the posterior pituitary (neurohypophysis; Lawrence, 2005).

   1. Infant suckling is the stimulus for the milk ejection reflex (MER).

   2. Milk ejection causes the suckling pattern to change from a non-nutritive to a nutritive pattern (Mizuno & Ueda, 2005).

E. Central nervous system (CNS) control of milk ejection contributes to MER occurring under circumstances that are conducive to effective milk removal (Lawrence, 2005).

F. Effective provision of milk requires:

   1. A storage system (alveoli).

   2. Exit channels (ducts).

   3. A prehensile appendage (areola).

   4. An expulsion mechanism (the MER).

   5. A retention mechanism (sympathetic activity; Lawrence, 2005).

IV. Non-Nutritive and Nutritive Patterns

A. Nutritive sucking is the process of obtaining nutrients.

B. Non-nutritive sucking occurs in the absence of nutrient flow and may be used to satisfy an infant's basic sucking urge or as a mechanism for regulating state (Wolf & Glass, 1992).

C. When human infants were observed sucking on an artificial nipple, two distinct sucking patterns were exhibited, a nutritive mode and a non-nutritive mode (Wolff, 1968; Woolridge, 1986a).

   1. When those same observations were made using a breastfeeding model, there was no difference between nutritive and non-nutritive suckling rates but rather a continuous variation of suckling rate in response to the rate of milk flow (Bowen-Jones, Thompson, & Drewett, 1982).

D. Non-nutritive sucking is characterized by a repetitive pattern of bursts and pauses.

   1. The number of sucks per burst and the duration of pauses are generally stable.
     a. Can vary with changes in state (Wolff, 1968, 1972).

E. Non-nutritive sucking such as the spontaneous sucking that occurs when a finger, pacifier, or dummy is placed in an infant's mouth can function as a mechanism for:

1. Increasing peristalsis of the gastrointestinal tract (Widstrom et al., 1988).

2. Enhancing secretion of digestive fluids (Widstrom et al., 1988).

3. Decreasing infant crying.

4. Reducing the risk for sudden infant death syndrome in pacifier-dependent infants (Hauck et al., 2003; Kahn et al., 2003).

F. Pacifiers.

1. While the use of pacifiers remains controversial, more data are needed before definitive statements can be made about the impact of pacifier use on breastfeeding, fertility, and dentition (Ingram et al., 2004; Ullah & Griffiths, 2003; Viggiano et al., 2004).

V. Mechanics of Suckling

Early data on suckling were collected using artificial nipples and bottles, but ultrasound imaging now allows researchers to visualize the lactating breast and the breastfeeding infant.

A. Historically, the baby sucked and the mother suckled. (Definitions have changed in modern times as noted previously.)

B. Suckling describes the removal of milk from the breast by the infant, that is, breastfeeding.

C. Mechanisms that facilitate milk removal.

1. Negative pressure within the oral cavity.

2. Positive pressure of the tongue against the teat (nipple and areola).

3. Peristaltic movement of the tongue along the teat.

4. Increased intraductal pressure.

D. Milk ejection is under neuroendocrine control.

1. Stimulation of tactile receptors for both oxytocin and prolactin release in the nipple is the most important factor in milk ejection (Meites, 1974).

2. Neither the negative or positive pressure exerted by suckling stimulate milk ejection.

E. Effective suckling.

1. Requires that the infant be able to coordinate three complex tasks: sucking, swallowing, and breathing.

2. Data show that while nasal breathing is preferred, it is not obligatory (Rodenstein, Perlmutter, & Stanescu, 1985).
   a. Infants were once categorized as obligate nose breathers, that is, that they were unable to breathe through their mouths.

      b. Infants have the ability to breathe through their mouth, albeit at the expense of respiratory efficiency (Miller, Martin, & Carlo, 1985).

   3. For many years it was believed that sucking and swallowing occurred in isolation from breathing.

      a. Wilson and colleagues (1980) were the first to report that swallowing coincided with cessation of nasal airflow, i.e., breathing stops when swallowing occurs.

      b. Weber and colleagues (1986) reported similar findings, i.e., the rhythmic swallowing accompanying sucking interrupts breathing.

      c. These findings support the current view that sucking, swallowing, and breathing must be coordinated in infant feeding.

F. Rate of suckling.

   1. Is variable up to 1 suck/swallow per second.

   2 The infant may exhibit interruptions (pauses) of various lengths.

      a. These interruptions may be part of the total suckling sequence (e.g., a few seconds of interruption after every 8 to 12 suck/swallow sequences) or they may be less predictable (Arvedson & Brodsky, 1993).

   3. The sucking rate is faster in non-nutritive sucking, averaging about 2 sucks per second (Wolf & Glass, 1992).

G. There is an inverse relationship between rate and flow. The higher the milk flow, the lower the rate of suckling (Bowen-Jones et al., 1982; Ramsay et al., 2004).

H. The rate of suckling may also be related to the size of the oral cavity. As the infant ages, the oral cavity enlarges, which may allow the infant to hold a greater amount of fluid before a swallow is needed (Wolf & Glass, 1992).

I. The volume of milk per suckle ranges from 0.14 to 0.21 mL at the beginning of a feed and 0.01 to 0.04 mL at the end of a feed (Woolridge, Baum, Drewett, 1980).

J. Milk volume intake is positively correlated with the number of milk ejections (Ramsay et al., 2004).

K. Milk ejection occurs on average 2.2 minutes after the infant begins to suckle (Bowen-Jones et al., 1982). This may explain why the highest level of energy during suckling activity occurs during the first 2 minutes (Voloschin et al., 1998).

L. Control of milk intake comes under intrinsic control of the infant during the first month (Woolridge et al., 1982).

M. Infants appear to feed more actively on high-fat milk, with longer bursts and fewer interruptions (Nysenbaum & Smart, 1982).

N. The wide range in breast milk volume in well-nourished populations is due more to variation in infant demand than to inadequacy of milk production (Dewey & Lonnerdal, 1986).

O. Sucking pressure plays an important role in modulating fluid flow. It appears that infants generate more pressure through negative intra-oral pressure (suction) than by positive pressure on the nipple (compression; Ellison, Vidyasagar, & Anderson, 1979).

P. Sucking pressures will also vary with state and behavioral factors. A sleepy infant will generate less pressure than an alert infant, and a hungry infant will generate more pressure than an infant who is full.

VI. Suckling Cycle (Figure 15-1) (Smith, Erenberg, & Nowak, 1988; Wolf & Glass, 1992; Woolridge, 1986a, 1986b)

A. The nipple, adjacent areola, and underlying tissue elongate to form a highly elastic teat two to three times its resting length and one-half its resting width.
B. Sucking fat pads in the cheeks provide stability and facilitate the formation of a passive seal and negative pressure in the oral cavity.
C. Negative pressure in the oral cavity functions to hold the nipple and areola in place.
D. The jaw provides a stable base for the movements of other structures including the tongue, lips, and cheeks. Slight downward movement of the jaw enlarges the oral cavity to produce suction.
E. The tongue plays a key role in all aspects of suckling. It works with the lips and the soft palate to seal the oral cavity.
F. Positive pressure of the tongue against the teat coupled with an increase in intraductal pressure facilitates milk removal. Suction does not appear to play a role in milk removal.

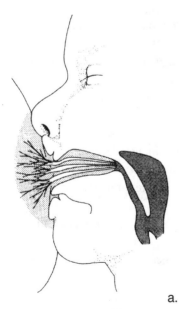

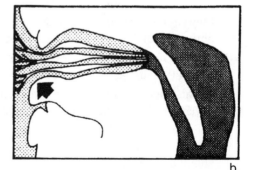

a.   b.

Figure 15-1 Complete suck cycle

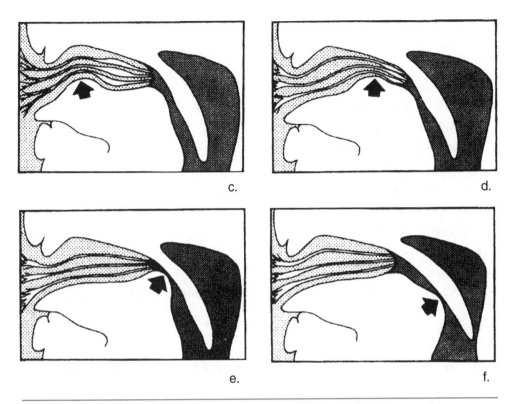

Figure 15-1   Complete suck cycle (continued)

G. The anterior portion of the tongue provides most of the compression, while the lowering of the posterior portion enlarges the space within the sealed oral cavity and creates negative pressure and suction.

H. The lateral margins of the tongue form a central trough or groove that channels milk to the posterior portion of the oral cavity. While some studies suggest distinct differences in tongue movements during breastfeeding and bottle-feeding, others report no difference (Ardran, Kemp, & Lind, 1958a, 1986b; Smith et al., 1988; Weber et al., 1986).

I. Accumulation of milk in the posterior oral cavity triggers a swallow.

VII. Factors That Influence Suckling and/or Contribute to Ineffective Suckling

Although it is difficult to list all the possible causes of dysfunction, several categories can be described along with examples of specific problems in each category.

A. Anomalies of the face, mouth, or pharynx.

1. Cleft lip/palate.

2. Macroglossia: excessively large tongue.

3. Micrognathia: recessed jaw and posteriorly placed tongue.

4. Ankyloglossia: short/tight frenulum ("tongue-tie").

5. High palatal arch: bubble palate.

B. Dysfunction of the central or peripheral nervous system or musculature.

1. Muscular dystrophy.

2. Cerebral palsy.

3. Prematurity.

4. Down syndrome.

5. Asphyxia.

6. Intracranial hemorrhage.

7. CNS infection (for example, toxoplasmosis, cytomegalovirus, or bacterial meningitis).

C. Miscellaneous.

1. Maternal analgesia/anesthesia.
   a. Rosen and Lawrence (1994) reported no effect of intrapartum anesthesia on ability to suckle or on initial weight loss.
   b. Riordan et al. (2000) reported lower suckling scores in infants whose mothers had epidural anesthesia, but the difference was not significant.
   c. Bader and colleagues (1995, 1992) concluded that even when maintained for many hours, continuous infusion labor analgesia does not appear to result in significant fetal drug accumulation. Measurable levels of bupivacaine were found in umbilical cord blood, the significance of which remains unclear.
   d. Murray reported measurable effects on neonatal neurobehavior in infants whose mothers had epidural anesthesia (Murray et al., 1981).
   e. Meperidine was associated with broad depression on most items on the Early Neonatal Neurobehavioral Scale (Hodgkinson, Bhatt, & Wang, 1978).
   f. Baumgarder and colleagues (2003) found that epidurals had a negative effect on breastfeeding during the first 24 hours.
   g. In a 2006 study, Torvaldsen et al. found links between epidurals and the following:
      i. Supplementation in the first week postpartum.
      ii. Reporting breastfeeding problems in the first week postpartum.
      iii. Cessation of breastfeeding before 24 weeks.

2. Maternal medications taken during the prenatal period.
   a. In addition to recreational drugs, some prescription medications can cause withdrawal symptoms and early feeding problems in the newborn, e.g., selective serotonin reuptake inhibitors (Nordeng et al., 2001).
   b. The widespread use of herbal drugs during pregnancy indicates an increased need for documentation about the safety of herbal drugs in pregnancy (Nordeng & Havnen, 2004).

3. Birth factors.
   a. Birth related factors including but not limited to duration of labor, mode of delivery, and vacuum extraction may contribute to early lactation failure (Dewey & Lonnerdal, 1986; Sievers et al., 2003; Vestermark, Hogdall, & Birch, 1990).
   b. Newborns delivered with vacuum extraction assistance have a higher rate of breastfeeding difficulties and an increased rate of weaning by 7 to 10 days of age (Hall et al., 2002).

4. Separation of mother and infant.
   a. Rooming-in facilitates exclusive breastfeeding (Buranasin, 1991; Centuori et al., 1999; Lindenberg, Cabrera Artola, & Jimenez, 1990; Perez-Escamilla et al., 1994; Yamauchi & Yamanouchi, 1990).

5. Hospital policies or practices that limit the length and/or frequency of breastfeeding.
   a. Hospital policies and practices impact the establishment of effective breastfeeding (Awi & Alikor, 2004; Braun et al., 2003; Philipp et al., 2003; Philipp & Merewood, 2004; Strembel et al., 1991; Widstrom et al., 1990; World Health Organization, 1998; World Health Organization/United Nations International Children's Emergency Fund, 1990).

6. Early introduction of artificial nipples and/or breast milk substitutes.
   a. Early use of supplement or pacifiers is associated with an increased risk for early weaning (Blomquist et al., 1994; Casiday et al., 2004; Hill et al., 1997; Howard et al., 2003; Kramer et al., 2001; Kurinij & Shiono, 1991).

7. Hyperbilirubinemia/kernicterus (Bertini et al., 2001; Hall, Simon, & Smith, 2000; Nylander et al., 1991).

8. Environmental temperature.
   a. Sucking pressure decreases as room temperature increases from 80 to 90 degrees F or 26.6 to 32.2 degrees C (Anderson, 1982).

9. Pain in the oral cavity.
   a. Herpes simplex lesions.
   b. Thrush.
   c. Oral trauma secondary to suctioning, intubation, etc.

Conclusion

Despite the available data, there is much to be learned about the complex activity of infant suckling. Through the use of advanced ultrasound technology, researchers are now able to visualize the breastfeeding infant and the lactating breast for sustained periods of time. Clear distinctions between the two mechanisms of infant feeding (breastfeeding and bottle-feeding) are emerging. Foremost among the findings is the remarkable adaptability of the human infant.

References

Anderson G. Development of sucking in term infants from birth to four hours post birth. *Res Nurs Health.* 1982;5:21–27.

Ardran G, Kemp F, Lind J. A cineradiographic study of bottle-feeding. *Br J Radiol.* 1958a;31:11–22.

Ardran G, Kemp F, Lind J. A cineradiographic study of breast-feeding. *Br J Radiol.* 1958b;31:156–162.

Arvedson J, Brodsky L. *Pediatric Swallowing and Feeding.* San Diego: Singular; 1993.

Awi DD, Alikor EA. The influence of pre- and post-partum factors on the time of contact between mother and her new-born after vaginal delivery. *Niger J Med.* 2004; 13:272–275.

Bader AM, Fragneto R, Terui K, et al. Maternal and neonatal fentanyl and bupivacaine concentrations after epidural infusion during labor. *Anesth Analg.* 1995;81:829–832.

Bader AM, Ray N, Datta S. Continuous epidural infusion of alfentanil and bupivacaine for labor and delivery. *Int J Obstet Anesth.* 1992;1:187–190.

Baumgarder D, Muehl P, Fischer M, Pribbenow B. Effect of labor epidural anesthesia on breastfeeding of healthy full-term newborns delivered vaginally. *J Am Board Fam Pract.* 2003;16:7–13.

Bertini G, Dani C, Tronchin M, Rubaltelli FF. Is breastfeeding really favoring early neonatal jaundice? *Pediatrics.* 2001;107:E41.

Blomquist HK, Jonsbo F, Serenius F, Persson LA. Supplementary feeding in the maternity ward shortens the duration of breast feeding. *Acta Paediatr.* 1994;83: 1122–1126.

Bosma K. Postnatal otogeny of performances of the pharynx, larynx and mouth. *Am Rev Respir Dis.* 1985;131:S10–S15.

Bowen-Jones A, Thompson C, Drewett RF. Milk flow and sucking rates during breast-feeding. *Dev Med Child Neurol.* 1982;24:626–633.

Brake S, Fifer W, Alfasi G, Fleischman A. The first nutritive sucking responses of premature newborns. *Infant Behav Dev.* 1988;11:1–9.

Braun ML, Giugliani ER, Soares ME, et al. Evaluation of the impact of the baby-friendly hospital initiative on rates of breastfeeding. *Am J Public Health.* 2003;93: 1277–1279.

Buranasin B. The effects of rooming-in on the success of breastfeeding and the decline in abandonment of children. *Asia Pac J Public Health.* 1991;5:217–220.

Casaer P, Daniels H, Devlieger H, et al. Feeding behavior in preterm neonates. *Early Hum Dev.* 1982;7:331–346.

Casiday RE, Wright CM, Panter-Brick C, Parkinson KN. Do early infant feeding patterns relate to breast-feeding continuation and weight gain? Data from a longitudinal cohort study. *Eur J Clin Nutr.* 2004;58:1290–1296.

Centuori S, Burmaz T, Ronfani L, et al. Nipple care, sore nipples, and breastfeeding: a randomized trial. *J Hum Lact.* 1999;15:125–130.

Dewey KG, Lonnerdal B. Infant self-regulation of breast milk intake. *Acta Paediatr Scand.* 1986;75:893–898.

Diamant N. Development of esophageal function. *Am Rev Respir Dis.* 1985; 131:S29–S32.

Ellison S, Vidyasagar V, Anderson G. Sucking in the newborn infant during the first hour of life. *J Nurse Midwifery.* 1979;24:18–25.

Fisher S, Painter M, Milmoe G. Swallowing disorders in infancy. *Pediatr Clin North Am.* 1981;28:845–853.

Hack M, Estabrook M, Robertson S. Development of sucking rhythms in preterm infants. *Early Hum Dev.* 1985;11:133–140.

Hall RT, Mercer AM, Teasley SL, et al. A breastfeeding assessment score to evaluate the risk for cessation of breastfeeding by 7 to 10 days of age. *J Pediatr.* 2002; 141:659–664.

Hall RT, Simon S, Smith MT. Readmission of breastfed infants in the first 2 weeks of life. *J Perinatol.* 2000;20:432–437.

Hauck FR, Herman SM, Donovan M, et al. Sleep environment and the risk of sudden infant death syndrome in an urban population: the Chicago Infant Mortality Study. *Pediatrics.* 2003;111:1207–1214.

Hill PD, Humenick SS, Brennan ML, Woolley D. Does early supplementation affect long-term breastfeeding? *Clin Pediatr.* (Phila) 1997;36:345–350.

Hodgkinson R, Bhatt M, Wang C. Double-blind comparison of the neurobehavior of neonates following the administration of different doses of meperidine to the mother. *Can Anaesth Soc J.* 1978;25:405–411.

Howard CR, Howard FM, Lanphear B, et al. Randomized clinical trial of pacifier use and bottle-feeding or cupfeeding and their effect on breastfeeding. *Pediatrics.* 2003;111:511–518.

Ianniruberto A, Tajani E. Ultrasonographic study of fetal movements. *Semin Perinatol.* 1981;5:175–181.

Ingram J, Hunt L, Woolridge M, Greenwood R. The association of progesterone, infant formula use and pacifier use with the return of menstruation in breast-feeding women: a prospective cohort study. *Eur J Obstet Gynecol Reprod Biol.* 2004;114:197–202.

Kahn A, Groswasser J, Franco P, et al. Sudden infant deaths: stress, arousal and SIDS. *Early Hum Dev.* 2003;75(Suppl):S147–S166.

Kennedy J, Kent R. Physiologic substrates of normal deglutition. *Dysphagia.* 1988;3:24–27.

Kramer MS, Barr RG, Dagenais S, et al. Pacifier use, early weaning, and cry/fuss behavior: a randomized controlled trial. *JAMA.* 2001;286:322–326.

Kurinij N, Shiono PH. Early formula supplementation of breast-feeding. *Pediatrics.* 1991;88:745–750.

Lawrence RA. *Breastfeeding: A Guide for the Medical Profession.* 6th ed. St. Louis: C.V. Mosby; 2005.

Lindenberg CS, Cabrera Artola R, Jimenez V. The effect of early post-partum mother-infant contact and breast-feeding promotion on the incidence and continuation of breast-feeding. *Int J Nurs Stud.* 1990;27:179–186.

Meites J. Neuroendocrinology of lactation. *J Invest Dermatol.* 1974;63:119–124.

Miller M, Martin R, Carlo W. Oral breathing in newborn infants. *J Pediatr.* 1985;107:465–469.

Mizuno K, Ueda A. Changes in sucking performance from nonnutritive sucking to nutritive sucking during breast- and bottle-feeding. *Pediatr Res.* 2005;59:728–731.

Morris S. *The Normal Acquisition of Oral Feeding Skills: Implications for Assessment and Treatment.* Central Islip: Therapeutic Media; 1982.

Murray A, Dolby R, Nation R, Thomas DB. Effects of epidural anesthesia on newborns and their mothers. *Child Dev.* 1981;52:71–82.

Nordeng H, Havnen GC. Use of herbal drugs in pregnancy: a survey among 400 Norwegian women. *Pharmacoepidemiol Drug Saf.* 2004;13:371–380.

Nordeng H, Lindemann R, Perminov KV, Reikvam A. Neonatal withdrawal syndrome after in utero exposure to selective serotonin reuptake inhibitors. *Acta Paediatr.* 2001;90:288–291.

Nylander G, Lindemann R, Helsing E, Bendvold E. Unsupplemented breastfeeding in the maternity ward. Positive long-term effects. *Acta Obstet Gynecol Scand.* 1991;70:205–209.

Nysenbaum A, Smart J. Sucking behavior and milk intake of neonates in relation to milk fat content. *Early Hum Dev.* 1982;6:205–213.

Perez-Escamilla R, Pollitt E, Lonnerdal B, Dewey KG. Infant feeding policies in maternity wards and their effect on breast-feeding success: an analytical overview. *Am J Public Health.* 1994;84:89–97.

Philipp BL, Malone KL, Cimo S, Merewood A. Sustained breastfeeding rates at a US baby-friendly hospital. *Pediatrics.* 2003;112:234–236.

Philipp BL, Merewood A. The baby-friendly way: the best breastfeeding start. *Pediatr Clin North Am.* 2004;51:761–783, xi.

Pritchard J. Fetal swallowing and amniotic fluid volume. *Obstet Gynecol.* 1966;28:606–610.

Ramsay DT, Kent JC, Owens RA, Hartmann PE. Ultrasound imaging of milk ejection in the breast of lactating women. *Pediatrics.* 2004;113:361–367.

Righard L, Alade MO. Effect of delivery room routines on success of first breast-feed. *Lancet.* 1990;336:1105–1107.

Riordan J, Gross A, Angeron J, et al. The effect of labor pain relief medication on neonatal suckling and breastfeeding duration. *J Hum Lact.* 2000;16:7–10.

Rodenstein D, Perlmutter N, Stanescu D. Infants are not obligatory nose breathers. *Am Rev Respir Dis.* 1985;131:343–347.

Rosen A, Lawrence R. The effect of epidural anesthesia on infant feeding. *Journal of the University of Rochester Medical Center.* 1994;6:3.

Sievers E, Haase S, Oldigs HD, Schaub J. The impact of peripartum factors on the onset and duration of lactation. *Biol Neonate.* 2003;83:246–252.

Smith WL, Erenberg A, Nowak A. Imaging evaluation of the human nipple during breast-feeding. *Am J Dis Child.* 1988;142:76–78.

Strembel S, Sass S, Cole G, Hartner J, Fischer C. Breast-feeding policies and routines among Arizona hospitals and nursery staff: results and implications of a descriptive study. *J Am Diet Assoc.* 1991;91:923–925.

Torvaldsen S, Roberts CL, Simpson JM, Thompson JF, Ellwood DA. Intrapartum epidural analgesia and breastfeeding: a prospective cohort study. *Int Breastfeed J.* 2006 Dec 11;1:24.

Tucker J. Perspective of the development of the air and food passages. *Am Rev Respir Dis.* 1985;131:S7–S9.

Ullah S, Griffiths P. Does the use of pacifiers shorten breastfeeding duration in infants? Br *J Community Nurs.* 2003;8:458–463.

Vestermark V, Hogdall C, Birch M. Influence of the mode of delivery on initiation of breastfeeding. *Eur J Obstet Gynecol Reprod Biol.* 1990;38:33.

Viggiano D, Fasano D, Monaco G, Strohmenger L. Breast feeding, bottle feeding, and non-nutritive sucking; effects on occlusion in deciduous dentition. *Arch Dis Child.* 2004;89:1121–1123.

Voloschin LM, Althabe O, Olive H, et al. A new tool for measuring the suckling stimulus during breastfeeding in humans: the orokinetogram and the Fourier series. *J Reprod Fertil.* 1998; 114:219–224.

Weber F, Woolridge M, Baum J. An ultrasonographic study of the organization of sucking and swallowing by newborn infants. *Dev Med Child Neurol.* 1986;28:19–24.

Widstrom AM, Marchini G, Matthiesen AS, et al. Nonnutritive sucking in tube-fed preterm infants: effects on gastric motility and gastric contents of somatostatin. *J Pediatr Gastroenterol Nutr.* 1988;7:517–523.

Widstrom AM, Wahlberg V, Matthiesen AS, et al. Short-term effects of early suckling and touch of the nipple on maternal behaviour. *Early Hum Dev.* 1990; 21:153–163.

Wilson S, Thach B, Brouillet R. Upper airway patency in the human infant: influence of airway pressure and posture. *J Appl Physiol.* 1980;48:500–504.

Wolf L, Glass R. *Feeding and Swallowing Disorders in Infancy Assessment and Management.* San Antonio: Therapy Skill Builders; 1992.

Wolff P. The serial organization of sucking in the young infant. *Pediatrics.* 1968; 42:943–956.

Wolff P. The interaction of state and non-nutritive sucking. In: Bosma J, ed. *Oral Sensation and Perception.* Springfield, MO: Charles C Thomas: 1972:293–312.

Woolridge MW. The anatomy of infant suckling. *Midwifery.* 1986a;2:164–171.

Woolridge MW. Aetiology of sore nipples. *Midwifery.* 1986b;2:172–176.

Woolridge MW, Baum JD, Drewett RF. Does a change in the composition of human milk affect sucking patterns and milk intake? *Lancet.* 1980;2:1292–1293.

Woolridge MW, How TV, Drewett RF, et al. The continuous measurement of milk intake at a feed in breast-fed babies. *Early Hum Dev.* 1982;6:365–373.

World Health Organization. *Evidence for the Ten Steps to Successful Breastfeeding,* (revised ed). Unpublished manuscript; 1998.

World Health Organization/United Nations International Children's Emergency Fund. (1990). Protecting, promoting and supporting breastfeeding: the special role of maternity services. A joint WHO/UNICEF statement. *Int J Gynaecol Obstet.* 1990; 31(Suppl 1):171–183.

Yamauchi Y, Yamanouchi I. The relationship between rooming-in/not rooming-in and breast-feeding variables. *Acta Paediatr Scand.* 1990;79:1017–1022.

Part

4

Nutrition and Biochemistry

NUTRITION FOR LACTATING WOMEN

Genevieve Becker, IBCLC, MSc, Reg Nutr
Revised by Michelle Scott, MA, RD/LD, CSP, IBCLC

OBJECTIVES

- Discuss the nutritional recommendations for pregnant women and breastfeeding women.
- Explain weight patterns during pregnancy and lactation.
- Describe the effects of the maternal diet on breast milk composition.
- Suggest suitable food choices, taking into account cultural practices and individual preferences.
- Evaluate the need for referral to a nutrition specialist or to another health care specialist.
- Discuss the value of food supplements and additives.

Introduction

A woman's nutrition can affect her health and the health of her child. Women might be particularly motivated to make nutritional changes during pregnancy and breast-feeding (Olson, 2005). Misconceptions abound regarding the amounts and types of foods to consume or avoid. Each mother presents with her own unique nutritional status and history, eating patterns, and food beliefs. The lactation consultant needs to provide information and suggestions that are compatible with the woman's lifestyle and beliefs, and that are within the woman's ability to understand and utilize. This chapter covers the basic information that the lactation consultant might need when assisting the mother. The goals are to provide appropriate nutrition information and recommendations, to identify women at nutritional risk, and to refer to a nutritionist or dietitian as necessary.

I. Assessment and Referral

The following risk factors that occur during pre-conception, pregnancy, or while breastfeeding indicate the need for the woman to be referred for detailed assessment and advice from a certified nutritionist or registered/licensed dietitian.

    A. *Body mass index (BMI).*

        1. A BMI of less than 19.8 (very underweight; Figure 16-1).

        2. BMI is calculated by weight divided by height squared.

        3. A BMI of > 26 (overweight is usually considered a BMI of 26–30; > 30 is considered obese).

    B. Teenagers who are within less than four years of menarche.

        1. Diets of teens are often low in iron and other nutrients, and they are still growing themselves (IOM, 1990).

    C. Medical conditions.

        1. Conditions such as: type 1 diabetes (insulin dependent), type 2 diabetes (non-insulin dependent), or gestational diabetes; women who have had bariatric surgery, gastrointestinal malabsorption conditions, metabolic diseases such as phenylketonuria (PKU), or eating disorders.

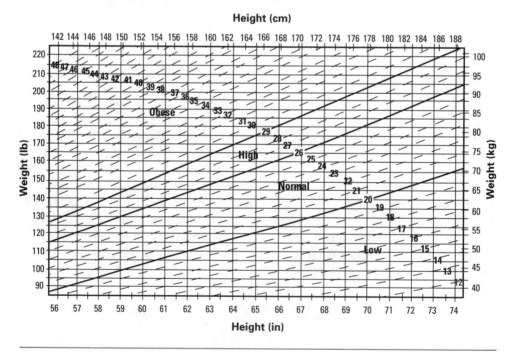

Figure 16-1   Chart for estimating BMI category and BMI

      a. Insulin requirements in a diabetic mother will change following delivery and during lactation.

      b. Type 1 diabetes can delay lactogenesis for up to three days (Neubauer et al., 1993).

      c. Postpartum mothers may need to increase their carbohydrate intake and/or their insulin dosage. Monitoring blood sugars is necessary for diabetic women and recommended for gestational diabetics based on their physician's recommendations (IOM, 1991).

      d. Blood sugar that is too low could lead to diabetic shock, releasing epinephrine into the mother's system and potentially inhibiting the milk ejection reflex and milk production.

  2. Self-diagnosed allergy or other special diets that exclude a major food group may create nutrient imbalances.

  3. Higher-order multiples.

  4. Excessive recent weight gain or weight loss.

  5. Teen pregnancies and closely spaced pregnancies ($<$ 18 months apart, including miscarriages; King, 2003).

  6. Poor nutrition intake might be a marker for other health problems.

  7. Poverty, cultural beliefs, physical disability, limited intellectual ability, or psychological problems might restrict food choices.

D. Refer mothers for dietary assessment to a nutritionist or dietitian, and/or refer to social service programs such as Women, Infants and Children (WIC) Program in the United States, food banks, and pregnancy/family programs.

II. General Nutritional Recommendations

A. Pre-conception.

  1. The lactation consultant might see a few women before their first pregnancy; however, the time after the birth of one child might be the pre-conception period before the next pregnancy. Therefore, because most lactating women have the possibility of becoming pregnant, the life cycle nutrition for women either pregnant or breastfeeding should be considered as a routine part of health care.

B. Recommendations to lactating women.

  1. Establish a healthy eating pattern that includes a variety of foods (Figure 16-2).

  2. Aim for the recommended normal weight range using BMI guidelines (Figure 16-1).

  3. Either severe underweight or overweight conditions can affect the ability to conceive.

  4. Low pre-pregnancy maternal weight is linked with low infant birth weight.

Anatomy of MyPyramid

One size doesn't fit all

USDA's new MyPyramid symbolizes a personalized approach to healthy eating and physical activity. The symbol has been designed to be simple. It has been developed to remind consumers to make healthy food choices and to be active every day. The different parts of the symbol are described below.

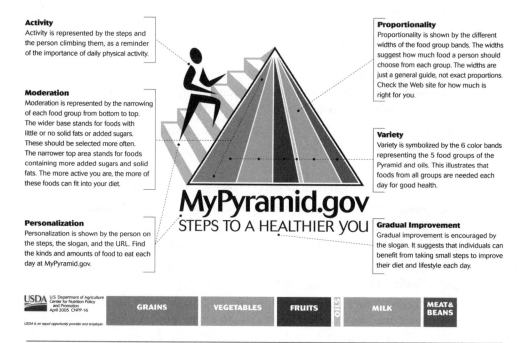

Activity
Activity is represented by the steps and the person climbing them, as a reminder of the importance of daily physical activity.

Moderation
Moderation is represented by the narrowing of each food group from bottom to top. The wider base stands for foods with little or no solid fats or added sugars. These should be selected more often. The narrower top area stands for foods containing more added sugars and solid fats. The more active you are, the more of these foods can fit into your diet.

Personalization
Personalization is shown by the person on the steps, the slogan, and the URL. Find the kinds and amounts of food to eat each day at MyPyramid.gov.

Proportionality
Proportionality is shown by the different widths of the food group bands. The widths suggest how much food a person should choose from each group. The widths are just a general guide, not exact proportions. Check the Web site for how much is right for you.

Variety
Variety is symbolized by the 6 color bands representing the 5 food groups of the Pyramid and oils. This illustrates that foods from all groups are needed each day for good health.

Gradual Improvement
Gradual improvement is encouraged by the slogan. It suggests that individuals can benefit from taking small steps to improve their diet and lifestyle each day.

MyPyramid.gov
STEPS TO A HEALTHIER YOU

USDA U.S. Department of Agriculture
Center for Nutrition Policy
and Promotion
April 2005 CNPP-16

USDA is an equal opportunity provider and employer.

GRAINS   VEGETABLES   FRUITS   OILS   MILK   MEAT & BEANS

Figure 16-2 The food guide pyramid. *Source:* Courtesy of the United States Department of Agriculture (USDA).

5. Reduce weight in advance of conception to lessen the risk of nutritional inadequacy that can be caused by women on a restricted diet. This can occur because of the mother's desire to comply with weight gain restrictions in pregnancy, or through a poor understanding of a nutritious diet.

6. The health care professional should accurately measure and weigh the mother and not strictly rely on the mother's self-report.

7. Ensure that blood iron levels are assessed and corrected if needed by dietary advice and/or supplementation. Hemoglobin below 12.0 g/dL or serum ferritin below 20 μg/dL are indications of iron deficiency anemia in the non-pregnant woman.

8. Ensure a folic acid supplement to reduce the risk of neural tube defects. This should be recommended for all women in their childbearing years, because about half of all pregnancies are unplanned, and folic acid is preventative in the immediate post-conception period.

9. Recommend steps to reduce risk of foodborne illness, such as *Lysteria, E. coli,* and *Salmonella.* The U.S. Food and Drug Administration (FDA) provides information on food safety for pregnant and postpartum women in English and Spanish at www.cfsan.fda.gov/~pregnant/pregnant.html.

C. Pregnancy

1. Good nutrition during pregnancy provides nutrients for optimum fetal growth as well as stores of some nutrients for lactation. Foods contain nutrients that are not captured in the vitamin/mineral supplements. Eating fortified nutrition bars and other fortified foods is not equivalent to eating a varied, healthy diet.

2. Pregnancy enhances fat deposition.

3. Fetal growth retardation, some congenital defects, and maternal anemia are linked to poor nutritional status during pregnancy.

4. Low maternal weight gain during pregnancy also has been associated with diminished milk production and lower fat concentration in breast milk (Figure 16-3).

5. Obesity is linked with maternal hypertension, greater risk of birth interventions, impaired glucose tolerance, and type 2 diabetes.

6. Excessive energy restriction during pregnancy might restrict other nutrient intakes and possibly lead to ketosis, which can compromise fetal mental development.

7. Most women store 2 to 4 kg (4.8–9.6 lb) of fat during pregnancy in preparation for lactation.

8. Recommendations.
   a. Eat a healthy diet of: two to three servings of protein; two to three servings of dairy or a calcium equivalent; five to nine servings of fruits/vegetables; and six or more servings of carbohydrates. Vegans will need a source of vitamin B_{12}; usually a prenatal vitamin is sufficient. Make sure women understand serving sizes if recommending following the food guide.
   b. Chart weight gain during pregnancy by referring to the guide in Figure 16-3.
   c. Take nutrition supplements, including folic acid, as recommended by health professionals.
   d. Avoid non-prescribed supplements, especially vitamin A (or retinol in skin preparations), since excess vitamin A is a known teratogen (mutagen that can cause birth defects). (Food and Nutrition Information Center at: www.nal.usda.gov/fnic/pubs/bibs/gen/dietsupp.html.)

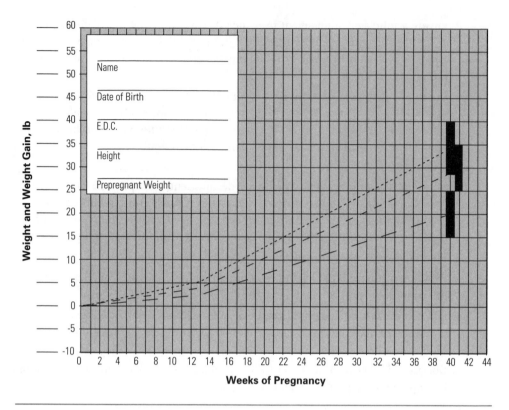

Figure 16-3 Prenatal weight gain chart

---

　　　　e. Reduce the intake of caffeine (if greater than 300 mg) and food additives if
　　　　 high.
　　　　f. Docosahexaenoic acid (DHA) supplements, either prenatally or postpartum,
　　　　 have not been shown to be necessary to ensure adequate DHA levels in
　　　　 breast milk.
　　　　g. Avoid smoking and smoky areas, alcohol, and non-prescribed medicines or
　　　　 street drugs.
　D. Labor, birth, and the hospital stay.
　　　1. Routine fasting during labor has not been shown by controlled trials to reduce
　　　　 the risk of Mendelson syndrome (a type of pneumonia caused by aspiration of
　　　　 fluids) and might have negative effects on the mother and her baby.
　　　2. Hospital menus might not reflect the cultural diets of all patients.
　　　3. Mothers should not have to choose between eating their own meal and feeding
　　　　 their infant; therefore, flexibility in the facility's meal service is needed,
　　　　 including ways to keep food cold or warm.

E. Lactation.

1. Lactation is a normal physiologic process for a woman who is generally healthy.

2. Special diets or foods are not needed.

3. Mothering is hard work, and all mothers who are caring for young children need to eat well, although not perfectly every single day.

4. Lactation increases the body's efficiency in its use of energy and the uptake of some nutrients.

5. Recommendations.
   a. Eat a varied and healthy diet (see C.8.a).
   b. Drink to satisfy thirst, using water as the main beverage. High-sugar content beverages are not recommended due to their low micronutrient content.
   c. Weight loss should be gradual, at not more than 1 lb (0.5 kg) per week. Calories used in making breast milk, healthy food choices (5 or more servings of fruits/vegetables), and gentle exercise will all help to achieve a weight loss (Hammer & Hinterman, 1998).
   d. Lactating women need a diet that is about 50% to 55% calories from carbohydrates, 12% to 15% from protein, and about 30% or less from fats.
   e. Avoid trans-fatty acids such as the ones in most processed foods (like crackers, baked goods, and snack products). These fatty acids appear in breast milk and can increase cardiovascular risk in the mother; little is known regarding their safety for infants (Mozaffarian et al., 2006).

F. Energy.

1. The caloric cost of producing one liter of milk is approximately 940 calories. This is based on an average mother's milk production of 750 mL/day. Each mL is about 0.67 calories plus some energy for the metabolic cost of milk synthesis.

2. Women often are told or read that breastfeeding a baby will require about 500 extra calories per day. However, in practice, most women have varied calorie needs based on their size, activity level, and age. About 300 to 400 calories a day can be used from fats stored prenatally, and the remaining calories will be taken in if the woman eats nutritious foods in response to hunger (Butte, 1984).

G. Protein.

1. The recommended intake is 65 grams/day during the first six months of lactation and 62 g/day during the second six months of lactation, with some individual variations in needs depending on age, level of activity, etc. (Example: 4 oz of meat at about 28 g + 24 oz milk at 24 g + 5 servings of carbohydrates at about 15 g = total of about 67 g of protein.)

2. Women typically get most of their protein from meat and dairy products.

3. Vegetarians and vegans should be getting their protein from a variety of the following foods: beans/legumes (includes soy), whole grains, nuts, and seeds. This assures them of getting all the necessary amino acids (Mangels, 2006).

H. Vitamins and minerals.
1. Refer to appropriate food guides, such as the 2006 recommended U.S. dietary intake guidelines (Web site: http://www.nal.usda.gov/fnic/etext/000105.html).
   a. Dietary reference intakes are a set of four nutrient-based reference values that expand upon and include the recommended dietary allowances (RDA).
   b. For most purposes and most nutrients, using the RDA will be sufficient to assess a woman's nutrition status.
   c. However, upper intake level may be needed to determine the possible danger of excess nutrient intake.
2. Iron.
   a. Ideally, anemia should be corrected pre-conception.
   b. Supplements should be used selectively because they have side effects, including teratogenicity, constipation, and nausea.
   c. Absorption of iron increases during pregnancy, so women with good iron stores prior to pregnancy do not need to be automatically supplemented.
   d. Hemodilution (increased blood volume) during pregnancy is normal and affects hemoglobin measurements; serum ferritin is a better indicator at this time.
   e. Iron levels in breast milk are not affected by maternal blood levels (WHO, 1998).
   f. Taking iron supplements with a source of vitamin C, or eating meats with foods such as broccoli, radishes, fresh cooked potatoes (not processed), or fruits such as citrus fruits, strawberries, kiwi, and others will enhance absorption.
3. Vitamin D.
   a. Vitamin D is necessary for calcium absorption.
   b. Food sources of vitamin D are limited to fortified milk, butter, eggs, and oily fish.
   c. Exposing the skin to sunlight causes the body to synthesize vitamin D. Normal exposure of sun to face and hands in all climates, and arms/legs during warmer weather, is usually enough to stimulate adequate stores of vitamin D.
   d. If sunlight is restricted due to climate, clothing, lifestyle, or beliefs, then a supplement of 400 IU should be taken by the mother. Large amounts of vitamin D, greater than 2000 IU is currently not recommended, but this may change. Babies whose mothers had adequate vitamin D stores during pregnancy will have a good start on their own vitamin D needs. Mother's milk and some sun exposure will continue to offer the necessary vitamin D.
   e. Dark-skinned babies and children who receive the minimum exposure to sun or live in a northern climate may still need a vitamin D supplement or their mothers may benefit from high dose vitamin D supplementation.

    f. Low maternal stores of vitamin D will result in low levels in the mother's milk. A typical multivitamin supplement will contain 400 IU of vitamin D, and, depending on the deficit, larger doses of vitamin D should be given if levels are assessed. Doses of 1,000 to 3,000 IU should be monitored every three to six months because higher levels can reduce the effectiveness of calcium–vitamin D bone building.

    g. High-dose supplementation of the breastfeeding mother with 6400 IU/day has been shown to elevate both maternal and infant circulating levels of 25(OH)D. Infant levels achieved exclusively through maternal supplementation were equivalent to levels in infants who received oral vitamin D supplementation (Basile et al., 2006; Wagner et al., 2006).

4. Calcium.

    a. Calcium absorption is reduced in a diet that is centered around whole unprocessed grains because the phytate in grains has this effect. It is rarely a problem for women who eat fewer than two to three whole grain servings per day, but may be a concern in countries where diets may be based on whole grains.

    b. Maternal intake has little effect on breast milk levels of calcium; there are mixed conclusions regarding requirements during lactation (Prentice, 1994).

    c. Women who avoid or are allergic or intolerant of dairy products might need other food choices that are high in calcium or, if this is not possible, 600 mg/day of elemental calcium may be necessary.

    d. Bone loss occurs during lactation even when dietary calcium is thought to be adequate. Remineralization takes place following the return of the menses, which ultimately results in more dense bones for well nourished, multi-para, breastfeeding women. The more babies and months a mother breastfeeds, the lesser the risk for osteoporosis.

5. Fluid.

    a. Increasing fluid intake does not increase milk supply unless the mother is severely dehydrated.

    b. Decreasing fluid intake does not reduce engorgement or suppress a high milk volume.

    c. Forcing fluids beyond what the body requires can decrease milk production (Dusdieker et al., 1990).

    d. If maternal urine is scant or dark colored, suggest an increase in fluid intake.

    e. Water is the best fluid for hydration. Sugary or salty fluids will increase thirst and are needed only in strenuous exercise of more than several hours.

    f. Remind mothers that it is not necessary to drink milk to make milk, but that two servings of dairy products provide protein, calcium, and some B vitamins as well as some fluid.

I. Recommended Intake.

1. A diet containing less than the recommended intake of calories is not necessarily deficient in a particular nutrient; however, it indicates a need for further assessment.

"Women living under a wide variety of circumstances in the United States and elsewhere are capable of fully nourishing their infants by breastfeeding them."

"Mothers are able to produce milk of sufficient quantity and quality to support growth and promote the health of infants—even when the mother's supply of nutrients and energy is limited."

(Nutrition During Lactation, Institute of Medicine, 1991)

J. Weight patterns.

1. In the past, mothers were advised to consume high levels of nutrients; however, it is now known that a lactating woman's body is very efficient at producing milk (Frigerio et al., 1991).

2. Body stores provide about 200 to 300 calories per day.

3. An increase of 300 to 500 calories per day (over non-pregnant requirements) is often recommended and can be met by nutritious snacks or additions to meals. Many women consume less than this amount and their babies grow well.

4. Weight is linked to culture. A thin nursing mother might be viewed as ideal or as indicating that her family did not care for her well, depending on the culture.

5. Return to pre-pregnant weight is influenced by the following:
   a. Previous weight.
   b. Weight gain during pregnancy.
   c. Parity.
   d. Lifestyle and beliefs.
   e. Maternal age.
   f. Level of physical activity.
   g. Caloric intake.

6. Breastfeeding mothers tend to lose more weight than non-breastfeeding women (Kac et al., 2004).

7. Weight loss greater than 6.5 lb (3 kg) in the early weeks might indicate that sufficient food is not being consumed.

8. Most mothers can safely lose 0.5 to 1 pound/week (0.45 kg/week).

9. Lactating mothers typically consume between 1800 to 2200 calories per day with minimal weight changes.

10. Mothers should avoid crash or fad diets and diet medications.

K. Special nutritional needs.

   1. Young mothers.
      a. Young mothers are often still growing and thus have higher nutrient requirements; sometimes they eat nutrient-poor diets.
      b. Counseling might be needed to discuss food choices. Refer young mothers to nutritionists or dietitians with experience in guiding teens during pregnancy/lactation (WIC and some teen programs).

   2. Malnourished women.
      a. Improve the maternal food and nutrient intake to benefit both the mother and the baby.
      b. Feeding the breastfeeding mother is less expensive than providing breast milk substitutes.
      c. Inadequate nutrition is linked to socioeconomic issues, and purely nutritional interventions are unlikely to succeed if these issues are not also addressed.
      d. Severely malnourished mothers might have reduced breast milk levels of water soluble vitamins, lactose, and fat concentrations; however, infants who are allowed to self-regulate their intake will usually take sufficient lower fat milk to meet their needs.
      e. Nutrients in breast milk that are not usually affected by maternal status are: zinc, iron, folate, calcium, and copper.

   3. Eating disorders.
      a. A woman who has anorexia or bulimia (or a history of either) needs to be under the care of suitable health care and counseling professionals.
      b. Anorexia: Breast milk composition might be affected (see 2. Malnourished women).
      c. Concern for her infant's well-being might motivate an anorexic mother to address her disorder.
      d. Bulimia: Wide variations in intake might affect the mother's nutritional status, and the breast milk. Little information is available regarding breast milk production and bulimia.

   4. Multiples.
      a. During pregnancy, the mother might need to eat very small, frequent meals because of the womb pushing upward and limiting stomach capacity at any one meal.

b. During breastfeeding, nutrient needs are increased above the needs of a mother who is breastfeeding a single infant, but doubling the vitamin/mineral supplement can be unsafe (vitamin A is too high), and there is no research to support such a recommendation. Nutrients will be increased by increasing foods to meet caloric needs. Monitor to avoid excessive or rapid weight loss.

c. The mother might need to discuss ways of finding time to eat.

5. Breastfeeding and pregnancy.

a. Nutrient needs are generally increased, but the advice of taking two prenatal vitamin pills per day is not evidence-based. Large doses of vitamin A are not safe for pregnant women, because it can cause birth defects.

b. The mother might need suggestions on coping with morning sickness and finding time to eat while also caring for other children.

6. Vegetarian women.

a. Vegetarians who are knowledgeable about their diet can have very healthy diets. An appropriate diet usually contains nuts and beans as well as soy protein. The following are typical types of vegetarians:

i. Vegan. No animal proteins, including egg and milk.

ii. Semi-vegetarian. Eats vegetables, milk products, seafood, and poultry (they basically just avoid red meat).

iii. Lacto-vegetarian. Consumes milk and milk products in addition to plant foods.

iv. Lacto-ovo-vegetarian. Consumes plant foods, dairy products, and eggs but no meat, poultry, or seafood.

v. Ovo-vegetarian. Consumes plant foods and eggs.

vi. Fruitarian. Consumes fruits, nuts, olive oil, and honey.

vii. Macrobiotic. Eats foods that are organic, fresh, and seasonal. The advanced diet form is not usually nutritionally adequate for lactating women but can be adapted if the mother is willing.

b. Vegetarian mothers who do not regularly receive some exposure to the sun might need a vitamin D supplement. This includes mothers who reside in northern latitudes, work indoors, wear cultural clothing that covers their skin, or have dark skin.

c. Pregnant vegetarians should be encouraged to eat foods or supplements that are rich in vitamin B_{12} in order to enhance lactation.

d. Alternative sources for vitamin B_{12} include:

i. A vitamin supplement.

ii. Nutritional yeast products.

iii. Fortified cereals (read the label because not all are fortified with vitamin B_{12}).

iv. Fortified soy milk and meat substitutes made from soy.

7. Exercise.
   a. The mother who exercises strenuously (> 1 hour per day) will have increased energy needs.
   b. Moderate exercise has no adverse effect on breast milk, and elevated levels of lactic acid are not seen with moderate exercise.
   c. The possibility of breast refusal by the baby following extremely heavy exercise has been suggested to be caused by elevated levels of lactic acid, but this has not been associated with harm.
   d. Mothers can feed the baby before exercising if this concern is present.
   e. Breastfeeding and exercising are compatible, and both should be encouraged.

8. Socioeconomic effects on food choices.
   a. Higher levels of education often correlate to better diets.
   b. A lack of money might limit the food that is available as well as the facilities to store and prepare the food. Ask questions such as: "Do you have a working stove, oven, microwave, refrigerator?"
   c. Provide phone numbers and information to the mother for food assistance programs (such as WIC in the United States or equivalent programs throughout the world), Food Stamps, local food banks, or other agencies that may include this kind of assistance. Provide follow-up contact to see if the family gained access to services.
   d. Much of the mother's information might come from product advertisements.
   e. An opinion of what a healthy diet consists of might vary considerably; ask what is eaten regularly rather than "do you eat well".
   f. Imposing healthy eating rules that must be followed can make breastfeeding seem too difficult for some women. A more supportive approach is to present options and suggestions.
   g. Refer mothers who lack cooking skills, or need help with meal planning to a dietitian, or to a community food assistance program that has skilled personnel who teach food classes.

9. Cultural and religious beliefs.
   a. Upbringing, habits, and beliefs affect food practices.
   b. Lactation consultants should educate themselves regarding the food practices of any special populations they will encounter in their practice.
   c. Food practices that are different than what the lactation consultant typically encounters should not be changed unless there is evidenced-based information to show that a practice is harmful.
   d. Galactogogues, foods that are supposed to enhance milk production, are common in many cultures.

10. Time.
   a. Time is needed to shop for food, prepare the food, and eat the food. A mother has many demands on her time and snacking on convenience foods might be how she manages her time.

b. Suggest foods that are easy, quick to prepare, and that fit with the other demands on her time. Soups, sandwiches, and raw fruits or vegetables can provide the same nutrition as a hot meal.

c. Explore the availability of in-home help for women who are at particular nutritional risk.

III. Effects of Maternal Food Intake on the Breastfeeding Infant

A. Milk volume/composition.

1. Increasing maternal energy intake and fluid does not increase milk volume unless the mother is very severely malnourished or dehydrated.

2. Major nutrients and minerals, such as iron, zinc, folate, calcium, and copper, are provided at a stable level in breast milk at the expense of the mother's nutrient stores.

3. In the chronically malnourished woman, vitamin A and the B group of vitamins are likely to be low; therefore, breast milk levels of these vitamins might be low. Supplements equaling 100% of the RDA can be given, with higher doses only if there is a thorough nutrition assessment performed.

4. Consuming fewer than 1500 calories per day has been shown to decrease milk volumes.

5. The types of fatty acids in milk but not the overall fat content are influenced by the maternal diet.

6. Carbohydrate levels of breast milk are not affected by maternal intake; maternal diabetes does not affect breast milk carbohydrate levels.

7. Factors other than nutrition, particularly nursing behavior and stress, have a greater effect on milk supply.

B. Immunological effects.

1. An adaptive mechanism keeps the iron level in milk at an optimum level to preserve the bacterostatic role of lactoferrin.

2. Severely malnourished women might have slightly reduced levels of immunoglobulins in their milk, although studies are not conclusive.

C. Colic and allergy.

1. There is little evidence to support the belief that gassy or spicy foods, when eaten in moderation by the mother, cause problems to most breastfeeding infants.

2. If a food is suspected of causing a problem, it can be eliminated for two weeks; if symptoms reappear when the food is reintroduced, it might be wiser to avoid it.

3. Mothers who avoid a major food (such as wheat or dairy products) must give consideration to replacing those nutrients; referral to a dietitian should be given.

4. A mother who has a strong family history of milk protein intolerance might pass more beta-lactoglobulin through her milk, which could cause colic-like symptoms in her baby (Jakobsson, 1991).

5. In high-risk allergic families, mothers might be advised to avoid peanuts and other potent allergens during pregnancy and breastfeeding (http://www.foodallergynetwork.net).

D. Caffeine.

1. Caffeine ingested by the mother in moderate amounts (< 300 mg/day) does not cause a problem for most babies because the amount of caffeine available to the baby is 0.06% to 1.5% of the maternal dose (Hale, 2006).

2. Preterm or ill infants might not metabolize caffeine well, leading to accumulation and wakefulness or irritability.

3. Coffee has 80 to 100+ mg of caffeine per 8 oz cup. Caffeine is also in black and green teas, and a wide variety of soft drinks. Chocolate contains theobromines that have a similar effect as caffeine. A few ounces of chocolate are not likely to bother a baby, especially after the first month of life.

E. Herbs and herbal teas.

1. Normal amounts of common herbs used in cooking do not usually affect the baby.

2. Herbal teas are used in many cultures for lactating women; however, caution should be exercised because some herbs such as chaparral, comfrey, germander, pennyroyal, and blue cohosh have been documented to cause problems in the baby, such as hepatotoxicity, anticholinergic symptoms, and cardiotoxicity (Hale, 2006).

3. Health care professionals and parents should exercise caution because sometimes neither the origin of the herbs is known nor the conditions under which they were grown, mixed, or packaged, and the FDA does not regulate these.

F. Alcohol (Anderson, 1995; Pengelley & Gyte, 1996).

1. High intakes may impair the milk ejection reflex. Doses of more than 2 g/kg (for a 132 pound woman this is about 4 oz of liquor) may completely block the milk ejection reflex.

2. A number of factors influence maternal blood alcohol concentrations, including body weight, amount of adipose tissue, stomach contents, how fast the alcohol is consumed, and the amount of alcohol consumed.

3. Peak alcohol levels in milk occur in 30 to 60 minutes on an empty stomach, and in 60-90 minutes when consumed with food. It takes approximately 1½ to 2 hours per ounce to metabolize alcohol in the adult. The alcohol content of milk falls as the blood levels fall due to back diffusion of alcohol from the milk to the maternal bloodstream.

4. Alcohol passes freely into the milk, and in large amounts it may cause drowsiness, slow growth, and neurodevelopmental delays in the infant.

5. Infants detoxify alcohol in the first four weeks of life at a rate approximately one-half that of an adult.

6. A high alcohol intake impairs the mother's ability to safely care for her child.

G. Taste.

1. Breast milk flavor changes depending on the foods and spices that the mother consumes.

2. Babies whose mothers eat a variety of foods, including highly flavored foods, are more accepting of a variety of solids when introduced (Sullivan & Birch, 1994).

3. Babies suckled for 50% longer when milk was garlic flavored, and even longer when exposed to vanilla-flavored milk (Mennella, 1995).

4. Some babies will suck more when a novel flavor is introduced.

H. Food additives.

1. Artificial sweeteners.
   a. Aspartame metabolizes into phenylalanine and aspartic acid.
   b. Aspartame would pose a risk to those with the inborn error of PKU.
   c. Moderate amounts of aspartame (NutraSweet) beverages or foods may not be harmful. Hale (2006) cites levels of 50 mg/kg for a woman as producing three to four times the normal dose used, which would still be a very low dose in the breast milk.
   d. Caution should be taken due to lack of research.

IV. Consultation

As a lactation consultant who is carrying out a consult with a nutritional focus, it is helpful to have the following.

A. Basic nutrition knowledge in order to assess the mother's intake.

B. Awareness of the diversity of cultural practices.

C. Counseling skills to gather information and discuss choices.

D. Simple charting to record information that is gathered.

E. Education strategies to provide information to the mother.

F. Knowledge of other services that are available and how to refer to them.

References

Anderson PO. Alcohol and breastfeeding. *J Hum Lact.* 1995;11:321–323.

Basile LA, Taylor SN, Wagner CL, et al. The effect of high-dose vitamin D supplementation on serum vitamin D levels and milk calcium concentration in lactating women and their infants. *Breastfeeding Med.* 2006;1:27–35.

Dusdieker LB, Stumbo PJ, Booth BM, et al. Prolonged maternal fluid supplementation in breast-feeding. *Pediatrics.* 1990;86:737–740.

Frigerio C, Schutz Y, Prentice A, et al. Is human lactation a particularly efficient process? *Eur J Clin Nutr.* 1991;45:459–462.

Hale, *Medications and Mothers' Milk.* Pharmasoft Medical Publishing; 2006.

Hammer RL, Hinterman C. Exercise and dietary programming to promote maternal health fitness and weight management during lactation. *J Perinat Educ.* 1998; 7:13–26.

Institute of Medicine. *Nutrition During Lactation. Cross-cultural Counseling—a Guide for Nutrition and Health Counselors.* Washington, DC: National Academy Press; 1991.

Institute of Medicine. *Nutrition During Pregnancy.* Washington, DC: National Academy Press; 1990.

Jakobsson I. Food antigens in human milk. *Eur J Clin Nutr.* 1991;(suppl 1):29–33.

Kac G, Benicio MH, Velasquez-Melendez G, et al. Breastfeeding and postpartum weight retention in a cohort of Brazilian women. *Am J Clin Nutr.* 2004;79:487–493.

King J. The risk of maternal nutrition and poor outcomes increases in early or closely spaced pregnancies. *J Nutr.* 2003;45(suppl 2):1732S–1736S.

Mangels R. *The Vegan Diet During Pregnancy and Lactation.* The Vegetarian Resource Group and Mangels R. Available at: http://www.vrg.org/nutrition/veganpregnancy. htm. Accessed December 12, 2006.

Mennella JA. Mother's milk: a medium for early flavor experiences. *J Hum Lact.* 1995; 11:39–45.

Mozaffarian D, Katan MB, Ascherio A, et al. Trans fatty acids and cardiovascular disease. *N Engl J Md.* 2006;354(13):1601–1613.

Neubauer S, Ferris A, Chase C, et al. Delayed lactogenesis in women with insulin dependent diabetes. *Am J Clin Nutr.* 1993;58:54–60.

Olson CM. Tracking food choices across the transition to motherhood. *Nutri Edu Behav.* 2005;37:129–136.

Pengelley L, Gyte G. *Eating and Drinking in Labour, a Summary of the Medical Research to Facilitate Informed Choice.* United Kingdom: National Childbirth Trust; 1996.

Prentice A. Maternal calcium requirements during pregnancy and lactation. *Am J Clin Nutr.* 1994;59(suppl 2):477S–483S.

Sullivan SA, Birch LL. Infant dietary experience and acceptance of solid foods. *Pediatrics.* 1994;93:271–277.

Wagner CL, Hulsey TC, Fanning D, et al. High-dose vitamin D_3 supplementation in a cohort of breastfeeding mothers and their infants: a 6-month follow-up pilot study. *Breastfeeding Med.* 2006;1:59–70.

World Health Organization. WHO/NUT 98.1. *Complimentary Feeding of Young Children in Developing Countries: A Review of Current Scientific Knowledge.* Geneva: WHO; 1998.

Suggested Readings

Food Allergy and Anaphylaxis Network. (A resource for information regarding foods to avoid, processed food contaminants, etc.) Available at: http://www.foodallergy.org. Accessed December 12, 2006.

Food and Nutrition Information Center, National Agricultural Library, U.S. Department of Agriculture, Agricultural Research Service. Extensive resource list on dietary supplements). Available at: http://www.nal.usda.gov/fnic/pubs/bibs/gen/dietsupp.html. Accessed December 12, 2006.

Food Safety Office, Centers for Disease Control and Prevention, Department of Health and Human Services. Available at: http www.cdc.gov/foodsafety. Accessed December 12, 2006.

Hattevig G, Sigurs N, Kjellman B. Effects of dietary avoidance during lactation on allergy in children at 10 years of age. *Acta Paediatr.* 1999;88:7–12.

Michaelsen KF, Larsen PS, Thomsen BL, Samuelson G. The Copenhagen Cohort Study on infant nutrition and growth: breast milk intake, human milk macronutrient content, and influencing factors. *Am J Clin Nutr.* 1994:59:600–611.

Office of Dietary Supplements. National Institutes of Health (NIH). Bethesda, MD: NIH. Available at: http://www.ods.od.nih.gov/. Accessed December 12, 2006.

Sadauskaiter-Kuehne V, Ludviqsson J, Padaiqa Z, et al. Longer breastfeeding is an independent protective factor against the development of type 1 diabetes mellitus in childhood. *Diabetes Metab Res Rev.* 2004;20:150–157.

BIOCHEMISTRY OF HUMAN MILK

Linda J. Smith, BSE, FACCE, IBCLC

OBJECTIVES

- Describe human milk synthesis and composition over the continuum of lactation.
- Discuss components of human milk and their functions.
- Discuss maternal nutrition in relation to milk volume and composition.
- Compare human milk with other products and manufactured milks.

Introduction

Human milk is a unique food designed specifically for the needs of a human infant. Nutritional and anti-infective components are woven into a tapestry of growth promoting elements, enzymes to aid in the digestion and absorption of nutrients, and a fatty acid profile that optimizes brain growth and development. The ingredients of breast milk are not interchangeable with manufactured milks or nutrients from other species. The protein and fat content of human milk reflect the identity of a species that requires close contact and frequent feedings. Human milk is not a means of supplying added benefits to an infant's diet. It is the reference food and the plan in nature for nourishing young humans. The lactation consultant will benefit from knowledge of human milk composition to educate parents in the importance of supplying breast milk for their baby.

I. Milk Synthesis and Milk Composition over the Continuum of Lactation

A. *Mammogenesis* is the development of duct structure from the woman's birth through her first pregnancy. Duct development begins in the embryonic stage; it slowly proliferates through young childhood and increases during puberty with fat deposition and duct development with each menstrual period.

B. *Lactogenesis I* is driven by the endocrine system during pregnancy and beyond.

1. Placental lactogen, prolactin, estrogen, and progesterone develop the cells. Cell growth continues for at least 6 weeks postpartum or longer; patterns of breast development vary widely and do not predict lactation success.

2. Lactocytes develop on duct structure (basement membranes) in a single layer, forming a hollow sphere (alveoli) of one layer of cells with a central lumen, surrounded by capillary vessels and myoepithelial cells.

3. Milk secretion begins in the first trimester at approximately 16 weeks of gestation.

4. There are five pathways for synthesis of milk components.
   a. Exocytosis: proteins, lactose, citrate; part of feedback system.
   b. Lipid (fat) released in droplets; lipases are released at the same time, aiding digestion.
   c. Osmosis through membrane contributes ions and water.
   d. Transport of immunoglobulins across cell membranes.
   e. Paracellular (junctures between cells) pathways for white cells and water-soluble compounds.

C. *Lactogenesis II* is the onset of copious milk secretion (so-called "milk coming in").

1. Trigger is delivery of placenta which withdraws progesterone; prolactin is now unopposed; insulin, cortisol, and citrate are permissive.

2. Changes begin 30 to 40 hours postpartum; the timing is not related to sucking stimulus and will occur regardless of the baby's status.

3. Unopposed prolactin turns on alpha-lactalbumin, which triggers lactose synthesis in lactocyctes; the increased lactose draws water into secretion via osmosis; milk volume often exceeds baby's needs.

D. *Lactogenesis III* (*galactopoiesis*) is ongoing maintenance of milk secretion.

1. Upper limit appears to be established in first two weeks or so. Oxytocin pushes out already-made milk. Prolactin surges finish cell growth and shift into a permissive (not regulatory) role.

2. Autocrine feedback takes on dominant role in short-term regulation of milk secretion. Three components have been identified to date, collectively referred to as feedback inhibitors of lactation (FIL): retained peptides (proteins) suppress the protein-producing exocytosis process; fatty acid accumulation slows fat synthesis; and prolactin in milk down-regulates prolactin receptors on lactocyctes.

3. Milk synthesis is controlled by the milk (autocrine control). As milk accumulates in the alveolar lumen, the rate of synthesis slows down due to chemical feedback from FIL components and physical pressure of retained milk, which changes the shape of the lactocyte.

4. The degree of fullness/emptiness of the breast determines rate of milk synthesis. "Empty" breasts try to refill quickly: up to 58 mL (2 oz) per hour; "full" breasts secrete milk slowly at about 11 mL (⅓ ounce) per hour. Babies consume an average of 67.3 % ± 7.8% of available milk per feed (Kent et al., 2006).

E. Changes over time.

1. Milk expressed in the second year of lactation has significantly increased fat and energy (Mandel, 2005).

2. Serotonin and lysozyme increase over time; zinc decreases over time.

3. As volume drops during weaning, the protective factors increase in importance and proportion to total fluid volume, providing protection to the child and the breast throughout the entire duration of lactation.

II. Components of Milk and Their Functions

A. Colostrum. Secretion begins at approximately 12 to 16 weeks of gestation.

1. High density; thick, almost gel-like; generally yellow-colored (beta-carotene).

2. Rapid increase in milk volume parallels newborn's increasing stomach capacity (Scammon & Doyle, 1920; Zangen et al., 2001).
   a. Day 1 volume: mean 37.1 mL (range 7–122.5 mL); stomach capacity 7 mL (2 mL/kg) (colostrum).
   b. Day 3 volume: mean 408 mL (range 98.3–775 mL); stomach capacity 27 mL (8 mL/kg) (transitional milk).
   c. Day 5 volume: mean 705 mL (range 425.5–876 mL); stomach capacity 57 mL (17 mL/kg) (mature milk).
   d. Calories, mean: 67 kcal/dL (18.76 kcal/oz; 2% fat).

3. Primary function is protective: coats gut to prevent adherence of pathogens; promotes gut closure.

4. Secretory immunoglobulin A (sIgA) is especially high immediately post-delivery.

5. White cells, especially polymorphonucleocytes (90% of cells in colostrum).

6. Lactoferrin, lysozyme epidermal growth factor, interleukin 10.

7. Laxative effect; clears meconium with its reservoir of bilirubin.

8. Growth factors stimulate infant's system; 2+ antioxidants.

9. Helps establish bifidus flora (non-pathogenic) in gastrointestinal (GI) tract.

10. Compared with mature milk: lower in lactose, fat, and water-soluble vitamins; higher in Vitamins A and E, carotenoids, protein, sodium, zinc, chloride, and potassium.

B. Water.

    1. Water makes up the majority (87.5%) of human milk.

    2. All other components are dissolved, dispersed, or suspended in water.

    3. Human milk provides all the water a baby needs, even in hot and arid climates.

C. Proteins and nonprotein nitrogen compounds in mature milk.

    1. Whey to casein ratio.

        a. Varies with stage of lactation from 90:10 in early lactation; 60:40 in mature milk; and 50:50 in late lactation (Kunz & Lonnerdal, 1992).

        b. Whey predominates in human milk and casein predominates in cow (bovine) milk.

    2. Total protein in mature milk is 0.8% to 1.0%; lowest of all mammals.

    3. Nineteen amino acids are essential to human development.

        a. Taurine: develops brain and retina, membrane stabilization, inhibitory neurotransmitter; not found in bovine milk.

        b. Tyrosine: low in human breast milk.

        c. Phenylalanine: much higher in cow's milk.

    4. Casein proteins.

        a. Phosphoproteins bind calcium, resulting in cloudy/opaque/white color.

        b. Forms soft, flocculent curds that are easily digested.

    5. Whey proteins are available for digestion and perform specific functions.

        a. Alpha-lactalbumin.

            i. Bovine milk is high in beta-lactoglobulin, which is not found in human milk.

            ii. Regulates milk synthesis.

            iii. Mucins bind pathogens; kill cancer cells in vitro.

        b. Lactoferrin.

            i. Iron transport and absorption.

            ii. Competes with bacteria to bind iron.

            iii. Antibacterial.

            iv. Essential growth factor for B- and T-cell lymphocytes.

            v. Promotes growth of lactobacilli.

            vi. Produced in mammary epithelial cells, milk ducts, and other regions of the body; speculated to have local as well as systemic protective properties.

        c. Secretory immunoglobulin A (SIgA).

            i. Other immunoglobulins are IgG, IgM, and IgE.

            ii. SIgA is most important immunoglobulin because it coats mucosal surfaces to prevent adherence and penetration by pathogens.

        d. Lysozyme aids in "digestion" of pathogens without triggering inflammation; increases over time.

e. Enzymes (40+ identified to date).
    i. Aid in digestion of the nutrients in milk.
    ii. Compensatory digestive enzymes.
    iii. Stimulate neonatal development.
    iv. Lipase digests fats; breaks down fatty acid chains.
    v. Bile salt-stimulated lipase is anti-protozoan; acts on *Giardia* and other organisms that cause diarrhea.
    vi. Lysozyme attacks cell walls of pathogens.
    vii. Amylase digests polysaccharides/starch.
    viii. Alkaline phosphatase.
    ix. Peroxidases act like hydrogen peroxide and oxidize bacteria.
       (1) Xanthine oxidase.
       (2) Sulfhydryl oxidase.
       (3) Glutathione peroxidase.
f. Hormones and hormone-like substances.
    i. Prolactin (different from mother's serum prolactin).
    ii. Prostaglandins, having anti-inflammatory properties.
    iii. Oxytocin.
    iv. Adrenal and ovarian steroids.
    v. Relaxin.
    vi. Insulin.
    vii. Thyroid hormones: TRH, TSH, thyroxine (T4) .
g. Growth factors.
    i. Epidermal growth factors aid gut and other tissue maturity.
    ii. Nerve growth factor may help heal central nervous system (CNS) from birth-related injury.
    iii. Insulin-like growth factor.

6. Nonprotein nitrogen compounds.
    a. Urea.
    b. Creatine.
    c. Creatinine.
    d. Uric acid.
    e. Glucosamine.
    f. Alpha-amino nitrogen.
    g. Nucleic acids.
    h. Nucleotides.
    i. Polyamines.

7. Carbohydrates.
    a. Principal carbohydrate in human milk is lactose: disaccharide (galactose + glucose) is found only in milk.
       i. Supplies 40% of baby's energy needs.

    ii. Synthesis begins at lactogenesis II, approximately 30 to 40 hours postpartum.
      (1) Rise in lactose secreted in cell draws water into secretion by osmosis and directly influences milk volume.
      (2) Colostrum is 4% lactose on day 1; rapidly increases.
    iii. Human milk is highest in lactose of all mammals.
      (1) Largest brain of all animals at birth.
      (2) 7.2 g/100 mL, and is the sweetest of all milks.
      (3) Component of galactolipids needed for CNS structural development.
    iv. Lactose is the primary carbohydrate in milk and least variable (most consistent).
      (1) Humans produce an abundance of lactase (the enzyme to digest the lactose) until age 2½ to 7 years or more.
      (2) Lactase is a brush border intestinal enzyme present by 24 weeks of fetal life.
      (3) Concentration at term is two to four times higher than at 2 to 11 months of age. Persistence of lactase production is genetically determined and decreases with age.
      (4) Lactose assists in the absorption of calcium and iron.
      (5) Primary lactose intolerance is extremely rare; infants of all races typically display a high degree of lactose tolerance.
  b. Oligosaccharides; 130+ specific compounds active against pathogens.
    i. Stimulate lactobacillus bifidus.
    ii. Blocks pathogens from attaching to gut.
    iii. Protect against enterotoxins in the gut, bind to bacteria.
  c. Bifidus factor: a combination of several different oligosaccharides.
    i. With lactose, growth of lactobacillus bifidus in infant gut is promoted, which occupies the intestine, crowds out pathogens, and produces an acid detrimental to pathogen growth.
    ii. Suppresses pathogens and is thought to contribute to unique aroma of exclusively breast milk stools.
  d. Other carbohydrates.
    i. Glycopeptides.
    ii. Fructose.
    iii. Galactose.
8. Fats (lipids): most variable compound in human milk and provides up to 50% of calories.
  a. Fat content of mature milk is 41.1 ± 7.8 g/L (range 22.3–61.6 g/L), which is independent of breastfeeding frequency (Kent et al., 2006), but is directly related to the relative fullness or emptiness of the breast. As a breast "empties" during an individual feed and/or over a day, the proportion of fat increases.

b. Ratio of saturated to unsaturated is relatively stable at 42% saturated; 57% unsaturated; smoking decreases the levels of some essential fatty acids in milk (Agostoni et al., 2003).
c. Lipases (enzymes) are released simultaneously.
  i. Break down long-chain fatty acids; aid digestion.
  ii. Free fatty acids kill bacteria and parasites, including *Giardia* and inactivates viruses.
d. Ninety-eight percent of lipids are encased in globules; membrane coating prevents clumping.
e. Variation in fat levels.
  i. Total fat is only somewhat related to mother's diet; profile of fatty acid chain-length varies with maternal diet (see below).
  ii. Fat levels increase within each feed (foremilk to hindmilk) and increase as breast "empties."
  iii. Approximately 70% of fat variation is related to relative "fullness" or emptiness of the breast
  iv. Fat levels significantly increase in second year of lactation.
f. Triglycerides predominate.
  i. Lipases break down triglycerides into free fatty acids.
g. Cholesterol in human milk.
  i. Unique metabolic effects.
  ii. Essential part of all membranes.
  iii. Cholesterol is an important constituent of brain tissue, being necessary for the laying down of the myelin sheath which is involved in nerve conduction in the brain, along with docosahexaenoic acid (DHA) and arachidonic acid (AA).
  iv. Breastfed babies have higher cholesterol levels than formula-fed infants.
h. Fatty acids.
  i. Long-chain polyunsaturated fatty acids specific to infant needs.
    (1) Central role in cognitive development, vision, nerve myelinization.
    (2) May be conditionally essential to newborns (Koletzko, Michaelson, & Hernell, 2000).
    (3) DHA and AA are especially important to brain maturation.
  ii. Can be synthesized from precursors (linolenic and linoleic acids).
  iii. Preformed dietary DHA is better synthesized into nervous tissue than that synthesized from linolenic acid.
i. Phospholipids.
j. Sterols, a component of lipid membranes.

9. Fat-soluble vitamins.
  a. Vitamin A and carotene.
  b. Vitamin D is a group of related fat-soluble compounds with antirachitic (rickets) activity and is also found in milk in an aqueous form.

      i. Exclusive breastfeeding results in normal infant bone mineral content when the maternal vitamin D status is adequate and the infant is regularly exposed to sunlight; breastfed infants require about 30 minutes of sunlight exposure per week if wearing only a diaper, or two hours per week if fully clothed without a hat; darkly pigmented infants require a greater exposure to sunlight (Sprecker et al., 1985). Only if the infant or mother (especially those with darker skin pigment or those who live in a geographic area with little sunlight) are not regularly exposed to sunlight, or if the mother's intake of vitamin D is low and cannot be raised would supplements to the mother or infant be indicated (Lawrence & Lawrence, 2005, p. 149). Supplementing the mother with high doses of Vitamin D is effective in raising Vitamin D levels in her milk (Hollis & Wagner, 2004; Basile et al., 2006).

    c. Vitamin E: functions as an antioxidant.

    d. Vitamin K: highest in colostrum; later manufactured in infant gut.

      i. Localized in the milk fat globule with hindmilk containing a twofold higher vitamin K concentration than milk from a full pumping.

10. Water-soluble vitamins. These vary because of the stage of lactation, maternal intake, and if delivery takes place before term; the breast does not synthesize these water-soluble vitamins, so their origin is maternal plasma derived from the maternal diet.

    a. Thiamin.

    b. Riboflavin.

    c. Niacin.

    d. Panthothenic acid.

    e. Biotin.

    f. Folate.

    g. Vitamin B_6.

    h. Vitamin B_{12}; needed by the baby's developing nervous system; Vitamin B_{12} occurs exclusively in animal tissue, is bound to protein, and is minimal to absent in plant protein; a vegetarian mother who consumes no animal products could have milk deficient in Vitamin B_{12} and need an acceptable source of intake.

    i. Vitamin C (higher in milk than maternal plasma).

    j. Inositol.

    k. Choline.

11. Cells.

    a. Macrophages.

      i. Contain IgA.

      ii. Ninety percent of cells in mature milk.

      iii. Phagocytosis.

      iv. Make/facilitate lactoferrin, complement.

b. Leukocytes.

c. Lymphocytes: 10% of cells; T-cells and B-cells; humoral immunity.

d. Epithelial cells.

e. Neutrophil granulocytes.

f. Chemical mediators released by cells and injured/inflamed tissue cause more white cells to move into the area to facilitate healing and prevent infection.

12. Minerals.

   a. Macronutrient elements.

      i. Numerous factors affect the levels of minerals in human milk; during pregnancy, involution, and mastitis, the junctions between the alveolar cells are open, allowing sodium and chloride to enter the milk space, drawing water with them; under these conditions, milk has much higher concentrations of sodium and chloride and decreased concentrations of lactose and potassium.

      ii. The presence of high sodium concentrations in human milk can be diagnostic of either mastitis or low milk volume secretion.

      iii. Calcium.

      iv. Phosphate.

      v. Magnesium.

      vi. Potassium.

      vii. Sodium.

      viii. Chloride.

      ix. Sulfate.

      x. Citrate.

   b. Trace elements.

      i. Copper.

      ii. Chromium.

      iii. Cobalt.

      iv. Iron

         (1) Full term infants are born with large physiologic stores of iron in the liver and hemoglobin, which along with the iron in breast milk is sufficient to meet the requirements for iron for about the first six months if babies are exclusively breastfed.

         (2) Approximately 50% of iron is absorbed from breast milk compared with 7% from fortified infant formulas, and 4% from fortified infant cereals.

         (3) Iron concentrations in breast milk are not influenced by the maternal iron status or intake; lactose, which promotes iron absorption, is higher in breast milk, especially compared to some commercial formulas, some of which contain no lactose at all.

      v. Iodine.

      vi. Fluoride.

       vii. Zinc.

      viii. Manganese.

       ix. Selenium.

13. Constituents have more than nutritive functions.

   a. "The unique feature of human milk is that virtually every component examined plays some extra-nutritional role. The elegance of the system is remarkable—the more so the more we learn about it." (Judy Hopkinson, PhD, Baylor College of Medicine).

   b. Alpha-lactalbumin.

       i. Nutrient synthesis.

      ii. Carries metals.

     iii. Prevents infection.

   c. Lactoferrin.

       i. Transports iron.

      ii. Prevents infection.

     iii. Prevents inflammation including necrotizing enterocolitis (NEC).

     iv. Promotes tissue growth and growth of lactobacilli in gut.

   d. sIgA, the most important immunoglobulin.

       i. Infant receives 0.5-2.5 g/dl in first month, which gradually decreases over time as the infant's own sIgA develops. sIgA concentration in colostrum is even higher in the first 24 hours (Goldman et al., 1982; Hennart et al., 1991).

      ii. Prevents inflammation.

     iii. Active against enveloped viruses, rotaviruses, polioviruses, respiratory syncytial, enteric and respiratory bacteria, and intestinal parasites.

     iv. Stimulates infant production of sIgA.

      v. General and specific protection against pathogens.

   e. Epidermal growth factor.

       i. Prevents inflammation.

      ii. Promotes growth.

     iii. Catalyzing reactions.

   f. Lipids: break down products (free fatty acids) active against enveloped viruses and intestinal parasites.

   g. Oligosaccharides: active against enteric and respiratory bacteria.

   h. Beta-carotene: antioxidant and nutrient.

   i. Anti-inflammatory and pharmacologically active components.

       i. Prostaglandins, ovarian steroids, gonadotropins, somatostatin, prolactin, insulin.

14. Anti-infectious agents are found in many components of milk.

   a. Lipids.

   b. Proteins.

            i. Lactoferrin, secretory IgA, lysozyme.
            ii. Enzymes. Bile salt-stimulated lipase active against protozoa.
        c. Nonspecific factors.
            i. Complement, interferon, bifidus factor, antiviral factors.
        d. Cells.
            i. T- and B-lymphocytes.
            ii. Macrophages.
            iii. Neutrophils.
    15. Variations in human milk composition.
        a. Changes within a feed (e.g., fat increases during each feed).
        b. Differences between breasts; changes over the 24-hour day.
            i. Fat levels increase as breast "empties."
            ii. Still maintain foremilk-to-hindmilk differential.
        c. Changes over short and long term of a lactation cycle (days to months to years).
            i. Zinc decreases slightly.
            ii. Whey-to-casein ratio changes, i.e., casein increases proportionally to whey.
            iii. Calcium decreases.
            iv. DHA levels change.
        d. Preterm milk.
            i. Higher protein, sodium, chloride than mature milk.
            ii. Lower lactose than mature milk.
            iii. Fatty acids parallel intrauterine levels and profiles.
        e. Colored milk.
            i. May be caused by something in maternal diet or medication.
            ii. No known harmful affect on infant.
            iii. If bright red or rusty colored, investigate the cause while continuing to breastfeed/provide milk to baby. Frank blood may need follow-up by the mother's physician.
        f. Odor and flavor influenced by mother's diet, which is considered helpful to the infant in adapting to the family nutrition styles and preferences.

III. Influence of Mother's Diet on Milk Volume and Composition

    A. Table 17-1 summarizes the influence of maternal diet on milk composition and volume.

IV. Comparison of Human Milk to Manufactured Milks (Human Milk Is Species-Specific)

    A. "Formula is adequate, not optimal, and is not perfectly acceptable. It does not resemble breast milk except that it contains protein, fat, and carbohydrates from

Table 17-1   Influence of Mother's Diet on Milk Volume and Composition

Milk Component	Affected by Mother's Diet?
Total milk volume	No, except possibly in maternal starvation conditions
Carbohydrates	No
Proteins	No
Lipids	Fatty acid profile only (total fats unaffected)
Cellular components	No
Immune factors	No
Fat-soluble vitamins	Slight variance related to fat levels in milk
Water-soluble vitamins	Yes, deficiencies can occur if maternal diet is inadequate (esp. Vitamin B_{12})
Minerals	No: macronutrient elements; iron, chromium, cobalt Slight/possible: iodine, fluoride; zinc, manganese, selenium, lead

bovine sources. It has none of the enzymes, ligands, immune properties or infection protection properties. It will stave off starvation and predispose to obesity" (Ruth A. Lawrence, MD, 2006).

B. Mother's milk matches much more than 50% of baby's genetic material. Milk from other species and plant-based fluids are genetically different from the infant. It has a unique balance of nutrients and other components; most closely matches milks of species with high maternal investment and frequent feedings.

C. Human milk composition is not static or uniform like artificial baby milks. Colostrum (1–5 days post-birth) evolves to transitional milk (6–13 days post-birth) and then into mature milk (14 days and beyond). The component called colostrum in the early weeks is more accurately described as an "immune layer" that persists throughout the duration of lactation.

D. Bioavailability is low for all other milks.

1. Human milk has little residue; low solute load; nutrients utilized efficiently.

2. Approximately 50% of human milk iron is utilized but < 7% of iron in cow-milk based formula is utilized.

3. Human milk contains the aromas and flavors of mother's diet, which baby tasted in utero, helping familiarize baby with the family's food preferences (Mizuno & Ueda, 2004).

E. Milk from other animals contains deficiencies and excesses of one or more components, only some of which can be modified for infant consumption.

   1. One hundred percent foreign proteins, derived from ruminant animals (cows, goats) or plants.

      a. Increased incidence of allergy; cow's milk protein and soy are known triggers for diabetes in genetically susceptible infants (Vaarala et al., 1999; AAP, 1994; AAP, 1998).

      b. Decreased arousability, which has been implicated in sudden infant death syndrome (Horne et al., 2004); compromises heart rhythms (Zeskind, Goff, & Marshall, 1991).

      c. Bovine milk is high in phenylalanine, which increases risks of complications of phenylketonuria, such as neurodevelopmental problems (Riva et al., 1996).

   2. Soy "milk" has bioactive components including phytoestrogens (13,000–20,000 higher), aluminum, and magnesium.

   3. Non-human fats with no capacity to protect myelin sheath, heal from injury, or develop CNS. Increased risk of multiple sclerosis (Pisacane et al., 1994), altered cholesterol metabolism, vision, and cognitive development.

   4. Absence or deficiency of lactose, which is needed for CNS and cognitive development.

   5. Unregulated components and special (unregulated) formulas and recalls for mistakes and contamination.

      a. Powdered formulas are not sterile; ~14% is contaminated with *enterobacter sakazakii*, which has caused fatal infections.

      b. Manufacturing errors.

      c. Experimental nature of product, including additions of DHA and AA from manufactured sources.

   6. Sub-optimum growth patterns (WHO, 2006).

      a. Formula-fed children are fatter per length, with smaller head circumference, and meet developmental milestones later.

      b. Increased incidence of short-term illness.

         i. GI and urinary tract infections.

         ii. Respiratory infections including wheezing, bronchitis, and asthma.

         iii. NEC, which can be fatal in vulnerable infants.

         iv. Meningitis.

      c. Increased incidence of long-term and chronic illness.

         i. Obesity.

         ii. Diabetes (both types 1 and 2).

         iii. Cancers, childhood and maternal including leukemia.

         iv. GI disorders such as Crohn's disease, pyloric stenosis, and appendicitis.

         v. Cardiovascular disorders including hypertension and atherosclerosis.

    d. Altered metabolism for women who do not sustain lactation.
      i. Postpartum obesity.
      ii. Osteoporosis.
      iii. Early return of fertility.
      iv. Higher stress levels.
  F. There are no "benefits" of human milk, but rather deficiencies of not being breastfed. Every other substance that may be used to feed human infants has deficiencies and documented problems.

References

Agostoni C, Marangoni F, Grandi F, et al. Earlier smoking habits are associated with higher serum lipids and lower milk fat and polyunsaturated fatty acid content in the first 6 months of lactation. *Eur J Clin Nutr.* 2003;57:1466–1472.

American Academy of Pediatrics Committee on Nutrition. *Soy Protein-based Formulas: Recommendations for Use in Infant Feeding.* 1998:148–153.

American Academy of Pediatrics Work Group on Cow's Milk Protein and Diabetes Mellitus. Infant feeding practices and their possible relationship to the etiology of diabetes mellitus. *Pediatrics.* 1994;94(5):572–574.

Basile LA, Taylor SN, Wagner CL, Horst RL, Hollis BW. The effect of high-dose vitamin D supplementation on serum vitamin D levels and milk calcium concentration in lactating women and their infants. *Breastfeeding Medicine.* 2006;1(1):27–35.

Goldman AS, Garza C, Nichols BL, Goldblum RM. Immunologic factors in human milk during the first year of lactation. *J Pediatr.* 1982;100(4):563–567.

Hennart PF, Brasseur DJ, Delogne-Desnoeck JB, Dramaix MM, Robyn CE. Lysozyme, lactoferrin, and secretory immunoglobulin A content in breast milk: influence of duration of lactation, nutrition status, prolactin status, and parity of mother. *Am J Clin Nutr.* 1991;53(1):32–39.

Hollis BW, Wagner CL. Vitamin D requirements during lactation: high-dose maternal supplementation as therapy to prevent hypovitaminosis D for both the mother and the nursing infant. *Am J Clin Nutr.* 2004;80(6):1752S–1758.

Horne RS, Parslow PM, Ferens D, et al. Comparison of evoked arousability in breast and formula fed infants. *Arch Dis Child.* 2004;89:22–25.

Kent JC, Mitoulas LR, Cregan MD, et al. Volume and frequency of breastfeedings and fat content of breast milk throughout the day. *Pediatrics.* 2006;117:e387–395.

Koletzko B, Michaelson KF, Hernell O. *Short and Long Term Effects of Breastfeeding on Child Health.* New York: Kluwer Academic/Plenum Publishers; 2000.

Kunz C, Lonnerdal B. Re-evaluation of the whey protein/casein ratio of human milk. *Acta Paediatr.* 1992;81:107–112.

Lawrence RA, Lawrence RM. *Breastfeeding, a Guide for the Medical Profession.* 6th ed. Philadelphia: Elsevier Mosby; 2005.

Mandel D, Lubetzky R, Dollberg S, et al. Fat and energy contents of expressed human breast milk in prolonged lactation. *Pediatrics*. 2005;116:e432–435.

Mizuno K, Ueda A. Antenatal olfactory learning influences infant feeding. *Early Hum Dev*. 2004;76:83–90.

Pisacane A, Impagliazzo N, Russo M, Valiani R, Mandarina A, Florio C, Vivo P. Breastfeeding and multiple sclerosis. *British Medical Journal*. 1994;308:1411–1412.

Riva E, Agostoni C, Biasucci G, et al. Early breastfeeding is linked to higher intelligence quotient scores in dietary-treated phenylketonuric children. *Acta Paediatr*. 1996; 85:56–58.

Scammon R, Doyle L. Observations on the capacity of the stomach in the first ten days of postnatal life. *Am J Dis Child*. 1920;20:516–538.

Specker BL, Valanis B, Hertzberg V, Edwards N, Tsang RC. Sunshine exposure and serum 25-hydroxyvitamin D concentrations in exclusively breast-fed infants. *J Pediatr*. 1985;107(3):372–376.

Vaarala O, Knip M, Paronen J, Hamalainen AM, Muona P, Vaatainen M, et al. Cow's milk formula feeding induces primary immunization to insulin in infants at genetic risk for type 1 diabetes. *Diabetes*. 1999;48(7):1389–1394.

World Health Organization (WHO), International Growth Standards. Geneva: World Health Organization 2006. http://www.who.int/childgrowth/en/. Accessed December 15, 2006.

Zangen S, Di Lorenzo C, Zangen T, et al. Rapid maturation of gastric relaxation in newborn infants. *Pediatr Res*. 2001;50:629–632.

Zeskind PS, Goff DM, Marshall TR. Rhythmic organization of neonatal heart rate and its relation to atypical fetal growth. *Dev Psychobiol*. 1991;24:413–429.

Suggested Readings

Cregan MD, De Mello TR, Kershaw D, et al. Initiation of lactation in women after preterm delivery. *Acta Obstet Gynecol Scand*. 2002;81:870–877.

Cregan MD, Hartmann PE. Computerized breast measurement from conception to weaning: clinical implications. *J Hum Lact*. 1999;15:89–96.

Daly SE, Kent JC, Huynh DQ, et al. The determination of short-term breast volume changes and the rate of synthesis of human milk using computerized breast measurement. *Exp Physiol*. 1992;77:79–87.

Daly SE, Kent JC, Owens RA, Hartmann PE. Frequency and degree of milk removal and the short-term control of human milk synthesis. *Exp Physiol*. 1996;81:861–875.

Global Strategy for Infant and Young Child Feeding: a Joint WHO/UNICEF Statement. Geneva: World Health Organization; 2003.

Goldman AS, Garza C. Immunologic components in human milk during the second year of lactation. *Acta Paediatr Scand*. 1983;72:461–462.

Hanson LA. *Immunobiology of Human Milk: How Breastfeeding Protects Babies*. Amarillo, TX: Pharmasoft Publishing; 2004.

Hartmann PE, Cregan MD, Ramsay DT, et al. Physiology of lactation in preterm mothers: initiation and maintenance. *Pediatr Ann.* 2003;32:351–355.

Hartmann PE, Rattigan S, Saint L, Supriyana O. Variation in the yield and composition of human milk. *Oxf Rev Reprod Biol.* 1985;7:118–167.

Hopkinson, Judy, PhD, Assistant Professor of Pediatrics, Baylor College of Medicine, Houston TX. Personal communication.

Jensen RG. *Handbook of Milk Composition.* San Diego: Academic Press; 1995.

Kent JC, Arthur PG, Retallack RW, Hartmann PE. Calcium, phosphate and citrate in human milk at initiation of lactation. *J Dairy Res.* 1992;59:161–167.

Kent JC, Mitoulas L, Cox DB, et al. Breast volume and milk production during extended lactation in women. *Exp Physiol.* 1999;84:435–447.

Kramer MS, Kakuma R. Optimal duration of exclusive breastfeeding. *Cochrane Database Syst Rev.* 2002(1):CD003517.

Labbok MH. Effects of breastfeeding on the mother. *Pediatr Clin North Am.* 2001; 48:143–158.

Mitoulas LR, Kent JC, Cox DB, et al. Variation in fat, lactose and protein in human milk over 24 h and throughout the first year of lactation. *Br J Nutr.* 2002;88:29–37.

Neville MC, Allen JC, Archer PC, et al. Studies in human lactation: milk volume and nutrient composition during weaning and lactogenesis. *Am J Clin Nutr.* 1991; 54:81–92.

Picciano MF. Nutrient composition of human milk. *Pediatr Clin North Am.* 2001; 48:53–67.

Saint L, Smith M, Hartmann PE. The yield and nutrient content of colostrum and milk of women from giving birth to 1 month post-partum. *Br J Nutr.* 1984;52:87–95.

ARTIFICIAL BABY MILKS (INFANT FORMULAS)

Marsha Walker, RN, IBCLC

OBJECTIVES

- Compare the components of breast milk and artificial baby milk (ABM), also known as infant formula.
- Identify the effect of artificial feeding on the brain, immune system, and acute and chronic diseases in an ABM-fed baby.
- Explain some of the hazards of ABM.
- Evaluate the criteria for the complementary feeding of infants.

Introduction

Many health care providers as well as the general public believe that the feeding of infant formula or ABM by bottle is equivalent to breastfeeding. Human milk is species-specific and has evolved throughout the millennia to facilitate the normal growth and development of human infants. Human milk is extremely complex, and its composition is most likely programmed by chemical communication between the mother and the infant, both pre- and postnatally. ABM does not duplicate the complexity, cannot provide the multiple tiers of disease protection, and cannot operate in the dynamic manner of human milk. Artificial baby milk simply fulfills the role of maintaining growth and development within normal limits.

I. Components of Artificial Baby Milk (ABM)

A. General concepts.

1. Human milk is used as a general guide for nutrient content in ABM.

2. While ABM contains similar categories of nutrients as in breast milk, such as proteins, fats, carbohydrates, vitamins, and minerals, it does not duplicate them.

3. ABM is an inert medium that has no bioactive components.
    a. ABM does not alter its composition to meet the changing needs of a growing infant.
    b. Unlike breast milk, ABM does not contain growth factors, hormones, live cells, immunologic agents, or enzymes.
4. The fatty acid profile of ABM does not resemble breast milk.
5. In general, the concentrations of nutrients in ABM are higher than those in human milk to compensate for their reduced bioavailability and to ensure their presence throughout the entire shelf life of the product.
6. Commercial ABMs have many similarities to each other but can differ significantly from each other in the quality and quantity of nutrients and in other additives.
7. There are a number of bodies worldwide that either oversee or make recommendations for the nutrient content of ABM.
    a. The American Academy of Pediatrics, Committee on Nutrition.
    b. The European Society of Paediatric Gastroenterology and Nutrition (ESPGHAN).
    c. The Food and Agriculture Organization, a part of the United Nations.
    d. Codex Alimentarius.
    e. European Communities.
    f. The United States Food and Drug Administration (FDA).
    g. Safety evaluations of new ingredients added to infant formulas in the United States have been found to be inadequate and lacking in rigor. The Institute of Medicine (2004) has recommended more thorough guidelines.
8. There are numerous types of artificial baby milks.
    a. Standard cow's milk-based.
    b. Cow's milk-based with reduced or no lactose.
    c. Soy.
    d. Follow-on.
    e. Extensively hydrolyzed (hypoallergenic).
    f. Partially hydrolyzed.
    g. Preterm.
    h. Special formulations for metabolic problems.
    i. Amino acid-based.
    j. With added soy fiber (for diarrhea).
    k. With added rice solids (for reflux).
    l. Follow-on preterm.
9. ABM is available in three forms: ready-to-feed, concentrated liquid, and powder.
    a. The composition of ABM within each of these forms can differ, even among those from the same manufacturer.

      b. The composition of ABM differs between manufacturers and varies from country to country, depending on the legal requirements for content.

10. ABM products frequently change composition, receive new labels, change scoop sizes in the powdered variety, are discontinued, or experience changes in their recommended usage (Walker, 2001).

11. ABM has an expiration date after which it should be discarded.

12. ABM labels state the minimum amount of ingredients that are supposed to be present at any one time.

13. Overages (additional amounts) of some components are added to compensate for their degradation over the shelf life of the product.

14. ABM is frequently recalled or withdrawn from the market due to health and safety issues.
      a. A list of recalled formulas in the United States can be found at www.naba-breastfeeding.org.

II. Selected Differences in Macronutrients

A. Protein.

1. ABM can have up to 50 percent more protein than human milk.

2. Protein intake per kg of body weight is 55% to 80% higher in formula-fed infants than in breastfed infants. High early protein intake enhances weight gain in infancy and can increase later obesity risk (Koletzko et al., 2005).

3. The whey-to-casein ratio of human milk changes over time from 90:10 in the early milk to 60:40 in mature milk, and to 50:50 in late lactation.

4. In ABM, cow's milk protein remains static and, depending on the brand, the levels could be 18:82, 60:40, or 100% whey.

5. Bovine casein is less-easily digested and forms a tough, rubbery curd in the infant's stomach, partially accounting for the slower gastric emptying time in ABM-fed babies.

6. There are compositional and functional differences between the casein and whey proteins in human milk and ABM. In ABM,
      a. Bovine alpha-lactalbumin is not well digested.
      b. There is no lactoferrin, a protein that aids in bacterial cell destruction (Hanson, 2004).
      c. There are no immunoglobulins, such as secretory immunoglobulin.
      d. There are no enzymes (digestive or defensive).
      e. There are few of the non-protein nitrogen components found in human milk.

7. Cow's milk ABM uses processing procedures that exclude colostrum, milk fat globule membranes, and fractions that contain DNA from the final product—components that provide disease protection that is species-specific to the calf.

B. Lipids (fat).

1. Lipids provide 40% to 50% of the energy in cow's milk ABM.

2. During processing, cow's milk fat (butterfat) is removed and replaced with vegetable oils or a mixture of vegetable and animal fats for better digestibility and absorption.

3. These fats include coconut oil, palm oil, soy oil, corn oil, safflower oil, palm olein, high oleic safflower oil, high oleic sunflower oil, oleo (de-stearinated beef fat), soy oil, and medium-chain triglycerides oil.

4. The fatty acid profile and stereo-specific structures differ significantly among various brands of ABM as well as between ABM and human milk (Straarup et al., 2006).

5. ABM fats do not contain docosahexaenoic (DHA) and arachidonic (AA) acids, the long-chain polyunsaturated fatty acids (LCPUFA) found in human milk that are thought to be necessary for normal brain growth and development.
   a. Addition of these LCPUFA to some ABM brands does not replicate the complex human milk fatty acid pattern.
   b. Sources of these additives include fish oils, egg yolks, evening primrose oil, micro algae, and fungal sources and must be provided in the correct ratio to avoid growth problems.
   c. Some infants who are fed ABM enriched with various combinations of these LCPUFA do not grow as well as with standard ABM or breast milk (Carlson et al., 1991).
   d. Clinical trials have failed to show efficacy in terms of improved mental and motor development, with little evidence to support any beneficial effects of adding DHA/AA to infant formulas relative to visual or general development (Simmer, 2003; Wright et al., 2006).
   e. The FDA does not approve infant formulas before they can be marketed. However, all formulas marketed in the United States must meet federal nutrient requirements, and infant formula manufacturers must notify the FDA prior to marketing a new formula (Guidance for Industry, 2006).

6. The brain composition of ABM-fed babies is measurably and chemically different than the brain of a breastfed baby, with DHA levels in ABM-fed term babies remaining static, decreasing in preterm infants, and increasing in breastfed babies (Cunnane et al., 2000).

7. ABM contains little to no cholesterol. Cholesterol is present in human milk and increases during the course of lactation. Cholesterol is an essential part of all membranes and is involved with the laying down of the myelin sheath, which facilitates nerve conduction in the brain.

C. Carbohydrates.

   1. Lactose is the principal sugar in human milk and in most other mammals' milk.

   2. Human milk lactose:

      a. Favors the colonization of the infant's intestine with microflora that compete with and exclude pathogens.

      b. Ensures a supply of galactocerebrosides that are major components of brain growth.

      c. Enhances calcium absorption.

   3. The use of cow's milk-based ABM with the lactose removed, all soy preparations, and some of the hydrolyzed ABM brands that have no lactose has an unknown effect on both brain development and disease outcomes in ABM-fed babies.

   4. There are approximately 130 oligosaccharides (non-lactose carbohydrates) in human milk. Cow's milk contains about 10% of this amount.

   5. Human oligosaccharides inhibit pathogens from binding to their receptor sites in the gut and on mucous membranes.

   6. Human oligosaccharides contain human blood group antigens, with women from different blood groups having distinct patterns contributing to the tailor-made disease protection within each mother/baby unit.

   7. Oligosaccharides in the milk of other species confer protection to the young of that species. Oligosaccharides in breast milk are unique to human milk and have not been replicated synthetically.

D. Vitamins and minerals.

   1. ABM is fortified with water- and fat-soluble vitamins.

   2. There are upper and lower limits for most of these vitamins.

   3. Most brands of ABM contain significantly higher amounts of vitamins than human milk in order to offset their reduced absorption.

   4. Excesses, deficiencies, and omissions of ingredients can and do occur in the manufacturing process.

   5. Approximately 50% of the iron in human milk is absorbed compared to 7% from iron-fortified ABM and 4% from iron-fortified cereals (AAP, 1999).

E. Defense agents.

   1. ABM contains no defense agents to protect human babies from acute and chronic disease.

   2. Some brands of ABM contain added nonhuman nucleotides or oligosaccharides, enabling the claim of enhanced immune response. The clinical significance of this addition has not been demonstrated.

III. Effects of Artificial Feeding on the Brain and Immune System

A. ABM-fed infants and children demonstrate less-advanced cognitive development compared with breastfed children (Anderson, Johnstone, & Remley, 1999).

B. Lower mental development and IQ scores are seen at all ages through adolescence in ABM-fed children.

C. Infants who are fed formula have significantly lower DHA in the gray and white matter of the cerebellum, the area of the brain that coordinates movement and balance (Jamieson et al., 1999).

D. A deficiency of 8 to 10 IQ points in ABM-fed subjects is reported in most studies (Angelsen et al., 2001).

E. Central to this discrepancy are particular fatty acids (DHA and AA) that are found in human milk but are absent in ABM.

F. DHA and AA are found in abundance as structural lipids in the brain, retina, and central nervous system of infants.

G. Unsupplemented ABM contains precursors of DHA and AA, linolenic and linoleic acid, from which an infant's immature liver is supposed to synthesize enough of these LCPUFA to meet the needs of the rapidly developing brain.

H. IQ studies are remarkably consistent in their demonstration of higher IQs that are dose dependant relative to the number of months that a child has been exclusively breastfed (Lucas et al., 1992).

I. Formula-fed one-week-old infants demonstrate suboptimal neurobehavioral organization (Hart et al., 2003).

J. Neural maturation of ABM-fed preterm infants shows a deficit compared to those who are fed human milk (Rao, 2002).

K. Delayed maturation in visual acuity can occur in both term and preterm ABM-fed infants (Birch et al., 1993; Williams et al., 2001).

L. Delayed maturation in visual acuity might affect other mental and physical functions later in development that are linked to the quality of early visual processing.

M. An IQ increase of as little as three points ($\frac{1}{5}$ of a standard deviation) from 100 to 103 would move a person from the 50th to the 58th percentile of the population and would potentially be associated with higher educational achievement, occupational achievement, and social adjustment.

    1. One IQ point has been estimated to be worth $14,500 in earning power and economic productivity (Grosse et al., 2002).

N. Defense agents are poorly represented in cow's milk (Jensen, 1995).

O. Bovine colostrum and its antimicrobial agents are specific for the cow and are removed from milk during processing.

P. Human milk not only provides passive protection, but also directly modulates the immunologic development of the recipient infant (Goldman, Chheda, & Garofalo, 1998).

Q. ABM-fed infants and children have increased risks and rates of:

1. Allergic disease (van Odijk et al., 2003).

2. Asthma (Oddy et al., 1999).

3. Crohn disease (Koletzko et al., 1989).

4. Ulcerative colitis (Corrao et al., 1998).

5. Type 1 (insulin-dependent) diabetes mellitus (Sadauskaite-Kuehne et al., 2004), and type 2 diabetes (Pettitt et al., 1997; Young et al., 2002).

6. Acute lymphoblastic leukemia and acute myeloblastic leukemia (Kwan et al., 2004; Shu et al., 1999); lymphomas (McNally & Parker, 2006).

7. Necrotizing enterocolitis (NEC) (Updegrove, 2004).

8. Diarrheal disease (Scariati et al., 1997).

9. Otitis media (Scariati et al., 1997).

10. Lower respiratory tract illness (bronchiolitis, croup, bronchitis, and pneumonia).

11. Obesity (Kvaavik, Tell, & Klepp, 2005; Von Kries et al., 1999).

12. Sudden infant death syndrome (Vennemann, 2005).

13. Sepsis (Hanson & Korotkova, 2002).

14. Urinary tract infections (Pisacane et al., 1992).

R. Humoral and cellular immune responses to specific antigens (such as vaccines) given during the first year of life appear to develop differently in breastfed and ABM-fed babies.

S. ABM-fed babies can show lower or absent antibody levels to their immunizations (Hahn-Zoric et al., 1990; Zoppi et al., 1983).

T. Infants who are fed soy ABM can have even lower antibody titers, with some showing no response at all to some of their vaccines.

IV. Hazards of Artificial Baby Milk

A. Genetically modified ingredients.

1. Genetically engineered corn and soy have been found in numerous brands of ABM.

2. Transgenic ingredients pose the risk of introducing novel toxins, new allergens, and increased antibiotic resistance in infants.

3. Labeling of genetically modified ingredients in the United States is not required, so parents are unaware of whether they are feeding their baby transgenic foods.

4. The long-term effects of these ingredients on ABM-fed infants are unknown.

B. Soy-based ABM.

1. Twenty-five percent of all ABM sold in the United States is soy.

2. Soy ABM is used much less extensively outside the United States.

3. Soy ABM might be allergenic in infants who are allergic to cow's milk protein. (ESPGHAN Committee on Nutrition, 2006).

4. Many soy preparations contain sucrose, which is a contributor to dental caries in babies who are fed soy ABM by bottle.

5. Soy is not recommended for preterm infants who have birth weights lower than 1800 g, for the prevention of colic or allergy, or with infants who have cow's milk protein-induced enterocolitis or enteropathy (ESPGHAN, 2006).

6. Infants who are fed soy ABM can have circulating phytoestrogen concentrations that are 13,000 to 22,000 times higher than normal levels in early life (Setchell et al., 1997).

7. This dose represents a 6- to 11-fold higher level of intake of isoflavones than that found to cause significant modifications to the hormonal regulation of the menstrual cycle in Western women.

8. The consumption of soy ABM was associated with an increased occurrence of premature thelarche (breast development in girls younger than eight years of age) in Puerto Rico and specifically in many girls before they were 18 months of age (Fremi-Titulaer et al., 1986).

9. It is unknown what other effects these bioactive compounds might produce by creating steroid hormone imbalances through competition with enzymes that metabolize steroids and drugs or by influencing gonadal function.

10. ABM, especially soy and some hydrolyzed ABM, contains 35 to 1,500 times the amount of aluminum as in breast milk.

11. Aluminum can accumulate in bones and in the brain, and the effect of large amounts in infancy is unknown.

12. A positive association has been found between feeding infants soy ABM and the development of autoimmune thyroid disease (Fort et al., 1990).

13. Soy ABM components can act against the thyroid by inhibition of thyroid peroxidase and can have the potential to disrupt thyroid function even in the presence of added iodine (Divi, Hebron, & Doerge, 1997).

C. Follow-on ABM.

1. Follow-on ABM is marketed for infants who are four months of age and older who are also receiving cereal and other solid foods.

2. The most significant difference in this category of products is that they are lower in fat than both breast milk and standard starter ABM.

3. Regular ABM and breast milk contribute 45% to 50% of the energy from fat.

4. Follow-on ABM can contribute as little as 37% energy from fat.

5. Current pediatric nutrition recommendations advise against lowering the fat intake of infants and children under the age of two years (Kleinman, 2004).

6. There are few additional sources of fat in the first year of life, and this period includes rapid growth and development with high energy requirements.

D. Neurotoxins and altered behavior patterns.

1. Toxic pollutants can affect the brain in different ways.

2. The manganese (Mn) concentration in breast milk is very low (4–8 mg/L). Cow's milk ABM is 10 times higher in Mn concentration (30–60 mg/L) than breast milk, while soy ABM has about a 50–75 times higher concentration than breast milk.

3. Mn lowers the levels of serotonin and dopamine–brain neurotransmitters that are associated with planning and impulse control.

4. Low levels of brain serotonin are known to cause mood disturbances, poor impulse control, and increased aggressive behavior.

5. There is little regulation of Mn uptake at young ages, and ABM-fed infants—especially those who are fed soy ABM—will have a much larger body burden of Mn.

6. Children who are raised from birth on ABM will absorb five times as much Mn as breastfed infants.

7. Altered brain chemistry combined with social stresses increases the risk of violent behavior.

8. Ingredients that contain processed free glutamic acid (monosodium glutamate) and free aspartic acid (known neurotoxins) are used in ABM.
   a. These are found in high levels in some hypoallergenic ABM brands and are cause for concern due to the underdeveloped blood-brain barrier that enables neurotoxins to be more accessible to the brain.

9. Schizophrenic patients are less likely to have been breastfed (McCreadie, 1997).

10. Some infants who were fed a chloride-deficient brand of ABM in 1978–1979 showed cognitive delays, language disorders, visual motor and fine motor difficulties, and attention deficit disorders at ages 8 to 9 years (Kaleita, Kinsbourne, & Menkes, 1991).

E. Contaminants in ABM and water used for reconstitution.

1. Silicon contamination can be seen in ABM with levels ranging from 746 to 13,811 ng/mL. Breast milk of women who do not have silicone implants contains approximately 51.05 ng/mL of silicon, while those who have implants show 55.45 ng/mL (Semple et al., 1998).

2. Lead intoxication can occur when hot tap water or lead-containing water is boiled and is used to reconstitute concentrated or powdered ABM (Shannon & Graef, 1992).

3. Boiling concentrates lead, arsenic, cadmium, and other contaminants in water.

4. Infants who are fed ABM that has been reconstituted with nitrate-contaminated water or untested well water are at risk for potentially fatal methemoglobinemia. The baby's system converts nitrates to nitrites, resulting in hemoglobin being converted to methemoglobin that cannot bind molecular oxygen (Dusdieker et al., 1994).

   a. Breastfed infants are not at risk of nitrate poisoning from mothers who ingest water with high nitrate content because nitrate does not concentrate in the milk (Greer & Shannon, 2005).

5. This risk increases if babies are younger than six months of age and are also fed baby food that has high concentrations of nitrates, such as green beans and bananas.

6. Atrazine is a weed killer found in the water supplies in agricultural areas; it is a carcinogen at high levels. ABM-fed infants can obtain a lifetime dose by age five. Most ready-to-feed ABM contains water that has atrazine filtered out of it before it is used for processing (Houlihan & Wiles, 1999).

7. Powdered infant formula is not sterile and has been implicated in a number of cases of meningitis, NEC, and sepsis in term and preterm infants (Centers for Disease Control, 2002). The formula can be contaminated with *Enterobacter sakazakii*, an emerging pathogen that is not seen in ready-to-feed or liquid concentrated formula.

   a. It has been recommended that no infant under the age of 4 weeks receive the powdered version of infant formula (Bowen & Braden, 2006; European Food Safety Authority, 2004).

   b. To reconstitute powdered infant formula, water should be brought to a rolling boil, then cooled to a temperature of 70°C (158°F) and added to the formula; this reconstituted formula should be further cooled to body temperature before feeding (Drudy et al., 2006).

F. Container hazards.

1. Phthalates are used as plasticizers and are testicular toxins and estradiol imitators; many tested brands of ABM have been shown to contain phthalates.

2. Bisphenol-A is used in the production of polycarbonate plastics and has been found in plastic baby bottles; this chemical can leach from the container and has been known to be estrogenic since 1938 (Larkin, 1995).

3. Bisphenol-A resins are used as lacquers to coat metal products such as food cans. This chemical can leach into the contents of cans during autoclaving. Some of the tested cans were concentrated milk-based ABM.

4. Bottle-fed babies are at risk for scald and burn injuries from bottles heated on the stove or in a microwave oven.

5. Babies who are fed by bottle have increased rates of malocclusion (Labbok & Krasovec, 1990). Muscles involved with breastfeeding are either immobilized (masseter and obicularis oris), overactive (chin muscle), or malpositioned (the tongue is pushed backwards) during artificial feeding (Inoue, Sakashita, & Kamegai, 1995), contributing to abnormal dentofacial development in the child (Palmer, 1998).

6. Bottle feeding is positively correlated with finger sucking, which can deform the maxillary arch and palate (Viggiano et al., 2004).

7. ABM is acidogenic and might play a significant role in the development of early dental caries in infants (Sheikh & Erickson, 1996).

8. Baby bottles that are decorated with name-brand soft drink logos, noncarbonated beverage logos, and juice logos encourage parents to give infants the respective beverage from the bottle.

G. Errors in ABM Preparation and Inappropriate Foods.

1. Babies who are fed powdered ABM are at risk for hyperosmolar (overconcentrated) feedings. Reports have been noted of mothers losing the measuring scoop, using graduated markings on a bottle that was brought home from the hospital, adding extra ABM to help a small baby grow faster, diluting formula to make it last longer, using warm tap water to reconstitute powdered formula, heating bottles in a microwave, leaving bottles out at room temperature, and so on (Fein & Falci, 1999).

2. Babies are also at risk for underconcentrated feedings if mothers use less powdered ABM per bottle to make the supply last longer.

3. Oral water intoxication can result not only from overly dilute ABM, but also from supplemental feedings of solute-free tap water, juice, tea, soda, and bottled drinking water marketed for infants (Keating, Schears, & Dodge, 1991).

4. Rapid ingestion of water over a short period of time can cause hyponatremic seizures and brain swelling.

5. Infants who ingest 260 mL to 540 mL (9 to 19 oz) of solute-free water can become symptomatic over a relatively short period of time (90 minutes to 48 hours).

H. Cardiorespiratory disturbances.

1. Both preterm and full-term infants who are fed by bottle are at an increased risk of cardiopulmonary disturbances, including prolonged airway closure and obstructed respiratory breaths due to repeated rapid swallowing (Koenig, Davies, & Thach, 1990).

2. Preterm infants have shown decreased oxygen saturations accompanied by apnea (an absent airflow for more than 20 seconds), bradycardia (a heart rate of

fewer than 100 beats per minute), and cyanosis (blue coloring) during bottle-feeding due to frequent swallowing and limited breathing time with high-flow nipples (Mathew, 1991).

I. Costs.

1. The direct cost of ABM to families for one year in the United States ranges from $1000 to $3,000 or more. In some developing countries, the cost of ABM can exceed 100% of the yearly family income.

2. The U.S. government is the single largest purchaser of ABM in the world for the Women, Infants, and Children supplemental food program.

V. Feeding: Breast Milk and Foods

A. Exclusive versus partial breastfeeding.

1. The absence of standard definitions for breastfeeding can prevent precision and comparability in research, causing inaccuracies and confusion at both policy-making and clinical levels.

2. A schema for defining breastfeeding has been devised. By using and describing the terms *full*, *partial*, and *token*, Labbok and Krasovec (1990) further subdivide these terms based on patterns of feedings.

3. These breastfeeding patterns might occur at any stage of the child's life and are not associated with age.

4. Precise definitions of breastfeeding in well-controlled research show that the protective effects of breast milk are afforded in a dose-response manner.

5. The less breast milk a baby receives, the higher the risk for disease and adverse cognitive development.

6. Even partial breastfeeding confers some measure of disease protection.

7. Exclusive breastfeeding is becoming an endangered practice.

8. Exclusive breastfeeding rates for infants who are younger than 4 months old range from 19% in Africa to 49% in Southeast Asia.

9. In the United States, about 59% percent of breastfed babies are breastfeeding exclusively at 7 days and 13.9% at 6 months of age (CDC, 2005).

10. Healthy, full-term breastfeeding infants should not be given supplements of water, glucose water, ABM, or other fluids unless ordered by a physician when a medical indication exists (AAP, 2005).

11. Supplements displace breast milk intake and can lead to increased morbidity, early cessation of breastfeeding, and interference with the bioavailability of certain key nutrients and disease-protective factors in breast milk.

12. Some babies will receive culturally valued supplements or ritual foods, such as tea, vitamin drops, honey, butter, and so on (but in very small amounts). While

these supplements and foods are not necessary, most pose no problem to breastfeeding. Honey can carry the possibility of infecting the infant with botulism, however, and should not be given to infants who are younger than one year of age.

B. Complementary feeding: starting solids.

1. For several decades, the World Health Organization (WHO) has issued recommendations regarding the appropriate age to begin complementary feeding (WHO, 1998).

2. These recommendations have varied and have sparked debate about whether recommendations should be the age range of 4 to 6 months or if the phrase "at about 6 months" expresses the desired flexibility and protection of infant health.

3. Studies show that in affluent populations, introducing solid foods before 6 months of age has little impact on the total energy intake or growth.

4. Studies show that there is no growth advantage in the complementary feeding of breastfed infants in developing countries prior to 6 months of age. The results of a WHO systematic review support the recommendation of exclusive breastfeeding for about 6 months.

5. The American Academy of Pediatrics states that exclusive breastfeeding is ideal nutrition and is sufficient to support optimal growth and development for approximately the first six months after birth (AAP, 2005).

6. At about 6 months of age, the normal infant begins using his or her iron stores.

7. Iron, energy, zinc, vitamin A, and calcium might be limiting nutrients with breast milk consumption alone sometime after 6 months of age.

8. The neuromuscular and gastrointestinal systems are beginning to mature around 6 months of age.

9. While infants at this age can physically manage food, the efficiency of consumption of different types of foods varies considerably with age.

10. It is practically impossible to supply enough iron from unmodified complementary foods to meet the calculated needs of an infant who is between 6 to 11 months of age without unrealistically high intakes of animal products.

11. Iron-fortified cereals or other iron-containing foods (such as meat) are usually introduced as the first solids where available.

12. Iron deficiency can result when using iron-fortified cereal and whole cow's milk during the second six months of life. This condition results from a combination of poor bioavailability of electrolytic iron in some cereals and the composition of cow's milk, which makes iron less available to the infant.

13. Giving infants coffee or tea can have a strong inhibitory effect on iron absorption from foods that are consumed in the same meal or from iron supplements.

14. Once complementary foods are introduced at about 6 months of age, special transitional foods (for example, with semi-solid consistency and adequate energy and nutrient densities) are recommended.

15. Breastfed infants from 6 to 8 months of age can receive (in addition to breast milk) two to three meals per day depending on the population's nutritional status and the energy density of the complementary foods.

16. Children who are older than 8 months can receive at least three meals per day.

C. Inappropriate foods (WHO/UNICEF, 2003).

1. The definition of *inappropriate foods* will vary with the population that is being discussed.

2. Generally, cow's milk or the fluid milk of other species is not recommended during infancy due to its displacement of breast milk, possible microbial contamination, an inappropriate blend of nutrients, and gastrointestinal blood loss when fresh milk is consumed.

3. Local foods that have a low nutrient density might need to be fortified.

4. Solid foods, such as cereals, should not be given to young babies to make them sleep through the night.

5. Solid foods should not be diluted and put in bottles for young babies to consume.

6. Acceptance of semi-solid food is not an indication of maturity.

7. Parents might need help in resisting the pressure from health care providers, baby food manufacturers, and grandparents to introduce solids before six months.

8. Water and fruit juices are unnecessary for exclusively breastfed babies during their first six months.

9. If commercial baby foods are used, parents should be counseled to avoid those that contain modified food starch or added sugar or salt, or those that have multiple ingredients.

10. Soy milk that is used in addition to or in place of ABM is inappropriate.

11. Coffee creamers, flour and water mixtures, adult beverages, and carbonated or alcoholic drinks are inappropriate.

References

American Academy of Pediatrics, Committee on Nutrition. Iron fortification of infant formula. *Pediatrics*. 1999;104:119–123.

American Academy of Pediatrics, Section on Breastfeeding. Breastfeeding and the use of human milk. *Pediatrics*. 2005;115:496–506.

Anderson JW, Johnstone BM, Remley DT. Breastfeeding and cognitive development: a meta-analysis. *Am J Clin Nutr*. 1999;70:525–535.

Angelsen NK, Vik T, Jacobsen G, Bakketeig LS. Breast feeding and cognitive development at age 1 and 5 years. *Arch Dis Child*. 2001;85:183–188.

Birch E, Birch D, Hoffman D, et al. Breastfeeding and optimal visual development. *J Pediatr Ophthalmol Strabismus*. 1993;30:30–38.

Bowen AB, Braden CR. Invasive *Enterobacter sakazakii* disease in infants. *Emerg Infect Dis*. 2006;12:1185–1189.

Carlson SE, Cooke RJ, Rhodes PG, et al. Long-term feeding of formulas high in linolenic acid and marine oil to very low birth weight infants: phospholipid fatty acids. *Pediatr Res*. 1991;30:404–412.

Centers for Disease Control and Prevention. *Enterobacter sakazakii* infections associated with the use of powdered formula-Tennessee, 2001. *MMWR*. 2002;51:297–300.

Corrao G, Tragnone A, Caprilli R, et al. Risk of inflammatory bowel disease attributable to smoking, oral contraception and breastfeeding in Italy: a nationwide case-control study. Cooperative Investigators of the Italian Group for the Study of the Colon and Rectum (GISC). *Int J Epidemiol*. 1998;27:397–404.

Cunnane SC, Francescutti V, Brenna JT, Crawford MA. Breastfed infants achieve a higher rate of brain and whole body docosahexaenoate accumulation than formula-fed infants not consuming dietary docosahexaenoate. *Lipids*. 2000;35:105–111.

Divi RL, Hebron CC, Doerge DR. Anti-thyroid isoflavones from soybean: isolation, characterization, and mechanisms of action. *Biochem Pharmacol*. 1997;54:1087–1096.

Drudy D, Mullane NR, Quinn T, et al. Enterobacter sakazakii: an emerging pathogen in powdered infant formula. *Clin Infect Dis*. 2006;42:996–1002.

Dusdieker LB, Getchell JP, Liarakos TM, et al. Nitrate in baby foods: adding to the nitrate mosaic. *Arch Pediatr Adolesc Med*. 1994;148:490–494.

ESPGHAN Committee on Nutrition. Agostoni C, Axelsson I, Goulet O, Koletzko B, Michaelsen KF, Puntis J, Rieu D, Rigo J, Shamir R, Szajewska H, Turck D. Soy protein infant formulae and follow-on formulae: a commentary by the ESPGHAN Committee on Nutrition. *J Pediatr Gastroenterol Nutr*. 2006;42:352–361.

European Food Safety Authority. Opinion of the Scientific Panel on Biological Hazards on a request from the Commission related to the microbiological risks in infant formulae and follow-on formulae. *Eur Food Safety Auth J*. 2004;13:1–34.

Fein SB, Falci CD. Infant formula preparation, handling, and related practices in the United States. *J Am Diet Assoc*. 1999;99:1234–1240.

Fort P, Moses N, Fasano M, Goldberg T, Lifshitz F. Breast and soy-formula feedings in early infancy and the prevalence of autoimmune thyroid disease in children. *J Am Coll Nutr*. 1990;9:164–167.

Fremi-Titulaer LW, Cordero JF, Haddock L, et al. Premature thelarche in Puerto Rico. A search for environmental factors. *Am J Dis Child*. 1986;140:1263–1267.

Goldman AS, Chheda S, Garofalo R. Evolution of immunologic functions of the mammary gland and the postnatal development of immunity. *Pediatr Res.* 1998; 43:155–162.

Greer FR, Shannon M. Infant methemoglobinemia: the role of dietary nitrate in food and water. *Pediatrics.* 2005;116:784–786.

Grosse SD, Matte TD, Schwartz J, Jackson RJ. Economic gains resulting from the reduction in children's exposure to lead in the United States. *Environ Health Perspect.* 2002;110:563–569.

Guidance for industry. Frequently asked questions about FDA's regulation of infant formula. Rockville, MD: Federal Drug Administration, Department of Health and Human Services. Available at: http://www.cfsan.fda.gov/~dms/infguid.html. Accessed December 15, 2006.

Hahn-Zoric M, Fulconis F, Minoli I, et al. Antibody responses to parenteral and oral vaccines are impaired by conventional and low protein formulas as compared to breastfeeding. *Acta Paediatr Scand.* 1990;79:1137–1142.

Hanson LA. *Immunobiology of Human Milk: How Breastfeeding Protects Babies.* Amarillo, TX: Pharmasoft Publishing; 2004.

Hanson LA, Korotkova M. The role of breastfeeding in prevention of neonatal infection. *Semin Neonatol.* 2002;7:275–281.

Hart S, Boylan LM, Carroll S, et al. Brief report: breastfed one-week-olds demonstrate superior neurobehavioral organization. *J Pediatr Psychol.* 2003;28:529–534.

Houlihan J, Wiles R. Into the mouths of babes: bottle-fed infants at risk from atrazine in tap water. Washington, DC: Environmental Working Group, 1999. Available at: http://www.ewg.org. Accessed December 15, 2006.

Inoue N, Sakashita R, Kamegai T. Reduction of masseter muscle activity in bottle fed babies. *Early Hum Dev.* 1995;42:185–193.

Institute of Medicine, Committee on the evaluation of the addition of ingredients new to infant formula, Food and Nutrition Board. Infant formula: evaluating the safety of new ingredients. Washington, DC: The National Academies Press; 2004.

Jamieson EC, Farquharson J, Logan RW, et al. Infant cerebellar gray and white matter fatty acids in relation to age and diet. *Lipids.* 1999;34:1065–1071.

Jensen RG, ed. *Handbook of Milk Composition.* San Diego, CA: Academic Press, Inc.; 1995.

Kaleita TA, Kinsbourne M, Menkes JH. A neurobehavioral syndrome after failure to thrive on chloride-deficient formula. *Dev Med Child Neurol.* 1991;33:626–635.

Keating J, Schears GJ, Dodge PR. Oral water intoxication in infants: an American epidemic. *Am J Dis Child.* 1991;145:985–990.

Kleinman RE, ed. *Pediatric Nutrition Handbook.* 5th ed. Elk Grove Village, IL: Committee on Nutrition, American Academy of Pediatrics; 2004.

Koenig JS, Davies AM, Thach BT. Coordination of breathing, sucking, and swallowing during bottle feedings in human infants. *J Appl Physiol.* 1990;69:1623–1629.

Koletzko B, Broekaert I, Demmelmair H, et al. Protein intake in the first year of life: a risk factor for later obesity? The EU childhood obesity project. *Adv Exp Med Biol.* 2005;569:69–79.

Koletzko S, Sherman P, Corey M, et al. Role of infant feeding practices in development of Crohn's disease in childhood. *BMJ.* 1989;298:1617–1618.

Kvaavik E, Tell GS, Klepp KI. Surveys of Norwegian youth indicated that breastfeeding reduced subsequent risk of obesity. *J Clin Epidemiol.* 2005;58:849–855.

Kwan ML, Buffler PA, Abrams B, Kiley VA. Breastfeeding and the risk of childhood leukemia: a meta-analysis. *Public Health Rep.* 2004;119:521–535.

Labbok M, Krasovec K. Toward consistency in breastfeeding definitions. *Stud Fam Plan.* 1990;21:226–230.

Larkin M. Estrogen: friend or foe? *FDA Consumer.* April 1995:25–29.

Lucas A, Morley R, Cole TJ, et al. Breast milk and subsequent intelligence quotient in children born premature. *Lancet.* 1992;339:261–264.

Mathew OP. Breathing patterns of preterm infants during bottle feeding: role of milk flow. *J Pediatrics.* 1991;119:960–965.

McCreadie RG. The Nithsdale schizophrenia surveys 16. Breast feeding and schizophrenia: preliminary results and hypotheses. *Br J Psychiatr.* 1997; 170:334–337.

McNally RJ, Parker L. Environmental factors and childhood acute leukemias and lymphomas. *Leuk Lymphoma.* April 2006;47(4):583–98.

Oddy WH, Holt PG, Sly PD, et al. Association between breastfeeding and asthma in 6-year-old children: findings of a prospective birth cohort study. *BMJ.* 1999;319: 815–819.

Palmer B. The influence of breastfeeding on the development of the oral cavity: a commentary. *J Hum Lact.* 1998;14:93–98.

Pettitt DJ, Forman MR, Hanson RL, Knowler WC, Bennett PH. Breastfeeding and incidence of non-insulin-dependent diabetes mellitus in Pima Indians. *Lancet.* 1997; 350:166–168.

Pisacane A, Graziano L, Mazzarella G, et al. Breastfeeding and urinary tract infections. *J Pediatr.* 1992;120:87–89.

Rao MR, Hediger ML, Levine RJ, et al. Effect of breastfeeding on cognitive development of infants born small for gestational age. *Acta Paediatr.* 2002;91:267–274.

Sadauskaite-Kuehne V, Ludvigsson J, Padaiga Z, et al. Longer breastfeeding is an independent protective factor against development of type 1 diabetes mellitus in childhood. *Diabetes Metab Res Rev.* 2004;20:150–157.

Scariati PD, Grummer-Strawn LM, Fein SB. A longitudinal analysis of infant morbidity and the extent of breastfeeding in the United States. *Pediatrics.* 1997;99:e5.

Semple JL, Lugowski SJ, Baines CJ, et al. Breast milk contamination and silicone implants: preliminary results using silicon as a proxy measurement for silicone. *Plast Reconstruct Surg.* 1998;102:528–533.

Setchell KDR, Zimmer-Nechemias L, Cai J, Heubi JE. Exposure of infants to phyto-estrogens from soy-based infant formula. *Lancet.* 1997;350:23–27.

Shannon MW, Graef JW. Lead intoxication in infancy. *Pediatrics.* 1992;89:87–90.

Sheikh C, Erickson PR. Evaluation of plaque pH changes following oral rinse with eight infant formulas. *Pediatr Dent.* 1996;18:200-204.

Simmer K. Longchain polyunsaturated fatty acid supplementation in infants born at term. *Cochrane Rev.* The Cochrane Library, 4, 2003.

Shu XO, Linet MS, Steinbuch M, et al. Breastfeeding and the risk of childhood acute leukemia. *J Natl Cancer Inst.* 1999;91:1765-1772.

Straarup EM, Lauritzen L, Faerk J, et al. The stereospecific triacylglycerol structures and fatty acid profiles of human milk and infant formulas. *J Pediatr Gastroenterol Nutr.* 2006;42:293-299.

Updegrove K. Necrotizing enterocolitis: the evidence for the use of human milk in prevention and treatment. *J Hum Lact.* 2004;20:335-339.

van Odijk J, Kull I, Borres MP, et al. Breastfeeding and allergic disease: a multidisciplinary review of the literature (1966-2001) on the mode of early feeding in infancy and its impact on later atopic manifestations. *Allergy.* 2003;58:833-843.

Vennemann MM, Findeisen M, Butterfass-Bahloul T, et al. Modifiable risk factors for SIDS in Germany: results of GeSID. *Acta Paediatr.* 2005;94:655-660.

Viggiano D, Fasano D, Monaco G, Strohmenger L. Breast feeding, bottle feeding, and non-nutritive sucking; effects on occlusion in deciduous dentition. *Arch Dis Child.* 2004;89:1121-1123.

von Kries R, Koletzko B, Sauerwald T, et al. Breastfeeding and obesity: cross sectional study. *BMJ.* 1999;319:147-150.

Walker M. *Selling Out Mothers and Babies: Marketing of Breast Milk Substitutes in the USA.* Weston, MA: National Alliance for Breastfeeding Advocacy; 2001.

Williams C, Birch EE, Emmett PM, Northstone K. Stereoacuity at age 3.5 y in children born full-term is associated with prenatal and postnatal dietary factors: a report from a population-based cohort study. *Am J Clin Nutr.* 2001;73:316-322.

World Health Organization (WHO). *Complementary Feeding of Young Children in Developing Countries: A Review of Current Scientific Knowledge.* WHO/NUT/98.1; Geneva, Switzerland, WHO, 1998.

World Health Organization/UNICEF. *Global Strategy for Infant and Young Child Feeding.* Geneva: WHO; 2003.

Wright K, Coverston C, Tiedeman M, Abegglen JA. Formula supplemented with docosahexaenoic acid (DHA) and arachidonic acid (ARA): a critical review of research. *J Spec Pediatr Nurs.* 2006;11:100-112.

Young TK, Martens PJ, Taback SP, Sellers EAC, Dean HJ, Cheang M, Flett B. Type 2 diabetes mellitus in children: Prenatal and early infancy risk factors among Native Canadians. *Arch Pediatr Adolesc Med.* 2002;156:651-655.

Zoppi G, Gasparini R, Mantovanelli F, et al. Diet and antibody response to vaccinations in healthy infants. *Lancet.* 1983;2:11-14.

Immunology, Infectious Disease, and Allergy Prophylaxis

Linda J. Smith, BSE, FACCE, IBCLC

OBJECTIVES

- Describe the components in human milk that contribute to disease protection and their actions.
- Discuss the role of breastfeeding in the long-term protection against chronic diseases and allergy.
- Identify maternal infectious diseases that are compatible with breastfeeding.
- Describe contraindications to breastfeeding.

Introduction

The mother serves as the baby's immune system, especially for the first six months during exclusive breastfeeding (Hanson, 2002). Breastfeeding and human milk fills an "immunologic gap" between the time when placentally-acquired immunity protects the fetus before birth, and approximately age three to four when the child's own immune system is robustly functional.

Current global recommendations are: immediate breastfeeding in the first half-hour after birth; exclusive breastfeeding for 6 months, followed by breastfeeding with complementary foods for two or more years. Three important policies underscore this recommendation: World Health Organization/United Nations Children's Fund's Global Strategy for Infant and Young Child Feeding (WHO, 2003); Systematic Review of the Optimum Duration of Exclusive Breastfeeding (Kramer & Kakuma, 2004); and WHO Child Growth Standards (WHO, 2006).

There are multiple mechanisms whereby milk components protect the nursling: active attack of pathogens, including: inactivation, binding, and destruction; binding nutrients needed by pathogens; creating an inhospitable milieu for pathogen growth and reproduction; and enhancing the growth, activity, effectiveness, and maturation of the infant's own immune system (Goldman, 1993). The mother's secretory immune system provides targeted protection against pathogens to which she (or the baby) has been exposed. Sensitized B-lymphocytes begin manufacturing targeted secretory immunoglobulin A (sIgA). The lymphocytes and the targeted sIgA migrate to the breast and pass into milk, where they are ingested by the baby and provide additional protection in the infant gut. Milk contains soluble components with immunologic properties, and living cells that are immunologically specific (Hanson, 2002; Hanson et al., 2003; Hanson, 2004).

"Non-breastfed human infants experience an acquired immunodeficiency that increases the risk of infections and other diseases. The antimicrobial, anti-inflammatory, and immunomodulating agents in human milk are multi-functional, act synergistically, and compensate for developmental delays in the infant" (Labbok, 2004).

Breastfeeding is strongly protective against allergy, delaying the onset and lessening the symptoms in the child. Dietary prophylaxis during pregnancy and exclusive breastfeeding for six months (not 4–6 months as previously recommended; Chantry Howard, & Auinger, 2006) has a strongly protective effect on illness prevention. Breastfeeding avoids infant exposure to dietary allergens, and slows or prevents absorption of allergens through the gut. Epidemiologic evidence of short- and long-term benefits of breastfeeding to the infant and mother continue to accumulate (Chen & Rogan, 2004; Dewey, Heinig, & Nommsen-Rivers, 1995). Lactation affects the woman's reproductive system, mediates her responses to stress, and reduces risk of several cancers. Breastfeeding protects the baby from numerous infections, improves cognitive and neurologic development, and reduces risk of many long-term and chronic diseases and conditions (Koletzko, Michaelson, & Hernell, 2000). Delaying breastfeeding increases the risk of neonatal mortality (Edmond et al., 2006). Breastfeeding is rarely contraindicated in cases of maternal infection (Lawrence & Lawrence, 2005, pp. 996–1012).

I. The Mother Serves as the Baby's Immune System (Hanson, 2000)

A. Prenatal and early postpartum.

1. The placenta passes maternal antibodies to the baby, and this protection persists for several weeks to months. The fetus also breathes and ingests/digests amniotic fluid, which provides significant amounts of protein.

2. Colostrum is exceedingly concentrated with anti-infective properties. Evolutionary evidence suggests that the earliest function of colostrum was to protect the young, with nutrition being a secondary purpose (Hennart et al., 1991; Goldman et al., 1982).

3. Human babies have a proportionally longer duration of colostrum feedings than other mammals.

B. Actions/features of milk components that protect the infant and the lactating breast.

1. Actively bind to pathogens, thus preventing their passage through the permeable infant gut mucosa. Components are highly targeted to foreign pathogens and ignore the infant's healthy gut flora (Hanson, 2000).

2. Bind and reduce availability of nutrients, vitamins, and/or minerals needed by pathogens.

3. Cellular components directly attack pathogens through phagocytosis.

4. Trigger and enhance development and maturation of infant's own immune system, including the increased effectiveness of immunizations.

5. Support optimal growth and maturation of the infant gut, respiratory, and urogenital tracts.

6. Prevent or reduce inflammation in infant organs and tissues, which protects them from infection.

7. Stimulate infant's immune system: Macrophages and T-lymphocytes provide immunologic maturation stimulus through cytokine production (Goldman & Goldblum, 1997; Goldman, Chheda, & Garofalo, 1998; Buescher, 1994).

C. Secretory immune system (entero-mammary and broncho-mammary pathways) provides protection against specific organisms to which the mother or infant has been exposed (Hanson, 2002).

1. Mother is exposed to a pathogen by ingestion, inhalation, or other contact, including pathogens that her baby has picked up. The pathogen comes in contact with the mucous membranes in her gut and bronchial tree, triggering an "alarm" in the mother's immune system.

2. T-lymphocytes located in mother's gut (in Peyer patches, or gut-associated lymphoid tissue) and bronchial tree (bronchus-associated lymphoid tissue) notice the new pathogen and pass on the specific message of "alarm" to nearby B-lymphocytes, which immediately begin production of sIgA targeted to that organism.

3. Sensitized B-lymphocytes migrate to mother's secretory organs or mucosal surfaces. There they secrete targeted sIgA into her blood, which is transported across the mammary secretory cells and released into the milk. (In addition, more sIgA appears to be synthesized in the mammary glandular cells.)

4. Targeted sIgA appears in milk shortly after maternal exposure to the original pathogen. Some sensitized B-lymphocytes also pass into milk and are ingested by the baby, and carry on their production of specific sIgA antibodies in the baby's gut.

5. The nursling ingests these targeted antibodies and sensitized live lymphocytes in the next breastfeed. The child may not get sick at all, or the illness is reduced in severity even if the mother becomes ill (Hanson, 2002).

II. Specific Protective Components of Milk (Butte et al., 1984).

A. Cellular components directly attack pathogens, mobilize other defenses, and activate soluble components. Although most live cells in the milk survive and continue to function in the infant gastrointestinal tract, they are usually destroyed by freezing, boiling, and other heat treatments.

  1. Immunologically specific: T-lymphocytes; B-lymphocytes.

  2. Accessory cells: neutrophils, macrophages, epithelial cells.

B. Soluble components have multiple protective functions including binding pathogens, secreting chemical markers, and binding nutrients needed by pathogens.

  1. Immunoglobulins: sIgA, IgE, IgG, IgM

  2. Nonspecific factors: complement, interferon, bifidus factor, antiviral factors.

  3. Carrier proteins: lactoferrin, transferrin.

  4. Enzymes: lysozyme, lipoprotein lipase, leukocyte enzymes.

  5. Cytokines including interferon and interleukins.

  6. Hormones and hormone-like substances: epidermal growth factor; prostaglandins; relaxin; somatostatin; gonadotropins and ovarian steroids; prolactin; and insulin.

C. Anti-inflammatory properties: Human milk lacks initiators of inflammation and destroys pathogens without triggering inflammation.

  1. Specific anti-inflammatory agents: lactoferrin; sIgA; lysozyme; prostaglandins; oligosaccharides; and epidermal growth factor.

D. Interaction of anti-inflammatory and anti-infective factors is synergistic, providing more protection in total than the sum of the parts, thus protecting both the mammary gland and infant from a vast array of pathogens.

E. Immunologic agents are "developmentally delayed" in infancy and are provided by human milk (Labbok, 2004).

  1. Antimicrobial: lactoferrin; lysozyme; sIgA; memory T cells; antibodies to T-cell-independent antigens.

  2. Anti-inflammatory: lactoferrin; lysozyme; sIgA; interleukin (IL)-10; platelet activating factor-acetylhydrolase.

  3. Immunomodulatory: sIgA; interferon-gamma (IF-γ); IL-8; IL-10.

III. Maternal Diseases and Breastfeeding

A. "Breastfeeding is rarely contraindicated in maternal infection." "Documenting transmission of infection from mother to infant by breastfeeding requires not only the exclusion of other possible mechanisms of transmission but also the demonstration of the infectious agent in the breast milk and a subsequent clinically significant infection in the infant caused by a plausible infectious process." (Lawrence & Lawrence, 2005, pp.629–630)

B. Standard precautions. "The CDC (Centers for Disease Control and Prevention) does not consider breast milk a body fluid with infectious risks for such policies." (Lawrence & Lawrence, 2005, p. 631; see Appendix C on universal precautions).

C. Contagious diseases.

  1. Bacterial infections: most bacteria are blocked.

      a. The mother should be treated and continue breastfeeding.

      b. Maternal Group B Streptococcal infections (GBS) are treated prenatally when identified or during the intrapartum period. Acquisition of GBS through breast milk or breastfeeding is rare. If a breastfed baby develops late onset GBS, milk is cultured, the mother is treated, and breastfeeding or breast milk feeding continues (Lawrence & Lawrence, 2005).

  2. Viral infections.

      a. Viral fragments for many diseases appear in mother's milk. These are not whole virus particles and do not appear to actually transmit disease. These fragments may act as a "vaccination" against the specific disease (e.g., cytomegalovirus).

      b. Human milk contains specific components active against many viruses, including poliovirus, respiratory syncytial virus, rotavirus, and influenza virus.

      c. Guidelines for breastfeeding or breast milk feeding when the mother is actively infected with a viral illness *at the time the baby is born* are published periodically.

          i. See Lawrence and Lawrence (2005) or similar references for treatment protocols for specific illnesses. In most, but not all, cases, breastfeeding can proceed normally. Even if viral fragments occur, the infant is generally asymptomatic.

          ii. Precautions are necessary when the mother is actively contagious with certain diseases *at the time of the baby's birth*. For example, the mother with an active tuberculosis or chickenpox infection on the day of birth must be isolated from her newborn until she has been treated or is not contagious. She can and should provide her milk for her infant since these diseases are not transmitted via breast milk.

          iii. Active infectious (i.e., herpes) lesions on the breast may require temporary separation of the mother from the baby until the lesions are dried. Careful hand washing, covering other lesions, and avoiding contact of lesions with the baby is necessary.

      d. As of late 2006, no information is available on risks or benefits of breastfeeding or breast milk feeding if the mother has a virus that causes highly fatal hemorrhagic fever, such as Ebola or Marburg. Consult current medical references and providers (Lawrence & Lawrence, 2005).

e. "Breastfeeding is even more important when disease exposures are common, and when there are other children or an immune-compromised individual in the household." (Labbok, 2004)

3. Human immunodeficiency virus/acquired immune deficiency syndrome (HIV/AIDS)

a. As of this writing, mother-to-child transmission of HIV/AIDS appears to occur mainly through direct blood contact at the time of birth or transplacentally in utero. Estimated rates of mother-to-child transmission range from 13% to 60% depending on the geographic area studied.

b. Some babies face additional risk of transmission of the virus through breastfeeding. The research has yet to be done to determine if the virus in breast milk is actually infectious or, if it is infectious, if it infects the baby. The data are not conclusive in this respect. As of this writing, the calculated incremental *additional* risk of transmission via breastfeeding ranges from 5% to 20% (WHO, 2004), depending on a multitude of contributing factors.

c. Individual countries and medical associations have published specific policies based on local economic, health, and other conditions.

d. HIV-1 transmission through breast milk may be more dependent on the pattern of breastfeeding or potential confounders such as breast disease, cracked nipples or Candida infection, rather than on the total amount or duration of all breastfeeding.

e. "Infants exclusively breastfed for 3 months or more had no excess risk of HIV transmission over 6 months than those never breastfed" (Coutsoudis et al., 2001; Iliff et al., 2005).

f. Exclusive breastfeeding for at least 3 months may carry half the risk of mother to child transmission of HIV-1 than mixed feeding (never breastfed, 18.8%; mixed fed, 24.1%; exclusive breastfed for 3 months, 14.6%; Coutsoudis et al., 2001).

g. WHO, UNICEF, and United Nations Programme on HIV/AIDS (UNAIDS) issued a joint Statement in 2003 containing these policy issues:

4. Human rights perspective.

a. Preventing HIV infection in women.

b. Health of mothers and children.

c. Elements of establishing a policy on HIV and infant feeding.

i. Supporting breastfeeding.

ii. Access to voluntary, individual, and confidential counseling and testing.

iii. Ensuring informed choice.

iv. Preventing commercial pressures for artificial feeding.

d. WHO/UNAIDS/UNICEF Basic Guidelines on HIV and Infant Feeding (WHO, 2006).

     i. "If status is unknown, or if tested and HIV negative (HIV−): Exclusive breastfeeding (EBF) for six months and continued breastfeeding for two years and beyond for HIV negative women and women of unknown status.

     ii. If tested and HIV positive (HIV+): If replacement feeding is affordable, feasible, acceptable, safe, and sustainable, avoidance of all breastfeeding is recommended. Otherwise EBF is recommended for the first months of the baby's life.

     iii. Women should have access to relevant infant feeding information, follow-up care, and support (including family planning and nutritional support).

e. Breastfeeding should continue to be promoted, protected, and supported in all populations worldwide. Health authorities consider the mother who is HIV+ to be an extraordinary circumstance. All women should have voluntary and confidential HIV testing and individualized counseling in order to make an informed decision regarding feeding their babies. There is no evidence to support better outcomes in terms of morbidity/mortality for abrupt weaning or early discontinuation of breastfeeding at this time (Thior, 2006).

f. Mothers who are HIV+ and decide not to breastfeed have been offered several options based on the assumption that HIV virus in breast milk is infectious. As of 2006, that assumption has not yet been verified by rigorous research.

     i. Mother's own modified milk, because heat treatment inactivates the virus.

     ii. Institutional pasteurization (Holder pasteurization).

     iii. Home pasteurization by hot water baths, flash heating, Pretoria pasteurization, or other methods that hold the milk at 60°C for 30 minutes (Hartman, Berlin, & Howett, 2006; Israel-Ballard et al., 2005, Jeffery & Mercer, 2000).

     iv. Antimicrobial treatment of the breastfeeding mother with anti-malarial drugs.

     v. Microbicidal treatment of milk with alkyl sulfates.

     vi. Banked donor human milk, because all banked milk is donated by screened donors and then pasteurized (HMBANA 2006).

     vii. Commercial infant formula.

     viii. Homemade formula.

g. The lactation consultant's role is to collect and compile current research, resources, and recommendations, and share these with the mother and her primary care provider(s). She/he may also assist with weaning or other breastfeeding-related issues. The lactation consultant does not have a decision-making role in caring for families with this disease.

5. Cross infection
   a. The baby/babies' mouth(s) and mother's breast(s) are in intimate physical contact many times a day during breastfeeding. Any communicable disease/infection on either the nipple surfaces or the infant's mouth is quickly transmitted to the other.
   b. The dyad needs to be treated simultaneously until both (or all) sites are healthy. Examples: oral thrush and nipple Candida; child with strep throat infects mother's nipple. Breastfeeding should continue during treatments.
   c. Standard precautions should be used by all health care providers. Concerning human milk:
      i. "Contact with breast milk does not constitute occupational exposure as defined by OSHA [Occupational Health and Safety Administration] standards" (U.S. Dept of Labor, 1992).
      ii. Gloves are not recommended for the routine handling of expressed human milk; but should be worn by health care workers in situations where exposure to breast milk might be frequent or prolonged, for example, in milk banking" (CDC, 1996).

6. Summary of maternal infectious diseases and compatibility with breastfeeding. Refer to Table 19-1. Caution: *Consult current medical references as new information becomes available. Each situation must be decided individually by the primary care provider(s). Contraindications to breastfeeding are rare.*

7. Immunizing the breastfeeding mother. Lactating women may be immunized as recommended for other adults to protect against (Lawrence & Lawrence 2005, pp. 420–421):
   a. Measles, mumps, rubella, tetanus, diphtheria, influenza, *Strep pneumoniae*, hepatitis A virus, hepatitis B virus, varicella, and may receive Rh immune globulin.
   b. Inactivated polio virus if traveling to a highly endemic area.
   c. No parents of infants are recommended to receive smallpox/cowpox vaccination; if needed, contact precautions must be observed.
   d. For current recommendations, visit "Breastfeeding During Travel" posted by the U.S. Centers for Disease Control at http://www.cdc.gov/breastfeeding/recommendations/travel_recommendations.htm.

IV. Protective Effects of Breastfeeding Against Allergy

A. Milk is species-specific. A baby is never allergic to its own mother's milk. The baby and the mother share 50% of the same genetic material. No antibody response to mother's milk has ever been documented. sIgA in milk binds with and prevents transport of dietary allergens until the infant gut is less permeable. This is most important in the early months until the baby begins producing its own sIgA.

Table 19-1   Summary of Maternal Infectious Diseases and Compatibility with Breastfeeding

Disease	OK to breastfeed in the United States?*	Conditions
Acute infectious disease	Yes	Respiratory, reproductive, GI infections
Active tuberculosis	Yes	If mother is actively infected at birth, separate until after mother has received treatment; milk is still OK.
Hepatitis A	Yes	
Hepatitis B	Yes	After infant receives HBIG, 1st dose before discharge.
Hepatitis C	Yes	If no co-infections (such as HIV).
Herpes simplex	Yes	Except if lesion is on breast where baby would contact; if lesion is on the infant's lips, there is no reason to suspend breastfeeding.
Herpes/cytomegalovirus	Yes	
Herpes/Epstein-Barr virus	Yes	
Herpes/Varicella-zoster (chickenpox)	Yes	If mother is actively infected at birth, separate until mother becomes non-infectious; baby can still receive her milk.
Lyme disease	Yes	As soon as mother begins treatment.
Mastitis (infectious)	Yes	Continue or increase breastfeeding; milk stasis will exacerbate the illness.
Toxoplasmosis	Yes	
Venereal warts	Yes	
HIV or HTLV-1	NO	*HIV positive—see WHO/UNICEF guidelines.

Source: Adapted from Table 7 in: Lawrence R. *A Review of the Medical Benefits and Contraindications to Breastfeeding in the United States* (Maternal and Child Health Technical Information Bulletin). Arlington, VA: National Center for Education in Maternal and Child Health, October 1997.

B. Breastmilk has multiple effects.

1. Prevents/avoids the infant's exposure to non-human proteins and pathogens.

2. Slows or prevents absorption of antigens through the infant gut.

C. Prophylactic management of children with a family history of atopic (allergic) disease.

1. Allergic disease has a strong hereditary basis.
   a. 47% incidence if both parents are allergic.
   b. 29% incidence if one parent is allergic.
   c. 13% incidence even if neither parent has a family history of allergy.

2. The only effective treatment is to reduce the allergenic load.

3. Dietary prophylaxis is clearly effective, especially in families with a strong history.
   a. Mothers have been advised to avoid common allergens during pregnancy, especially dairy products, fish, eggs, and peanuts with mixed results.
   b. Exclusive breastfeeding for about six months.
   c. Longer exclusive breastfeeding may be advantageous to the infant with a family history of allergy.

D. Allergic disease is responsible for ⅓ of pediatric office visits, ⅓ of chronic conditions of children under age 17, and ⅓ of lost school days due to asthma (Lawrence & Lawrence, 2005, p. 695). Allergic diseases are strongly linked to artificial feeding, including eczema, asthma, hay fever, gut and respiratory infection, ulcerative colitis, and even sudden death.

E. All non-human milks currently available, including hydrolyzed or "hypoallergenic" products, have been shown to cause anaphylactic reactions in sensitive babies (AAP, 2000; Ellis, Short, & Heiner, 1991; Saylor & Bahna, 1991).

1. Severe reactions have occurred, even at the "first" exposure. It was discovered that the infants who reacted so strongly had received undocumented feeds of cow's milk formula in a hospital nursery (Host, Husby, & Osterballe, 1988).

2. Hypoallergenic formulas are not completely non-allergic; they have the capacity to provoke anaphylactic shock in susceptible infants; hypoallergenic means that 90% of affected individuals will not be allergic to the product.

3. "Between 17% and 47% of milk allergic children can have adverse reactions to soy" (ASCIA, 2006). The American Academy of Pediatrics (AAP) does not recommend the use of soy formula when a documented allergy to cow's milk formula exists because soy formula has not been demonstrated to reduce development of atopy in infancy and childhood (AAP, 1998).

F. Food allergies occur in ~5.8% to 6% of children; cow's milk allergy ranges from .5% to 7.5% (Lawrence & Lawrence, 2005).

1. Solid foods introduced before 15 weeks are associated with increased probability of wheezing, respiratory illness, and eczema. Any substance other than mother's own milk can provoke a reaction, and reactions are dose-related.

2. According to the Food Allergy and Anaphylaxis Network, the eight most common food allergens are:
   a. Milk and other dairy products (cow's milk protein).
   b. Eggs.
   c. Peanuts.
   d. Tree nuts (walnuts, cashews, etc.).
   e. Fish.
   f. Shellfish.
   g. Soy and soy products (tofu, soy milk, soy nuts, etc.).
   h. Wheat.

3. If a mother suspects that her child is having a problem with food allergies or intolerances, and the baby's health care provider is dismissive of these concerns, the mother can be advised to ask for a referral to an allergist. Symptoms that would indicate a problem include:
   a. Chronic eczema: long periods of scaly and itchy skin rashes.
   b. Hives often show up as itchy red welts on the surface of the skin.
   c. Chronic unexplained digestive or respiratory problems.
   d. Colic: chronic, unexplained, excessive crying.
   e. **Caution:** Anaphylaxis is a severe allergic reaction that can be fatal. Call Emergency Services (9-1-1 in the United States) immediately if you see signs of anaphylaxis: severe hives or hives in conjunction with another reaction, facial swelling, swelling of mouth and throat (constriction of the throat is especially dangerous because as the throat swells shut, the child will stop breathing and turn blue from the lack of oxygen), vomiting, diarrhea, cramping, drop in blood pressure, fainting, death.

4. Gut closure affects allergic sensitization.
   a. Age at which other milks are introduced rather than total breastfeeding length is more closely associated with atopy at six years of age.
   b. Arbitrary, inadvertent, or unnecessary cow's milk-based formula supplementation given to susceptible breastfed babies during the first three days of life can sensitize these babies and provoke allergic reactions to cow's milk protein later in the first year of life (Walker, 2006, pp. 159–160).
      i. Cow's milk proteins are usually the first foreign antigens encountered by newborn infants in their diet. Intestinal absorption of macromolecules is greatest during the first two months of life, which is the critical time period for induction of a specific immune response to dietary antigens. An incomplete mucosal barrier and increased gut permeability are seen in altered immunologic responses.

ii. For infants prone to developing cow's milk allergy, short exposure to cow's milk-based formula in the hospital or exclusive breastfeeding combined with infrequent intake of small amounts of cow's milk-based formula may stimulate specific IgE antibody production. However, frequent feeding of large volumes of cow's milk-based formula induces development of non-IgE mediated delayed-type hypersensitivity to cow's milk.

iii. Cow's milk proteins (beta-lactoglobulin) do transfer to human milk, sensitizing predisposed babies to cow's milk (Jakobsson et al., 1985).

iv. Introduction of cow's milk protein in the first 8 days is a significant risk factor for type I diabetes in genetically susceptible populations. The AAP recommends no cow's milk protein for the first year of life if there is a family history of type I diabetes (Lawrence & Lawrence, 2005, pp. 580–581).

5. **Even small allergen exposures (doses)** may be sensitizing in allergy prone people. Prevalence of eczema and food allergy is highest between 1 and 3 years, and respiratory allergy is highest between 5 to 17 years.
   a. Breastfeeding also confers long-term protection against allergic sensitization.
      i. Breastfeeding for longer than one month with no other milk supplements offers significant prophylaxis against food allergy at three years and respiratory allergy at 17 years (Saarinen & Kajosaari, 1995).
      ii. Six months of breastfeeding significantly reduces eczema during the first three years and at adolescence (Saarinen & Kajosaari, 1995).
      iii. Allergic manifestations include: recurrent wheezing, elevated IgE levels, eczema, atopic dermatitis, GI symptoms of diarrhea, vomiting, and blood in the stool.
      iv. Exclusive breastfeeding for six months is more protective than the former recommendation of exclusive breastfeeding for four to six months, especially for respiratory tract infections (Kramer et al., 2001).

6. A dose-response relationship exists between the amount of breast milk as the percentage of the infant's feed, with babies receiving exclusive breast milk for longer periods of time showing the least amount of short- and long-term disease and allergy. The more breast milk an infant receives during the first six months of life, the less likely he/she is to develop illness or allergy. The largest difference in health outcomes is found in exclusively breastfed compared with exclusively formula-fed children.

7. WHO recommendations for infant feeding, in order of preference:
   a. Direct breastfeeding (expressed mother's own milk is next best).
   b. Milk of another woman (wet-nursing).
   c. Pasteurized donor human milk from a milk bank.
   d. Manufactured infant formula.
      i. Animal-based milks (cow-milk based).
      ii. Plant-based "milks" (soy-based).

e. Babies who demonstrate an allergic reaction to hydrolyzed formula may need to be fed with elemental or amino acid-derived formulas.

V. Breastfed Infants Have Different Health, Growth, and Developmental Outcomes Than Formula-Fed Babies

A. WHO published new Growth Standards in early 2006.

1. "The World Health Organization is launching new global Child Growth Standards for infants and children up to the age of five. With these new WHO Child Growth Standards it is now possible to show how children *should* grow. They demonstrate for the first time ever that children born in different regions of the world and given the optimum start in life, have the potential to grow and develop to within the same range of height and weight for age" (WHO, 2006).

2. The 2006 WHO Growth Standards are standards (prescriptive: how children should grow in optimum conditions) and not references (descriptive: how children do grow in certain situations). The data were compiled from six regions of the world.

3. Chapter 28 has more information on the WHO Growth Standards.

B. Formula-fed babies have an increased risk and incidence of the following (AAP, 2005; Labbok, Clark & Goldman, 2004; Scariati, Grummer-Strawn, & Fein, 1997; Walker, 2001):

1. GI disease.
   a. Diarrhea: bacterial, viral, parasitic (Newburg, Ruiz-Palacios, & Morrow, 2005).
   b. Necrotizing enterocolitis.

2. Respiratory disease.
   a. Otitis media.
   b. Upper and lower respiratory infections (Howie et al., 1990).
   c. Wheezing.
   d. Asthma (Oddy, 2004).
   e. Allergies (Oddy, 2004; Oddy, 2006; Zieger, 2000).

3. Urinary tract infections.

4. Deficient response to childhood immunizations (Hahn-Zoric et al., 1990; Zopp et al., 1983).

C. Formula-fed babies have a different brain composition than breastfed babies with half the docosahexaenoic acid (DHA) as in the brain of a breastfed infant, and can experience: (Lanting et al., 1994; Walker, 2006, p. 9).

1. Discrepancy in visual acuity.

2. Lower IQ.

3. Poorer school performance.

4. Increased risk for neurologic dysfunction (Tanoue & Oda, 1989).

5. Increased risk for specific language impairment.

6. Lower DHA in the gray and white matter of the cerebellum, which coordinates movement and balance.

7. Increased risk for multiple sclerosis.

D. Long-term and chronic diseases are more common in artificially fed children, such as:

1. Obesity (Oddy, 2006)

2. Sudden infant death syndrome (Horne et al., 2004).

3. Juvenile rheumatoid arthritis.

4. Childhood cancers, especially lymphomas and leukemia.

5. Diabetes: type 1 and type 2 (Stuebe et al., 2005).

6. GI disorders: Crohn disease, ulcerative colitis, reflux (Cavataio et al., 1996; Iacono et al., 1996; Machida et al., 1994).

7. Autoimmune thyroid disease.

8. Dental caries and dental fluorosis.

9. Structural changes.
   a. Inguinal hernia.
   b. Bone mineralization.
   c. Gastro-esophageal reflux.
   d. Pyloric stenosis.
   e. Smaller thymus gland (Hasselbalch et al., 1996).

E. Differences due to the physical act of breastfeeding (sucking at breast).

1. Orthodontic changes affecting bite, alignment; malocclusion; deformed maxillary arch (Davis & Bell, 1991; Labbok & Hendershot, 1987).

2. Oral muscle changes affecting speech, articulation (Inoue, Sakashita, & Kamegai, 1995).

3. Visual development, because bottle-feeding consistently in one position can reduce visual stimulation of one eye.

F. Mothers who do not breastfeed have higher levels of stress (Groer, 2005; Montgomery, Ehlin, & Sacker, 2006).

References

American Academy of Pediatrics Committee on Nutrition. Hypoallergenic Infant Formulas. *Pediatrics*. 2000;106:346-349.

American Academy of Pediatrics Committee on Nutrition. Soy Protein-based Formulas: Recommendations for Use in Infant Feeding. *Pediatrics*. 1998;101(1):148-153.

American Academy of Pediatrics Section on Breastfeeding. Breastfeeding and the Use of Human Milk. *Pediatrics.* 2005;115(2):496–506.

Australasian Society of Clinical Immunology and Allergy (ASCIA). Balgowlah, NSW, Australia. Available at http://www.allergy.org.au/. Accessed December 27, 2006.

Buescher ES. Host defense mechanisms of human milk and their relations to enteric infections and necrotizing enterocolitis. *Clin Perinatol.* 1994;21:247–262.

Butte NF, Goldblum RM, Fehl LM, et al. Daily ingestion of immunologic components in human milk during the first four months of life. *Acta Paediatr Scand.* 1984; 73:296–301.

Cavataio F, Iacono G, Montalto G, et al. Clinical and pH-metric characteristics of gastro-oesophageal reflux secondary to cow's milk protein allergy. *Arch Dis Child.* 1996;75:51–56.

Centers for Disease Control and Prevention. Perspectives in Disease Prevention and Health Promotion Update: Universal Precautions for Prevention of Transmission of Human Immunodeficiency Virus, Hepatitis B Virus, and Other Bloodborne Pathogens in Health-Care Settings. *MMWR.* June 24, 1988;37(24):377–388; updated 1996.

Chantry CJ, Howard CR, Auinger P. Full breastfeeding duration and associated decrease in respiratory tract infection in US children. *Pediatrics.* 2006;117:425–432.

Chen A, Rogan WJ. Breastfeeding and the risk of postneonatal death in the United States. *Pediatrics.* 2004;113:e435–439.

Coutsoudis A, Pillay K, Huhn L, et al. Method of feeding and transmission of HIV-1 from mothers to children by 15 months of age: prospective cohort study from Durban, South Africa. *AIDS.* 2001;15:379–387.

Davis D, Bell PA. Infant feeding practices and occlusal outcomes: A longitudinal study. *J Can Dent Assoc.* 1991;57:593–594. Abstract.

Dewey KG, Heinig J, Nommsen-Rivers L. Differences in morbidity between breastfed and formula-fed infants. *J Pediatr.* 1995;126:696–702.

Edmond KM, Zandoh C, Quigley MA, et al. Delayed breastfeeding initiation increases risk of neonatal mortality. *Pediatrics.* 2006;117:e380–386.

Ellis MH, Short JA, Heiner DC. Anaphylaxis after ingestion of a recently introduced hydrolyzed whey protein formula. *J Pediatr.* 1991;118(1):74–77.

Goldman AS, Cheda S, Garofalo R. Evolution of immunologic functions of the mammary gland and the postnatal development of immunity. *Pediatr Res.* 1998; 43:155–162.

Goldman AS, Garza C, Nichols BL, Goldblum RM. Immunologic factors in human milk during the first year of lactation. *J Pediatr.* 1982;100:563–567.

Goldman AS, Goldblum RM. Transfer of maternal leukocytes to the infant by human milk. *Curr Top Microbiol Immunol.* 1997;222:205–213.

Goldman AS. The immune system of human milk: antimicrobial, antiinflammatory and immunomodulating properties. *Pediatr Infect Dis J.* 1993;12:664–671.

Groer MW. Differences between exclusive breastfeeders, formula-feeders, and controls: a study of stress, mood, and endocrine variables. *Biol Res Nurs.* 2005;7:106–117.

Hahn-Zoric M, Falconis F, Minoli I, et al. Antibody responses to parenteral and oral vaccines are impaired by conventional and low protein formulas as compared to breastfeeding. *Acta Paediatr Scand.* 1990;79:1137–1142.

Hanson LA, Ceafalau L, Mattsby-Baltzer I, et al. The mammary gland-infant intestine immunologic dyad. *Adv Exp Med Biol.* 2000;478:65–76.

Hanson LA, Korotkova M, Haversen L, et al. Breast-feeding, a complex support system for the offspring. *Pediatr Int.* 2002;44:347–352.

Hanson LA, Korotkova M, Lundin S, et al. The transfer of immunity from mother to child. *Ann N Y Acad Sci.* 2003;987:199–206.

Hanson LA, Korotkova M. The role of breastfeeding in prevention of neonatal infection. *Semin Neonatol.* 2002;7:275–281.

Hanson LA, Silfverdal SA, Korotkova M, et al. Immune system modulation by human milk. *Adv Exp Med Biol.* 2002;503:99–106.

Hanson LA. *Immunobiology of Human Milk: How Breastfeeding Protects Babies.* Amarillo, TX: Pharmasoft (Hale) Publishing; 2004a.

Hanson LA. Protective effects of breastfeeding against urinary tract infection. *Acta Paediatr.* 2004b;93:154–156.

Hanson LA. The mother-offspring dyad and the immune system. *Acta Paediatr.* 2000; 89:252–258.

Hartmann SU, Berlin CM, Howett MK. Alternative modified infant-feeding practices to prevent postnatal transmission of human immunodeficiency virus type 1 through breast milk: past, present, and future. *J Hum Lact.* 2006;22:75–88; quiz 89–93.

Hasselbalch H, Jeppesen DL, Engelmann MDM, et al. Decreased thymus size in formula-fed infants compared with breastfed infants. *Acta Paediatr.* 1996;85:1029–1032.

Hennart PF, Brasseur DJ, Delogne-Desnoeck JB, Dramaix MM, Robyn CE. Lysozyme, lactoferrin, and secretory immunoglobulin A content in breast milk: influence of duration of lactation, nutrition status, prolactin status, and parity of mother. *Am J Clin Nutr.* 1991;53(1):32–39.

Horne RS, Parslow PM, Ferens D, Watts AM, Adamson TM. Comparison of evoked arousability in breast and formula fed infants. *Arch Dis Child.* 2004;89(1):22–25.

Host A, Husby S, Osterballe O. A prospective study of cow's milk allergy in exclusively breast-fed infants. Incidence, pathogenetic role of early inadvertent exposure to cow's milk formula, and characterization of bovine milk protein in human milk. *Acta Paediatr Scand.* 1988;77(5):663–670.

Howie PW, Forsyth JS, Ogston SA, et al. Protective effect of breastfeeding against infection. *Br Med J.* 1990;300:11–16.

Iacono G, Carroccio A, Vatataio F, et al. Gastroesophageal reflux and cow's milk allergy in infants: a prospective study. *J Allergy Clin Immunol.* 1996;97:822–827.

Iliff PJ, Piwoz EG, Tavengwa NV, et al. Early exclusive breastfeeding reduces the risk of postnatal HIV-1 transmission and increases HIV-free survival. *AIDS.* 2005; 19:699–708.

Inoue N, Sakashita R, Kamegai T. Reduction of masseter muscle activity in bottle-fed babies. *Early Hum Dev.* 1995;42:185–193.

Israel-Ballard K, Chantry C, Dewey K, et al. Viral, nutritional, and bacterial safety of flash-heated and pretoria-pasteurized breast milk to prevent mother-to-child transmission of HIV in resource-poor countries: a pilot study. *J Acquir Immune Defic Syndr.* 2005;40:175–181.

Jakobsson I, Lindberg T, Benediktsson B, Hansson BG. Dietary bovine beta-lactoglobulin is transferred to human milk. *Acta Paediatr Scand.* 1985;74(3):342–345.

Jeffery BS, Mercer KG. Pretoria pasteurization: a potential method for the reduction of postnatal mother-to-child transmission of the human immunodeficiency virus. *J Trop Pediatr.* 2000;46:219–223.

Koletzko B, Michaelson KF, Hernell O. *Short and Long Term Effects of Breastfeeding on Child Health.* New York: Kluwer Academic/Plenum Publishers; 2000.

Kramer M, Chalmers B, Hodnett E, et al. Promotion of Breastfeeding Intervention Trial (PROBIT): a randomized trial in the Republic of Belarus. *JAMA.* 2001;285:463–464; 2001:285:2446–2447.

Kramer MS, Kakuma R. The optimal duration of exclusive breastfeeding: a systematic review. *Adv Exp Med Biol.* 2004;554:63–77.

Labbok MH, Hendershot GE. Does breastfeeding protect against malocclusion? An analysis of the 1981 child health supplement to the National Health Interview Survey. *Am J Prev Med.* 1987;3:227–232.

Labbok MH, Clark D, Goldman AS. Breastfeeding: maintaining an irreplaceable immunological resource. *Nat Rev Immunol.* 2004;4:565–572.

Labbok MH. The Immunological Secrets of Breastfeeding: Implications for Policy and Practice. Presentation. International Lactation Consultant Association Annual Conference; 2004.

Lanting CE, Fidler V, Huisman M, et al. Neurological differences between 9-year-old children fed breastmilk or formula-milk as babies. *Lancet.* 1994;344:1319–1322.

Lawrence RA, Lawrence RM. Breastfeeding. *A Guide for the Medical Profession.* 6th ed. Philadelphia: Elsevier/Mosby; 2005.

Machida HM, Catto Smith AG, Gall DG, et al. Allergic colitis in infancy: clinical and pathologic aspects. *J Pediatr Gastroenterol Nutr.* 1994;19:22–26.

Newburg DS, Ruiz-Palacios GM, Morrow AL. Human milk glycans protect infants against enteric pathogens. *Annu Rev Nutr.* 2005;25:37–58.

Oddy WH, Li J, Landsborough L, et al. The association of maternal overweight and obesity with breastfeeding duration. *J Pediatr.* 2006a;149:185–191.

Oddy WH, Pal S, Kusel MM, et al. Atopy, eczema and breast milk fatty acids in a high-risk cohort of children followed from birth to 5 yr. *Pediatr Allergy Immunol.* 2006b;17:4–10.

Oddy WH, Scott JA, Graham KI, Binns CW. Breastfeeding influences on growth and health at one year of age. *Breastfeed Rev.* 2006c;14:15–23.

Oddy WH, Sherriff JL, de Klerk NH, et al. The relation of breastfeeding and body mass index to asthma and atopy in children: a prospective cohort study to age 6 years. *Am J Public Health.* 2004;94:1531–1537.

Oddy WH. A review of the effects of breastfeeding on respiratory infections, atopy, and childhood asthma. *J Asthma.* 2004;41:605–621.

Saarinen UM, Kajosaari M. Breastfeeding as prophylaxis against atopic disease: prospective follow-up study until 17 years old. *Lancet.* 1995;346:1065–1069.

Saylor JD, Bahna SL. Anaphylaxis to casein hydrolysate formula. *J Pediatr* 1991;118(1): 71–74.

Scariati PD, Grummer-Strawn LM, Fein SB. A longitudinal analysis of infant morbidity and the extent of breastfeeding in the US. *Pediatrics.* 1997;99:e5.

Stuebe AM, Rich-Edwards JW, Willett WC, et al. Duration of lactation and incidence of type 2 diabetes. *JAMA.* 2005;294:2601–2610.

Tanoue Y, Oda S. Weaning time of children with infantile autism. *J Autism Dev Disord.* 1989;19:425–434.

Thior I, Lockman S, Smeaton LM, et al. Breastfeeding plus infant zidovudine prophylaxis for 6 months vs formula feeding plus infant zidovudine for 1 month to reduce mother-to-child HIV transmission in Botswana: a randomized trial: the Mashi Study. *JAMA.* 2006;296:794–805.

U.S. Department of Labor. Breast milk does not constitute occupational exposure as defined by standard (Policy Interpretation). 1992. Washington, DC; United States Department of Labor. Available at http://www.osha.gov/pls/oshaweb/owadisp. show_document?p_table=INTERPRETATIONS&tp_id=20952. Accessed January 5, 2007.

Walker M. *Selling Out Mothers and Babies: Marketing Breastmilk Substitutes in the USA.* Weston, MA; NABA REAL; 2001.

Walker M. *Breastfeeding Management for the Clinician: Using the Evidence.* Sudbury, MA: Jones and Bartlett Publishers; 2006.

World Health Organization (WHO). Global Strategy on Infant and Young Child Feeding. Geneva: WHO; 2003. Available at: http://www.who.int/nutrition/topics/global_strategy/ en/index.html. Accessed December 27, 2006.

World Health Organization (WHO). HIV and Infant Feeding: Infant Feeding Options and Guidelines for Decision-Makers. Geneva: WHO; 2003.

World Health Organization (WHO). HIV Transmission through breastfeeding: A review of the evidence. Geneva: World Health Organization 2004. Available at: http://www. who.int/nutrition/publications/HIV_IF_Transmission.pdf. Accessed January 5, 2007.

World Health Organization (WHO). HIV and infant feeding: framework for priority action. Geneva: World Health Organization; 2003.

World Health Organization (WHO). WHO Child Growth Standards. Geneva: World Health Organization; 2006. Available at: http://www.who.int/childgrowth/en. Accessed December 27, 2006.

Zieger RS. Dietary aspects of food allergy prevention in infants and children. *J Pediatr Gastroenterol Nutr.* 2000;30:S77–S86.

Zoppi G, Gasparini R, Mantovanelli F, et al. Diet and antibody response to vaccinations in healthy infants. *Lancet.* 1983;7:11–14.

Suggested Readings

Asthma information. Centers for Disease Control and Prevention. Atlanta, GA: CDC. Available at: http://www.cdc.gov/asthma/children.htm. Accessed December 27, 2006.

Ball TM, Wright AL. Health care costs of formula-feeding in the first year of life. *Pediatrics.* 1999;103:870–876.

Basile LA, Taylor SN, Wagner CL, et al. The effect of high-dose vitamin D supplementation on serum vitamin D levels and milk calcium concentration in lactating women and their infants. *Breastfeeding Med.* 2006;1:27–35.

Beaudry M, Dufour R, Marcoux S. Relation between infant feeding and infections during the first six months of life. *J Pediatr.* 1995;126:191–197.

Burr ML, Limb ES, Maguire MJ, et al. Infant feeding, wheezing, and allergy: a prospective study. *Arch Dis Child.* 1993;68:724–728.

Businco L, Bruno G, Giampietro PG. Soy protein for the prevention and treatment of children with cow-milk allergy. *Am J Clin Nutr.* 1998;68(6 suppl):1447S–1452S.

DiPietro J, Larson S, Porges S. Behavioral and heart rate pattern differences between breastfed and bottle-fed neonates. *Dev Psychol.* 1987;23:467–474.

Duncan B, Ey J, Holberg CJ, et al. Exclusive breast-feeding for at least 4 months protects against otitis media. *Pediatrics.* 1993;91:867–872.

Falth-Magnusson K. Breast milk antibodies to foods in relation to maternal diet, maternal atopy and the development of atopic disease in the baby. *Int Arch Allergy Appl Immunol.* 1989;90:297–300.

Food Allergy and Anaphylaxis Network. Fairfax, VA. Available at: http://www.foodallergy.org/. Accessed December 27, 2006.

Gerstein HC. Cow's milk exposure and type I diabetes mellitus: a critical overview of the clinical literature. *Diabet Care.* 1994;17:13–18.

Goldman AS. Immunologic system in human milk. *J Pediatr Gastroenterol Nutr.* 1986; 5:343–345.

Hanson LA, Ahlstedt S, Andersson B, et al. Protective factors in milk and the development of the immune system. *Pediatrics.* January 1985;75(1 Pt 2):172–176.

Hanson LA, Ahlstedt S, Andersson B, et al. The immune response of the mammary gland and its significance for the neonate. *Ann Allergy.* December 1984;53(6 Pt 2):576–582.

Hanson LA, Korotkova M, Telemo E. Breast-feeding, infant formulas, and the immune system. *Ann Allergy Asthma Immunol.* 2003;90(6 sSuppl 3):59–63.

Host A. Importance of the first meal on the development of cow's milk allergy and intolerance. *Allergy Proc.* 1991;10:227–232.

Host A, Halken S. Hypoallergenic formulas—when, to whom and how long: after more than 15 years we know the right indication! *Allergy.* 2004;59(suppl 78):45–52.

Host A, Halken S, Jacobsen HP, Christensen AE, Herskind AM, Plesner K. Clinical course of cow's milk protein allergy/intolerance and atopic diseases in childhood. *Pediatr Allergy Immunol.* 2002;13 Suppl 15:23–28.

Institute of Medicine (Subcommittee on Nutrition during Lactation, Food and Nutrition Board). Nutrition during Lactation. Washington, DC: National Academy of Sciences; 1991.

Kostraba JH, Cruickshanks KJ, Lawler-Heavner J, et al. Early exposure to cow's milk and solid foods in infancy, genetic predisposition, and risk of IDDM. *Diabetes.* 1993; 42:288–295.

Lawrence R. A review of the medical benefits and contraindications to breastfeeding in the United States (Maternal and Child Health Technical Information Bulletin). Arlington, VA: National Center for Education in Maternal and Child Health; October 1997.

Lawrence RA, Howard CR. Given the benefits of breastfeeding, are there any contraindications? *Clin Perinatol.* 1999;26:479–490, viii.

Liles C, Tompson M. Breastfeeding in the context of HIV/AIDS: where is the evidence base supporting policy recommendations? Toronto, ON: XVI Int AIDS Conference; 2006. Poster.

Lucas A, Morley R, Cole TJ, Gore SM. A randomized multicentre study of human milk versus formula and later development in preterm infants. *Arch Dis Child.* 1994; 70;F141–F146.

Merrett TG, Burr ML, Butland BK, et al. Infant feeding and allergy: twelve-month prospective study of 500 babies in allergic families. *Ann Allergy.* 1988;61:13–20.

Mestecky J, ed. *Immunology of Milk and the Neonate.* New York: Plenum Press; 1991.

Montgomery SM, Ehlin A, Sacker A. Breast feeding and resilience against psychosocial stress. *Arch Dis Child.* 2006;91:990–994.

Paradise JL, Elster BA, Tan L. Evidence in infants with cleft palate that breast milk protects against otitis media. *Pediatrics.* 1994;94:853–860.

Raisler J, Alexander C, O'Campo P. Breastfeeding and infant illness: a dose-response relationship? *Am J Pub Health.* 1999;89:25–30.

Rapp D. *Is This Your Child? Discovering and Treating Unrecognized Allergies in Children and Adults.* New York: Quill William Morrow; 1991.

Riordan J. *Breastfeeding and Human Lactation.* 3rd ed. Sudbury, MA: Jones and Bartlett Publishers; 2005.

Schwartz RH, Amonette MS. Cow milk protein hydrolysate infant formulas not always "hypoallergenic." *J Pediatr.* 1991;118:839. Letter.

Setchell KDR, Zimmer-Nechemias L, Cai J, Heubi JE. Exposure of infants to phyto-oestrogens from soy-based infant formula. *Lancet.* 1997;350:23–27.

Wilson AC, Forsyth JS, Greene SA, et al. Relation of infant diet to childhood health: 7 year follow-up of cohort of children in Dundee infant feeding study. *Br Med J.* 1998;316:21–25.

PROTECTION AGAINST CHRONIC DISEASE FOR THE BREASTFED INFANT

Carol A. Ryan, MSN, RN, IBCLC

OBJECTIVES

- List selected chronic diseases that are affected by breastfeeding.

- Discuss long-term outcomes of those who receive breast milk.

- Provide evidence-based support for the World Health Organization (WHO) and American Academy of Pediatrics' (AAP) recommendations to exclusively breastfeed for the first six months of life, throughout the first year, and hopefully into the second year of life as a preventative measure in reducing the incidence of chronic disease.

Introduction

Both medical research and clinical practice have long acknowledged the immediate benefit of human milk for the human infant. Longitudinal research has explored and studied breastfed infants into their adulthood. Research findings support many long-term benefits for the world's children to consume human milk, and this evidence has improved the medical community and general public's support of breastfeeding. Some of the most notable and life-sustaining outcomes are in studies that examine Crohn's disease, ulcerative colitis, type 1 diabetes (formerly known as insulin dependent diabetes mellitus), type 2 diabetes (formerly known as non-insulin dependent diabetes mellitus) in later life, obesity, and some childhood lymphomas and leukemia. Because these diseases can have a devastating impact on the child, his/her family, the community, and the health care system, a lactation consultant's working knowledge of these disease entities is essential in health care planning and counseling both pre- and postnatally. Those who are not breastfed demonstrate an increased incidence of these diseases as lifelong conditions, underscoring the importance of human milk for human infants (Riordan, 2005).

I. Crohn's Disease, an Inflammatory Bowel Disease

A. Crohn's disease has increased in incidence since its recognition.

B. Noted in Western populations with Northern European and Anglo-Saxon cultures.

C. Found also in developing African-American and Hispanic populations.

D. Will occur equally in both sexes.

E. Most common in Jewish populations.

F. Follows a familial tendency and can overlap with ulcerative colitis.

G. Peak incidences occur at ages 14 and 24 years of age.

H. Appears as patchy inflammatory ulcerations on the mucosa of the intestinal walls with a combination of longitudinal and transverse ulcers and intervening mucosal edema.

I. Creates inflammation of the small intestine, most often in the ileum, though this can affect the digestive system from the mouth to the anus.

J. The inflammation can extend into the deepest layers of the intestinal wall.

K. Most common signs and symptoms include diarrhea with abdominal pain, fever, anorexia, weight loss, bleeding, and a right lower mass or fullness.

L. Children with Crohn's disease may experience delayed development and stunted growth.

M. Breast milk is essential to the development of normal immunological competence of the intestinal mucosa (Bergstrand & Hellers, 1983; Lawrence & Lawrence, 2005).

N. Individuals with Crohn's disease are more prevalent in groups presenting with little or no breastfeeding as infants (Bergstrand & Hellers, 1983; Calkins & Mendeloff, 1986).

II. Ulcerative Colitis, an Inflammatory Bowel Disease

A. A chronic, nonspecific inflammatory and ulcerative disease process arising in the colonic mucosa.

B. Characterized frequently as periods of bloody, mucus-filled diarrhea, and abdominal cramping varying in intensity and duration, and with intermittent exacerbations and emissions.

C. Complications can be life-threatening.

D. Etiology is similar to Crohn's disease.

E. It has a nonspecific microbial etiology.

F. A familial tendency is less evident than Crohn's disease.

G. Peak incidences are noted at 15 to 30 years of age and a smaller peak between ages 50 to 70.

H. The disease process usually begins in the recto-sigmoid area, extending proximally, eventually amassing the whole colon (or the entire large bowel). Included is ulceration and inflammation of the inner rectum and colon linings.

I. Human milk develops normal immunological competence of the intestinal mucosa, protecting it from adhesion and penetration of bacteria, viruses, and foreign proteins that compromise mucosal integrity and provoke inflammatory responses (Klement et al., 2004, Lebenthal & Leung, 1987).

J. Human milk is therapeutic to a damaged gastrointestinal (GI) tract (Howie et al., 1990).

III. Diabetes

A. Type 1 diabetes represents 10% to 15% of all incidences of diabetes mellitus before 30 years of age.

B. Type 1 diabetes is clinically significant due to hyperglycemia (high blood sugar), infinity to diabetic ketoacidosis (coma), infections, nephropathy, atherosclerotic coronary and peripheral vascular disease, neuropathy, and retinopathy (Gerstein, 1994).

C. Type 1 diabetes requires insulin intake for life, and occurs most often in childhood or in adolescence (AAP, 1994).

D. Type 1 diabetes is caused by a genetically conditioned, immune-mediated, selective destruction of more than 90% of the insulin-secreting pancreatic B cells.

E. Children with diabetes are more likely to have been formula fed.

　　1. Infants who are breastfed at least three months are significantly less at risk for type 1 diabetes and type 2 diabetes (Virtanen et al., 1992; Pettitt et al., 1997; Pettitt & Knowler, 1998; Young et al., 2002).

　　2. Increased rates of breastfeeding duration are associated with lower rates of type 1 diabetes (Malcova et al., 2006).

　　3. Longer, exclusive and total breastfeeding appears to be an independent protective factor with regards to type 1 diabetes (Sadauskaite-Kuehne et al., 2004).

　　4. Longer duration of breastfeeding was associated with reduced incidence of type 2 diabetes in young and middle-aged women by improving glucose homeostasis (Stuebe et al., 2005).

F. Higher weight gain later in life is associated with type 1 diabetes (Johansson, Samuelsson, & Ludvigsson, 1994).

G. Mechanisms that may lead to a more protective effect by breastfeeding are not well understood.

　　1. A permissive factor in the development of type 1 diabetes may be diet.

　　2. Newly diagnosed children have increased immunoglobulin (Ig)A and IgG antibodies to bovine beta-lactoglobulin (Savilahti et al., 1993).

3. Autoimmune destruction of pancreatic cells occurs (Vaarala et al., 1999).

4. One or more environmental factors trigger type 1 diabetes, though several recessive genes map the risk of diabetes.

5. Bovine milk is a major environmental trigger (Karjalainen et al., 1992).

6. Whey protein bovine serum albumin may be a trigger. Its antibodies can cross-react with a pancreatic beta cell surface protein, destroying it in an immune reaction attack.

7. A specific immune memory may be established at the time of dietary exposure to bovine milk (Wasmuth & Kolb, 2000).

8. The timing of gut closure, the presence of digestive enzymes such as trypsin, GI infections, and oral tolerance mechanisms may all collaborate in provoking an autoimmune response.

9. Clinical manifestations develop in about 5 to 6 per 1,000 hosts with relevant genetic predisposition.

10. Exposure to bovine milk and solid foods before three months of age may be particularly important in terms of diabetic risk (Monte, Johnston, & Roll, 1994).
    a. Introduction of alternative infant milks and weaning solid foods are etiologically important.
    b. Antigens may cross the gut barriers and cause irritation when early introduction of bovine milk occurs before gut cellular juncture closure or when infection causes GI alteration.

11. Children with type 1 diabetes have a higher incidence of more frequent feeding of soy-based infant formulas, demonstrating anti-thyroid antibody levels that are twice as high as breastfed children (Minchin, 1987).

12. Increased risk of type 1 diabetes is associated with a high weight gain during the first 30 months of life.
    a. Overfeeding formula causes an increased demand for insulin, which may result in an increased beta cell antigen presentation and help explain the tendency to develop type 1 diabetes during periods of increased insulin demand.

13. Insufficient breastfeeding of genetically susceptible newborn infants may lead to B-cell infections and type 1 diabetes later in life (Lawrence & Lawrence, 2005).

IV. Childhood Cancers

A. Lymphoma, a heterogeneous group of neoplasms arising in the reticuloendothelial and lymphatic systems.

1. Children with immune deficiencies, regardless of socioeconomic status, have an increased risk for lymphomas due to an altered immunoregulation

(disturbed immune competence), which might contribute to an increased risk of lymphoproliferative disease (Kwan et al., 2004).

2. A 2005 metaanalysis suggested that "increasing breast-feeding from 50% to 100% would prevent at most 5% of cases of childhood acute leukemia or lymphoma" (Martin et al., 2005).

B. Hodgkin's disease, a complex cellular immune disorder with chronic infection.

1. This is a chronic disease with lymphoreticular proliferation of an unknown cause that may present itself in a localized or disseminated manner.

2. Peaks first around 15 to 34 years of age and again around 60 years of age.

3. Signs and symptoms vary depending on the disease progression, though not necessarily inclusive: intense pruritis, fever, night sweats, weight loss, lymph node compression, and internal organ obstructions.

4. Clinical symptoms appear as the disease spreads from one site to another.

5. Progression rate can vary from slowly to very aggressively.

6. Children who were never breastfed or who were breastfed for only a short time have a higher risk of developing Hodgkin's disease but *not* non-Hodgkin's lymphoma than those who were breastfed for six months or more (Martin et al., 2005).

C. Leukemia.

1. Leukemia is the most common childhood malignancy in Western countries; it accounts for one-third of all cancers occurring in children younger than 15 years of age.

2. Longer breastfeeding duration has been associated with a reduction of childhood acute lymphocytic leukemia (Guise, Austin, & Morris, 2005; Lawrence & Lawrence, 2005; Svanborg et al., 2003).

3. Specific or nonspecific anti-infectious effects and early immune stimulation effects of breast milk may work synergistically or independently to protect children against acute leukemia (Shu et al., 1995, 1999).

V. Obesity

A. Overweight and obesity in industrialized countries represent the most common nutritional disorders in children and adolescents.

B. Overweight and obesity in children are increasing, raising worldwide concern.

C. A clear dose-dependent effect of the duration of breastfeeding on overweight or obesity prevalence at the time of school entry is evidence-based (Burdett et al., 2006; Dubois & Girard, 2006; Koletzko et al., 2005; Owen et al., 2005a; Tulldahl et al., 1999; Von Kries et al., 2000).

D. The protectiveness of breastfeeding may have a cell programming effect in reducing overweight conditions and obesity later in life (Gillman et al., 2001; Knip & Akerblom, 2005).

E. Formula-fed infants have higher plasma concentrations of insulin, which may stimulate fat deposition and development of early adipocytes or fat cells (Knip & Akerblom, 2005).

F. Breastfed infants do not consume as much energy and protein as formula-fed infants, which may contribute to a decreased body mass index of children and adolescents who were breastfed (Gillman et al., 2001; Weyermann, Rothenbacher, & Brenner, 2006).

G. Weaning foods, behavioral modeling, and exercise are intregal to lifetime eating habits.

H. Breastfed infants are leaner than formula-fed infants at one year of age, weighing one to two pounds less (Dewey et al., 1993).

I. Universally, children grow similarly when their health and basic care needs are optimally met (WHO, 2006; See chapter 28).

J. Exclusive breastfeeding for six months and continued breastfeeding with appropriate weaning and complementary foods contribute to optimal infant and child growth and development (AAP, 2005).

VI. Long-term Health Care Risks Associated with the Lack of or Very Short-Term Breastfeeding

A. Hypercholesterolemia, diabetes, hypertension, coronary heart and artery disease at a population level (Schack-Neilsen & Michaelson, 2006; Turck, 2005).

B. Type 2 diabetes in young and middle-aged women who have lactated may be reduced because of improved glucose homeostasis (Knip & Akerblom, 2005; Stuebe et al., 2005; Taylor et al., 2005).

C. Respiratory infections are reduced for children up to 7 years of age, if these children were breastfed at least 15 weeks (Wilson, 1998).

D. Introduction of gluten while the child is still breastfeeding may optimize the protective effects of breast milk. (Ivarsson, 2000; Ivarsson et al., 2002).

E. Breast and ovarian cancer are reduced with long-term lactation in the pre-menopausal period (Zheng et al., 2000).

F. Hip fractures and osteoporosis are reduced in the post-menopausal period (Dursun et al., 2006; Turck, 2005).

G. There are fewer occurrences of dental caries for breastfed children (Erickson & Mazhari, 1999).

H. Cholesterol levels may be improved in adults who were breastfed (Owen, 2002).

I. Type 2 diabetes in adults may be reduced if they were exclusively breastfed for at least two months (Pettitt et al., 1997; Pettitt & Knowler, 1998).

References

American Academy of Pediatrics (AAP). Breastfeeding and the use of human milk. *Pediatrics*. 2005;115:496–506.

American Academy of Pediatrics (AAP). Work Group on Cow's Milk Protein and Diabetes Mellitus. Infant feeding practices and their possible relationship to the etiology of diabetes mellitus. *Pediatrics*. 1994;94:752–755.

Bergstrand O, Hellers G. Breastfeeding during infancy and later development of Crohn's disease. *Scand J Gastroenterol*. 1983;18:903–908.

Burdette HL, Whitaker RC, Hall WC, Daniels SR. Breastfeeding, introduction of complementary foods and adiposity at 5 years of age. *Am J Clin Nutr*. 2006, 83:550–558.

Calkins BM, Mendeloff AI. Epidemiology of inflammatory bowel disease. *Epidemiol Rev*. 1986;8:60–91.

Dewey KG, Heninq MJ, Nommensen LA, et al. Breastfed infants are leaner than formula fed infants at one year of age: The DARLING study. *Am J Clin Nutr*. 1993;57:140–145.

Dubois L, Girard M. Early determinants of overweight at 4.5 years in a population-based longitudinal study. *Int J Obesity*. 2006;30:610–617.

Dursun N, Akin S, Dursun E, et al. Influence of duration of total breastfeeding on bone mineral density in a Turkish population: does the priority of risk factors differ from society to society? *Osteoporos Int*. 2006;17:651–655.

Erickson PR, Mazhari E. Investigation of the role of human breastmilk in caries development. *Pediatr Dent*. 1999;21:86–90.

Gerstein HC. Cow's milk exposure and type I diabetes mellitus: a critical overview of the clinical literature. *Diabetes Care*. 1994;17:13–18.

Gillman MW, Rifas-Shiman SL, Cumargo CA, et al. Risk of overweight among adolescents who were breastfed as infants. *JAMA*. 2001;283:2461–2466.

Guise JM, Austin D, Morris CD. Review of case-control studies related to breastfeeding and reduced risk of childhood leukemia. *Pediatrics*. 2005;116:724–731.

Howie PW, Forsyth JS, Ogston SA, et al. Protective effect of breastfeeding against infection. *Br Med J*. 1990;300:11–16.

Ivarsson A, Hernell O, Stenlund H, et al: Breastfeeding provides protection against celiac disease. *Am J Nutr*. 75:914-921, 2002.

Johansson C, Samuelsson U, Ludvigsson J. A high weight gain early in life is associated with an increased risk of Type I (insulin dependent) diabetes mellitus. *Diabetologia*. 1994;37:91–94.

Karjalainen J, Martin J, Knip M, et al. A bovine albumin peptide as a possible trigger of insulin dependent diabetes mellitus. *N Engl J Med*. 1992;327:302–307.

Klement E, Cohen RV, Boxman J, et al. Breastfeeding and the risk of inflammatory bowel disease: a systtematic review with meta-analysis. *Am J Clin Nutr*. 2004; 80:1342–1352.

Knip M, Akerblom HK. Early nutrition and later diabetes. *Adv Exp Med Biol*. 2005; 569:142–150.

Koletzko B, Broekaert I, Demmelmair H, et al. Protein intake in the first year of life: a risk factor for later obesity? The E.U. childhood obesity project. *Adv Exp Med Biol.* 2005:569:69–79.

Kwan ML, Buffler PA, Abrams B, Kiley VA. Breastfeeding and the risk of childhood leukemia: a meta-analysis. *Public Health Rep.* 2004;119:521–535.

Lawrence RA, Lawrence RM. *Breastfeeding: A Guide for the Medical Profession.* 6th ed. Philadelphia: Elsevier Mosby; 2005:Chapts 5, 15, 16.

Lebenthal E, Leung YK. The impact of development of the gut on infant nutrition. *Pediatr Ann.* 1987;16(3):211, 215–216, 218 passim.

Malcova H, Sumnik Z, Drevinek P, et al. Absence of breastfeeding is associated with the risk of type 1 diabetes: a case control study in a population with rapidly increasing incidence. *Eur J Pediatr.* 2006;165:114–119.

Martin RM, Gunnell D, Owen CG, Smith GD. Breastfeeding and childhood cancer: a systematic review with meta-analysis. *Int J Cancer.* 2005;117:1020–1031.

Minchin M. Infant formula: a mass uncontrolled trial in perinatal care. *Birth.* 1987; 14:25–35.

Monte WD, Johnston CS, Roll LE. Bovine serum albumin detected in infant formula is a possible trigger for insulin dependent diabetes mellitus. *J Am Diet Assoc.* 1994; 94:314–316.

Owen, CG. Breastfeeding linked to improved cholesterol levels later in life. *Pediatrics.* 2002;110:597–608.

Owen CG, Martin RM, Whincup PH, et al. Effect of infant feeding on the risk of obesity across the life course: a quantitative review of published evidence. *Pediatrics.* 2005a: 115:1367–1377.

Pettitt DJ, Forman MR, Hanson RL, et al. Breastfeeding and incidence of noninsulin dependent diabetes mellitus in Pima Indians. *Lancet.* 1997;350:166–168.

Pettitt DJ, Knowler WC. Long term effects of the intrauterine environment, birth weight, and breastfeeding in Pima Indians. *Diabetes Care.* 1998;21(suppl 2):B138–B141.

Riordan J. *Breastfeeding and Human Lactation.* 3rd ed. Sudbury, MA: Jones and Bartlett Publishers; 2005;97–135.

Sadauskaite-Kuehne V, Ludvigsson J, Padaiga Z, Jasinskiene E, Samuelsson U. Longer breastfeeding is an independent protective factor against development of type 1 diabetes mellitus in childhood. *Diabetes Metab Res Rev.* 2004;20:150–157.

Savilahti E, Saukkonen TT, Virtala ET, et al. Increased levels of cow's milk and betalactoglobulin antibodies in young children with newly diagnosed IDDM. *Diabetes Care.* 1993;16:984–989.

Schack-Neilson L, Michaelson KF. Breastfeeding and future health. *Curr Opin Clin Nutr Metab Care.* 2006;9:289–296.

Shu XO, Clemens J, Zheng W, et al. Infant breastfeeding and the risk of childhood lymphoma and leukaemia. *Int J Epidemiol.* 1995;24:27–32.

Shu XO, Linet M, Steinbuch M, et al. Breastfeeding and risk of childhood acute leukemia. *J Natl Cancer Inst.* 1999;91:1765–1772.

Stuebe AM, Rich-Edwards JW, Willett WC, et al. Duration of lactation and incidence of type 2 diabetes. *JAMA*. 2005;294:2601–2610.

Svanborg, C, Agerstam, H, Aronson A, et al, HAMLET kills tumor cells by an apoptosis-like mechanism: cellular, molecular, and therapeutic aspects. *Adv Cancer Res*. 2003;88:1-29.

Taylor, JS, Kacmar JE, Nothnagle M, Lawrence RA. A systematic review of the literature associating breastfeeding with type 2 diabetes and gestational diabetes. *J Am Coll Nutr*. 2005;24:320–326.

Tulldahl J, Pettersson K, Andersson SW, Hulthen L. Mode of infant feeding and achieved growth in adolescence: early feeding patterns in relation to growth and body composition in adolescence. *Obesity Res*. 1999;7:431–437.

Turck D. [Breastfeeding: health benefits for the child and mother]. Committee on Nutrition, French Pediatric Society. *Arch Paediatr*. 2005;12(suppl 3):S145–S165 [in French].

Vaarala O, Knip M, Paronen J, et al. Cow's milk formula feeding induces primary immunization to insulin in infants at genetic risk for type I diabetes. *Diabetes*. 1999; 48:1389–1394.

Virtanen SM, Rasanen L, Aro A, et al. Feeding in infancy and the risk of type 1 diabetes mellitus in Finish children. Childhood Diabetes in Finland Study Group. *Diabet Med*. 1992;9:815–819.

Von Kries R, Koletzko B, Sauerwald T, et al. Does breastfeeding protect against childhood obesity? *Adv Exp Med Biol*. 2000;478:29–39.

Wasmuth HE, Kolb H. Cow's milk and immune-mediated diabetes. *Proc Nutr*. 2000; 59:573–579.

Weyermann M, Rothenbacher D, Brenner H. Duration of breastfeeding and risk of overweight in childhood: a prospective birth cohort study from Germany. *Int J Obes*. 2006;30:1281–1287.

World Health Organization. WHO Child Growth Standards. Available at: http://www.who.int/childgrowth. Accessed December 27, 2006.

Young TK, Martens PJ, Taback SP, et al. Type-2 diabetes in Canadian aboriginal children: prenatal and early infancy risk factors. *Arch Pediatr Adolesc Med*. 2002; 156:651–655.

Zheng T, Duan L, Liu Y, et al. Lactation reduces breast cancer risk in Shandong Province, China. *Am J Epidemol*. 2000:152:1129–1135.

Suggested Readings

Akre J, ed. *Infant Feeding: The Physiologic Basis*. Geneva: World Health Organization; 1989.

Chen Y, Yu S, Li W. Artificial feeding and hospitalization in the first 18 months of life. *Pediatrics*. 1988;81:58–62.

Clavano NR. Mode of feeding and its effect on infant mortality and morbidity. *J Trop Pediatr*. 1982;28:287–293.

Dewey KG, Heinig J, Nommensen-Rivers LA. Differences in morbidity between breastfed and formula fed infants. *J Pediatr.* 1995;126:697–702.

Dewey KG, Peerson JM, Brown KH. Growth of breastfed infants deviates from current reference data: a pooled analysis of US, Canadian, and European data sets. *Pediatrics.* 1995;96:495–503.

Gulick EE. The effect of breastfeeding on toddler health. *Pediatr Nuts.* 1986;12:51–54.

Hanson, LA. *Immunobiology of Human Milk: How Breastfeeding Protects Babies.* Texas, 2004, 123-194.

Ivarsson A, et al. Epidemic of celiac disease in Swedish children. Acta Paediatr 2000; 89:165–271. *Comments in Acta Paediatr.* 2000;89:140–141 and 2000;89:749–750.

Koletzko S, Sherman P, Corey M, et al. Role of infant feeding practices in development of Crohn's disease in childhood. *Br Med J.* 1989;298:1617–1618.

Koopman JS, Turkish VJ, Monto AS. Infant formulas and gastrointestinal illness. *Am J Public Health.* 1985;75:477–480.

Kostraba JH, Cruickshanks KJ, Lawler-Heavner J, et al. Early exposure to cow's milk and solid foods in infancy, genetic predisposition, and risk of IDDM. *Diabetes.* 1993; 42:288–295.

Mathur GP, Gupta N, Mathur S, et al. Breastfeeding and childhood cancer. *Indian Pediatr.* 1993:30:651–657.

McKinney PA, Parslow R, Gurney KA, et al. Perinatal and neonatal determinants of childhood type I diabetes. A case control study in Yorkshire, UK. *Diabetes Care.* 1999; 22:928–932.

Merck Manual of Diagnosis and Therapy. 16th ed. Rahway, NJ: Merck Research Laboratories; 1992.

Miller RW, Fraumeni JF. Does breastfeeding increase the child's risk of breast cancer? *Pediatrics.* 1996;49:645. Abstract.

Rennie J. Formula for diabetes? *Sci Am.* 1992;267:24.

Riordan J. The cost of not breastfeeding. *J Hum Lact.* 1997;13:93–97.

Scott FW. Cow milk and insulin dependent diabetes mellitus: is there a relationship? *Am J Clin Nutr.* 1990;51:489–491.

Walker M. A fresh look at the risks of artificial infant feeding. *J Hum Lact.* 1993; 9:97–107.

Whorwell PJ, Hodstack G, et al. Bottlefeeding, early gastroenteritis, and inflammatory bowel disease. *BMJ.* 1979;1:382. Abstract.

Wilson JV, Self TW, Hamburger R. Severe cow's milk induced colitis in an exclusively breastfed neonate. *Clin Pediatr.* 1990;29:77–80.

Wilson AC, Forsyth JS, Greene SA, et al. Relation of infant diet to childhood health: seven year follow up of cohort of children in Dundee infant feeding study. *BMJ.* 1998;316:21–25.

World Health Organization. Working Group on Infant Growth and Nutrition Unit. An evaluation of infant growth. Geneva: World Health Organization; 1994.

World Health Organization, Growth Charts (Breastfed infant as the norm). Available at: www.who.org.

LACTATIONAL PHARMACOLOGY

Thomas W. Hale, RPh, PhD
Revised by Frank J. Nice, RPh, DPA, CPHP

OBJECTIVES

- Describe the entry of medications into human milk.
- List the effect of postpartum timing on drug entry.
- Describe the chemistry of medications that enables or prevents their entry into human milk.
- Describe drug kinetic parameters that are important in breastfeeding mothers.
- Describe the milk/plasma ratio and its importance for evaluating drug risks in the breastfeeding mother.

Introduction

Safely using medications in breastfeeding mothers requires a certain basic knowledge of how drugs enter breast milk, which drugs are of potential risk, and factors that might increase or decrease the infant's sensitivity to the medication. The amount of drug entering breast milk is largely determined by its maternal plasma kinetics, its lipid solubility, its molecular mass, and other factors. The use of these kinetic parameters makes determining the risks of medications much less difficult, particularly with newer medications. Although there are many exceptions, a simple rule of thumb is that less than 1% of the maternal dose will ultimately find its way into the milk (and subsequently, to the baby). Also, the infant's daily dose (from ingested breast milk), adjusted for the infant's weight, can be compared to the mother's weight-adjusted daily dose. If the infant's weight-adjusted dose is less than 10% of the mother's, the drug is generally considered safe for the infant.

I. Determine the Need for Medication

A. Is this medication really necessary, and could the mother do without the medication?

1. Just how effective is the drug?
   a. Some antihistamines are only minimally effective and may not be necessary.
   b. If a medication is not efficacious, then its use might not be advisable.
   c. An example is the use of antihistamines for colds, etc.

2. Could the mother wait several months before undergoing therapy, such as for a toenail fungus or a cosmetic surgical procedure?

3. If the drug is an herbal medication, is it really necessary?
   a. Could the mother wait to use the drug until after she has discontinued breastfeeding?
   b. Is its use really justified?

4. Extremely high doses of vitamins could be potentially harmful and are not really necessary; thus, their risks might outweigh the benefits of their use.

II. Use the Stepwise Approach to Minimizing Infant Drug Exposure

A. Table 21-1 contains strategies for minimizing opportunities for the infant to be exposed to drugs.

Table 21-1   Stepwise Approach to Minimize Infant Drug Exposure

A. Withhold the drug.

1. Avoid the use of nonessential medications by enlisting the mother's cooperation.

B. Try non-drug therapies.

1. Instead of analgesics: relaxation techniques, massage, warm baths.
2. Instead of cough, cold, or allergy products: saline nose drops, cool mist, steam.
3. Instead of anti-asthmatics: avoid known allergens, particularly animals.
4. Instead of antacids: eat small meals, sleep with head propped, avoid head-bending activities, avoid gas-forming foods.
5. Instead of laxatives: eat high fiber cereal, prunes; drink hot liquids with breakfast and more water throughout the day.

Table 21-1   Stepwise Approach to Minimize Infant Drug Exposure (continued)

    6. Instead of antidiarrheals: discontinue solid foods for 12 to 24 hours, and increase fluid intake; eat toast/saltine crackers.

C. Delay therapy.

    1. Mothers who are ready to wean the infant might be able to delay elective drug therapy or elective surgery.

D. Choose drugs that pass poorly into milk.

    1. Within some drug classes, there are large differences among class members in drug distribution into milk.

E. Choose more breastfeeding-compatible dosage forms.

    1. Take the lowest recommended dose, avoid extra-strength and long-acting preparations, avoid combination ingredient products.

F. Choose an alternative route of administration.

    1. Local application of drugs to the affected maternal site may minimize drug concentrations in milk and subsequently the infant's dose.

G. Avoid breastfeeding at times of peak drug concentrations in milk.

    1. Breastfeeding before a dose is given may avoid the peak drug concentrations in milk that occur about one to three hours after an oral dose.

    2. This works best for drugs with short half-lives.

H. Administer the drug before the infant's longest sleep period.

    1. This will minimize the infant's dose and is useful for long-acting drugs that can be given once daily.

I. Temporarily withhold breastfeeding.

    1. Depending on the estimated length of drug therapy, nursing can be temporarily withheld.

    2. Mothers may be able to pump a sufficient quantity of milk beforehand for use during therapy.

    3. The pharmacokinetics of the drug must be examined to determine when the resumption of breastfeeding is advisable.

J. Discontinue breastfeeding.

    1. A few drugs are too toxic to allow breastfeeding but may be necessary for the mother's health.

III. Maternal Factors That Affect Drug Transfer

A. Dose of medication.

1. Is the dose of the medication greater or lesser than the normal range?

2. How is the plasma level of the medication changed by the dose used in the mother? (For example, if a mother is using 25,000 units of vitamin A, that is significantly more risky than a 5,000-unit dose).

3. Is the medication formulation a rapid or sustained-release product?
   a. How does this medication change the mother's plasma levels and the risk to the infant?
   b. Sustained-release drugs should be considered as if they are long half-life drugs.

4. When is the medication dosed, and how does the dosing interval affect plasma levels and milk levels?
   a. If a mother takes a medication at night and does not breastfeed until the morning, this situation is significantly different than if she breastfeeds every two hours.

5. Is the dose of medication absorbed orally by the mother?
   a. Thus, what are her plasma levels? Are they high or really low?
   b. Plasma levels are generally in equilibrium with the milk at all times.
   c. Higher plasma levels mean higher milk levels.

6. Most asthma medications are used via inhalation; thus, maternal plasma levels of the medication are virtually nil and are not likely to produce milk levels at all.

7. Plasma levels of most topical and ophthalmic preparations are virtually nil and are not likely to produce milk levels at all.

IV. Entry of Drugs into Human Milk

A. The amount of drug excreted into milk depends on a number of factors.

1. The lipid solubility of the drug.

2. The pH (acidity) of the drug.

3. The molecular size of the drug.

4. The blood level attained in the maternal circulation.

5. The maternal volume of distribution of the drug.

6. Protein binding in the maternal circulation.

7. Oral bioavailability in the infant and mother.

8. The half-life in the maternal and infant plasma compartments.

B. Although this description is somewhat simplistic for a sophisticated and somewhat obscure system, these pharmacokinetic terms provide a reasonably complete system for evaluating drug penetration into milk and the degree of exposure of the infant.

V. Drug Entry into the Milk Compartment

A. Drugs enter the breast milk primarily by diffusion driven by equilibrium forces between the maternal plasma compartment and the maternal milk compartment.

1. Medications enter the milk by transferring from the maternal plasma, through the capillary walls, past the alveolar epithelium, and into the milk compartment.

2. During the first four days postpartum, large gaps exist between alveolar cells.

3. These gaps might permit enhanced drug entry into human milk during the colostral period, but the absolute amount of the drug in the milk might still be quite low (see Figure 21-1).

4. After 4 to 14 days, the alveolar cells enlarge—shutting off many of the intercellular gaps—and the amount of drug entry into the milk is reduced.

5. Because the alveolar epithelium has rather tight junctions, most drugs dissolve through the bilayer membranes of the alveolar cells.

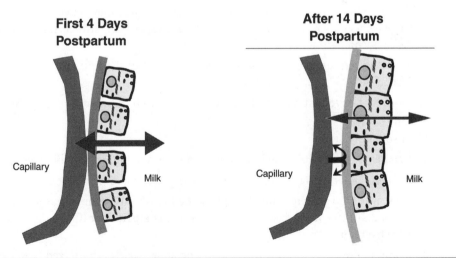

Figure 21-1   Alveolar cell gaps as a function of days postpartum. *Source:* Courtesy Thomas Hale, *Medications and Mother's Milk*, 9th ed., 2000.

6. Dissolving through the bilayer lipid membranes is difficult for most medications, particularly those that are ionic or polar.

7. The more lipid-soluble a drug, the greater the capability of the drug to penetrate into the milk.

8. Drugs that are active in the central nervous system (CNS) generally attain higher levels in the milk compartment simply because their chemistry is ideal for entry.

9. Drugs in the maternal plasma compartment are in complete equilibrium with the milk compartment; there might be more or less in the milk compartment, but they are still in equilibrium.

10. Several drug pumping systems exist, one of which is most important.
    a. For example, iodine has a rather high milk/plasma ratio and is readily pumped into the milk compartment.
    b. Therefore, high doses of iodine should be avoided.
    c. Includes vaginal povidone iodide (Betadyne®) and radioactive sodium iodine-131a (^{131a}I).

11. Many electrolytes (such as sodium chloride, magnesium, etc.) are tightly controlled by the alveolar cell; even high maternal levels might not produce significant changes in milk-electrolyte composition.

B. Protein binding and its effect on drug levels in milk.

1. As a general rule, most drugs are transported in blood that is bound to plasma albumin, which is a large molecular-weight protein that resides in the plasma.

2. The more the drug is bound to plasma protein, the less that is available free in the plasma compartment to enter into various other compartments, particularly the milk compartment.

3. As the percent of drug binding increases, the level of the drug in the milk decreases.

4. Drugs that have high protein binding can be chosen in order to attempt to reduce milk levels.

C. Lipid solubility.

1. As a general rule, the more lipid-soluble a drug, the higher the milk levels.

2. The more polar or water-soluble a drug, the less the milk levels will be.

3. While it is hard to determine the lipid solubility of most compounds, a good rule is that if the drug readily enters the brain compartment (CNS), then it is more likely to enter the milk.

4. A drug that is active in the brain should be more closely scrutinized than one that is not active. Examples of these types of drugs would include those to treat epilepsy, psychotherapeutic drugs, and narcotic analgesics.

D. Half-life of the medication.

1. Elimination half-life of the medication generally describes the time interval that is required after administration of the medication until one-half of the drug is eliminated from the body.

2. It is better to choose drugs that have shorter half-lives, because the length of exposure of the infant to the medication (via milk) is generally reduced.

3. Milk levels during the day will generally be lower if the maternal peak is avoided by waiting several half-lives to breastfeed the infant.

4. Long half-life drugs might have a tendency to build up in an infant.
   a. In many instances, the half-life of the medication might be much longer in a newborn infant than in the adult.

5. Prolonged exposure to long half-life medications might lead to increasing plasma levels of the medication in the infant (refer to the drug fluoxetine [Prozac®] as an example).

6. In essence, long half-life medications really become a problem only if they are ingested by the mother over a long period, because the infant builds up higher and higher plasma levels of the medications.
   a. Acute use of long half-life medications is not generally a problem.

7. Long half-life medications cannot always be avoided.
   a. In these instances, become aware of the clinical dose provided to the infant via milk.
   b. If this dose is still low, then accumulation is not as likely to occur in the infant.

8. A general guideline is that it takes approximately five half-lives before a drug is virtually eliminated from the system.

E. Bioavailability.

1. *Bioavailability* of a medication is a measure of how much medication reaches the plasma of that individual.

2. While there is not a large amount of good bioavailability data regarding infants, it is thought that it does not differ greatly from that of an adult.

3. Measured in percentage, a drug that has 50% bioavailability generally means that only 50% of the medication administered actually reaches the plasma compartment of the mother or infant.

4. Drugs that have poor bioavailability fail to reach the plasma compartment for a variety of reasons.
   a. They are sequestered in the liver and cannot exit.
   b. They are destroyed in the gut (proteins, peptides, aminoglycosides, etc.).
   c. They are not absorbed in the small intestine (vancomycin).

5. The drug that has the lowest bioavailability should be chosen for breastfeeding mothers because it will greatly reduce the exposure of the infant to the medication.

F. Molecular size of the medication (mass is measured in Daltons [D]).

1. In general, the larger the molecular size of the medication, the less likely it is to enter into the milk compartment.
   a. While some medications might enter the milk, their levels are reduced.

2. Drugs that have molecular sizes greater than 800 to 1,000 D have greater difficulty in passing through the alveolar cell and entering the milk.

3. Drugs that have huge molecular sizes (25,000–200,000 D) are virtually excluded from milk in clinically relevant amounts.

4. Drugs that have huge molecular sizes include heparin, insulin, interferons, and low-molecular-weight heparins.

G. Milk/plasma ratio.

1. Scientifically, the milk/plasma ratio is a useful tool to evaluate the relative concentration of medication in the maternal plasma compared to the maternal milk compartment.

2. High milk/plasma ratio drugs like to enter milk, while low milk/plasma ratio drugs are less attracted to the milk compartment.
   a. Unless both levels (plasma and milk) are known in the specific patient, the milk/plasma ratio might not indicate the true risk of using the medication.

3. In the case where a medication has a high milk/plasma ratio (for example, 5) and an extremely low maternal plasma level, then five times a very low level is still very low (bupropion: Wellbutrin, Zyban®).

4. Unless a great deal is known about the maternal plasma level, the milk/plasma ratio might give the clinician the wrong impression.

5. It is helpful if the health care provider knows the dose per unit of milk.
   a. This way, he or she can calculate the dose to the infant via the breast milk and obtain a realistic view of the clinical dose that will be transferred to the infant via milk.

VI. Evaluating the Infant

A. Assume that the preterm infant is more susceptible to maternal drugs.

1. While many medications are often used in these situations, increased attentiveness to the risks is warranted.

2. Using a medication in an 8-month-old infant is significantly less risky than with a preterm infant or even a full-term newborn.

B. Be aware of the health and well-being of the infant.

C. What medication(s) is the infant ingesting?

1. Drug–drug interactions might occur between medications that the mother is ingesting and medications that the infant is ingesting.

D. Sedating medications should be avoided.

1. These include diazepam-like drugs (such as Valium®), barbiturates, and older antihistamines, particularly in infants who have apnea or who are susceptible to sudden infant death syndrome.

2. However, their use in acute, one-time situations is significantly less problematic.

E. Over-the-counter (OTC) medications.

1. OTC medications and herbals are also drugs.

2. Many mothers self-medicate without consulting a health care professional.

3. Mothers should avoid medications that are labeled as extra strength, maximum strength, or long acting.
   a. Usually, the lowest possible dose is recommended and is marked or labeled as regular strength.

4. Mothers should avoid (if possible) medications that contain a variety of ingredients (see Tables 21-2 through 21-4).

F. Minimizing the effect of maternal medication on the infant.

1. Avoid the use of long-acting forms of medications; the infant might have difficulty excreting it due to the requirement of detoxification by an immature infant's liver.

2. Doses can be scheduled so that the minimum amount of drug enters the milk; medications can be taken right before or right after a breastfeeding.

3. Infants should be watched for unusual or adverse signs or symptoms, such as a change in feeding patterns, level of alertness, sleeping patterns, fussiness, rash, and bowel changes.

4. Drugs can be chosen that produce the least amount in the milk.

G. Radioactive drugs.

1. Administration of any radiopharmaceutical will result in at least some excretion of radioactivity into milk.
   a. The amount and time course of excretion varies among radiopharmaceuticals.
   b. Any period of breastfeeding interruption depends upon the total radioactivity ingested by an infant having been reduced to an acceptable level.

Table 21-2 Herbal Products Used as Galactagogues

Common Name	Evidence for Efficacy	Possible Adverse Reactions
Alfalfa; *Medicago sativa*	No scientific or clinical evidence for efficacy as a galactogogue	Large quantities may cause pancytopenia
Caraway; *Carun carvi*	No scientific or clinical evidence for efficacy as a galactogogue	None
Dill; *Anethum graveolens*	No scientific or clinical evidence	None
Fennel; *Foeniculum vulgare*	Historical use	Allergic reaction, photo dermatitis, and contact dermatitis
Fenugreek; *Trigonella foenum*	Historical use	None when ingested in usual quantities
Rosemary; *Rosmarinus officinalis*	No scientific or clinical evidence for efficacy as a galactagogue	Ingestion of large amounts of the oil can result in gastrointestinal distress, kidney damage has been reported
Watercress; *Nasturtium officinale*	No scientific or clinical evidence	Gastrointestinal upset
Chaste tree; *Vitex angus-castus*	Animal studies have found an increase in lactation and mammary enlargement	Gastrointestinal reactions, itching, rash, headaches, and increased menstrual flow
Lettuce Opium; *Lactuca virosa*	No scientific or clinical evidence	
Milk Thistle; *Silybum marianum*	Historical use	Allergic reaction, mild laxative effects have been reported

Table 21-3 Herbal Products to Avoid During Breastfeeding

Common Name	Potential Uses	Reason
Aloe vera; *Aloe ferrox; Aloe perryi; Aloe vera*	*Used orally as a stimulant laxative*	*Contains anthranoid derivatives*
Basil; *Ocimum Basilicum*	Delayed menstruation	The concerns of this herb are based on therapeutic use and not use as a spice. The herb contains estragole, which is a procarcinogen. Long-term use is not recommended; not recommended for use during lactation.
Black cohosh; *Cimicifuga racemosa*	Uterine stimulant, PMS, Menopause	Safety data lacking
Bladderwrack; *Fucus Vesiculosus*	Thyroid deficiency	Contains iodine
Borage; *Borago officinalis*	Mild expectorant, diuretic	Contains pyrrolizidine alkaloids. There is no evidence for effectiveness.
Buckthorn berry and bark; *Rhamnus catharticus*	Stimulant laxative	Contains anthranoids, which are contraindicated in breastfeeding. Lack of toxicological information.
Coltsfoot; *Tussilago farfara*	Coughs, bronchial congestion	Contains pyrrolizidine alkaloids
Comfrey; *Symphytum officinale*	Heal stomach ulcers, purify the blood; only topical use is recommended	Contains pyrrolizidine alkaloids

continues

343

Table 21-3 Herbal Products to Avoid During Breastfeeding (continued)

Common Name	Potential Uses	Reason
Ginseng; Panax ginseng; *Panax quinquefolium*	Increased mental capacity	May cause estrogenic side effects; also can cause diminished platelet adhesiveness. Some texts recommend avoiding during breastfeeding until more information is available.
Goldenseal; *Hydrastis canadensis*	Travelers diarrhea, topical antiseptic	Some texts recommend avoiding during lactation.
Kava Kava; *Piper methysticum*	Sedation	Sedative effects possibly pass into milk.
Licorice; *Glycyrrhiza glabra*	Flavoring	Excessive consumption can result in pseudoaldosteronism.
Male fern; *Drypteris filix-mas*	Topical use only	Poisonings have occurred. Use by German E Commission not recommended.
Podophyllum; *Podophyllum peltatum*	Topical use only	Although there are no documented adverse reactions during breastfeeding, it is systematically absorbed and toxic; use is discouraged during breastfeeding.
Purging buckthorn; *Rhamnus catharticus*	Stimulant laxative	Contains anthranoid derivatives
Rhubarb Root; *Rheum officinale; Rheum palmatum*	Stimulant laxative	Lack of sufficient data
Uva Uris; *Arctostaphylos uva-ursi*	Urinary antiseptic, diuretic	Hydroquinone primary antiseptic portion of the plant can be toxic. Lack of information on transfer into milk; German E Commission recommends against use in lactation. Other compounds work just as well and may not be absorbed.

Table 21-4 Over-the-Counter Medications

Analgesics

Acetaminophen 325 mg–Y

Acetaminophen 500 mg–N

Actron (ketoprofen)–Y

Advil (ibuprofen)–Y

Aleve (naproxen)–Y

Alka-Seltzer Effervescent Antacid and Pain Reliever (aspirin, sodium bicarbonate)–N

Anacin (aspirin, caffeine)–N

Anacin Maximum Strength (aspirin, caffeine)–N

Anacin-3 Regular Strength (acetaminophen)–Y

Anacin-3 Maximum Strength (acetaminophen)–N

Anodynos (aspirin, salicylamide, caffeine)–N

Arthritis Pain Formula (aspirin, aluminum-magnesium hydroxide)–N

Arthritis Foundation (ibuprofen)–Y

Arthritis Foundation Aspirin Free (acetaminophen)–N

Arthritis Foundation Nighttime (acetaminophen, diphenhydramine)–N

Arthritis Foundation Safety Coated Aspirin (aspirin)–N

Arthropan (choline salicylate)–N

Ascriptin Arthritis Pain (aspirin, aluminum-magnesium hydroxide, calcium carbonate)–N

Ascriptin Regular Strength (aspirin, aluminum-magnesium hydroxide, calcium carbonate)–N

Aspercin (aspirin)–N

Aspercin Extra (aspirin)–N

Aspergum (aspirin)–N

Aspermin (aspirin)–N

Aspirin 81 mg–N

Aspirin 325 mg–N

Aspirin 500 mg–N

Aspirin Free Pain Relief (acetaminophen)–Y

Azo-Diac (phenazopyridine)–Y

Azo-Standard (phenazopyridine)–Y

Backache Caplets (magnesium salicylate)–N

Back-Quell (aspirin, ephedrine sulfate, atropine sulfate)–N

Bayer Adult Low Strength (aspirin)–N

Bayer Arthritis Extra Strength (aspirin)–N

Bayer Aspirin (aspirin)–N

Bayer Aspirin Extra Strength (aspirin)–N

Bayer Regular Strength (aspirin)–N

Bayer Plus Extra Strength (aspirin)–N

Bayer PM Aspirin Plus Sleep Aid (aspirin, diphenhydramine)–N

BC Arthritis Strength (aspirin, salicylamide, caffeine)–N

Note: Y = usually safe when breastfeeding; Y* = usually safe when breastfeeding, monitor infant for drowsiness; Y** = usually safe when breastfeeding, monitor for decreased milk production, mother should drink extra fluids; Y*** = use of loperamide should not exceed two days; N = avoid when breastfeeding; N* = less than 150 mg two to three times a day has no apparent effect on breastfeeding infant. Probably better to drink a cup of coffee than to take the drug; x = consultation with a physician is highly recommended prior to use.

continues

Table 21-4　Over-the-Counter Medications (continued)

BC Powder (aspirin, salicylamide, caffeine)–N

Bromo-Seltzer (acetaminophen, sodium bicarbonate, citric acid)–N

Bufferin Analgesic Tablets (aspirin)–N

Bufferin Arthritis Strength (aspirin)–N

Bufferin Extra-Strength (aspirin)–N

Cope (aspirin, caffeine, aluminum-magnesium hydroxide)–N

Datril Extra Strength Non-Aspirin (acetaminophen)–N

Doan's Extra Strength (magnesium salicylate)–N

Doan's PM Extra Strength (magnesium salicylate, diphenhydramine)–N

Doan's Regular Strength (magnesium salicylate)–N

Dynafed EX (acetaminophen)–N

Dynafed IB (ibuprofen)–Y

Dyspel (acetaminophen, ephedrine sulfate, atropine sulfate)–N

Ecotrin Low, Regular, or Maximum Strength (aspirin)–N

Emagrin (aspirin, caffeine, salicylamide)–N

Empirin Aspirin (aspirin)–N

Empirin Free (acetaminophen, caffeine)–N

Excedrin Aspirin Free (acetaminophen, caffeine)–N

Excedrin Extra Strength (acetaminophen, aspirin, caffeine)–N

Excedrin PM (acetaminophen, diphenhydramine)–N

Feverall Adult Strength Suppository (acetaminophen)–Y

Goody's Extra Strength (acetaminophen, aspirin, caffeine)–N

Goody's Extra Strength Headache (acetaminophen, aspirin, caffeine)–N

Haltran (ibuprofen)–Y

Healthprin Brand Aspirin (aspirin)–N

Heartline (aspirin)–N

Ibuprohm (ibuprofen)–Y

Legatrin (acetaminophen, diphenhydramine)–N

Midol IB Cramp Relief Formula (ibuprofen)–Y

Midol Menstrual Maximum Strength (acetaminophen, caffeine, pyrilamine)–N

Midol Menstrual Regular Strength Multisymptom Formula (acetaminophen, pyrilamine)–N

Midol PMS Maximum Strength (acetaminophen, pamabrom, pyrilamine)–N

Midol Teen Maximum Strength (acetaminophen, pamabrom)–N

Mobigesic (magnesium salicylate, phenyltoloxamine)–N

Momentum (magnesium salicylate)–N

Motrin IB (ibuprofen)–Y

Nuprin (ibuprofen)–Y

Orudis KT (ketoprofen)–Y

P-A-C (aspirin, caffeine)–N

Panadol Maximum Strength (acetaminophen)–N

Percogesic (acetaminophen, phenyltoloxamine)–N

Premsyn PMS (acetaminophen, pamabrom, pyrilamine)–N

Prodium (phenazopyridine)–Y

Re-Azo (phenazopyridine)–Y

St. Joseph Adult Aspirin (aspirin)–N

Stanback AF Extra Strength Powder
(acetaminophen)–N

Stanback Original Formula Powder
(aspirin, salicylamide, caffeine)–N

Supac (acetaminophen, aspirin, calcium
gluconate, caffeine)–N

Tapanol Extra Strength (acetaminophen)–N

Tempra (acetaminophen)–Y

Tempra Quicklet (acetaminophen)–Y

Tylenol Arthritis Extended Relief
(acetaminophen)–N

Tylenol Extra Strength (acetaminophen)–N

Tylenol PM (acetaminophen,
diphenhydramine)–N

Tylenol Regular Strength
(acetaminophen)–Y

Ultraprin (ibuprofen)–Y

Unisom with Pain Relief Nighttime
(acetaminophen, diphenhydramine)–N

Uristat (phenazopyridine)–Y

UroFemme (phenazopyridine)–Y

Valorin (acetaminophen)–Y

Valorin Extra (acetaminophen)–N

Valorin Super (acetaminophen, caffeine)–N

Valprin (ibuprofen)–Y

Vanquish (aspirin, acetaminophen,
caffeine, aluminum-magnesium
hydroxide)–N

XS Hangover Relief (acetaminophen,
calcium citrate, magnesium trisilicate,
calcium carbonate, caffeine)–N

Cough, Cold, Allergy Preparations

Actifed (tripolidine, pseudoephedrine)–Y*,
Y**

Actifed Allergy Daytime
(pseudoephedrine)–Y**

Actifed Allergy Nighttime (pesudoephedrine,
diphenhydramine)–Y**

Actifed Plus (acetaminophen,
pseudoephedrine, tripolidine)–N

Actifed Sinus Daytime (acetaminophen,
pseudoephedrine)–N

Actifed Sinus Nighttime (acetaminophen,
pseudoephedrine, diphenhydramine)–N

Advil Cold and Sinus (ibuprofen,
pseudoephedrine)–N

Alcomed 2-60 (dexbrompheniramine,
pseudoephedrine)–Y*, Y**

Alka-Seltzer Plus Cold & Cough Medicine
(aspirin, chlorpheniramine,
phenylpropanolamine,
dextromethorphan)–N

Alka-Seltzer Plus Cold & Cough Medicine
Liqui-Gels (aspirin, chlorpheniramine,
phenylpropanolamine,
dextromethorphan)–N

Alka-Seltzer Plus Cold & Flu Medicine
(acetaminophen, dextromethorphan,
phenylpropanolamine,
chlorpheniramine)–N

Alka-Seltzer Plus Cold & Flu Medicine
Liqui-Gels (acetaminophen,
dextromethorphan,
phenylpropanolamine,
chlorpheniramine)–N

continues

Table 21-4   Over-the-Counter Medications (continued)

Alka-Seltzer Plus Cold Medicine (aspirin, chlorpheniramine, pseudoephedrine, acetaminophen)–N

Alka-Seltzer Plus Cold Medicine Liqui-Gels (aspirin, chlorpheniramine, pseudoephedrine, acetaminophen)–N

Alka-Seltzer Plus Cold & Sinus Medicine (aspirin, phenylpropanolamine)–N

Alka-Seltzer Plus Cold & Sinus Medicine Liqui-Gels (pseudoephedrine, acetaminophen)–N

Alka-Seltzer Plus Night-Time Cold Medicine (aspirin, phenylpropanolamine)–N

Alka-Seltzer Plus Night-Time Cold Medicine Liqui-Gels (dextromethorphan, doxylamine, pseudoephedrine, acetaminophen)–N

Allerest Headache Strength (acetaminophen, chlorpheniramine, pseudoephedrine)–N

Allerest Maximum Strength (chlorpheniramine, pseudoephedrine)– Y*, Y**

Allerest No Drowsiness (acetaminophen, pseudoephedrine)–N

Allerest Sinus Pain Formula (acetaminophen, pseudoephedrine)–N

Allerest 12 Hour (chlorpheniramine, phenylpropanolamine)–N

Bayer Select Sinus Pain Relief Formula (acetaminophen, pseudoephedrine)–N

BC Allergy Sinus Cold Powder (aspirin, phenylpropanolamine, chlorpheniramine)–N

BC Sinus Cold Powder (aspirin, phenylpropanolamine)–N

Benadryl Allergy/Congestion (diphenhydramine, pseudoephedrine)– Y*, Y**

Benadryl Allergy/Cold (diphenhydramine, pseudoephedrine, acetaminophen)–N

Benadryl Allergy Liquid or Dye-Free Liquid (diphenhydramine)–Y*

Benadryl Allergy Sinus Headache Caplets & Gelcaps (diphenhydramine, pseudoephedrine, acetaminophen)–N

Benadryl Allergy Ultratab Tablets, Ultratab Kapseals, Chewables, or Dye-Free Liqui-Gels (diphenhydramine)–Y*

Benylin Adult Formula (dextromethorphan)–Y*

Denylin Cough Syrup (diphenhydramine)– Y*

Benylin Expectorant (dextromethorphan, guaifenesin)–Y*

Benylin Multisymptom (guaifenesin, pseudoephedrine, dextromethorphan)–N

Buckley's Mixture (dextromethorphan, ammonium carbonate, camphor, balsam, glycerin, menthol, pine needle oil)–N

Cerose DM (dextromethorphan, chlorpheniramine, phenylephrine, alcohol 2.4%)–N

Cheracol-D (dextromethorphan, guaifenesin)–Y*

Cheracol Plus (phenylpropanolamine, dextromethorphan, chlorpheniramine)–N

Cheracol Sinus (dexbrompheniramine, pseudoephedrine)–N

Chlor-Trimeton 4-Hour Allergy (chlorpheniramine)–Y*

Chlor-Trimeton 4-Hour Allergy/
Decongestant (chlorpheniramine,
pseudoephedrine)–Y*, Y**

Chlor-Trimeton 8- and 12-Hour Allergy
(chlorpheniramine)–N

Chlor-Trimeton 12-Hour
Allergy/Decongestant
(chlorpheniramine, pseudoephedrine)–N

CoADVIL (ibuprofen, pseudoephedrine)–N

COMTREX Deep Chest Cold and
Congestion Relief (acetaminophen,
guaifenesin, phenylpropanolamine,
dextromethorphan)–N

COMTREX Maximum Strength Multi-
Symptom Acute Head Cold & Sinus
Pressure Relief (acetaminophen,
brompheniramine, pseudoephedrine)–N

COMTREX Maximum Strength Multi-
Symptom Cold & Cough Relief Caplet or
Tablet (acetaminophen,
pseudoephedrine, chlorpheniramine,
dextromethorphan)–N

COMTREX Maximum Strength Multi-
Symptom Cold & Cough Relief Liquid
(acetaminophen, pseudoephedrine,
chlorpheniramine, dextromethorphan)–N

COMTREX Maximum Strength Multi-
Symptom Cold & Cough Relief
Liqui-Gels (acetaminophen,
phenylpropanolamine, chlorpheniramine,
dextromethorphan)–N

Contac Severe Cold & Flu
(phenylpropanolamine, chlorpheniramine,
acetaminophen, dextromethorphan)–N

Contac 12-Hour Caplets
(phenylpropanolamine,
chlorpheniramine)–N

Contac 12-Hour Capsules
(phenylpropanolamine,
chlorpheniramine)–N

Coricidin D Decongestant (acetaminophen,
chlorpheniramine,
phenylpropanolamine)–N

Coricidin HBP Cold & Flu (acetaminophen,
chlorpheniramine)–N

Coricidin HBP Cough & Cold
(chlorpheniramine, dextromethorphan)–N

Coricidin HBP Nighttime Cold & Cough
Liquid (acetaminophen,
diphenhydramine)–N

Delsym Cough Formula
(dextromethorphan)–N

Dimetapp Cold & Allergy Chewable
Tablets or Quick Dissolving Tablets
(brompheniramine,
phenylpropanolamine)–N

Dimetapp Cold & Cough Liqui-Gels
(brompheniramine,
phenylpropanolamine,
dextromethorphan)–N

Dimetapp Cold and Fever Suspension
(acetaminophen, pseudoephedrine,
brompheniramine)–N

Dimetapp DM Elixir (brompheniramine,
phenylpropanolamine,
dextromethorphan)–N

Dimetapp Elixir (brompheniramine,
phenylpropanolamine)–N

Dimetapp Extentabs (brompheniramine,
phenylpropanolamine)–N

Dimetapp Tablets and Liqui-Gels
(brompheniramine,
phenylpropanolamine)–N

continues

Table 21-4   Over-the-Counter Medications (continued)

Dristan (phenylephrine, chlorpheniramine, acetaminophen)–N

Dristan Maximum Strength (pseudoephedrine, acetaminophen)–N

Drixoral Allergy/Sinus (pseudoephedrine, dexbrompheniramine, acetaminophen)–N

Drixoral Cold & Allergy (pseudoephedrine, dexbrompheniramine)–N

Drixoral Cold & Flu (acetaminophen, dexbrompheniramine, pseudoephedrine)–N

Drixoral Nasal Decongestant (pseudoephedrine)–N

Efidac-24 (pseudoephedrine)–N

Expressin 400 (guaifenesin, pseudoephedrine)–Y**

4-Way Cold Tablets (acetaminophen, phenylpropanolamine, chlorpheniramine)–N

Guaifed (guaifenesin, pseudoephedrine)–Y**

Guaitab (guaifenesin, pseudoephedrine)–Y**

Hyland's Cough Syrup with Honey (ipecac, potassium antimony tartrate)–N

Hyland's C-Plus Cold Tablets (herbs, potassium iodide)–N

Isoclor Timesule (chlorpheniramine, phenylpropanolamine)–N

Isohist 2.0 (dexbrompheniramine)–Y*

Motrin IB Sinus Pain Reliever (ibuprofen, pseudoephedrine)–N

Nasalcrom A Tablets (chlorpheniramine)–Y*

Nasalcrom CA Caplets (pseudoephedrine, acetaminophen)–N

Novahistine (chlorpheniramine, phenylephrine)–Y*, Y**

Novahistine-DMX (dextromethorphan, guaifenesin, pseudoephedrine)–N

Oscillococcinum Pellets (herbs)–N

Pertussin DM Extra Strength (dextromethorphan)–N

Pyrroxate (chlorpheniramine, phenylpropanolamine, acetaminophen)–N

Robitussin (guaifenesin)–Y

Robitussin-CF (guaifenesin, phenylpropanolamine, dextromethorphan)–N

Robitussin-DM (guaifenesin, dextromethorphan)–Y*

Robitussin-PE (guaifenesin, pseudoephedrine)–Y**

Robitussin Cold–Cold, Cough, & Flu Liqui-Gels (acetaminophen, guaifenesin, pseudoephedrine, dextromethorphan)–N

Robitussin Cold–Night-Time Liqui-Gels (acetaminophen, pseudoephedrine, dextromethorphan)–N

Robitussin Cold–Severe Congestion Liqui-Gels (guaifenesin, pseudoephedrine)–Y**

Ryna Liquid (chlorpheniramine, pseudoephedrine)–Y*, Y**

Ryna-C Liquid (codeine)–N

Ryna-CX Liquid (codeine, pseudoephedrine, guaifenesin)–N

Scot-Tussin DM (dextromethorphan, chlorpheniramine)–N

Scot-Tussin Expectorant (guaifenesin)–Y

Scot-Tussin Sugar Free, Alcohol Free Expectorant (guaifenesin)–Y

Scot-Tussin Sugar-Free Allergy Relief Formula (diphenhydramine)—Y*

Scot-Tussin Sugar-Free DM (dextromethorphan, chlorpheniramine)—N

Sinarest No Drowsiness (acetaminophen, pseudoephedrine)—N

Sinarest Regular and Extra Strength (acetaminophen, chlorpheniramine, phenylpropanolamine)—N

Sine-Aid Maximum Strength Sinus Medication (acetaminophen, pseudoephedrine)—N

Sine-Off No Drowsiness Formula (acetaminophen, pseudoephedrine)—N

Sine-Off Sinus Medicine (chlorpheniramine, pseudoephedrine, acetaminophen)—N

Singlet (pseudoephedrine, chlorpheniramine, acetaminophen)—N

Sinutab Non-Drying Liquid Caps (pseudoephedrine, guaifenesin)—Y**

Sinutab Sinus Allergy Medication Maximum Strength (acetaminophen, chlorpheniramine, pseudoephedrine)—N

Sudafed Cold & Allergy Tablets (chlorpheniramine, pseudoephedrine)—Y*, Y**

Sudafed Cold & Cough Liquid Caps (acetaminophen, guaifenesin, pseudoephedrine, dextromethorphan)—N

Sudafed Cold & Sinus Liquid Caps (acetaminophen, pseudoephedrine)—N

Sudafed Nasal Decongestant (pseudoephedrine)—Y**

Sudafed Non-Drying Sinus Liquid Caps (guaifenesin, pseudoephedrine)—Y**

Sudafed Severe Cold Formula (acetaminophen, pseudoephedrine, dextromethorphan)—N

Sudafed Sinus (acetaminophen, pseudoephedrine)—N

Sudafed 12-Hour Tablets (pseudoephedrine)—N

Sudafed 24-Hour Tablets (pseudoephedrine)—N

Suppressin DM (dextromethorphan, guaifenesin)—Y*

TAVIST Allergy Tablets (clemastine)—Y*

TAVIST-D Caplets or Tablets (clemastine, phenylpropanolamine)—N

TAVIST Sinus Caplets or Gelcaps (acetaminophen, pseudoephedrine)—N

Theraflu Flu and Cold Medicine (acetaminophen, pseudoephedrine, chlorpheniramine)—N

Theraflu Maximum Strength Flu, Cold and Cough Medicine (acetaminophen, dextromethorphan, pseudoephedrine, chlorpheniramine)—N

Theraflu Maximum Strength Flu and Cold Medicine (acetaminophen, pseudoephedrine, chlorpheniramine)—N

Theraflu Maximum Strength Nighttime (acetaminophen, pseudoephedrine, chlorpheniramine)—N

Theraflu Maximum Strength Non-Drowsy (acetaminophen, pseudoephedrine, dextromethorphan)—N

Triaminic AM Cough and Decongestant (pseudoephedrine, dextromethorphan)—N

Triaminic AM Decongestant (pseudoephedrine)—Y*

continues

Table 21-4   Over-the-Counter Medications (continued)

Triaminic Cold & Allergy Softchews (pseudoephedrine, dextromethorpham, chlorpheniramine)–Y*, Y**

Triaminic Cold & Cough Softchews (pseudoephedrine, dextromethorphan, chlorpheniramine)–N

Triaminic DM Syrup (phenylpropanolamine, dextromethorphan)–N

Triaminic Expectorant (guaifenesin, phenylpropanolamine)–N

Triaminic Night Time (pseudoephedrine, dextromethorphan, chlorpheniramine)–N

Triaminic Severe Cold & Fever (acetaminophen, pseudoephedrine, dextromethorphan, chlorpheniramine)–N

Triaminic Sore Throat (acetaminophen, dextromethorphan)–N

Triaminic Syrup (phenylpropanolamine, chlorpheniramine)–N

Triaminic Throat Pain & Cough Softchews (acetaminophen, pseudoephedrine, dextromethorphan)–N

Triaminicin Tablets (acetaminophen, phenylpropanolamine, chlorpheniramine)–N

Triaminicol Cold & Cough (phenylpropanolamine, dextromethorphan, chlorpheniramine)–N

Tylenol Allergy Sinus Maximum Strength (acetaminophen, chlorpheniramine, pseudoephedrine)–N

Tylenol Allergy Sinus NightTime Maximum Strength (acetaminophen, pseudoephedrine, diphenhydramine)–N

Tylenol Cold Medication Multi-Symptom Formula (acetaminophen, chlorpheniramine, pseudoephedrine, dextromethorphan)–N

Tylenol Cold Medication No Drowsiness Formula (acetaminophen, pseudoephedrine, dextromethorphan)–N

Tylenol Cold Multi-Symptom Severe Congestion (acetaminophen, dextromethorphan, guaifenesin, pseudoephedrine)–N

Tylenol Flu NightTime Maximum Strength Gelcap (acetaminophen, diphenhydramine, pseudoephedrine)–N

Tylenol Flu NightTime Maximum Strength Hot Medication (acetaminophen, diphenhydramine, pseudoephedrine)–N

Tylenol Flu NightTime Maximum Strength Liquid (acetaminophen, dextromethorphan, doxylamine, pseudoephedrine)–N

Tylenol Severe Allergy (acetaminophen, diphenhydramine)–N

Tylenol Sinus Maximum Strength (acetaminophen, pseudoephedrine)–N

Tylenol Sinus NightTime Maximum Strength (acetaminophen, doxylamine, pseudoephedrine)–N

Ursinus (pseudoephedrine, aspirin)–N

Vicks DayQuil LiquiCaps, Liquid (pseudoephedrine, acetaminophen, dextromethorphan)–N

Vicks DayQuil Sinus Pressure & Pain Relief (ibuprofen, pseudoephedrine)–N

Vicks 44 Cough Relief (dextromethorphan, alcohol 5%)–Y*

Vicks 44D Cough & Head Congestion
Relief (dextromethorphan,
pseudoephedrine, alcohol 5%)—N

Vicks 44E Cough & Chest Congestion
Relief (dextromethorphan, guaifenesin,
alcohol 5%)—Y*

Vicks 44M Cough, Cold & Flu Relief
(dextromethorphan, pseudoephedrine,
chlorpheniramine, acetaminophen,
alcohol 10%)—N

Vicks NyQuil Liquid (doxylamine,
destromethorphan, acetaminophen,
pseudoephedrine, alcohol 10%)—N

Cough and Cold Lozenges and Sprays

Celestial Seasonings Soothers Herbal
Throat Drops (menthol, pectin)—Y

Cepacol Maximum Strength Sore Throat
Lozenges (menthol, cetylpyridinium,
benzocaine)—Y

Cepacol Maximum Strength Sore Throat
Spray (dyclonine, cetylpyridinium)—Y

Cepacol Regular Strength Sore Throat
Lozenges (menthol, cetylpyridinium)—Y

Cepastat Cherry Lozenges (phenol,
menthol)—N

Cepastat Extra Strength Lozenges (phenol,
menthol eucalyptus oil)—N

Cepastat Lozenges (phenol)—N

Cheracol Sore Throat Spray (phenol)—N

Halls Mentho-Lyptus Drops (menthol)—Y

Halls Plus Cough Suppressant Drops
(menthol, pectin)—Y

HOLD Lozenges (dextromethorphan)—Y*

Listerine Lozenges (hexylresorcinol)—N

N'ICE Lozenges (menthol)—Y

Robitussin Cough Drops (menthol, pectin,
eucalyptus)—Y

Scot-Tussin Sugar-Free Cough Chasers
(dextromethorphan)—Y*

Sucrets 4-Hour Cough Suppressant
Lozenges (menthol,
dextromethorphan)—Y*

Sucrets Maximum Strength lozenges
(dyclonine)—Y

Sucrets Regular Strength
(hexylresorcinol)—N

Sucrets Regular Strength Vapor
(dyclonine)—Y

Vicks Chloraseptic Lozenges (benzocaine,
menthol)—Y

Vicks Cough Drops (menthol)—Y

Nasal Preparations

Afrin Allergy Spray (phenylephrine)—Y**

Afrin Extra Moisturizing Spray
(oxymetazoline)—Y**

Afrin Moisturizing Saline Mist (sodium
chloride)—Y

Afrin Original Spray, Nose Drops and
Pump Mist (soxymetazoline)—Y**

Afrin Saline Mist with Eucalyptol and
Menthol (Sodium chloride)—Y

continues

Table 21-4   Over-the-Counter Medications (continued)

Afrin Severe Congestion Spray (oxymetazoline)—Y**

Afrin Sinus Nasal Spray (oxymetazoline)—Y**

Alconefrin (phenylephrine)—Y**

AYR Saline Mist and Drops (sodium chloride)—Y

Benzedres Inhaler (propylhedrine)—N

Cheracol Spray (oxymetazoline)—Y**

Dristan Long Lasting Spray (oxymetazoline)—Y**

Dristan Spray (phenylephrine, pheniramine)—N

Duration 12-Hour Spray (oxymetazoline)—Y**

4-Way Fast Acting Nasal Spray (phenylephrine)—Y**

4-Way Long Acting Spray (oxymetazoline)—Y**

4-Way Saline Moisturizing Mist (sodium chloride)—Y

HuMIST Saline (sodium chloride)—Y

Little Noses Saline (sodium chloride)—Y

Nasalcrom Nasal Spray (cromolyn sodium)—Y

Nasal Moist Gel (aloe vera)—Y

Nasal Moist Solution (sodium chloride)—Y

Neo-Synephrine Drops (phenylephrine)—Y**

Neo-Synephrine Extra Strength Drops (phenylephrine)—Y**

Neo-Synephrine Mild, Regular, and Extra Strength Spray (phenylephrine)—Y**

Neo-Synephrine 12-Hour Extra Moisturizing Spray (oxymetazoline)—Y**

Neo-Synephrine 12-Hour Spray (oxymetazoline)—Y**

Nose Better Natural Mist (glycerin, sodium chloride)—Y

Nostril Nasal Decongestant (phenylephrine)—Y**

NTZ Spray and Drops (oxymetazoline)—Y**

Ocean Nasal Mist (sodium chloride)—Y

Otrivin Nasal Drops and Spray (xylometazoline)—N

Pretz (glycerin)—Y

Priviner Nasal Spray and Solution (naphazoline)—N

St. Joseph Nasal Decongestant (phenylephrine)—Y**

Salinex Nasal Mist and Drops (sodium chloride)—Y

Vicks Sinex Nasal Spray and Ultra Fine Mist (phenylephrine, camphor, eucalyptol, menthol)—N

Vicks Vapor Inhaler (leumetamfetamine, menthol, camphor)—N

Asthma Preparations

Asthmahaler (epinephrine)—x

Asthmanephrin (racepinephrine)—x

Bronkaid Caplets (ephedrine, guaifenesin, theophylline)—x

Bronkaid Mist (epinephrine)—x

Bronkoelixir (ephedrine, guaifenesin, theophylline, phenobarbital)—x

Primatene Mist (epinephrine)—x

Antacids and Digestive Aids

Alka-Mints (calcium carbonate)–Y

Alka-Seltzer (aspirin, sodium bicarbonate)–N

Alka-Seltzer Extra Strength (aspirin, sodium bicarbonate)–N

Alka-Seltzer Gas Relief (simethicone)–Y

Alka-Seltzer Gold (sodium, potassium bicarbonate)–N

Alkets/Alkets Extra Strengh (calcium carbonate)–Y

Almora (magnesium gluconate)–Y

AlternaGEL (aluminum hydroxide)–Y

Alu-Cap (aluminum hydroxide)–Y

Aludrox (aluminum-magnesium hydroxide)–Y

Alu-Tab (aluminum hydroxide)–Y

Amitone (calcium carbonate)–Y

Amphogel (aluminum hydroxide)–Y

Axid AR (nizatidine)–Y

Basaljel (aluminum carbonate)–Y

Beano (enzymes, sorbitol)–Y

BeSure (food enzymes)–Y

Chooz Antacid Gum (calcium carbonate)–Y

Citrocarbonate (sodium bicarbonate-citrate)–N

Creamalin (aluminum-magnesium hydroxide)–Y

Dairy Ease (lactase)–Y

DDS-Acidophilus (lactobacillus acidophilus)–Y

Dicarbosil (calcium carbonate)

DiGel (simethicone, calcium carbonate, magnesium hydroxide)–Y

Eno (sodium tartrate-citrate)–N

Gas-X (simethicone)–Y

Gas-X Extra Strength (simethicone)–Y

Gaviscon Extra Strength (aluminum hydroxide, magnesium carbonate)–Y

Gaviscon Regular Strength Liquid (aluminum hydroxide, magnesium carbonate)–Y

Gaviscon Regular Strength Tablets (aluminum hydroxide, magnesium trisilicate)–Y

Gaviscon-2 (aluminum hydroxide, magnesium trisilicate, sodium bicarbonate)–N

Gelusil (aluminum-magnesium hydroxide, simethicone)–Y

Kudrox (simethicone, aluminum-magnesium hydroxide)–Y

Lactaid Original, Extra Strength, and Ultra (lactase)–Y

Lactinex (lactobacillus culture)–Y

Lactrase (lactase)–Y

Maalox Anti-Gas (simethicone)–Y

Maalox Anti-Gas Extra Strength (simethicone)–Y

Maalox Heartburn Relief (aluminum hydroxide, magnesium-calcium carbonate, potassium bicarbonate)–N

Maalox Magnesia and Alumina Oral Susp. (magnesium-aluminum hydroxide)–Y

Maalox Maximum Strength (magnesium-aluminum hydroxide, simethicone)–Y

Maalox Quick Dissolve Tablets (calcium carbonate)–Y

continues

Table 21-4　Over-the-Counter Medications (continued)

Marblen (magnesium-calcium carbonate)–Y

Mylanta AR (famotidine)–Y

Mylanta Fast-Acting (aluminum-magnesium hydroxide, simethicone)–Y

Mylanta Maximum Strength (aluminum-magnesium hydroxide, simethicone)–Y

Mylanta Supreme (calcium carbonate, magnesium hydroxide)–Y

Mylanta Tablets and Gelcaps (calcium carbonate, magnesium hydroxide)–Y

Nephrox (aluminum hydroxide)–Y

Pepcid AC (famotidine)–Y

Pepto-Bismol Original (bismuth subsalicylate)–N

Pepto-Bismol Maximum Strength (bismuth subsalicylate)–N

Phazyme-125 Softgels (simethicone)–Y

Phazyme-166 Maximum Strength (simethicone)–Y

Phillips Milk of Magnesia (magnesium hydroxide)–Y

Riopan (magaldrate)–Y

Riopan Plus (magaldrate, simethicone)–Y

Riopan Plus 2 (magaldrate, simethicone)–Y

Rolaids (calcium carbonate, magnesium hydroxide)–Y

Sodium Bicarbonate (sodium bicarbonate)–N

Tagamet HB (cimetidine)–Y

Tempo (calcium carbonate, aluminum-magnesium hydroxide)–Y

Titralac (calcium carbonate)–Y

Titralac Extra Strength (calcium carbonate)–Y

Titralac Plus Antacid (calcium carbonate, simethicone)–Y

Tums E-X Antacid (calcium carbonate)–Y

Tums Regular (calcium carbonate)–Y

Tums ULTRA Antacid (calcium carbonate)–Y

Zantac 75 (ranitidine)–Y

Laxatives, Stool Softeners

Bisacodyl–N

Cascara Sagrada–Y

Ceo-Two Evacuant Suppository (sodium bicarbonate, potassium bitartrate)–Y

Citrucel (methylcellulose)–Y

Colace (docusate)–Y

Correctol Laxative (bisacodyl)–N

Correctol Stool Softener (docusate)–Y

Dialose (docusate)–Y

Doxidan (casanthranol, docusate)–N

Dulcolax Tablets and Suppositories (bisacodyl)–N

Effer-Syllium (psyllium)–Y

Emulsoil (caster oil)–N

Epsom Salt (magnesium sulfate)–Y

Evac-Q-Kwik (bisacodyl)–N

Ex-Lax Chocolate or Regular (sennosides)–Y

Ex-Lax Maximum (sennosides)–N

Fiberall (psyllium)–Y

Fibercon (calcium polycarbophil)–Y

Fiber Naturale (methylcellulose)–Y

Fleet Enema Regular (sodium biphosphate, phosphate)–Y

Fleet Laxative (bisacodyl)–N

Garfield's Tea (senna)–Y

Gentlax S (senna concentrate, docusate)–N

Gentle Nature (sennosides)–Y

Glycerin Suppositories–Y

Haley's M-0 (magnesium hydroxide, mineral oil)–N

Herb-Lax (senna)–Y

Hydrocil (psyllium)–Y

Innerclean Herbal (senna, psyllium)–N

Kellogg's Tasteless Castor Oil (castor oil)–N

Kondremul (mineral oil)–N

Konsyl Fiber (polycarbophil)–Y

Konsyl Powder (psyllium)–Y

Maalox Daily Fiber (psyllium)–Y

Maltsupex (barley malt extract)–Y

Metamucil (psyllium)–Y

Milkinol (mineral oil)–N

Mitrolan (polycarbophil)–Y

Mylanta Natural Fiber Supplement (psyllium)–Y

Nature's Remedy Tablets (cascara sagrada, aloe)–N

Neoloid (castor oil)–N

Perdiem Fiber (psyllium)–Y

Perdiem Overnight Relief (psyllium, senna)–N

Peri-Colace (casanthranol, docusate)–N

Phillips Gelcaps (docusate)–Y

Phillips Milk of Magnesia (magnesium hydroxide)–Y

Phospho-Soda (sodium phosphate)–Y

Purge Concentrate (castor oil)–N

Regulace (casanthranol, docusate)–N

Regulax SS (docusate)–Y

Regutol (docusate)–Y

Senokot (sennosides)–Y

Senokot-S (sennosides, docusate)–N

SenokotXTRA (sennosides)–N

Surfak (docusate)–Y

Syllact (psyllium)–Y

Anti-Diarrheal Preparations

Dairy Ease (lactase)–Y

Diar Aid (loperamide)–Y***

Diarrid (loperamide)–Y***

Diasorb (attapulgite)–Y

Donnagel (attapulgite)–Y

Equalactin (polycarbophil)–Y

Hylant's Diarrex (arsenicum, podophyllum, phosphorus, mercurius)–N

Imodium A-D (loperamide)–Y***

Imodium Advanced (loperamide, simethicone)–Y***

Kao-Paverin (kaolin, pectin)–Y

Paopectate (attapulgite)–Y

Pepto-Bismol (bismuth subsalicylate)–N

Rheaban (attapulgite)–Y

continues

Table 21-4   Over-the-Counter Medications (continued)

Nausea and Vomiting, Motion Sickness Preparation

Benadryl (diphenhydramine)–Y*

Bonine (meclizine)–N

Calm-X (dimenhydrinate)–Y*

Dramamine (dimenhydrinate)–Y*

Dramamine Less Drowsy (meclizine)–N

Emetrol (phosphorated carbohydrates)–Y

Pepto-Bismol (bismuth subsalicylate)–N

Nauzene (diphenhydramine)–Y*

Triptone (dimenhydrinate)–Y*

Hemorrhoidal Preparations

Americaine (benzocaine)–Y

Anusol HC-Ointment (hydrocortisone)–Y

Anusol Ointment (pramoxine, mineral oil, zinc oxide)–Y

Anusol Suppositories (starch)–Y

Balneol (mineral oil, lanolin oil)–Y

Calmol 4 (zinc oxide, cocoa butter)–Y

Fleet Medicated Wipes (witch hazel)–Y

Fleet Pain-Relief (pramoxine)–Y

Hemorid for Women (pramoxine, phenylephrine)–Y

Hydrosal Hemorrhoidal (benzyl alcohol, ephedrine, zinc oxide)–Y

Nupercainal (dibucaine)–Y

Nupercainal Anti-Itch Cream (hydrocortisone)–Y

Nupercainal Suppositories (cocoa butter, zinc oxide)–Y

Pazo (benzocaine, ephedrine, zinc oxide, camphor)–Y

Peterson's Ointment (phenol, camphor)–Y

Preparation H Hydrocortisone Cream (hydrocortisone)–Y

Preparation H Ointment, Suppositories, and Cream (phenylephrine, shark liver oil)–Y

Procto Foam Non-Steroid (pramoxine)–Y

Rectacaine Ointment (petrolatum, shark liver oil, mineral oil)–Y

Rectacaine Suppositories (phenylephrine)–Y

Tronolane Cream (pramoxine)–Y

Tronothane Hydrochloride (pramoxine, glycerin)–Y

Tronolane Suppository (zinc oxide)–Y

Tucks Pads (witch hazel)–Y

Wyanoids (cocoa butter, shark liver oil, glycerin)–Y

Sleep Preparations

Alka-Seltzer PM Pain Reliever & Sleep Aid Medicine (aspirin, diphenhydramine)–N

Anacin PM Aspirin Free (acetaminophen, diphenhydramine)–N

Bayer PM Extra Strength Aspirin Plus Sleep Aid (aspirin, diphenhydramine)–N

Benadryl (diphenhydramine)–Y*

Compoz (diphenhydramine)–Y*

Doan's PM Extra Strength (magnesium salicylate, diphenhydramine)–N

Dormarex and Dormarex 2 (diphenhydramine)–Y*

Dormin (diphenhydramine)–Y*

Excedrin PM (acetaminophen, diphenhydramine)–N

Goody's PM (acetaminophen, diphenhydramine)–N

Legatrim PM (diphenhydramine, acetaminophen)–N

Melatonex (melatonin)–N

Melatonin (melatonin)–N

Melatonin (pyridoxine, melatonin)–N

Melatonin Lozenge (melatonin, xylitol)–N

Melatonin PM Dual Release (calcium, vitamin B6, magnesium, niacin, melatonin, xylitol)–N

Midol PM Night Time Formula (diphenhydramine, acetaminophen)–N

Nervine Nightime Sleep Aid (diphenhydramine)–Y*

Nite Gel (doxylamine, acetaminophen, pseudoephedrine, dextromethorphan)–N

Nytol Natural (ignatia amara, aconitum radix)–N

Nytol Quickcaps and Quickgels (diphenhydramine)–Y*

Restyn 76 (diphenhydramine)–Y*

Sleep-Ettes D (diphenhydramine)–Y*

Sleep-Eze 3 (diphenhydramine)–Y*

Sleepinal (diphenhydramine)–Y*

Sleepiness (diphenhydramine)–Y*

Sleep Rite (diphenhydramine)–Y*

Snooze Fast (diphenhydramine)–Y*

Sominex Original (diphenhydramine)–Y*

Sominex Pain Relief Formula (diphenhydramine, acetaminophen)–N

Tranquil (diphenhydramine)–Y*

Tranquil Plus (diphenhydramine, acetaminophen)–N

Unisom Maximum Strength (diphenhydramine)–Y*

Unisom with Pain Relief (acetaminophen, diphenhydramine)–N

Stimulants

No Doz (caffeine 200 mg)–N*

Vivarin (caffeine 200 mg)–N*

Appetite Suppressant Products

Acutrim (phenylpropanolamine)–N

Amfed T.D. (phenylpropanolamine)–N

Dexatrim (phenylpropanolamine)–N

Dieutrim T.D. (phenylpropanolamine, benzocaine)–N

Mini Slims (phenylpropanolamine)–N

Mini Thin Diet Aid (phenylpropanolamine)–N

Permathene (phenylpropanolamine)–N

Protrim (phenylpropanolamine)–N

Thinz Back to Nature and Thinz-Span (phenylpropanolamine)–N

continues

Table 21-4   Over-the-Counter Medications (continued)

Insulin Preparations

All insulin-containing products are safe in breastfeeding; however, it is recommended that the insulin dose be reduced by 25 percent of the prepregnancy dose.

Artificial Sweetners

Equal (aspartame)—Y***	Sweet 'N Low (saccharin)—Y
NutraSweet (aspartame)—Y***	

References for Table 21-4

1. Wilkes D. The international perspective on the OTC market. *IMS Health Self Medication/OTC Bulletin.* December 9, 1998.

2. Findlay J, DeAngelis R, Kearney M, et al. Analgesic drugs in breast milk and plasma. *Clin Pharmacol Ther.* 1981;29:625–633.

3. Anderson PO. Drug use during breast-feeding. *Clin Pharm.* 1991;10:594–624.

4. Rathmell JP, Viscomi CM, Ashburn MA. Management of nonobstetric pain during pregnancy and lactation. *Anesth Analg.* 1997;85:1074–1087.

5. Britt R, Pasero C. Using analgesics during breastfeeding. *Am J Nurs.* 1999;99:20. Abstract.

6. American Academy of Pediatrics Committee on Drugs. The transfer of drugs and other chemicals into human milk. *Pediatrics.* 1994;13:137–150.

7. Kok TH, Taitz LS, Bennett MJ, et al. Drowsiness due to clemastine transmitted in breast milk. *Lancet.* 1982;1:914–915.

8. Briggs G, Freeman R, Yaffe S. *Drugs in Pregnancy and Lactation: A Reference Guide to Fetal and Neonatal Risk.* 5th ed. Baltimore: Williams & Wilkins; 1998:72–73, 217, 222, 407–408, 548, 661–662, 958–959.

9. Nice FJ. Breastfeeding and OTC medications. *Pharm Times.* 1992;58:114–124, 126–127.

10. Kanfer I, Dowse R, Vuma V. Pharmacokinetics of oral decongestants. *Pharmacotherapy.* 1993; 13:116S–128S.

11. Scariati P, Grummer-Strawn L, Fein S. A longitudinal analysis of infant morbidity and the extent of breastfeeding in the United States. *Pediatrics.* 1997;99:E5. Abstract.

12. Briggs G, Freeman R, Yaffe S. *Drugs in Pregnancy and Lactation Update.* Baltimore: Williams & Wilkins; 1998.

13. Redetzki HM. Alcohol. In: Wilson JT, ed. *Drugs in Breast Milk.* Balgowlah, Australia: ADIS Health Science Press; 1981:46–49.

14. Hornby P, Abrahams T. Pulmonary pharmacology. *Clin Obstet and Gynecol.* 1996;39:17–35.

15. Meny RG, Naumburg EG, Alger LS, et al. Codeine and the breastfed neonate. *J Hum Lact.* 1993;9:237–240.

16. Covington T, Pau A. Oxymetazoline. *Am Pharm.* 1985;NS25:21–26.

17. Yurchak AM, Jusko WJ. Theophylline secretion into breast milk. *Pediatrics.* 1976;57:518–520.

18. Stewart JJ. Gastrointestinal drugs. In: Wilson JT, ed. *Drugs in Breast Milk.* Balgowlah, Australia: ADIS Health Science Press; 1981:65–71.

19. Hagemann T. Gastrointestinal medications and breastfeeding. *J Hum Lact.* 1998;14:259–262.

20. Nikodem VC, Hofmeyr GJ. Secretion of the antidiarrhoeal agent loperamide oxide in breast milk. *Eur J Clin Pharmacol.* 1992;42:695–696.

21. Figueroa-Quintanilla D, Lindo E, Sack B, et al. A controlled trial of bismuth subsalicylate in infants with acute watery diarrheal disease. *N Engl J Med.* 1993;328:1653–1658.

22. Oo C, Kuhn R, Desai N, McNamara P. Active transport of cimetidine into human milk. *Clin Pharmacol Ther.* 1995:58:548–555.

23. Somogyi A, Gugler R. Cimetidine excreation into breast milk. *Br J Clin Pharmacol.* 1979;7:627–629.

24. Kearns G, McConnell R, Trang J, Lkuza R. Appearance of ranitidine in breast milk following multiple dosing. *Clin Pharm.* 1985;4:322–324.

25. Obermeyer B, Bergstrom R, Callaghan J, et al. Secretion of nizatidine into human breast milk after single and multiple dosing. *Clin Pharmacol Ther.* 1990;47:724–730.

26. Courtney T, Shaw R, Cedar E, et al. Excretion of famotidine in breast milk. *Br J Pharmacol.* 1988;26:639P.

27. Stoukides C. Topical medications and breastfeeding. *J Hum Lact.* 1993;9:185–187.

28. Committee on Drugs, American Academy of Pediatrics. The transfer of drugs and other chemicals into human breast milk. *Pediatrics.* 1983;72:375–383.

29. Juszczak M, Stempniak B. The effect of melatonin on suckling-induced oxytocin and prolactin release in the rat. *Brain Res Bull.* 1997;44:253–258.

30. Ryu J. Effect of maternal caffeine consumption on heart rate and sleep time of breast-fed infants. *Dev Pharmacol Ther.* 1985;8:355–363.

31. Davies H, Clark J, Dalton K, Edwards O. Insulin requirements of diabetic women who breastfeed. *BMJ.* 1989;298:1357–1358.

32. Steqink LD, Filer LJ, Baker GL. Plasma, erythrocyte, and human milk levels of free amino acids in lactating women administered aspartame or lactose. *J Nutr.* 1979;109:2173–2181.

33. Egan PC, Marx CM, Heyl PS, et al. Saccharin concentration in mature human milk. *Drug Intell Clin Pharm.* 1984;18:511. Abstract.

    c. The ideal method would be to assay the breast milk for radioactivity and resume breastfeeding when levels are safe.

  2. Basically, three options exist in a radiopharmaceutical/breastfeeding situation.
    a. Discontinue breastfeeding.
        i. Breastfeeding should probably be discontinued following the use of radioactive I^{131} due to the enhanced risk of thyroid carcinoma in the infant.
        ii. This also may be necessary for extended interruptions when milk production is already waning.
    b. Interrupt breastfeeding for a short period.
        i. A breast pump can be used to express milk and store for use during interruptions.
    c. Do not interrupt breastfeeding.
        i. Interruptions are not always necessary depending upon the type of radiopharmaceutical administered.

  3. The Office of Nuclear Regulatory Research's guide contains instructions and recommendations on the use of radiopharmaceuticals during breastfeeding. In addition, objective mathematically-derived guidelines for the administration of radiopharmaceuticals in nursing mothers have been developed (Hale, 2006).

Reference

Hale T. Medications and Mothers' Milk: *A Manual of Lactational Pharmacology.* 12th ed. Amarillo, TX: Hale Publishing; 2006.

Suggested Readings

American Academy of Pediatrics Committee on Drugs. The transfer of drugs and other chemicals into human milk. *Pediatrics.* 2001;108:776–789 (see also: American Academy of Pediatrics Policy Statement: The Transfer of Drugs and Other Chemicals into Human Milk. Available at: http://aappolicy.aappublications.org/cgi/content/full/pediatrics%3b108/3/776. Accessed December 28, 2006.

Briggs GG, Freeman RK, Yaffe SJ. *Drugs in Pregnancy and Lactation.* 7th ed. Baltimore: Lippincott Williams & Wilkins; 2005.

Hale T. *Clinical Therapy in Breastfeeding Mothers.* Amarillo, TX: Pharmasoft Publishing; 2000.

Lawrence RA, Lawrence RM. *Breastfeeding: A Guide for the Medical Profession.* 6th ed. St. Louis: C.V. Mosby; 2005:377–426.

Nice FJ, Snyder JL, Kotansky BC. Breastfeeding and over-the-counter medications. *J Hum Lact.* 2000;16:319–331.

Nice FJ, DeEugenio D, DiMino TA, et al. Medications and breast-feeding: a guide for pharmacists, pharmacy technicians, and other healthcare professionals, Part I. *J Pharm Tech.* 2004;20:17–27.

Nice FJ, DeEugenio D, DiMino TA, et al. Medications and breast-feeding: a guide for pharmacists, pharmacy technicians, and other healthcare professionals, Part II. *J Pharm Tech.* 2004;20:85–95.

Nice FJ, DeEugenio D, DiMino TA, et al. Medications and breast-feeding: a guide for pharmacists, pharmacy technicians, and other healthcare professionals, Part III. *J Pharm Tech.* 2004;20:165–177.

LACTATIONAL TOXICOLOGY

Marsha Walker, RN, IBCLC
Revised by Marsha Walker, RN, IBCLC and
Frank J. Nice, RPh, DPA, CPHP

OBJECTIVES

- Discuss the issue of environmental chemicals in human milk.

- Discuss recreational and illegal drug use in lactating women.

Introduction

With rare exception—usually on the occasion of a large environmental contamination—chemical agents have not been shown to adversely affect breastfeeding infants. Only in exceptional circumstances would the benefits derived from breastfeeding fail to outweigh the possible toxic consequences of chemical exposure through human milk (Rogan et al., 1991; Rogan & Ragan, 1994). Data relating to chemical contaminants in human milk are often conflicting, inaccurate, or speculative, which has resulted in uncertainty and less clarity. Data concerning the toxicity of chemicals in humans are often sparse and limited to high-dose or mixed chemical exposures, often as a result of occupational exposure or accidents. The presence of environmental contaminants in human milk is also used in the political arena as a justification to clean up the environment or as a weapon against breastfeeding. Because many environmental contaminants can be transported across the placenta to the fetus, it is difficult to separate the effects of prenatal exposure from those of exposure through human milk. If the infant and mother are exposed to the same environmental contaminants in the home (such as lead), then human milk might not be the chief route of exposure. Furthermore, exposure to environmental chemicals varies from country to country (and even in each country from region to region), which makes it difficult to generalize information to all populations. The lactation consultant will benefit from a general overview of this topic and from an understanding of the multiple contributors to lactational toxicology and governmental recommendations.

I. General Considerations (Jensen & Slorach, 1991)

A. Based on the growth patterns of breastfed and formula-fed infants, a breastfed baby acquires more body fat during the first three months of life and theoretically would be more susceptible to lipophilic (having an affinity for fat) compound toxicity during this time period than a formula-fed infant.

B. From 3 to 12 months of age, a breastfed baby becomes leaner than a formula-fed baby, and hence would be theoretically less susceptible during this time period.

C. If a breastfed infant is switched to formula at three months of age, there would be an increase in the risk of toxicity to lipophilic agents between 3 and 12 months because these infants possess more fat and thus potentially store more toxins.

D. Growth or weight gain is frequently used as an index of toxicity in animals and humans and should not be the sole parameter used to establish toxicity in the first year of life, due to the differences in growth between breastfed and formula-fed babies.

E. Lipophilic contaminants can be present in human milk, stored in mammary fat, or stored in body fat (with adverse effects related to the concentration and release from fat).

F. The fats in human milk arise from three sources (Schreiber, 1997).

1. 30% from the current maternal diet.

2. 60% from maternal adipose tissue stores.

3. 10% from synthesis in the mammary gland itself.

G. Even with adequate maternal fat intake in the diet, adipose tissue stores still contribute 60% of the fats to the milk.

H. Exposure to chemicals is generally over a period of years; these chemicals are mobilized during lactation and might represent a route of elimination (Schreiber, 1997).

I. Women who lose a large amount of weight rapidly can release greater amounts of lipophilic contaminants into the breast milk.

J. The number of children previously nursed by a mother will affect the chemical levels in her milk for her next baby.

K. Subsequent children will consume milk containing lower concentrations of persistent chemicals.

L. Obese women can have up to 50% more body fat than women who are at or near their optimal weight.

1. The extra fat provides a greater reservoir for chemical contaminants, diluting their presence.

2. If the obese woman ingests greater amounts of food containing contaminants, then contaminant levels within the fat will equal or exceed the general population.

M. Compounds that have a molecular size (mass) of below 200 Daltons are likely to be found in milk, especially if they are lipophilic.

N. Many of the chemicals under consideration are ubiquitous, making it difficult to find control samples for exposure comparisons.

O. Analytical techniques have become very sophisticated, permitting the detection of extremely low levels of chemicals that previously have been reported to be below the limit of detection.

P. Conclusions based on a single subject or a small sample size might be misleading when translating outcomes from studies with small numbers into public health policy.

Q. Human milk levels of contaminants are used as epidemiologic markers of human exposure within a community because of the correlation between human milk levels and levels in the fat stores.

R. Unless the circumstances are unusual, however, breastfeeding should not be abandoned on the basis of chemical presence alone; only extreme levels of contaminants in human milk represent more of a hazard than the failure to breastfeed.

S. In most cases, the levels of pesticides in human milk are less than those in cow's milk.

II. Halogenated Hydrocarbons

A. DDT [(1,1-bis(p-chlorophenyl)-2,2,2-trichloroethane] and its related compounds and metabolites, mirex, polychlorinated biphenyls (PCBs), heptachlor, aldrin/dieldrin, chlordane, and hexachlorobenzene.

1. Most of the early studies until 1980 showed detectable levels of DDT in nearly all women who were tested.

2. Adverse effects on infants were not shown at the levels detected.

3. Because DDT was banned in the United States in 1972, the average woman in the United States is not considered at risk for excessive levels of DDT in her milk.

4. In some developing countries, however, mothers might continue to be at risk in rural or agricultural areas.
   a. In utero exposure to DDT and dichlorodiphenyldichloroethylene (DDE) has been shown to adversely affect the neurodevelopment of exposed infants. Breastfeeding these infants helps to offset the potential neurodevelopmental deficit caused by exposure of the developing fetus (Eskenazi et al., 2006).

5. The World Health Organization does not consider human milk to be a major source of DDT.

6. DDE is a major metabolite of DDT and has been associated with a shortened duration of breastfeeding; this effect is thought to arise from the weak estrogen

activity of DDE and related isomers possibly contributing to a reduced milk supply.

7. No adverse effects have been noted in the recipient infants.

B. PCB and polybrominated biphenyl (PBB).

1. Formerly used as insulation media in electrical systems, lubricants, and as paint additives, these components are now used only in closed systems to prevent air, soil, and water contamination.

2. These compounds can exert neurotoxic effects on the infant's developing brain.

3. Except in cases of unusually heavy exposure, there is no contraindication to breastfeeding (Jensen & Slorach, 1991).

4. If there is a question about environmental exposure and the safety of breastfeeding, the respective state health department (in the United States) can be consulted for specific advice or to measure plasma and breast milk levels.
   a. Long-term studies following groups of babies exposed in utero have found that breastfed infants appear to be less impacted by these chemical exposures than their formula-fed counterparts, showing fewer neurologic effects of PCB exposure (Dekoning & Karmaus, 2000; Jacobson & Jacobson, 2002).

5. Polybrominated diphenyl ethers are flame retardants used in upholstered furniture, electronics, automobile interiors, and plastics.
   a. Research on animals shows that fetal exposure to minute doses of brominated fire retardants at critical points in development can cause deficits in sensory and motor skills, learning, memory, and hearing.
   b. Even women with very high levels of fire retardants in their milk should continue to breastfeed their babies. Effects on learning and behavior are strongly associated with *fetal* exposure to persistent pollutants, not with human milk exposure (LaKind et al., 2005).
   c. Breastfeeding appears to overcome some of the harmful effects of high fetal exposure to persistent chemicals.

C. Dioxins and benzofurans.

1. Dioxins are a group of related compounds that are both man-made and occur naturally in low levels in the environment.

2. Dioxins are released into the air from combustion processes such as commercial or municipal waste incineration, burning fuels such as wood, coal, or oil, burning household trash, and forest fires; chlorine bleaching of pulp and paper, and certain other types of chemical and manufacturing processes can create small amounts of dioxins, as does cigarette smoking.

3. One of the best known dioxins is Agent Orange.

4. The U.S. Environmental Protection Agency (EPA) released a draft report on a reassessment of dioxin exposure and hazards (EPA, 2004).

a. This document was reviewed by the U.S. National Academies of Science (NAS, 2006).

5. Data within this report show that it is safe to breastfeed infants in the United States relative to dioxin, because dioxin levels in the environment have decreased.

6. The findings in the EPA (2004) document include the following statements: "We believe there are overwhelming benefits of breastfeeding and encourage women to continue the practice . . . Findings in the draft EPA dioxin report do NOT suggest that women should stop breastfeeding. Women are encouraged to continue the practice of breastfeeding given its overall benefits to mother and child."

7. Perchlorate is both naturally occurring and a man-made chemical used in the manufacturing of rubber, paint, enamel products, fireworks, car air bags, highway flares, and as an explosive propellant in rocket fuel.
   a. Human exposure sources include drinking water, cow's milk, and vegetables.
   b. Perchlorate competitively inhibits iodine uptake in the thyroid gland, which could potentially reduce thyroid function.
   c. Impaired thyroid function in pregnant women may affect the fetus and newborn with delayed development and decreased learning capacity.
   d. High perchlorate levels in mothers may potentially reduce iodine levels in their milk.
   e. Mothers with high perchlorate levels can take iodine supplements to offset reduced iodine levels (Kirk et al., 2005).
   f. Mothers should continue to breastfeed, with infants evaluated for hypothyroidism at routine well-child visits.

D. Organochlorine insecticides.

   1. These include aldrin, dieldrin, endrin, naphthalene derivatives, lindane, heptachlor, and chlordane; many of these have been banned in industrialized countries.

   2. Lindane (used in shampoos and treatment of head lice in children) appears in milk, but no reports of adverse effects on breastfeeding infants have been reported.

   3. Heptachlor and chlordane are used for control of the cotton boll weevil; levels can be measured in milk but no adverse effects in breastfed infants have been reported (Berlin & Kacew, 1997).

E. Organophosphorous insecticides.

   1. Chlorpyrifos and malathion have both been identified in breast milk.

   2. Toxicity is theoretically possible in severe exposure conditions.

F. Solvents and solvent abuse.

   1. Organic solvents are aromatic compounds that are present in paint, glue, resins, dyes, stain removers, polishes, paint thinner, gasoline, and aerosol propellants.

   2. Benzene and butane are widespread, but most of the solvent present in frequently abused substances is toluene.

3. Heavy exposure to the dry cleaning solvent perchloroethylene has been associated with jaundice in the breastfed infant (Schreiber, 1997).

4. Mothers can be exposed in occupational settings (shoe repair, furniture refinishers, printing shops, etc.).

5. Inhaled volatile organic chemicals can be deposited into adipose tissue and occur in breast milk.

6. Exposure to organic solvents during pregnancy has the potential to result in toxemia and anemia in the mother.

7. Organic solvents have a high affinity for lipid-rich tissues, including the brain and central nervous system.

8. Deliberate inhalation of organic solvents is a popular form of drug abuse.

9. They are properly classified as anesthetics and typically produce a short period of stimulation before central nervous system depression.

10. When deliberately concentrated and inhaled, these highly volatile compounds are rapidly absorbed in the lungs and lead to a rapid brief "high."

11. Toluene might not be detected on routine drug screens.

12. The release of organic solvents from breast milk fat needs to be considered among solvent abusers in light of what is known about adverse effects to the fetus during pregnancy.

G. Heavy metals.

1. Little information is available concerning the effects in babies of heavy metal exposure through human milk.

2. Heavy metal exposure is related to water supplies, ingestion of cow's milk, intake of infant formula, consuming certain foods, etc.

3. Breastfed infants are exposed to lower amounts of heavy metals because formula is often mixed with water that can contain the heavy metal; boiling contaminated water concentrates the heavy metal.

4. Lead is still present in the environment despite the lowered lead levels resulting from the elimination of leaded gasoline, lead solder from cans, and lead in paint.

5. Lead intake still arises from lead water pipes or lead solder, leaded paint chips in older housing, and lead in the soil.

6. Less lead passes into human milk than across the placenta.

7. Human milk levels are one-tenth to one-fifth of maternal levels.

8. Formula-fed infants have higher lead levels than breastfed babies.

9. Breastfeeding is not contraindicated unless the maternal lead level exceeds 40 micrograms/deciliter (Lawrence & Lawrence, 2005).

10. Cadmium exposure through human milk has not been clearly reported; the major route of cadmium intake is through cigarette smoke.

11. Maternal malnutrition in cadmium-exposed, lactating women could increase toxicity in the breastfeeding baby.

12. Mercury levels in breast milk are usually very low.

13. Exposure of the general public is usually from industrial sources or from seafood sources; rare environmental disasters have contributed mercury to the general environment.

14. Only if maternal serum levels of mercury were extremely high would the milk need to be tested.

15. Any woman who has been exposed should be evaluated by her physician.

16. Heavy metals are rarely a contraindication to breastfeeding and then only under extreme exposure circumstances (Lawrence & Lawrence, 2005).

H. Recreational and illegal drugs (Nice et al., 2004a; Nice et al., 2004b; Nice et al., 2004c).

1. Generally, recreational and illegal drugs are contraindicated for breastfeeding mothers; however, there is not universal agreement on some drugs.
   a. Typically contraindicated are amphetamines (misuse and/or abuse), cocaine, heroin, and phencyclidine.
   b. Cocaine may produce tachycardia, tachypnea, hypertension, irritability, and tremulousness in breastfed infants.
   c. Heroin may cause dependence and withdrawal symptoms in nurslings.
   d. Phencyclidine may cause hallucinogenic effects in infants.
   e. Reports disagree about the effects of marijuana and nicotine (smoking).
   f. Tetrahydrocannabinol from smoking marijuana is concentrated in human milk; long-term effects on nursing babies are not yet known.
   g. Tobacco smoking is not a contraindication to breastfeeding.
   h. Smoking can decrease milk volume and fat content as well as depress the milk ejection reflex immediately prior to breastfeeding (Hopkinson et al., 1992; Vio, Salazar, & Infante, 1991).
   i. If a woman smokes, her baby is at risk for respiratory infection; however, the risk of respiratory infection in breastfed babies in smoking environments is equivalent to that of breastfed babies in nonsmoking environments if the baby is breastfed at least 6 months (Nafstad et al., 1996). It remains more advantageous to infants to be breastfed in the presence of a smoking mother who is unable or unwilling to quit.
   j. Nicotine absorbed from milk is less than 5% of the average daily dose of the adult.
   k. Other contaminants from tobacco smoking are also present in human milk.
   l. Nicotine patches as an alternative to smoking are an acceptable alternative for smoking mothers who are breastfeeding.
   m. The risk of sudden infant death syndrome (SIDS) is significantly higher in infants who are formula-fed and whose mothers smoke; breastfeeding is protective against SIDS when mothers smoke.

n. Approximately two servings of caffeine-containing products per day is a reasonable intake for nursing mothers.

o. Decrease or eliminate caffeine in diet if breastfed infant exhibits hyper-excitability or irritability.

p. Adult metabolism of alcohol is approximately 1 oz in three hours. With moderate alcohol ingestion, mothers can breastfeed as soon as they feel that the effects of the alcohol have worn off (Hale, 2006).

   i. Amount of alcohol ingested in a specified period of time as well as the weight of the mother affects how quickly alcohol exits from human milk (Ho et al., 2001).

   ii. Alcohol has been noted to adversely affect milk production (Mennella, 2001a) and diminish lactational performance (Giglia & Binns, 2006).

   iii. The rate of milk consumption by the infant during the 4 hours immediately after alcohol ingestion has been shown to be reduced (Mennella, 2001b). The alcohol equivalent of one can of beer has been shown to reduce breast milk production by 23% when the mean concentration of alcohol in breast milk was 320 mg/L (Mennella & Beauchamp, 1991).

q. Intoxicated and/or chronic alcoholics should not breastfeed.

I. Silicone breast implants (Levine, 1997).

1. Silicone is the second most abundant element in the Earth's crust.

2. Certain foods and beverages contain significant levels of silicon (vegetables, rice, grains, and beer).

   a. Silicon is also found in large amounts in simethicone preparations for infant colic, with no identifiable problems related to the silicone content.

   b. Artificial nipples and pacifiers, some nipple shields, and some breast pump parts contain silicone.

3. Silicone is a synthetic compound that is a polymer of 40% silicon by weight; it is used in items such as prostheses, medical devices, and pharmaceutical products.

4. Silicone breast implants were widely used until their restriction in 1992 by the U.S. Food and Drug Administration (FDA) to be available only through clinical trials; concerns arose regarding silicone gel leakage and connective tissue disease in some women who have implants.

   a. In certain situations, women were able to still obtain these implants if they agreed to enroll in a clinical trial and be followed for a period of five to ten years.

   b. The FDA has recently approved silicone breast implants for use again.

5. Suggestions that there was an association between the silicone implants and an esophageal disease in breastfed infants have been seriously questioned because of problematic methodology and involvement with the plaintiffs in a lawsuit against the implant maker (Levine & Ilowite, 1999).

6. Studies of silicon levels in the milk of mothers with and without implants show no significant differences between the two groups (Semple et al., 1998).
    a. Human milk silicon levels of mothers who do not have silicone implants: 51.05 ng/mL.
    b. Human milk silicon levels of mothers who have silicone implants: 55.45 ng/mL.
    c. Cow's milk silicon levels: 708.94 ng/mL (range 666.5–778.3 ng/mL).
    d. Mean silicon level in 26 brands of infant formula; mean 4402.5 ng/mL (range 746.0–13,811.0 ng/mL).
7. Biologic effects of circulating silicone remain unknown, and silicone implants do not present a contraindication to breastfeeding.
J. Primary environmental contaminants are listed in Table 22-1.

Table 22-1   Summary of Medical Contraindications to Breastfeeding in the United States*

Problem	Okay to Breastfeed in the U.S.?	Conditions
Infectious Diseases		
Acute infectious disease	Yes	Respiratory, reproductive, gastrointestinal infections
HIV	No	HIV-positive
Hepatitis		
Hepatitis A	Yes	As soon as the mother receives gamma globulin
Hepatitis B	Yes	After infant receives HBIG, first dose of hepatitis B vaccine should be given before hospital discharge
Hepatitis C	Yes	If no co-infections (e.g., HIV)
Venereal warts	Yes	
Herpes viruses		
Cytomegalovirus	Yes	
Herpes simplex	Yes	Except if lesion on breast
Varicella-zoster (Chickenpox)	Yes	As soon as mother becomes noninfectious
Epstein-Barr	Yes	

continues

Table 22-1   Summary of Medical Contraindications to Breastfeeding in the United States* (continued)

Problem	Okay to Breastfeed in the U.S.?	Conditions
Toxoplasmosis	Yes	
Mastitis	Yes	
Lyme disease treatment	Yes	As soon as mother initiates
HTLV-1	No	
Medication/Prescription Drugs and Street Drugs		
Antimetabolites	No	
Radiopharmaceuticals		
Diagnostic dose	Yes	After radioactive compound has cleared mother's plasma
Therapeutic dose	No	
Drugs of abuse	No	Exceptions: cigarettes, alcohol
Other medications	Yes	Drug-by-drug assessment
Environmental Contaminants		
Herbicides	Usually	Exposure unlikely (except workers heavily exposed to dioxins)
Pesticides		
DDT, DDE	Usually	Exposure unlikely
PCBs, PBBs	Usually	Levels in milk very low
Cyclodiene pesticides	Usually	Exposure unlikely
Heavy metals		
Lead	Yes	Unless maternal level is > 40 mg/dL
Mercury	Yes	Unless mother is symptomatic and levels are measurable in breast milk
Cadmium	Usually	Exposure unlikely
Radionuclides	Yes	Risk is greater to bottle-fed infants

Note: This table provides a brief summary. Each situation must be decided individually. Contraindications are rare in the United States.

Source: Lawrence RA. A review of the medical benefits and contraindications to breastfeeding in the United States. *Maternal and Child Health Technical Information Bulletin.* Arlington, VA: National Center for Education in Maternal and Child Health; 1997.

References

Berlin CM, Kacew S. Environmental chemicals in human milk. Chapt 4. In: Kacew S, Lambert GH, eds. *Environmental Toxicology and Pharmacology of Human Development*. Washington, DC: Taylor and Francis; 1997.

Dekoning EP, Karmaus W. PCB exposure in-utero and breast milk: a review. *J Expo Anal Environ Epidemiol*. 2000;10:285–293.

Environmental Protection Agency. Exposure and human health reassessment of 2,3,4,8-tetrachlorodibenzo-p-dioxin (TCDD) and related compounds. Available at: http://www.epa.gov/ncea/dioxin.htm. Accessed December 29, 2006.

Eskenazi B, Marks AR, Bradman A, et al. In utero exposure to dichlorodiphenyltrichloroethane (DDT) and dichorodiphenyldichloroetheylene (DDE) and neurodevelopment among young Mexican-American children. *Pediatrics*. 2006;118:233–241.

Giglia R, Binns C. Alcohol and lactation: a systematic review. *Nutrition & Dietetics*. 2006;63:103–116.

Hale TW. *Medications and Mothers' Milk*. Amarillo, TX: Hale Publishing; 2006.

Ho E, Collantes A, Kapur BM, et al. Alcohol and breastfeeding: calculation of time to zero level in milk. *Biol Neoante*. 2001;80:219–222.

Hopkinson JM, Schanler RJ, Fraley JK, Garza C. Milk production by mothers of premature infants: influence of cigarette smoking. *Pediatr*. 1992;90:934–938.

Jacobson JL, Jacobson SW. Association of prenatal exposure of environmental contaminant with intellectual function in childhood. *J Toxicol Clin Toxicol*. 2002;40:467–475.

Jensen AA, Slorach SA, eds. *Chemical Contaminants in Human Milk*. Boca Raton, FL: CRC Press; 1991.

Kirk AB, Martinelango PK, Tian K, et al. Perchlorate and iodide in dairy and breast milk. *Environ Sci Technol*. 2005;39:2011–2017.

LaKind JS, Brent RL, Dourson ML, et al. Human milk biomonitoring data: interpretation and risk assessment issues. *J Toxicol Environ Health A*. 2005;68:1713–1769.

Lawrence RA. A review of the medical benefits and contraindications to breastfeeding in the United States. *Maternal and Child Health Technical Information Bulletin*. Arlington, VA: National Center for Education in Maternal and Child Health; 1997.

Lawrence RA, Lawrence RM. *Breastfeeding: A Guide for the Medical Profession*. Philadelphia: Elsevier Mosby, 2005.

Levine JJ. Breast silicone implants and pediatric considerations. Chapt 7. In: Kacew S, Lambert GH, eds. *Environmental Toxicology and Pharmacology of Human Development*. Washington, DC: Taylor and Francis; 1997.

Levine JJ, Ilowite NT. Sclerodermalike esophageal disease in children breastfed by mothers with silicone breast implants. *JAMA*. 1999;271:213–216.

Mennella J. Alcohol's effect on lactation. *Alcohol Res Health*. 2001a;25:230–234.

Mennella JA. Regulation of milk intake after exposure to alcohol in mothers' milk. *Alcohol Clin Exp Res.* 2001b;25:590–593.

Mennella JA, Beauchamp GK. The transfer of alcohol to human milk. Effects on flavor and the infant's behavior. *N Engl J Med.* 1991;325:981–985.

Nafstad P, Jaakkola JJ, Hagen JA, et al. Breastfeeding, maternal smoking and lower respiratory tract infections. *Eur Respir J.* 1996;9:2623–2629.

National Academies of Science (NAS). Health risks from dioxin and related compounds. Evaluation of the EPA Reassessment. Available at: http://www.ejnet.org/dioxin/nas2006.pdf. Accessed December 29, 2006.

Nice FJ, DeEugenio D, DiMino TA, et al. Medications and Breast-Feeding: A Guide for Pharmacists, Pharmacy Technicians, and Other Healthcare Professionals, Part I. *J Pharm Tech.* 2004a;20:17–27.

Nice FJ, DeEugenio D, DiMino TA, et al. Medications and Breast-Feeding: A Guide for Pharmacists, Pharmacy Technicians, and Other Healthcare Professionals, Part II. *J Pharm Tech.* 2004b;20:85–95.

Nice FJ, DeEugenio D, DiMino TA, et al. Medications and Breast-Feeding: A Guide for Pharmacists, Pharmacy Technicians, and Other Healthcare Professionals, Part III. *J Pharm Tech.* 2004c;20:165–177.

Rogan W, Blanto P, Portier C, Stallard E. 1991. Should the presence of carcinogens in breast milk discourage breastfeeding? *Regul Toxicol Pharmacol.* 1991;13:228–240.

Rogan WJ, Ragan NB. Chemical contaminants, pharmacokinetics, and the lactating mother. *Environ Health Perspect.* 1994;102(suppl II):89–95.

Schreiber JS. Transport of organic chemicals to breast milk: Tetrachloroethene case study. Chapt 5. In: Kacew S, Lambert GH, eds. *Environmental Toxicology and Pharmacology of Human Development.* Washington, DC: Taylor and Francis; 1997.

Semple JL, Lugowski SJ, Baines CJ, et al. 1998. Breast milk contamination and silicone implants: Preliminary results using silicon as a proxy measurement for silicone. *Plast Reconstr Surg.* 1998;102:528–533.

Vio F, Salazar G, Infante C. Smoking during pregnancy and lactation and its effects on breast milk volume. *Am J Clin Nutr.* 1991;54:1011–1016.

Breastfeeding Management

Breastfeeding Technique

Assessment of Infant Oral Anatomy

Barbara Wilson-Clay, BSEd, IBCLC

OBJECTIVES

- Identify key aspects of assessment of infant oro-facial structures and oral motor functions.
- Identify abnormal infant oral anatomy and discuss its effect upon breastfeeding.
- List the oral feeding reflexes and describe their abnormal presentations.
- Discuss coordination of the suck-swallow-breathe (SSB) triad and its importance in breastfeeding.
- Discuss the issue of the "fit" between the infant's oral anatomy and the mother's breast.

Introduction

This chapter provides an overview of the structures and function of the face and mouth that influence feeding behavior and later dentition, speech, and appearance. An understanding of normal appearance and function clarifies abnormal presentations (Bosma, 1977; Merkel-Piccini & Rosenfeld-Johnson, 2003; Ogg, 1975).

I. Overview

A. Oral assessment of the breastfeeding infant.

1. Observation of the infant's oro-facial anatomy.
   a. Lips, cheeks, jaws, tongue, palate, and nasal passages.

2. Identification of abnormal infant oral anatomy with knowledge of how this may contribute to dysfunctional feeding behavior.

3. Observation of infant feeding reflexes and their abnormal presentations.
   a. Review the rooting reflex, the sucking reflex (including absent suck, weak suck, and uncoordinated suck), the swallowing reflex, the gag reflex, and the cough reflex.

b. Describe the nutritive suck (NS) and non-nutritive suck (NNS).

4. Observation of rhythmicity and effectiveness of feeding (coordination of the SSB triad).

5. Observation of the "fit" between the infant's mouth and the mother's nipple.

B. Lactation counseling for the parents of an infant who breastfeeds poorly.

1. Awareness of the connection between feeding success and maternal self-esteem.

2. Identification of safe methods of alternate feeding to protect infant intake.

3. Protection of the maternal milk supply.

4. Protection of "breast focus" (that is, the development of an intervention with eventual full breastfeeding as the goal).

II. Anatomy of the Infant's Oral Cavity

A. Importance.

1. Feeding, respiration, dentition, and speech are influenced by the anatomy of the mouth.

2. The tone and functioning of the muscles of the face, neck, and trunk affect feeding.

3. Some aspects of oral anatomy change with maturation and growth, or may be surgically corrected (Bosma, 1977).

4. Sometimes oro-facial structures change as the infant recovers from minor injury (for example, bruising during birth, or trauma related to instrument delivery (Caughey et al., 2005).

5. Oro-facial structure and function can be impaired by injury (Smith, Crumley, & Harker, 1981), congenital malformation, neurological deficits, prematurity, or illness.
   a. Impairment may negatively impact breastfeeding.
   b. The presence of these factors in a case signal the need for more focused assessment and may identify a dyad in need of greater lactation support (Ogg, 1975; Wolf & Glass, 1992).

B. Lips (Morris, 1977; Ogg, 1975; Wolf & Glass, 1992).

1. The infant uses the lips to draw in the nipple and stabilize it in the mouth.

2. Lips are normally intact, with no evidence of a cleft, and appear mobile, well defined, and expressive.

3. The lips flange and seal smoothly around the breast during breastfeeding.

4. Abnormal presentations.
   a. Weak lip tone.
      i. *Hypotonic* lip tone results in weak ability of the lips to seal around the breast. This can impair the amount of suction that the infant is able to

generate. Because the infant keeps losing the seal and having to re-form it, the work of feeding increases. Feeding becomes inefficient and tiring, resulting in reduced infant intake.

   ii. Weak lip seal may result in a loss of liquid during feeding (milk spilling).

   iii. Weak lip tone reflects poor motor/muscular control of the lips, and may be revealed as intermittent breaks in suction (smacking sounds).

   iv. Low muscle tone or weakness (owing to prematurity, muscular weakness, or illness) creates stamina deficits that impair the baby's ability to maintain lip seal. Ideally, an entire feeding is observed to detect stamina-related problems that may only occur late in the feeding.

b. Abnormal tongue movements.

   i. Abnormal tongue movements can cause breaks in the lip seal.

   ii. This problem is related to the tongue but affects the lips.

c. Abnormally wide jaw excursions.

   i. Poorly graded jaw excursions also can cause breaks in the lip seal.

d. Tight *labial frenum* (a growth of the tissue that attaches the upper lip to the upper gum).

   i. Classified (similarly to tongue-tie) as a minor mid-line congenital defect, a tight labial frenum may affect dentition.

   ii. The forward attached frenum creates a gap between the front teeth.

   iii. If the upper labial frenum is non-elastic, it may contribute to lip retraction during breastfeeding. The retracted lips may cause friction trauma that damages the mother's nipples. The inability to normally flange the upper lip was reported in one case as a factor contributing to breastfeeding difficulty (Wiessinger & Miller, 1995).

e. Excessive lip tone.

   i. *Hypertonic* lip tone or reliance on increased lip activity to hold the breast in the mouth may reflect neurological abnormality, or injury of the tongue jaws, or facial nerves (Smith et al., 1981).

   ii. If tongue or jaw function is impaired, or facial nerves are injured, the baby may compensate by using increased lip activity to hold onto the breast.

f. "Purse string lips" inhibit the inability of the infant to open the lips to allow objects into the mouth.

   i. They are also revealed as a pulling up at the corners of the mouth and increased tension around the lips.

   ii. Hypertonic lips may be a marker for neurologic involvement (Wilson-Clay & Hoover, 2005).

g. Cleft lip.

   i. A relatively common congenital mid-line defect generally repaired in the early postpartum.

ii. While disfiguring, cleft lip does not significantly interfere with successful breastfeeding (Garcez & Giugliani, 2005).

5. Assessment of the lips.
   a. Visually assess a feeding (ideally an entire feeding) to observe whether the infant can seal the lips smoothly around the breast and maintain the seal during feeding without evidence of early fatigue.
   b. Observe the shape of the lips. A bow-shaped upper lip with a well-defined philtrum generally indicates normal lip tone.
   c. Observe for the presence of a tight upper labial frenum.
   d. Listen for breaks in the seal while the infant feeds.
   e. Observe for lip retraction and lip tremors.
   f. Observe for leaking milk (during both breast and alternative feeding).
   g. Apply gentle digital pressure against the lips; some resistance to this pressure should be felt.
   h. Note uncommon events such as drooling.
      i. In infants younger than 3 months of age, drooling is associated with weak control of swallowing (even of the infant's own saliva) or may reveal pharyngeal or esophageal obstruction (Riordan, 2005).
   i. Identify the presence of sucking blisters.
      i. Sucking blisters are caused by friction abrasion resulting from retracted lips during breastfeeding (or by a tight upper labial frenum that restricts upper lip flanging).

6. Methods of assisting when the feeding problem results from structural abnormalities or abnormal tone of the lips.
   a. Use firm pressure stimulus (tapping, stretching) of the lips prior to feeding to improve tone and strengthen lip seal (Alper & Manno, 1996).
   b. Use a clean finger or a round, somewhat firm pacifier to play tug-of-war with the baby. This exercises the ability of the lips to grip objects.
   c. Mimic "open wide" mouth positions to encourage the infant to imitate lip movement.
   d. Observe the infant for stress cues when engaging in these activities and discontinue when the infant becomes fatigued.
   e. Teach the mother to use a finger or breast tissue to seal a cleft of the lip.
   f. Refer to speech and language pathologists or occupational therapists for assessment and remediation.
      i. Dialogue with cleft lip/palate teams to facilitate support for human milk feeds, including the use of special palatal obturators that increase feeding efficiency in infants with cleft palate (Turner et al., 2001).
   g. Share research that documents the fact that postoperative breastfeeding after cleft lip repair is safe and results in better weight gain than does bottle-feeding (Darzi, Chowdri, & Bhat, 1996; Weatherly-White et al., 1987).

h. Demonstrate to the mother how to use her finger tip to gently pull back on the skin above the baby's upper lip to correct lip retraction. The mother can manually flange the lip as often as needed, especially if lip retraction causes nipple pain. Refer to appropriate specialists for evaluation in the (rare) event that a tight labial frenum appears to require release.

i. Reassure parents that lip tone typically improves as the infant matures and grows. This tends to be the case even if the underlying cause is an enduring neurologic disorder or is related to a structural abnormality.

C. Cheeks (Wolf & Glass, 1992).

1. Facial tone influences oral function.

   a. Subcutaneous fat deposits in the cheeks help provide structural support for infant oral and pharyngeal activity.

   b. Fat pads give the baby a "puffy cheek" appearance and should be visible for six to eight months (Wolf & Glass, 1992).

2. Poorly developed fat pads (owing to prematurity or low birth weight) and thin cheeks affect facial tone.

   a. Low or weak tone may cause the infant to experience difficulty in creating and sustaining adequate levels of suction.

3. Abnormal presentation of the cheeks.

   a. Weak cheek tone/thin cheeks.

      i. Facial hypotonia (low tone) and weakness contribute to poor cheek stability.

      ii. The cheeks influence lip seal; low facial tone makes it harder for the infant to use the lips normally.

      iii. Thin cheeks mean that the infant's intraoral space is larger than would normally be the case. The infant must therefore create a larger vacuum to generate and sustain suction, so the work of feeding is increased. The infant may fatigue early before finishing feedings.

4. Assessment of the cheeks (Wilson-Clay & Hoover, 2005; Wolf & Glass, 1992).

   a. Digitally assess the subcutaneous fat deposits in the cheeks by placing a gloved finger inside the infant's mouth and a thumb on the outside of the cheek to sense the thickness of the fat pads.

      i. Performing this examination on a number of babies gives the examiner the awareness that dimensions of fat pads vary, but in babies with thin cheeks, the fingers almost touch.

   b. Observe the shape of the cheeks at rest and during feeding.

      i. Identify deep creases under the infant's eyes as a marker for thin cheeks.

   c. If the cheeks are weak, thin, or unstable, they will collapse while sucking. Identify cheek collapsing (revealed by *dimpling*).

    d. Observe the duration of feeds for infant fatigue.

       i. Early discontinuation of feeds owing to fatigue is a risk factor for poor infant intake and poor stimulation of milk production. (Test weights are confirmatory; Sachs & Oddie, 2002.)

  5. Methods of assisting when feeding problems or slow growth result from thin cheeks or low facial muscle tone (Wilson-Clay & Hoover, 2005).

    a. Use external counter-pressure applied to the cheeks during feeding (the so-called *Dancer's hand technique*) to improve cheek stability (Danner, 1992; Wilson-Clay & Hoover, 2005:175, Figs. 357–358).

    b. Supplement (ideally with own mother's milk) to improve infant growth. As the fat pads develop in the cheeks, facial stability will improve, contributing to improvement in breastfeeding ability.

D. Jaws (Palmer, 1993b; Wilson-Clay & Hoover, 2005; Wolf & Glass, 1992).

  1. The jaws provide stability for the movements of the tongue, lips, and cheeks.

  2. *Mandibular retrognathia* (receding lower jaw) is characteristic in infants. Dramatic forward growth usually occurs during the first four months postpartum (Ranley, 1998).

  3. Normal jaw movements are neither too wide nor too narrow during feeding; opening and closing motions are smooth, graded, and regular.

  4. Preterm infants often have jaw instability owing to immature muscles and low muscle tone (which is characteristic for preterm babies; Palmer, 1993b).

  5. Abnormal presentations of the jaw.

    a. *Micrognathia*, an abnormally receding chin that can be familial, associated with chromosomal disorders, or can result from intrauterine positioning that prevents the jaw from growing forward (as in certain breech presentations).

       i. Severe micrognathia positions the tongue posteriorly, where it may obstruct the airway as in Pierre Robin syndrome (Bull & Givan, 1990).

      ii. A receding jaw may contribute to sore nipples unless the infant's head is tipped back in a slightly extended position to bring the chin closer to the breast.

     iii. Jaw asymmetry contributes to poor jaw function and unstable feeding, including inability to breastfeed. It can be caused by birth injury, asymmetrical muscle tone (i.e., torticollis), injury, paralysis, breech position, or structural deformity (Wall & Glass, 2006). Note how the face of the infant in Figure 23-1 droops to the right. Her jaw asymmetry and low facial tone contributed to inefficient feeding and failure to thrive.

    b. Abnormally wide jaw excursions.

       i. Poor grading of the jaw movements can cause breaks in the seal formed at breast, resulting in loss of suction and increased work of feeding. Intake may be decreased.

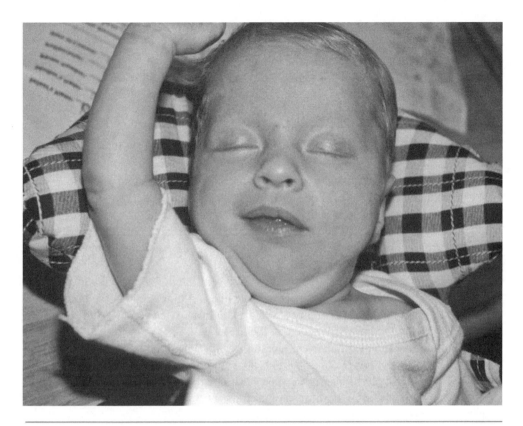

Figure 23-1   Facial asymmetry and low facial tone. *Source:* Reproduced with permission from Barbara Wilson-Clay.

     c. Jaw clenching.
       i. Sometimes infants clench their jaws as a strategy to manage rapid milk flow. If clenching to manage milk flow is ruled out, jaw clench or thrusting generally reflects hypertonia. It also may be a *compensatory action* resulting from weakness in another area (for example, poor tongue function or low lip tone that forces the baby to overuse the jaws to hold in the nipple). Clenching contributes to sore nipples/breasts.
   6. Assessment of the jaws.
     a. Observe for asymmetry.
     b. Identify micrognathia.
     c. Observe breastfeeding to identify jaw grading, clenching, or tremors.

     d. Insert a gloved (pinkie, or "little") finger in the corner of the infant's mouth between the gum pads.

         i. Count the number of reflexive bites (chews) elicited.

         ii. The infant should respond with approximately 10 little chews on each side.

         iii. Observe for difficulty producing these reflexive bites or for infant stress cues during this assessment.

         iv. Weakness of the jaw is revealed by inability to perform the activity (Palmer, 1993b).

  7. Methods of assisting when the feeding problem relates to abnormalities, weakness, or injury involving the jaws.

     a. Provide external jaw support with a finger placed under the *bony part* of the lower jaw to control and stabilize the distance of jaw excursions.

     b. Hip flexion and stabilization of the infant's trunk facilitates stable feeding (Redstone & West, 2004).

     c. Exercise the jaws (using the same assessment method described above to elicit an increased number of reflexive bites). Avoid stressing the infant.

     d. Position the infant carefully and maintain head extension as a strategy for bringing the lower jaw closer to the breast.

     e. Refer the infant for physical therapy, occupational therapy, or infant massage if issues relating to abnormal muscular tension impinge upon jaw activity.

     f. Work carefully to identify feeding positions that emphasize postural stability. Side-lying feeding positions are useful.

E. Tongue (Palmer, 1993; Wolf & Glass, 1992).

  1. Normally soft, thin, and mobile, with a rounded tip and good tone. The infant uses the tongue with the lips to draw in the nipple.

  2. Assists the lips in helping to seal the oral cavity. When the infant cheek is pulled back, a small section of cupped tongue is visible at the corners of the mouth during breastfeeding.

  3. In relation to the hard tissue of the mouth, the rest position of the tongue shapes the structures around it. Therefore, the tongue affects dentition and speech (Merkel-Piccini & Rosenfeld-Johnson, 2003).

  4. Ultrasound studies suggest that suction is the primary mechanism of milk extraction during breastfeeding. Mobility of the tongue is critical to creating adequate levels of suction (Ramsay et al., 2004a).

  5. The tongue must be able to lift freely and thin the mother's nipple against the hard palate so that with each subsequent drop of the tongue, there is an adequate enlargement of the oral cavity to create negative pressure (Ramsay et al., 2004b).

  6. The tongue forms a central groove that provides a channel that organizes the bolus of milk for safe swallowing.

7. The tongue tip extends over the lower gum ridge, providing a degree of padding during breastfeeding that helps protect the mother's nipples.

8. When the tongue moves improperly, the baby cannot suck, swallow, or breathe efficiently. The work of feeding increases in such instances, putting the baby at risk for early discontinuation of feeds and limited intake; there is also a risk of poor breast emptying.

9. Limitations in the mobility or strength of the tongue require the infant to use compensatory activities to feed. Compensations may involve increased jaw activity (clenching) or lip retraction. The mother may describe the suck as "strong" when actually it is weak. *It is the baby's compensations that often damage the nipples.*

10. Abnormal presentations of the tongue.
    a. *Ankyloglossia* (tongue-tie).
        i. A congenital mid-line anomaly in which the bottom of the tongue is attached to the floor of the mouth by a membrane (the *lingual frenulum*) that limits the range of motion of the tongue (Fernando, 1998; Lalakea & Messner, 2003; Messner et al., 2000).
        ii. Typically there is a "heart shaped" appearance to the tongue tip; however, one variety of tongue-tie consists of a non-elastic posterior adhesion of the tongue to the floor of the mouth. This is more difficult to visualize (Coryllos, Genna, & Salloum, 2004).
        iii. Incidence of ankyloglossia ranges between 2% and 5% of infants, occurring somewhat more commonly in males. Typically it is an isolated anatomic variation and may run in families. It appears with increased frequency in association with various congenital syndromes (Flinck et al., 1994; Lalakea & Messner, 2003; Ricke et al., 2005).
        iv. Some infants are able to breastfeed without difficulty (Messner et al., 2000).
        v. May affect infant intake, maternal comfort during breastfeeding, and may impair effective milk removal with resultant ill effect on milk production (Ballard, Auer, & Khoury, 2004; Neifert, 1999; Powers, 1999).
        vi. Either frenotomy (simple release achieved by clipping the lingual frenulum) or frenulectomy/frenuloplasty (resectioning of the tongue) is curative and changes the sucking dynamics of the breastfeeding infant (Ramsay et al., 2004b).
            (1) Frenotomy is often performed without anesthesia as an office procedure and has a high satisfaction rate and few complications (Amir, James, & Beatty, 2005).
            (2) Frenulectomy and frenuloplasty are more involved surgical procedures with a longer recovery period, but appear to be successful in remediating significant ankyloglossia (Ballard et al., 2004).

  b. A bunched or retracted tongue.

   i. May be caused by abnormally high muscle tone or by ankyloglossia.

  c. Tongue protrusion.

   i. May result from low muscle tone (as in Down syndrome) and contribute to poor coordination of sucking and swallowing.

  d. Tongue-tip elevation.

   i. Tongue tip elevation can make insertion of the nipple frustrating and difficult.

   ii. Touch to the tongue tip results in reflexive tongue extrusion, causing the baby to keep pushing objects out of the mouth.

  e. Tongue asymmetry.

   i. Tongue asymmetry may result from injury (such as forceps trauma that damages the nerves controlling the tongue (Smith et al., 1981).

   ii. Also may be associated with syndromic conditions.

11. Assessment of the tongue.

  a. Sometimes poor infant head position during feeding negatively influences tongue position. Correct the feeding position before evaluating the tongue during feeding.

  b. Visual assessment identifies the shape and position of the tongue, and rules out tongue-tie and other abnormal presentations.

  c. Digital exam consists of gentle pressure with a clean, gloved, fingertip to the surface of the tongue at midsection. There should be some resistance and the examiner should sense the tongue pressing up against the finger.

  d. Insertion of a finger should elicit sealing and sucking. The lactation consultant should sense the tongue cupping around the finger. The examiner must be careful not to insert the finger too deeply (to avoid triggering a gag reflex).

  e. While the infant is breastfeeding, gently pull the breast away from the cheek and observe the corners of the lips. The side of the tongue should be visible, helping the lips form the seal that preserves suction.

  f. Listen for breaks in seal (revealed by smacking noises).

   i. A weak tongue may interfere with maintaining a seal at breast.

   ii. A normal infant who is struggling with rapid milk flow may deliberately break the seal at breast (with resultant smacking noises).

   iii. In a compromised infant, such sounds often mean that the jaw has dropped so far that the tongue has lost contact with the breast.

   iv. Too-wide jaw excursions and frequent loss of seal usually result in poor milk transfer.

  g. Observe the ability of the infant to lift the tongue past the midline of the mouth with the mouth open wide.

   i. The tongue should lift to the palate.

      ii. Limited lift reveals ankyloglossia, even without the sign of an obviously forward-placed lingual frenulum (Coryllos et al., 2004).

    h. Observe tongue extension by tapping the tongue tip to elicit tongue protrusion.

      i. Can the infant extend the tongue beyond the gum, and ideally the lower lip line? Inhibition of extension may reveal ankyloglossia.

    i. Can the infant lateralize the tongue?

      i. This is another assessment of mobility.

      ii. The tongue should seek the examiner's finger as it moves from side to side.

      iii. Limited lateralization may reveal ankyloglossia.

12. Methods of assisting when the feeding problem results from dysfunction or anomalies of the tongue.

    a. The same exercises that can be used to strengthen the lips may assist in exercising a weak tongue (such as "tug-of-war" with a finger or pacifier, mimicking tongue extension).

    b. Short, frequent feedings allow the baby recovery time if the tongue gets tired.

    c. Positioning the baby with the head in extension brings the lower jaw close in to the breast.

      i. Reducing the distance a short or restricted tongue must reach (to extend over the lower gum ridge) may help protect the nipples from trauma.

    d. Inform the mother of ways to manage nipple trauma (topical cleansing of open cuts, alternating pumping with breastfeeding, etc.).

    e. Refer infant to the pediatrician, family practice doctor, pediatric ear, nose, and throat (ENT) specialist, or to a pediatric dentist for evaluation for release of tongue-tie.

    f. Occupational therapy or speech and language therapy may facilitate improved function if the tongue is injured, affected by paralysis, recovering from frenuloplasty, or is weak owing to a syndromic condition.

    g. Reassure parents that while some infants will feed well immediately following simple clips of a tongue-tie, other infants may not breastfeed well until the tongue fully heals.

    h. Supplement with pumped milk if needed to stabilize infant growth and protect milk production with pumping as long as necessary.

F. Palates (Cleft Palate Foundation, 2006; Glenny et al., 2004; Goldman, 1993; Gorski et al., 1994; Kogo et al., 1997; Paradise, Elster, & Tan, 1994; Snyder, 1997; Turner et al., 2001; Wilson-Clay & Hoover, 2005; Wolf & Glass, 1992).

1. The shape of the palates can be influenced by hereditary and genetic factors, or result from circumstances that prevent the normal shaping of the hard palate by the tongue during gestation (such as ankyloglossia or by breech position).

    a. Figure 23-2 shows an infant after a simple frenotomy to clip a forward-placed lingual frenulum. However, baby still demonstrates limited ability to lift the tongue to the upper gum ridge (Coryllos et al., 2004).

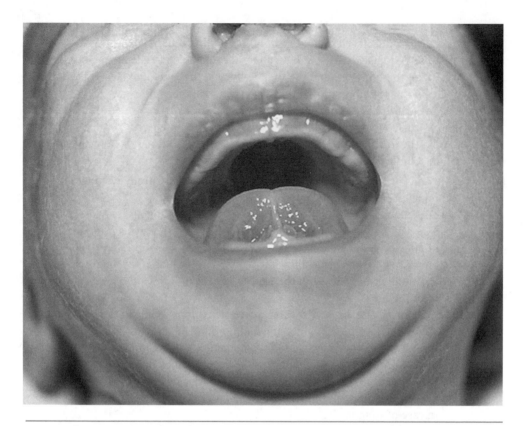

Figure 23-2 Bubble palate (note limited tongue elevation). *Source:* Reproduced with permission from Barbara Wilson-Clay and Kay Hoover. *The Breastfeeding Atlas.* Austin, TX; LactNews Press; 2005.

     b. Note bubble shape of the hard palate that has resulted from ankyloglossia.

2. Hard palate.
    a. The bony hard palate opposes the tongue, helping to compress the nipple and maintain nipple position in the mouth.
    b. It should be intact with no evidence of a cleft.
    c. The slope should be moderate and smooth, and should approximate the shape of the tongue (Merkel-Piccini & Rosenfeld-Johnson, 2003).
    d. Small, round, white cysts (*Epstein's pearls*; Figure 23-3) are often observed along the ridge of the hard palate (also the gums, where they may be identified as teeth). While sometimes also mistaken for oral thrush, these cysts are benign, resolve around two months postpartum, and do not interfere with feeding (Riordan, 2005).

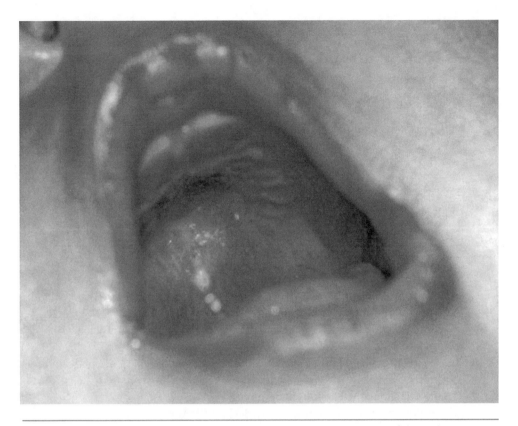

Figure 23-3   Epstein's pearls on the palate (sometimes mistaken for thrush). *Source:* Reproduced with permission from Barbara Wilson-Clay and Kay Hoover. *The Breastfeeding Atlas.* Austin, TX; LactNews Press; 2005.

3. Soft palate.
   a. The soft palate is a muscle that works with the tongue to create a posterior seal of the oral cavity, permitting the creation of suction.
   b. It should be intact and elevate during swallowing.
4. Abnormal presentations of the hard and soft palates.
   a. Abnormalities of the palate make breastfeeding difficult (Lawrence & Lawrence, 2005).
   b. Familial high arched, grooved, or bubble-shaped hard palate makes it difficult for the infant to properly position the nipple and to compress it with the tongue.

    c. Long periods of intubation or syndromic conditions (for example, Down or Turner syndrome) can create grooves in the hard palate. Later, food or other chewed objects may become trapped in the channel or bubble (Rovet, 1995).

5. Cleft palate.

    a. A common congenital mid-line defect with an incidence of one in 600 to 800 births. Clefts are more common in Native Americans, Maoris, and Chinese.

    b. Clefts may be unilateral or bilateral and are classified as *partial* or *incomplete*, or *complete*.

      i. A partial or incomplete cleft is isolated.

      ii. A complete cleft extends from the lip to the soft palate and may also involve the nose.

    c. Regardless of the size, clefts of the hard or soft palates make it difficult or impossible for the infant to fully breastfeed because the baby is unable to seal the oral cavity to generate suction, which negatively affects infant growth and milk production.

    d. Some infants with wide palatal clefts have additional swallowing problems owing to problems with intra-oral muscular movements. There is no palatal back guard for tongue movements (Lawrence & Lawrence, 2005). Palatal obturators are a prosthetic device that can increase feeding efficiency in infants with clefts (Kogo et al., 1997; Turner et al., 2001).

    e. An infant with a cleft may feed constantly, mostly sleeping at breast. Intake must be empirically assessed with test weights on an accurate scale, and growth should be carefully monitored.

    f. Feeding tube devices and specially designed bottles may assist, but considerable experimentation is often needed to find a method of feeding that ensures adequate growth. Feedings are slow and often stressful, owing to aspiration (Glenny et al., 2004).

    g. Submucosal clefts.

      i. Defects of the closure of the shelves of the hard palate are difficult to identify, owing to the presence of a layer of skin that has grown over the cleft.

      ii. Shining a light on the palate reveals a translucent area on the palate that identifies a submucosal cleft (that is, one can see the cleft under the skin).

    h. A family history of cleft lip or cleft lip and palate should cue the lactation consultant to examine the palate more carefully.

6. Weak soft palate.

    a. Because the palate is a muscle, generalized low muscle tone (resulting from prematurity or a syndromic condition) may affect soft palate function.

    b. Poor infant stamina may influence soft palate function. As the infant tires and loses muscle control, the soft palate fails to work with the tongue to effectively seal off the mouth as the baby swallows and breathes.

      c. Adversely affects control of safe swallowing, creating an increased risk of choking known as *fatigue aspiration* (Wolf & Glass, 1992).

  7. Assessment of the hard and soft palates.

      a. Visual assessment of the palates should identify intact structures and the presence of a *uvula*.

      b. *Bifid* (forked) uvula or absent uvula reveal abnormal formation of the soft palate (that is, a cleft of the soft palate).

      c. With a gloved finger, gently slide a fingertip along the hard palate starting just behind the upper gum ridge.

         i. Assess the slope of the hard palate for bony prominences, clefts, or abnormally prominent *rugae* (ridges).

      d. Observe a feeding and elicit information regarding nasal regurgitation. Nasal regurgitation of milk or excessive nasal stuffiness might reveal a weak soft palate seal (or, more rarely, the presence of a submucosal cleft; Morris, 1977).

  8. Methods of assisting when the feeding problem results from abnormalities of the hard and/or soft palates.

      a. Feeding problems related to the abnormal formation of the palates are difficult to correct.

      b. Cleft defects can be corrected surgically at various ages.

      c. Monitor infant intake carefully and supplement with mother's pumped milk or banked milk; the incidence of chronic otitis media (a risk for infants with cleft defects) is reduced when infants are exclusively human-milk fed (Paradise et al., 1994).

      d. Help the mother position the baby for breastfeeding in upright positions such as the seated straddle. Demonstrate chin support to stabilize the latch. Teach breast compression as a method of expressing milk into the baby's mouth (Mohrbacher & Stock, 2003).

      e. Assist the mother in finding a method of alternative feeding that is effective and does not stress the infant (Wilson-Clay, 2005).

      f. Teach the mother to observe for infant stress cues that will help her feed in a manner that protects the baby from developing feeding aversions (Abadie et al., 2001).

      g. Protect the milk supply by establishing an appropriate pumping schedule.

      h. Refer to appropriate specialists, including cleft palate teams.

G. Nasal passages (Alper & Manno, 1996; Bosma, 1977; Wilson-Clay, 2005; Wilson-Clay & Hoover, 2005; Wolf & Glass, 1992).

  1. While infants typically are nose breathers, they can adapt to mouth breathing if the nasal passages are occluded.

  2. If nasal breathing is impaired, the infant will resist feeding, owing to his or her need to protect mouth breathing.

3. Nasal congestion (in the absence of symptoms of respiratory illness) may reveal dried accumulations of milk aspirated during feedings.

4. Nasal stuffiness may be the result of fluid aspirated during reflux episodes.

5. Abnormal presentations of the nasal passages.
   a. Rarely, abnormally small nasal openings are observed.
      i. *Choanal atresia* is a congenital condition in which the openings of one or both of the nasal cavities are partially or completely blocked by a bony or membranous occlusion.
   b. Facial bruising (resulting from birth trauma or instrument-assisted delivery) can create swelling of the nose and impair breathing.

6. Assessing the nasal passages.
   a. The nasal passages should be visually assessed if the infant's breathing sounds congested or if the infant struggles and pulls away gasping while being fed.
   b. Elicit information about birth trauma, instrument-assisted delivery, bruising, nasal regurgitation, etc.

7. Methods to assist an infant with feeding problems related to the nasal passages.
   a. Baby-strength saline nose drops may be useful to help clear the nasal passages. Bulb syringes used to extract nasal debris may increase internal swelling.
   b. Employ external pacing methods during feeding to protect respiratory stability (Wilson-Clay, 2005).
   c. Refer the infant to the primary medical care provider, or pediatric ENT specialist for further assessment if a problem related to the nasal passages interferes with feeding.

III. Infant Feeding Reflexes

A. Rooting reflex (Wolf & Glass, 1992).

1. Helps the baby to locate the nipple.

2. It is stimulated by touch to any part of the head.
   a. Pushing on the head during latch-on can distract the baby from turning toward the nipple.

3. It is present at birth and extinguishes between two and four months of age, although it can persist longer in breastfed infants.

4. An absent or diminished rooting reflex may signal poor tactile receptivity or poor neural integration.

5. If excessive, a hypersensitive (hyper-reactive) rooting reflex can interfere with latching on.

a. Possible management strategies to assist might include decreasing the other stimuli in the environment, avoiding touching the infant's head, feeding when the infant is sleepy and less aware.

B. Sucking reflex (Premji & Paes, 2000; Wolf & Glass, 1992).

1. Observed *in utero* as early as 15 to 18 weeks gestation.

2. Categorized into two modes: NS and NNS (see also Chapter 15, Part IV).
   a. NS can be effective or ineffective.

3. It is stimulated by pressure (and perhaps chemical receptors) along the tongue and stroking near the junctions of the hard and soft palates.

4. Some infants can sustain effective feeding at 34 to 35 weeks gestational age for brief periods of time. However, preterm infants are at risk for fatigue during feeding and for hospital re-admittance secondary to poor feeding (Kramer et al., 2000).

5. Inadequate breast emptying owing to a weakly sucking infant creates a risk of rapid, early down-regulation of milk production (Kent et al., 1999).

6. When a weakly sucking infant is identified, careful infant growth monitoring is required.
   a. The infant may require supplementation (ideally with own mother's pumped hindmilk).
   b. Protect the milk supply with pumping (Alper & Manno, 1996; Hill, Aldag, & Chatterton, 2001; Kavanaugh et al., 1995; Scanlon et al., 2002; Valentine, Hurst, & Schanler, 1994).

7. Absent or diminished sucking might indicate central nervous system (CNS) immaturity, prematurity, delayed maturation, CNS mal-development (various trisomies), prenatal CNS insults (drugs in labor, asphyxia, trauma), or systemic congenital problems (heart disease, sepsis, infant hypothyroidism) (McBride & Danner, 1987).

8. A weak suck might indicate CNS abnormalities associated with hypotonia, medullary lesions, Myasthenia gravis or botulism, or abnormalities of the muscles resulting in weak oral and *buccal* (cheek) musculature (McBride & Danner, 1987).

9. Discoordinated sucking is marked by a mis-timing of normal movements or is marked by interference by hyperactive reflexes.
   a. It can result from asphyxia, perinatal cerebral insults, and CNS mal-development (McBride & Danner, 1987).

10. NS (Alper & Manno, 1996; Palmer, 1993; Wolf & Glass, 1992).
    a. NS is highly organized into a series of sucking bursts and pauses and occurs solely in the presence of oral fluid.

      b. Because breathing must be interspersed with swallowing, the sucking rate is slower during NS than it is during NNS. The breathing rate increases during pauses between sucking bursts (Geddes et al., 2006).

      c. New technologies will hopefully better elucidate the SSB relationships more accurately (Geddes et al., 2006).

      d. It is useful to count sucking bursts.

         i. Infants who are unable to sustain long bursts (taking fewer than 10 SSBs per burst) manifest weak or immature sucking (Palmer & Heyman, 1993).

      e. If short sucking bursts result from prematurity, maturation will normalize the stability of sucking (Palmer & Heyman, 1993).

      f. Other sucking problems (see above) may prove enduring and more difficult to resolve.

    11. NNS (Alper & Manno, 1996; Palmer & Heyman, 1993).

      a. NNS is not the same thing as *ineffective suck*; it is simply sucking that occurs for reasons other than feeding, that is, state regulation, management of infant pain, etc. (Gray et al., 2002; Premji & Paes, 2000).

      b. Characterized by fast, shallow sucks, with more sucking than swallowing.

      c. Swallowing is infrequent and consists primarily of swallowing saliva or pooled milk.

      d. There is a 6 to 8 suck:1 swallow ratio in NNS.

C. Swallowing reflex (Wolf & Glass, 1992).

    1. Develops early in fetal life (12–14 weeks gestation).

    2. Triggered by the delivery of a bolus of fluid to the back of the tongue.

    3. Also triggered by chemical receptors in the tongue.

    4. Abnormalities of the tongue and palate can create problems with swallowing that may lead to a risk of aspiration.

    5. Swallowing dysfunction may result in poor weight gain and aversive feeding responses.

    6. *Reflux* is classified as a swallowing disorder.

      a. While most infants experience some degree of reflux, serious cases can create significant problems for the infant.

      b. Because the infant begins to associate eating with pain, feeding aversion results.

      c. The baby with severe reflux may self-limit intake, contributing to a diagnosis of failure to thrive.

      d. Respiratory illness may also be present, owing to aspiration of ascending fluids that cause inflammation of the airways and nasal passages.

D. Gag reflex (Morris, 1977).

    1. The function of the gag reflex is to protect the airway from large objects.

    a. The gag is generally triggered by pressure to the rear of the tongue, but may be stimulated at a more shallow depth in the mouths of young infants (Wolf & Glass, 1992).

2. The gag reflex may be hyperactive.

3. Constant activation by long nipples or invasive procedures may create feeding aversion.

4. Observe the infant during latch for gagging.

5. Gentle digital exam with a gloved finger can identify a gag reflex that is triggered by shallow oral penetration.

    a. Infants with easily triggered gag reflexes may simply be immature, or they may require occupational therapy to facilitate acceptance of objects in the mouth.

E. Cough reflex (Wolf & Glass, 1992).

1. Protects against the aspiration of fluids into the airways.

2. May be immature in preterm and even in some term newborns.

3. The immature response to fluids in the airways is *apnea* (breath-holding) followed by attempts to swallow with a delayed cough.

4. *Silent aspiration*, which is prolonged apnea and aspiration of fluids without the signal of coughing, can occur in immature infants (Law-Morstatt et al., 2003).

5. Coughing *during* feeding is generally in response to aspiration of descending fluids.

6. Coughing *between* feedings might be in response to aspirating ascending fluids (reflux).

IV. Coordination of the Suck-Swallow-Breathe Triad

A. The normal, full-term infant sucks, swallows, and breathes in a well-regulated, rhythmic manner (Bosma, 1977).

B. Feeding evaluation must consider all three aspects of the SSB triad (Glass & Wolf, 1994).

C. Sucking, swallowing, and breathing are functionally and anatomically interrelated (overlapping function of cranial nerves and structures).

D. Observation of feeds in compromised infants should include observation of the *entire* feed to permit identification of fatigue, loss of rhythmicity, evidence of respiratory distress, and so on (Alper & Manno, 1996; Wolf & Glass, 1992).

E. Dysrhythmic sucking and poor coordination of SSB are common even in term infants during the first few days postpartum.

1. Observe feedings for:

    a. *Stridor*: a raspy, respiratory noise heard upon inspiration (as with laryngomalacia or upon expiration as with tracheomalacia) caused by narrowing or obstruction of the airway.

    b. *Wheezing*: a high-pitched noise occurring during exhalation (caused by airway constriction due to inflammation or reactive airway disease caused by silent microaspiration during feeding).

    c. *Apnea* during feeding: periodic breath-holding while attempting to manage swallows (Law-Morstatt et al., 2003).

    d. *Fatigue* during feeding: falling asleep too early during a feeding as the result of the infant being unable to accomplish the work of feeding or owing to stress.

    e. *Poor intake*: Test weights on reliable scales are critical when assessing the intake of the unstable feeder (Sachs & Oddie, 2002; Scanlon et al., 2002).

    f. *Poor growth*: Newborn infant weight loss > 8% and failure to promptly recover birth weight are markers for suboptimal infant feeding behavior. Prompt, careful lactation assessment is required (Dewey, Nommsen-Rivers, & Heinig, 2003).

    g. *Feeding aversion:* May result owing to aspiration, respiratory compromise, choking, reflux, or sensory-based problems (Palmer & Heyman, 1993).

V. The "Fit" Between the Infant's Oral Anatomy and Maternal Breast/Nipple Anatomy (Gunther, 1955; Neifert, 1999; Wilson-Clay & Hoover, 2005)

A. The breastfeeding mother and baby form a dyad.

B. Evaluation involves the assessment of both.

C. The diameter, consistency, length, elasticity, and shape of the maternal nipple might or might not be a good fit with the baby's mouth.

    1. Flat, inverted, or non-elastic nipples may frustrate infant latch and lead to breast refusal (Gunther, 1955; Neifert, Lawrence, & Seacat, 1995; Wilson-Clay, 1996).

    2. The elasticity of the nipples can be improved by softening an engorged breast.
       a. Over time, pumping may help nipples to be easier to grasp.
       b. Older, stronger babies can more easily adapt to challenging nipple configurations, including non-elastic nipples.

    3. Nipple shields can assist breastfeeding when flat or inverting nipples frustrate latch or fail to give the infant adequate intra-oral stimulation to initiate sucking (Wilson-Clay, 1996).

    4. Long maternal nipples.
       a. Infant growth will eventually accommodate for long maternal nipples.

    b. At first, if long maternal nipples activate the infant's gag reflex, alternate methods of feeding will be required.

5. Large diameter, non-compressible nipples.

    a. Increased infant size, strength, and stamina will accommodate the infant's initial inability to manipulate meaty, non-compressible nipples.

6. Creative positioning can somewhat accommodate for challenging nipple shapes.

7. Certain configurations of breasts/nipples might be more or less easy for infants with certain oral anomalies.

    a. A mother with soft, elastic breast tissue might be able to use her breast tissue to plug a cleft lip.

    b. A mother with taut breast tissue might not be able to assist her infant in this way.

References

Abadie V, Andre A, Zaouche A, et al. Early feeding resistance: a possible consequence of neonatal oro-esophageal dyskinesia. *Acta Pediatr.* 2001;90:738–745.

Alper M, Manno S. Dysphagia in infants and children with oral-motor deficits: assessment and management. *Semin Speech Language.* 1996;17:283–305, 309.

Amir L, James J, Beatty J. Review of tongue-tie release at a tertiary maternity hospital. *J Paediatr Child Health.* 2005;41:243–245.

Ballard J, Auer C, Khoury, JC. Ankyloglossia: assessment, incidence, and effect of frenuloplasty on the breastfeeding dyad. *Pediatrics.* 2004;110:e63.

Bosma J. Structure and function of the infant oral and pharyngeal mechanisms. In: Wilson J, ed. *Oral-Motor Function and Dysfunction in Children.* Chapel Hill, NC: University of North Carolina at Chapel Hill; 1977:25–28, 39, 52, 69.

Bull M, Givan D. Improved outcome in Pierre Robin sequence: effect of multidisciplinary evaluation and management. *Pediatrics.* 1990;86:294–301.

Caughey A, Sandberg, P, Zlatnik M, et al. Forceps compared with vacuum: rates of neonatal and maternal morbidity. *Obstet Gynecol.* 2005;106:908–912.

Cleft Palate Foundation. Information for Families. Pittsburgh: Cleft Palate Foundation; 2006. Available at: http://cleftline.org/what_we_do/publications. Accessed January 21, 2007.

Coryllos E, Genna C, Salloum A. Congenital tongue-tie and its impact on breastfeeding. American Academy of Pediatrics, Section on Breastfeeding. *Breastfeeding: Best for Baby and Mother*; Summer 2004:1–6.

Danner SC. Breastfeeding the neurologically impaired infant. NAACOG's Clinical Issues in Perinatal and Women's Health Nursing. *Breastfeeding.* 1992;3:640–646.

Darzi M, Chowdri N, Bhat A. Breast feeding or spoon feeding after cleft lip repair: a prospective, randomized study. *Br J Plast Surg.* 1996;49:24–26.

Dewey K, Nommsen-Rivers L, Heinig MJ. Risk factors for suboptimal infant breastfeeding behavior, delayed onset of lactation, and excess neonatal weight loss. *Pediatrics*. 2003;112:607–619.

Fernando C. *Tongue Tie: From Confusion to Clarity*. Sydney, Australia: Tandem Publications; 1998.

Flinck A, Paludan A, Matsson L, et al. Oral findings in a group of Swedish children. *Int J Paediatr Dent*. 1994;2:67–73.

Garcez L, Giugliani E. Population-based study on the practice of breastfeeding in children born with cleft lip and palate. *Cleft Palate Craniofac J*. 2005;42(6):687–693.

Geddes D, McClellen H, Kent J, et al. Patterns of respiration in infants during breastfeeding. 13th International Conference of the International Society for Research in Human Milk and Lactation (ISRHML). September 22–26, 2006. Niagara-on-the-Lake, Ontario, Canada.

Glass R, Wolf L. Incoordination of sucking, swallowing, and breathing as an etiology for breastfeeding difficulties. *J Hum Lact*. 1994;10:185–189.

Glenny A, Hooper L, Shaw W, et al. Feeding interventions for growth and development in infants with cleft lip, cleft palate or cleft lip and palate. *Cochrane Database Syst Rev*. 2004; (3): CD003315.

Goldman A. The immune system of human milk: antimicrobial, anti-inflammatory and immunomodulating properties. *Pediatric Infect Dis J*. 1993;12:664–671.

Gorski S, Adams K, Birch PH, et al. Linkage analysis of X-linked cleft palate and ankyloglossia in Manitoba Mennonite and British Columbia native kindreds. *Hum Genet*. 1994;94:141–148.

Gray L, Miller L, Philipp B, et al. Breastfeeding is analgesic in healthy newborns. *Pediatrics*. 2002;109:590–593.

Gunther M. Instinct and the nursing couple. *Lancet*. 1955;1:575–578.

Hill P, Aldag J, Chatterton R. Initiation and frequency of pumping and milk production on non-nursing preterm infants. *J Hum Lact*. 2001;17(1):9–13.

Jones N. The protective effects of breastfeeding for infants of depressed mothers. *Breastfeeding Abstracts*. 2005;24:19–20.

Kavanaugh K, Mead L, Meier P, et al. Getting enough: mothers' concerns about breastfeeding a preterm infant after discharge. *J Obstet Gynecol Neonatal Nurs*. 1995; 24:23–32.

Kent J, Mitoulas L, Cox D, et al. Breast volume and milk production during extended lactation. *Exp Physiol*. 1999;84:435–447.

Kogo M, Okada G, Ishii S, et al. Breast feeding for cleft lip and palate patients, using the Hotz-type plate. *Cleft Palate Craniofac J*. 1997;34(4):351–353.

Kramer M, Demissie K, Yang H, Platt R, et al. The contribution of mild- and moderate preterm birth to infant mortality. *JAMA*. 2000;284:843–849.

Lalakea M, Messner A. Ankyloglossia: does it matter? *Pediatr Clin N Am*. 2003;50:381–397.

Lawrence RA, Lawrence RM. *Breastfeeding: A Guide for the Medical Profession.* Philadelphia: Elsevier Mosby; 2005:540–546.

Law-Morstatt L, Judd D, Snyder P, et al. Pacing as a treatment technique for transitional sucking patterns. *J Perinatol.* 2003;23:483–488.

McBride M, Danner S. Sucking disorders in neurologically impaired infants: assessment and facilitation of breastfeeding. *Clin Perinatol.* 1987;14:109–130.

Merkel-Piccini R, Rosenfeld-Johnson S. Connections between tongue placement and dental alignment. *ADVANCE for Speech-Language Pathologists and Audiologists.* 2003;13:9.

Messner A, Lalakea L, Aby J, et al. Ankyloglossia: incidence and associated feeding difficulties. *Arch Otolaryngol Head Neck Surg.* 2000;126:36–39.

Mohrbacher N, Stock J. *The Breastfeeding Answer Book.* 3rd ed. Schaumburg, IL: La Leche League International; 2003:84.

Morris S. A glossary of terms describing the feeding process. In: Wilson J, ed. *Oral-Motor Function and Dysfunction in Children.* Chapel Hill, NC: University of North Carolina at Chapel Hill; 1977:160.

Neifert M. Clinical aspects of lactation. *Clin Perinatol.* 1999;26:282–283.

Neifert M, Lawrence R, Seacat J. Nipple confusion: toward a formal definition. *J Pediatr.* 1995;126:S125–S129.

Ogg L. Oral-pharyngeal development and evaluation. *Physiol Ther.* 1975;55:235–241.

Palmer M. Identification and management of the transitional suck pattern in premature infants. *J Perinat Neonatal Nurs.* 1993;7:66–75.

Palmer MM, Heyman MB. Assessment and treatment of sensory-versus motor-based feeding problems in very young children. *Infants Young Child.* 1993;6:67–73.

Paradise J, Elster B, Tan L. Evidence in infants with cleft palate that breast milk protects against otitis media. *Pediatrics.* 1994;94:853–860.

Powers N. Slow weight gain and low milk supply in the breastfeeding dyad. In: Wagner C, Purohit D, eds. *Clinics in Perinatology.* 1999;26(2):399–430.

Premji S, Paes B. Gastrointestinal function and growth in premature infants: is non-nutritive sucking vital? *J Perinatol.* 2000;1:46–53.

Ramsay D, Mitoulas L, Kent J, et al. Ultrasound imaging of the sucking mechanics of the breastfeeding infant. Abstract. Proceedings of the 12th International Conference of the International Society for Research in Human Milk and Lactation, Queens College, Cambridge, UK; Sept. 10–14, 2004a.

Ramsay D, Langton D, Gollow I, et al. Ultrasound imaging of the effect of frenulotomy on breastfeeding infants with ankyloglossia. Abstract. Proceedings of the 12th International Conference of the International Society for Research in Human Milk and Lactation., Queens College, Cambridge, UK; September 10–14, 2004b.

Ranley D. Early orofacial development. *J Clin Pediatr Dent.* 1998;22:267–275.

Redstone F, West J. The importance of postural control for feeding. *Pediatr Nurs.* 2004; 30:97–100.

Ricke L, Baker N, Madlon-Kay D, et al. Newborn tongue-tie: prevalence and effect on breastfeeding. *J Am Board Fam Pract.* 2005;18:1–7.

Riordan J. *Breastfeeding and Human Lactation.* 3rd ed. Sudbury, MA: Jones and Bartlett Publishers; 2005.

Rovet J, ed. *Turner Syndrome Across the Lifespan.* Markham, Ontario, Canada. Kelin Graphics; 1995; iv.

Sachs M, Oddie S. Breastfeeding—weighing in the balance: reappraising the role of weighing babies in the early days. *MIDIRS Midwifery Digest.* 2002;12:296–300.

Scanlon K, Alexander M, Serdula M, et al. Assessment of infant feeding: The validity of measuring milk intake. *Nutrition Reviews.* 2002;60(8):235–251.

Smith J, Crumley R, Harker L. Facial paralysis in the newborn. *Otolaryngol Head Neck Surg.* 1981;89:1021–1024.

Snyder J. Bubble palate and failure to thrive: a case report. *J Hum Lact.* 1997;13:139–143.

Turner L, Jacobsen C, Humenczuk M, et al. The effects of lactation education and a prosthetic obturator appliance on feeding efficiency in infants with cleft lip and palate. *Cleft Palate Craniofac J.* 2001;38(5):519–524.

Valentine C, Hurst N, Schanler R. Hindmilk improves weight gain in low-birth-weight infants fed human milk. *J Pediatr Gastroent Nutr.* 1994;474–477.

Wall V, Glass R. Mandibular asymmetry and breastfeeding problems: experience from 11 cases. *J Hum Lact.* 2006;22:328–334.

Weatherly-White R, Kuehn D, et al. Early repair and breast-feeding for infants with cleft lip. *Plast Reconstr Surg.* 1987;79:879–885.

Wiessinger D, Miller M. Breastfeeding difficulties as a result of tight lingual and labial frena: a case report. *J Hum Lact.* 1995;11:313–316.

Wilson-Clay B. *External Pacing Techniques: Protecting Respiratory Stability During Feeding.* Pharmasoft Publishing Independent Study Module (ISM). Amarillo, TX: Pharmasoft Publishing; 2005.

Wilson-Clay B. Clinical use of nipple shields. *J Hum Lact.* 1996;12:279–285.

Wilson-Clay B, Hoover K. The *Breastfeeding Atlas.* Austin, TX: LactNews Press; 2005.

Wolf L, Glass R. *Feeding and Swallowing Disorders in Infancy.* Tucson, AZ: Therapy Skill Builders; 1992.

Breastfeeding Assessment

Marie Davis, RN, IBCLC

OBJECTIVES

- Describe the criteria for comfortable maternal positioning.

- List three types of breast support.

- Demonstrate four infant positions for breastfeeding.

- Demonstrate three special positions for breastfeeding difficulties.

- List three objective findings that contribute to poor maternal and infant positioning for breastfeeding.

- Describe the components of proper latch-on.

- List the signs of milk transfer.

- Describe three criteria for assessing sufficient milk intake.

- List three signs of swallowing.

- Document a breastfeeding assessment.

Introduction

Proper maternal and infant positioning forms the cornerstone of the breastfeeding experience. Comfortable, pain free, and effective breastfeeding can be achieved through exploring what works best for each mother/baby pair. Numerous options and variations exist for positioning. Mothers do not need to know all of these positions, and their positioning preference should be respected. Lactation consultants must be able to assess positioning, latch-on, and milk transfer/swallowing as well as appropriately document a complete breastfeeding assessment in the medical record.

I. Maternal and Infant Breastfeeding Positions (Minchin, 1989; Renfrew, Fisher, & Arms, 2000)

A. Provide for mother's physical and emotional (psychological) comfort.

   1. Structure the environment for privacy.
      a. Assess the mother's comfort with visitors and family.
      b. If indicated, ask them to leave and return after the feeding.

   2. Ensure a comfortable room temperature and quiet environment.

   3. Turn off the television, radio, and telephone. Have an answering machine or family member answer phone calls.

   4. Give pain medication prior to feedings if necessary.

   5. Cushion for episiotomy if needed.

   6. The mother should empty her bladder if needed and wash her hands.

   7. Washing the nipples and areolae are unnecessary.

B. If the mother is seated on a straight-backed chair.

   1. Knees should be slightly higher than the hips.

   2. Provide a footstool to raise the mother's knees so that the baby faces mother's body, which prevents back strain.

   3. Use pillows as needed for comfort and support.
      a. Pillows can be placed behind her back.
      b. A firm pillow (or commercial nursing pillow) can be placed in the mother's lap to raise the baby to the level of the breasts if necessary.
      c. The mother should not lean back or hunch forward over the baby.

C. If the mother is seated in a bed.

   1. Raise the head of the bed to a 90 degree angle or to the comfort of the mother.

   2. Use pillows behind her back if necessary.

   3. Place a pillow under her knees and/or under her arms if needed.

   4. A pillow can be placed on her lap to raise the baby to the level of the breast if needed or to protect a cesarean incision.

D. If the mother is lying down.

   1. Mothers may experience less fatigue if breastfeeding while lying down.

   2. Some mothers express concern over the number of pillows needed to nurse in a side lying position (suffocation hazard or too cumbersome for them to arrange by themselves).

   3. Mothers can be assisted onto their side if necessary, with the baby placed facing toward the breast to be used for the feeding.

   4. A pillow can be placed between her legs lengthwise to level the hips and to relieve lower back pain.

5. Place a pillow behind her back if needed.

6. A rolled baby blanket or towel can be used if needed behind the infant to prevent him from rolling onto his back.

7. The mother can cradle the infant with her lower arm or place the arm behind her head.

E. If the mother is flat on her back.

1. Not an optimum position for breastfeeding.

2. The weight of the infant against her breast might be painful.

3. The infant's face might become buried in the breast.

4. Might be needed if the mother has complications from an epidural or spinal.

5. Might help the infant cope with a fast milk flow (see prone position).

F. Positioning the infant.

1. The infant should be well supported so that the baby is flexed and the limbs are tucked into the body.

2. The infant should face the mother's body with the ear, shoulder, and hip in a straight line.

3. Calling it "tummy-to-tummy" positioning is misleading and might cause the mother to hold the baby's body too low.

4. The baby's body should be level.

5. The baby's lower end should not drift into the mother's lap.
   a. In the cradle hold, the mother's elbow should be at a 90 degree angle.
   b. Cradle position is illustrated in Figure 24-1.

6. Avoid positions that cause the infant's neck to twist to the side.

7. Avoid pressure against the back of the infant's head (occipital area), because this action will cause the baby to arch away from the breast.

G. Madonna or cradle hold (Figure 24-1).

1. Most commonly used position.

2. Feels the most natural to the mother.

3. Offers the least amount of control over the infant's head.

4. The baby lies across the mother's forearm on the side that the mother will be using for the feeding.

5. The baby's head is either in the bend of the mother's elbow or midway down her forearm, whichever results in the best positioning.

6. The mother holds the baby's buttocks with her hand.

7. The mother's arm should be level.

8. The mother avoids dropping the baby's bottom toward her lap. A pillow in her lap can help keep baby level.

Figure 24-1 Cradle
position

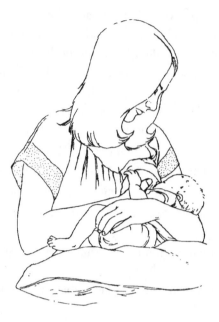

9. If the baby is not level, this situation might put downward pressure on the
   breast, which might alter the latch, pulling the breast out of the baby's mouth.
10. The baby's lower arm can be placed around the mother's back or tucked down
    along next to his or her body.
11. The baby's legs can be wrapped around the mother's waist if needed to bring
    the baby closer to the breast.
H. Clutch or football hold (Figure 24-2).
   1. Often preferred when a new mother is having difficulty with latch-on.
   2. Gives the mother better control of the infant's head.
   3. Improves the mother's view of her nipple and areola and of the baby's mouth.
   4. Place two pillows beside the mother if needed.
   5. Place the infant on the pillows with the baby's hips flexed, baby's bottom
      against the back of the chair/couch/bed, the feet aiming toward the ceiling.
   6. The feet should not touch the back of the chair.
   7. Pressure on the feet can trigger arching and the stepping reflex.
   8. The baby's arms can be placed across his or her chest or around the breast.
   9. Slide the arm under the infant's back with the hand at the base of the baby's
      head.

Figure 24-2 Clutch or
football hold

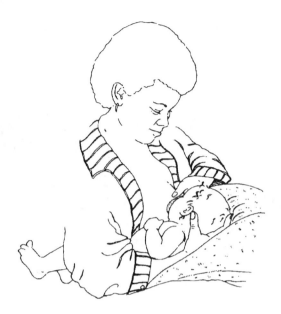

I. Elevated clutch hold.

   1. Use approximately the same positioning as for the clutch hold except the baby is elevated into a sitting position next to the mother.

   2. Place one or two pillows beside the mother if needed.

   3. Place the infant's bottom on the pillow(s) with the baby's hips flexed (legs tucked up) with knees flexed in an upright "seated" position.

   4. Infant's arms can be folded across the chest or tucked under the mother's breast or to the sides of the breast.

   5. Use arm to support baby's back with hand placed at the base of the baby's head.

J. Cross-cradle hold (Figure 24-3).

   1. Principles are the same as for the cradle hold.

   2. The baby lies across the forearm of the opposite arm from the breast being used for the feeding (the left arm for the right breast).

   3. The baby's head is held just below the ears at the nape of the neck.

   4. The breast is supported with the hand on the same side as the breast to be used for the feeding.

   5. Also used for preterm infants.

Figure 24-3   Cross-cradle
hold

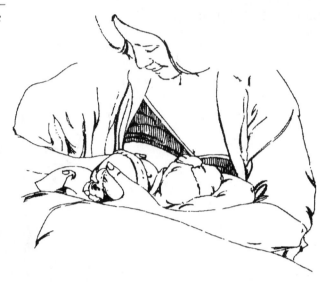

K. Side-lying feeding position (Figure 24-4).

   1. Position the mother on her side and slightly rolled toward her back.

   2. Lying completely on her side will make her baby's latch-on difficult.
      a. Breast turned too far into bed, may not be accessible.
      b. May be difficult to hold position due to back pain.

Figure 24-4   Side-lying
position

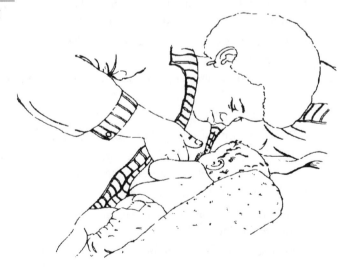

3. The baby is placed on the bed turned toward the breast.

4. The mother can use her arm to hold the infant in position.

5. The breast is held by the mother's upper hand.

L. Australian or posture feeding (prone oblique).

1. The baby is placed on his or her abdomen across the mother's chest with the mother lying back.

2. The mother might need to support the forehead of the baby with the heel of her hand to prevent the baby's head from falling forward.

3. Used for mothers who have a forceful milk ejection reflex that is overwhelming the baby.

4. Also used for babies who:
   a. Bite or retract their tongue; helps the jaw and tongue move down and forward.
   b. Have upper airway disorders such as tracheomalacia and laryngomalacia.

5. Care must be taken that the breasts are adequately drained when using this position.

M. Table 24-1 is a summary of the various advantages and disadvantages of the basic positions.

II. Latch-on

A. Key points.

1. A good latch-on will prevent many breastfeeding problems.
   a. Essential to the prevention of nipple pain.
   b. Essential for adequate milk transfer.

2. Things to avoid during latch-on.
   a. Moving the breast out of its resting position.
   b. Taking the breast to the baby.
   c. Twisting of the mother's or infant's body.
   d. Pushing down on the baby's chin to force the mouth open.
   e. Pushing the baby's head into the breast.
   f. Flexing the baby's neck (chin to chest).
   g. Extending the baby's neck.
   h. Allowing the baby's arms and legs to flail.

B. Breast support.

1. Hand and finger placement.
   a. Fingers need to be far enough back to allow full access to the mother's areola.
      i. Many women grasp the breast with the thumb well up on the breast but the fingers too close to the areola on the underside of the breast.

Table 24-1   Advantages and Limitations of Basic Positions

Position	Advantages	Limitations	Pertinent Points
Cradle hold	• Women are most likely to have seen this position used • Works best for most situations	• Difficult to achieve good sitting position in hospital bed; use chair if possible • Requires sitting; cesarean incision or hemorrhoids may make sitting a less desirable position • Poor control of infant's head	• Be sure that infant is chest-to-chest rather than chest-to-ceiling • Infant should be at the level of the nipple
Side-lying	• Helpful after cesarean birth • Great for nighttime feedings	• Difficult to visualize latch	• Be sure that infant is chest-to-chest rather than chest-to-ceiling • Use folded receiving blanket behind infant to maintain chest-to-chest position • Mother's body should be at a slight angle to the mattress, leaning backward just a bit against a pillow
Football	• Helpful after cesarean birth • Helpful for women with especially large breasts • Provides better visualization of latch-on process • Good control of infant's head	• Often difficult to do sitting up in hospital bed	• Be sure that infant is chest-to-chest rather than chest-to-ceiling

     ii. The mother cannot easily see her finger position on the breast.

     iii. Suggest that the mother practice holding her breast in front of a mirror.

  b. The weight of the breast should be supported with the mother's hand.

     i. Large-breasted women may benefit from a rolled washcloth or towel placed under the breast to elevate it and to prevent the baby from pulling down on the nipple.

     ii. Small-breasted women might not need to support the breast but will need to place the heel of the hand against the chest so that the infant's access is not obstructed.

  c. C-hold (thumb on top of the breast with all four fingers below) is preferred.

     i. Gentle compression of the breast tissue between the thumb and fingers, making the areola more oblong than round.

     ii. Pushing slightly back into the chest wall will cause the nipple to protrude.

     iii. Gentle pressure applied with the thumb so the nipple points slightly upward.

  d. The scissors hold (breast grasped between the index and middle fingers) might work for some mothers as long as the fingers are well away from the areola.

  e. The dancer hold (breast grasped from below with the hand in a U shape with the baby's chin resting in the fleshy part between the thumb and index finger) might be needed for preterm infants or for infants who have poor jaw support or control.

2. Attachment: bringing baby to the breast.

  a. Brush the lips lightly with the nipple.

     i. The mother should do this by gently moving her breast up and down.

     ii. Caution the mother to keep her fingers away from the baby's mouth.

       (1) Some mothers are tempted to "pry" the mouth open with the index finger.

       (2) Touching the baby's mouth may cause clamping (bite reflex).

  b. Some babies might respond better when the upper lip is stimulated.

3. The baby will open his or her mouth slightly at first, drop the head back slightly, then gape and move toward the breast.

  a. Mouth open wide, tongue to the floor of the mouth.

     i. A crying baby might open the mouth wide but the tongue will be at the roof of the mouth.

     ii. Verbal and visual cues given to the baby might assist with latch-on, such as the mother saying "open" and opening her own mouth wide.

     iii. The mother may need to gently depress the tongue with her clean index finger, stroking the tongue down and forward.

  b. With baby's mouth open wide, the mother should quickly pull the baby into the breast.

      i. Avoid the rapid arm movement technique, because this action often startles the baby and is counterproductive.

     ii. A baby should never be pushed or shoved into the breast.

4. The baby's chin should touch the breast first, with both the chin and the tip of the nose touching the breast.

   a. The baby's mouth should be brought "up and over" the areola with the baby leading with his or her chin.

   b. Sometimes helps to tell the mother to envision trying to eat a sandwich larger than her mouth and go through the steps she would make to take the first bite.

C. Concerns over the infant's nose.

1. Many mothers naturally push into the breast to keep it away from the baby's nose.

   a. This action will alter the latch-on, pulling the breast out of the baby's mouth.

   b. Might be a cause for nipple pain and/or plugged ducts.

   c. If the mother cannot see the baby's nose, she should alter the baby's body position or the position of her hand.

      i. Raising the infant's bottom half so that it is more level with the head might clear the nose.

     ii. Wrapping the baby's legs around the mother's waist might also work.

   d. Lifting up slightly on the breast might clear the nose.

D. Mouth position.

1. Opinions differ as to the position of the baby on the areola.

   a. Some say centered.

   b. Some say asymmetrical, with the lower jaw covering more of the areola than the upper jaw (Newman & Pittman, 2000).

   c. The most important things are maternal comfort and good milk transfer.

2. The baby's mouth should be wide open.

3. The angle at the corner of the mouth should be 130–150 degrees or better (Hoover, 1996).

4. The baby should not have a dimple in the cheek (indicates that the tongue is drawn behind the lower gum and that the baby is sucking, as if from a straw).

5. Both lips should be flared outward.

   a. Common for baby to have the upper lip pulled in.

   b. Flip upper lip out or re-latch if this occurs.

   c. Tight labial frenulum may keep the upper or lower lip from rolling outward (Wiessinger & Miller, 1995).

6. The nipple and approximately one-fourth to one-half inch of the areola should be in the mouth; it is unnecessary for the baby to draw an entire areola into his or her mouth.

7. The breast is not placed into the baby's ̶̶ ̶̶ ̶̶
   his/her mouth.

E. Signs of swallowing (milk transfer).

   1. Puff of air from the nose.

   2. "Ca" sound from the throat.

   3. Deeper jaw excursion preceding each swallow.

   4. Slight vibration or movement can be seen near the

   5. Can hear the swallow with a stethoscope placed on t̶

   6. Top of the areola moves inward toward baby's mouth.

III. Breastfeeding Assessment Tools

A. A number of tools are used to assess and document various aspects of breastfeeding.

   1. The validity and reliability of some tools have been studied showing advantages and disadvantages of each (Adams & Hewell, 1997; Jenks, 1991; Riordan, 1998; Riordan et al., 2001; Riordan & Koehn, 1997; Schlomer, Kemmerer, & Twiss, 1999).

   2. For more information and examples of various latch assessment tools, please visit www.ilca.org and look under Resources.

B. Systematic Assessment of the Infant at Breast (Shrago & Bocar, 1990).

   1. Assesses the mechanics of positioning, latch-on, and swallowing.

   2. Easy to use.

   3. Validity and reliability have not been thoroughly studied.

C. Infant Breastfeeding Assessment Tool (Matthews, 1988).

   1. Looks at the readiness to feed.

   2. Lacks a measurable criterion for swallowing or milk transfer.

D. LATCH (Jensen, Wallace, & Kelsay, 1994).

   1. Evaluates the amount of help a mother needs to physically breastfeed.

   2. Does not clearly evaluate the latch-on component.

E. Mother–Baby Assessment (Mulford, 1992).

   1. Has a strong evaluation component of the mother's developing skills in both recognizing when it is time to feed the baby and how to feed the baby.

F. Potential Early Breast Feeding Problem Tool (Kearney, Cronenwett, & Barrett, 1990).

   1. Developed to determine which breastfeeding problems are rated highest among breastfeeding mothers.

tions that use a four-point Likert scale.

gher the score, the more breastfeeding problems occurred.

ternal Breast Feeding Evaluation Scale (Leff, Jeffries, & Gagne, 1994).

1. Consists of three subscales: maternal enjoyment/role attainment, infant satisfactions/growth, and lifestyle/maternal body image.

2. Designed to measure positive and negative aspects of breastfeeding that mothers have identified as important in defining successful lactation.

IV. The Lactation Consultant's Assessment (Walker, 1989a; Walker, 1989b)

A. The purpose of the lactation consultation is to gather enough data to be able to conduct a reasonable assessment of the feeding difficulty and to offer suggestions for overcoming that difficulty.

B. Data collection.

1. Accurate and complete history taking is especially important for the lactation consultant.

   a. Breastfeeding problems can be a manifestation or symptom of another problem.

   b. The lactation consultant cannot form a hypothesis or feeding plan if the data collected are incomplete.

2. Data collection is done by obtaining both subjective and objective data.

   a. Subjective data.

      i. Details are related by the mother to the lactation consultant, gathered from her verbal history.

      ii. Data are based upon the interpretation of the facts by the person relating the history.

      iii. Under most circumstances, this type of data cannot be verified.

   b. Objective data.

      i. Details are based on direct observation or measurement.

      ii. Evaluation of infant (for example, weight, gestational age, skin color, bilirubin or blood glucose level, presence of cephalohematoma, etc.).

      iii. Evaluation of maternal breasts (for example, size, nipple shape/ protractility, presence of swelling or erythema, surgical scars, etc.).

      iv. Suckling/milk transfer.

      v. Assessment of entire breastfeeding session.

3. Assessment is drawn from the data collected and the lactation consultant's knowledge base.

C. History taking.

1. Previous breastfeeding experience.

   a. Has the mother breastfed previous children? If so, then for how long?

  b. Did she have sore nipples or other problems?
  c. When and reason for weaning.

2. Previous breastfeeding education (classes, reading, videos, etc.).

3. Cultural influences.

4. Assess the mother's concerns regarding modesty.
   a. What are her feelings about breastfeeding in front of other people and in public places?

5. Who functions as her support system?

6. Intrapartum.
   a. Did she have a vaginal delivery?
      i. Episiotomy pain will influence the mother's comfort and position.
      ii. What type (if any) labor medications did she receive? Some might cause sedation or poor responsiveness in the infant (Walker, 1997).
      iii. Is she taking pain medication? Pain medication 20 minutes prior to feedings might increase her comfort level but large dosages might sedate both her and her baby.
   b. Assisted delivery (were vacuum extraction or forceps used?).
   c. Did she have a cesarean delivery?
      i. Type and location of incision.
      ii. Pain might limit her early positions.
   d. What type of medications did she have during labor and for subsequent pain control?

7. Is she on any other regular medications, supplements, and /or herbs?

8. Are there any complications from childbirth?
   a. Extension of episiotomy.
   b. Bladder, cervical, uterine, rectal, or perineal problems.
   c. Fever.

9. Level and location of pain.
   a. Perineum.
   b. Back.
   c. Legs, arms, neck, shoulders.
   d. Wrist and hand (such as carpal tunnel syndrome).
   e. Breasts or nipples.

10. What are her limitations?
    a. Physical.
    b. Psychological/social.
       i. Feelings of inadequacy.
       ii. Lack of self-confidence.
       iii. Sensitivity to comments and criticism.
       iv. Is she on medications for depression?

   v. Overwhelmed.

   vi. Fatigued.

  c. Medical.

 11. Environmental concerns.

  a. Where will she breastfeed at home?

  b. Who else is in the household?

 12. Breasts and nipples.

  a. Size and shape of breasts.

  b. Large, pendulous breasts might require that a rolled up towel or receiving blanket be placed under them for support.

  c. The direction that the nipple points will influence where the baby's mouth is placed.

  d. Anomalies (tubular, asymmetric).

  e. Condition of the nipples and areola.

   i. Everted, flat, retracted/inverted.

   ii. Edematous areola from intravenous fluids can flatten a normal nipple as it is enveloped with swollen areolar tissue.

  f. Nipple anomalies, supernumerary nipples.

D. Behavioral state of the baby.

 1. Deep sleep.

  a. Limp extremities, no body movement.

  b. Placid face.

  c. Quiet breathing.

  d. Cannot be easily aroused.

 2. Light or active sleep.

  a. Resistance in extremities when moved.

  b. Mouthing or suckling motions.

  c. Facial grimaces.

  d. More easily awakened, more likely to remain awake if disturbed.

  e. If left undisturbed, will easily fall back asleep.

 3. Drowsy.

  a. Eyes open and close intermittently.

  b. Might make sounds (murmur or whisper).

  c. Might yawn and stretch.

 4. Quiet alert.

  a. Looks around; interacts with environment.

  b. Body still and watchful.

  c. Breathing even and regular.

  d. Excellent time for breastfeeding.

 5. Active alert.

  a. Moves extremities.

   b. Wide eyed, irregular breathing.

   c. More sensitive to discomfort (wet diaper or excessive stimulation).

6. Crying.

   a. Agitated, disorganized.

   b. Needs comforting.

   c. Poor state to attempt breastfeeding.

V. Planning and Implementation by the Lactation Consultant

A. Obtains signed consent form from the mother before the consultation if in private practice.

B. Systemically evaluates the mother and infant's positioning.

C. Avoids positioning and latching the baby for the mother; rather, this process is facilitated so that the mother learns to do this action herself.

D. Avoids pushing on the back of the baby's head, compressing the mother's areola, or inserting the areola into the baby's mouth.

E. Notes how the nipple appears immediately after feeding.

   1. The nipple comes out of the infant's mouth round and of equal color with the areola.

   2. The nipple shows no evidence of trauma.

   3. Notes abnormal nipple shape, blisters, and/or blanching.

F. Will note the following after a feed:

   1. The baby should be calm, satiated, and relaxed.

   2. Note irritability and/or fussiness.

   3. The mother reports the absence of shoulder, neck, or back pain.

   4. The mother appears relaxed.

   5. The mother verbalizes confidence in positioning herself and her infant.

G. Corrects positioning and latch-on techniques only as needed.

H. Observes a return demonstration of skills learned by mother.

 I. Documents the consultation.

J. Completes lactation consultation chart.

K. Gives written instructions to mother for ongoing self-care.

L. Arranges for follow-up care:

   1. In person follow-up within a reasonable amount of time.

   2. Telephone follow-up if appropriate.

M. Consults with another health care provider if needed.

   1. Immediate contact of the medical provider where warranted.

   2. Provides a written report to the mother's and baby's health care provider.

References

Adams D, Hewell SD. Maternal and professional assessment of breastfeeding. *J Hum Lact.* 1997;13:279–283.

Hoover K. Visual assessment of the baby's wide open mouth. *J Hum Lact.* 1996;12:9.

Jenks MA. LATCH assessment in the hospital nursery. *J Hum Lact.* 1991;7:19–20.

Jensen D, Wallace S, Kelsay P. LATCH: a breastfeeding charting system and documentation tool. *J Obstet Gynecol Neonatal Nurs.* 1994;23:27–32.

Kearney M, Cronenwett L, Barrett J. Breastfeeding problems in the first week postpartum. *Nurs Res.* 1990;39:90–95.

Leff E, Jeffries S, Gagne M. The development of the maternal breastfeeding evaluation scale. *J Hum Lact.* 1994;10:105–111.

Matthews MK. Developing an instrument to assess infant breastfeeding behavior in the early neonatal period. *Midwifery.* 1988;4:154–165.

Minchin M. Positioning for breastfeeding. *Birth.* 1989;16:67–73.

Mulford C. The Mother-Baby Assessment (MBA): an "Apgar score" for breastfeeding. *J Hum Lact.* 1992;8:79–82.

Newman J, Pitman T. *The Ultimate Breastfeeding Book of Answers.* Roseville, CA: Prima; 2000:60–65.

Renfrew M, Fisher C, Arms S. *Breastfeeding: Getting Breastfeeding Right for You.* Revised ed. Berkeley, CA: Celestial Arts; 2000.

Riordan J. Predicting breastfeeding problems. *AWHONN Lifelines.* December 1998: 31–33.

Riordan J, Bibb D, Miller M, Rawlins T. Predicting breastfeeding duration using the LATCH breastfeeding assessment tool. *J Hum Lact.* 2001;17:20–23.

Riordan JM, Koehn M. Reliability and validity testing of three breastfeeding assessment tools. *J Obstetr Gynecol Neonatal Nurs.* 1997;26:181–187.

Schlomer JA, Kemmerer J, Twiss JJ. Evaluating the association of two breastfeeding assessment tools with breastfeeding problems and breastfeeding satisfaction. *J Hum Lact.* 1999;15:35–39.

Shrago L, Bocar D. The infant's contribution to breastfeeding. *J Obstetr Gynecol Neonatal Nurs.* 1990;19:209–215.

Walker M. Management of selected early breastfeeding problems seen in clinical practice. *Birth.* 1989a;6:148–158.

Walker M. Functional assessment of infant feeding patterns. *Birth.* 1989b;16:140–147.

Walker M. Do labor medications affect breastfeeding? *J Hum Lact.* 1997;13:131–137.

Wiessinger D, Miller M. Breastfeeding difficulties as a result of tight lingual and labial frena: a case report. *J Hum Lact.* 1995;11:313–316.

GUIDELINES FOR INFANT BREASTFEEDING

Marie Davis, RN, IBCLC

OBJECTIVES

- Identify two things that will aid the baby in his or her transition to extra-uterine life.
- Give at least two examples of physiological and psychological benefits to the mother and baby related to early first contact.
- Identify at least two routine hospital procedures that disrupt the normal first attachment needs of both mother and baby.
- List at least three things parents should be made aware of in the prenatal setting that can enhance first contact and that should be incorporated into the birth plan.
- State the significance of amniotic fluid transfer in relation to first contact.
- State one rationale for skin-to-skin (STS) contact between the mother and the neonate.

Introduction

The establishment of lactation begins with the separation of the placenta. Birth interventions that disrupt the natural interaction between the mother and the infant in the immediate postpartum period can impact long-term breastfeeding success. For the past several decades, hospitals have used "an intensive care approach" during the transition period to extra-uterine life, treating all newborns as "recovering patients until they have demonstrated evidence of smooth transition" (Thureen et al., 1999, p. 91). The medicalization of birth and postpartum processes has created additional barriers to successful breastfeeding (Lawrence & Lawrence, 2005).

The World Health Organization and the United Nations Children's Fund's *Baby Friendly Hospital Initiative*, the U.S. *Healthy People 2010* goals, and the breastfeeding statements from the American Academy of Pediatrics (2005) are directing maternity care away from an antiquated treatment model that applies to fewer than 10% of all newborns. A mother's breastfeeding experience can be "profoundly affected by what happens during the first hours after birth" (Newman & Pitman, 2000, p. 43). The lactation consultant might not be present for the first mother–infant breastfeeding contact. However, she or he can educate parents and medical providers about how critical this first step is toward successful breastfeeding and how to handle it safely and effectively.

I. Teaching Points

A. Encourage parents to have a written birth plan and feeding plan (Riordan, 2005) before hospital admission.

B. Encourage hospitals and birth centers to limit nonessential routine interventions in labor and birth (Lauwers & Swisher, 2005).

   1. More natural birth processes enhance the instinctual and reflexive aspects of breastfeeding.

   2. Labor medications and interventions dull breastfeeding and bonding processes (Powers & Slusser, 1997).

   3. Mothers who initiate breastfeeding within an hour of birth breastfeed longer than those who have delayed contact (Mikiel-Kostyra, Mazur, & Boltruszko, 2002).

C. Encourage parents and health care providers to recognize and facilitate the baby's reflexes for self-attachment.

D. Human imprinting is not discussed in pediatric texts. "Comfort sucking and formation of nipple preference are genetically determined behaviors for imprinting on the mother's nipple" (Lawrence & Lawrence, 2005, pp. 223–224; Mohrbacher and Stock, 2003, p. 83).

E. The baby recognizes his or her mother by oral, tactile, and olfactory modes. (Marlier, Schaal, & Soussignan, 1997).

   1. The baby learns the smell of amniotic fluid in utero and shows a preference for objects that are coated with amniotic fluid (Schaal, Hummel, & Soussignan, 2004; Varendi & Porter, 2001).

   2. This preference changes to a preference for the smell of the mother's milk four or five days after birth.

   3. Babies who are exposed to the amniotic fluid smell cried less than those who were exposed to no odor or to the odor of the mother's breast (Varendi et al., 1998).

   4. Odors play an important role in the mediation of an infant's early behavior (Varendi et al., 1998).

F. Most babies from unmedicated births will self-attach and suckle correctly in fewer than 50 minutes (Righard & Alade, 1990).

1. If left undisturbed with the mother, the baby responds with an unlearned pattern of attachment; the process is innate (Righard & Alade, 1990).

2. When a baby self-attaches, he or she will attach correctly to the areola and not to the nipple alone (Righard & Alade, 1990).

3. If separated from the mother for newborn procedures, the baby's initial suckling attempts are disturbed (AAP, 2005).

4. Delayed gratification of the early sucking reflex might make it more difficult for the infant to suckle later on (Riordan, 2005).

G. Organized breastfeeding behavior develops in a predictable way during the first hours of life; the pre-feeding sequence of behaviors include the following (Kennell & Klaus, 1998):

1. Licking movements precede and follow the rooting reflex in alert infants.

2. The tongue is placed on the floor of the mouth during this distinct rooting.

3. "Mouth and lip smacking movements begin, and the infant begins to drool. The baby then begins to move forward slowly, starts to turn the head from side to side, and open the mouth widely upon nearing the nipple. After several attempts, the lips latch on to the areola and not the nipple" (Kennell & Klaus, 1998, p. 6).

H. A healthy infant should be given the opportunity to show hunger and optimal reflexes and attach to the areola by him- or herself (Lawrence & Lawrence, 2005).

I. Forcing the infant to the breast can be counterproductive in that it might disturb the rooting reflex and alter the tongue position as the infant reflexively raises his or her tongue to protect the airway.

J. Birth plans and hospital protocols should include the following:

1. Provision for labor support.

2. Support of the mother in labor has been shown to have positive effects on birth, bonding, and breastfeeding success (Kennell et al., 1991; Langer et al., 1998).
   a. Family/primary support person, usually the baby's father.
   b. Doula.
      i. Powerful force intrapartum; mother receives one-to-one support from the doula throughout labor (Berg & Terstad, 2006).
      ii. Medical care cost reduction: a reduced need for medical interventions including pitocin, epidural anesthesia, and cesarean sections (Gordon et al., 1999; Klaus, Kennell, & Klaus, 1993; Perez, 1998; Rosen, 2004).
      iii. Shortened labors (averaging slightly less than six hours for the first time mother).
      iv. The level of support has the greatest influence on successful labor and breastfeeding outcomes (Klaus et al., 1993).

a. Postpartum doula facilitates breastfeeding (Bonaro & Kroeger, 2004).

3. "Women rank partners or husbands after doulas, midwives, and other family members in terms of the quality of supportive labor care" (Rosen, 2004).

4. A combination of doula support and female family support appears to be the most effective in a positive birth experience (Rosen, 2004).

K. Limit the use of labor interventions.

1. Artificial Rupture of Membranes.

2. Induction and augmentation (pitocin/prostaglandins).

3. Analgesics: mothers who have been medicated during labor are more likely to leave the hospital without having established breastfeeding.

a. Narcotics, barbiturates can sedate the baby.

b. Epidural analgesia; epidurals increase the risk of intrapartum maternal fever, leading to separation, septic workup for the baby, and the use of antibiotics (Dashe et al., 1999; Gross et al., 2002; Leighton & Halpern, 2002; Lieberman et al., 1997; Lieberman & O'Donoghue, 2002; Negishi et al., 2001).

i. In mothers who develop a fever from the epidural, babies have an increased risk of seizures (Lieberman et al., 2000a).

ii. Mothers who have had epidurals spend less time with their baby during the hospital stay (Sepkoski et al., 2005).

iii. Medications can depress the efficacy of early suckling and interfere with state and motor control (Lieberman et al., 2000b; Perlman, 1999; Petrova et al., 2001; Phillip et al., 1999).

c. Numerous analgesics might disturb and delay important newborn behaviors such as breast-seeking, latch-on, and suckling. Analgesics can depress these developing breastfeeding behaviors that stimulate the mother's breast (Ransjo-Arvidson et al., 2001; Walker, 1997).

4. Excessive intravenous (IV) fluids: large amounts of IV fluids (especially with the addition of pitocin) increase the risk of maternal fluid retention, an edematous areola, and an inflated infant birth weight; diuresis of the excess fluid by the infant might be misconstrued as abnormal weight loss (Cotterman, 2004; Merry & Montgomery, 2000; Walker, 2006).

5. Routine episiotomy can be extremely painful for seven to ten days or more, making it difficult to become comfortable (Stainton et al., 1999).

6. Limit the use of/need for instrument-assisted delivery by facilitating more natural birthing positions.

a. Vacuum extraction; increases the risk for intracranial hemorrhage and subdural hematoma, which are serious and can be fatal (FDA,1998; Towner et al., 1999).

i. Infants delivered by vacuum extraction may have impaired suckling reflexes, delaying successful breastfeeding initiation (Hall et al., 2002; Vestermark et al., 1991).

b. Forceps increases the risk for intracranial hemorrhage and subdural hematoma, which are serious and can be fatal.

c. The infant may suffer headaches in the first few days after birth that can be exaggerated by instrument-assisted delivery.

L. Delay, minimize, or eliminate postpartum procedures that interfere with first contact; stress on the neonate from procedures can result in sensory overload and cause the baby to temporarily shut down in order to reorganize his or her nervous system (Karl, 2004).

1. Keep the mother and infant together after birth; separation of the mother and the infant after birth has been shown to interfere with breastfeeding and bonding.

   a. The baby should be allowed to self-attach.

   b. Provide for STS contact (also called *kangaroo care*), with the mother immediately after birth and for the first few hours after birth.

      i. "The most appropriate position for the healthy full term newborn is in close body contact with the mother" (Christensson et al., 1995).

      ii. If contact with the mother is not possible because of cesarean delivery or maternal condition, then STS contact with the father should be provided (Christensson, 1996).

      iii. STS also has been shown to assist preterm infants (34–36 weeks gestation) with recovering from birth-related fatigue (Ludington-Hoe et al., 1999).

      iv. STS contact has been shown to help the infant regulate his or her body temperature (Chiu, Anderson, & Burkhammer, 2005), breathing, and heart rate faster than radiant warmers and incubators.

   c. Babies might be genetically encoded against separation from their mothers (Christensson et al., 1995).

      i. Babies who are separated from their mothers display "separation distress calls" (Michelsson et al., 1996).

      ii. When separated from the mother, a baby's crying occurs in pulses and stops upon reunion.

2. Minimize suctioning.

   a. Bulb and DeLee mucus suctioning of the mouth and/or nares might cause physical injury and/or cause nasal edema and stuffiness, making latch-on and breathing difficult.

   b. Routine suctioning of gastric contents can result in electrolyte imbalances.

   c. Can result in injury to the oropharynx.

   d. Can cause retching.

   e. Can cause physiological changes, such as increased blood pressure and changes in heart rate.

   f. Disrupts pre-feeding behavior or cueing (Widstrom et al., 1987).

g. Might affect the baby's desire to latch on for several days due to pain/injury to the oropharynx; might demonstrate oral defensiveness (AAP, 2005).

3. In situations where intubation, visualization, and deep suctioning of the trachea and bronchial tree below the vocal cords are required due to possible meconium aspiration, suctioning should be done as gently as possible.

4. Bathing should be delayed until after the initial bonding period.
   a. The vernix should be allowed to soak into the skin to lubricate and protect it.
   b. Dry the infant except for the hands and forearms; leave some amniotic fluids on the hands and forearms; amniotic fluid transferred to the breast when the baby is placed STS on the mother's chest might be beneficial for latching-on (Mennella, Jagnow, & Beauchamp, 2001).
   c. Delay bathing to prevent the loss of amniotic fluid odors and thermal losses (with resultant hypoglycemia).

5. Delay giving eye treatments, which can cause blepharospasm (will prevent the infant from opening the eyes); the mother has a high emotional need for eye-to-eye contact with the infant immediately after birth.

6. Delay vitamin K injection until after first contact.

7. Delay painful procedures such as circumcision until the baby has had several good feedings.

II. Clinical Practice Implications

A. First contact should occur as soon as possible after birth, usually within the first hour (AAP, 2005).

1. Mother and baby are in a heightened state of readiness (Riordan, 2005, p.186).

2. Quiet alert state might last up to two hours after birth; following this quiet alert period, the baby might be sleepy and not willing to nurse for as long as 24 hours (Riordan, 2005, p.187).

3. First contact can last as long as 120 minutes.

4. The baby might only lick or nuzzle the breast.

5. The mother might need reassurance if she is concerned because the infant does not breastfeed as vigorously as expected.

B. Physiological effects of first contact.

1. For the human female, the window of time in the first few hours after delivery is the sensitive period for bonding. "Sensitive periods in biologic phenomena are times when events can alter later behaviors" (Lawrence & Lawrence, 2005, p. 201).

2. Maternal hormonal release.
   a. Maternal estrogen, progesterone, oxytocin, and prolactin are believed to be responsible for many mothering behaviors.

   b. Oxytocin.
      i. Induces uterine contractions.
      ii. Helps expel placenta.
      iii. Prevents excessive bleeding.
      iv. Levels are significantly elevated at 15, 30, and 45 minutes post-birth.
      v. Known as the "cuddle hormone" (Lauwers & Swisher, 2005), it has been associated with maternal bonding; thus, it is appropriate to optimize mother-infant interaction at this highest point of oxytocin by facilitating infant suckling (Kennell & Klaus, 1998, p. 8; Lawrence & Lawrence, 2005, p. 249).
      vi. Helps mold maternal behavior. Oxytocin not only participates in a reflex arc to the target myoepithelial cells in the breast, but also disperses into a closed system within the brain, bathing the area that is responsible for social preferences and affiliative behavior.
      vii. Oxytocin deficiency has been reported with epidural block.
      viii. Opiates can inhibit the sucking-induced oxytocin release.
      ix. Morphine administration can significantly reduce the oxytocin response to suckling (Lindow et al., 1999).
      x. Stimulates the release of gastrointestinal (GI) hormones such as insulin, cholecystokinin, somatostatin, and gastrin.
      xi. Causes the mother to feel relaxed or sedated and calmer.
      xii. Increases skin temperature (flushing).
      xiii. Increases thirst.
   c. Prolactin release.
      i. The amount is proportional to the amount of nipple stimulation; prolactin is released in pulses directly related to nipple stimulation.
      ii. Often called "the milk-making hormone."
      iii. Often called the "mothering hormone," it stimulates a feeling of yearning for her baby (Lauwers & Swisher, 2005) and a calming, relaxing, even euphoric effect (Riordan, 2005) during the feeding.
      iv. Release can be inhibited by ergot preparations that are used to control postpartum bleeding.
   d. Other supporting hormones are released: gastrointestinal (19 hormones released by vagal signals alter gut hormones in mother and infant, coordinating their metabolisms (Kennell & Klaus, 1998).

3. Baby's response.
   a. Oxytocin contained in the mother's milk is destroyed in the baby's stomach.
   b. Oxytocin found in neonatal serum is produced by the baby; whether oxytocin has a physiological effect on the neonatal gut or other systems is unknown (Lawrence & Lawrence, 2005).
   c. Prolactin.

          i. Present in milk; might be soothing/calming to the baby.

          ii. Biologically potent and absorbed by the infant; affects intestinal fluid and electrolyte absorption as well as sodium, potassium, and calcium in the newborn (Lawrence & Lawrence, 2005; Riordan, 2005).

    d. Early mother and infant contact helps the baby adapt to the new nonsterile environment by colonizing skin, respiratory, and gastrointestinal tracts with the mother's microorganisms and immunological factors, such as sIgA.

    e. The mother's normal body flora, which tends to be nonpathogenic, will colonize her baby's body, but only if she is the first person to hold him rather than a nurse, physician, or others (Lauwers & Swisher, 2005).

    f. Swallowing causes digestive peristalsis and early passing of the bilirubin-laden meconium stool, reducing neonatal jaundice.

    g. Meconium is the first medium for *lactobacillus bifidus*, which is introduced through colostrum.

C. Early mother-infant contact has emotional effects.

    1. Mother: boosts mothering confidence.

    2. Baby: calms, relaxes, and stops crying.

III. Planning and Implementation

A. For the first feeding immediately after birth, an atmosphere of tranquility is desirable.

B. The role of the lactation consultant and medical providers is one of observant noninterference.

    1. Assist the mother into a comfortable position.

    2. Dry the infant except for his or her hands and forearms; the infant only needs to be clothed in a diaper.

    3. Place the baby near the breast or between the breasts on the mother's bare chest and cover both with a light blanket.

    4. Maternal and neonatal vital signs can be monitored with minimal interruption.

C. Concerns in the immediate postpartum period.

    1. Mother.

      a. Comfort, level of pain.

      b. Effects of medications (narcotics/sedatives).

      c. Epidural effects.

      d. Bleeding often controlled by uterine massage.

        i. Normally done by staff.

        ii. Painful and intrusive.

        iii. Lessens when breastfeeding (see *Oxytocin* above).

      e. Positioning issues.

        i. IV lines can obstruct use of hands and arms.

        ii. Shaking/chills: Cover the mother and baby with a warm blanket, and place the radiant warmer over the mother and baby.

        iii. Unable to change position because of epidural or operative delivery.

     f. Fatigue.

  2. Infant.

     a. Breathing.

     b. Circulation.

     c. Temperature regulation.

        i. Best accomplished by STS contact with the mother.

        ii. Prevent thermal stress on the infant by adjusting the temperature of the birthing room.

        iii. Chilling an infant sets off a cascade of events, from hypothermia to hypoglycemia, tachypnea and mild acidosis, to the extent of requiring a septic workup.

        iv. Hypothermia can be more easily prevented than treated.

D. Recognize the emotional needs of the family unit; provide time for the mother and father to be alone to get acquainted with their newborn.

  1. Hidden cameras in research studies have revealed that some intimate attachment behaviors occur only in complete privacy, including kissing, licking, and tasting the infant.

  2. Keep in mind that bonding comprises the attachment of both the mother and the father to their infant.

  3. Fathers find touching and talking to their newborn babies pleasing and necessary for forming close emotional ties.

E. Allow the baby to take the lead in first contact; it is unnecessary to force the baby to the breast.

  1. Mother and infant can remain in STS contact until they are both ready to nurse.

  2. When the baby begins to show an interest in latching on:

     a. The baby will assume whatever position is natural to him or her.

     b. Provide for the infant's safety.

F. Provide positional support only as needed.

  1. The mother should be encouraged to use the most natural and comfortable position for her.

  2. Give instructions/demonstrations of hand placement and/or positioning only when requested.

  3. Use positive reinforcement and praise the mother's mothering abilities.

  4. Avoid "take over" behaviors (Fletcher & Harris, 2000).

References

American Academy of Pediatrics. Breastfeeding and the use of human milk. *Pediatrics.* 2005;115:496–506. Available at: http://aappolicy.aappublications.org/cgi/content/full/pediatrics;115/2/496. Accessed February 1, 2007.

Berg M, Terstad A. Swedish women's experiences of doula support during childbirth. *Midwifery.* 2006;22:330–338.

Bonaro, D, Pascali MK. Continuous female companionship during childbirth: a crucial resource in times of stress or calm. *J Midwifery Women's Health.* 2004;49(suppl 1): 19–27.

Chiu SH, Anderson GC, Burkhammer MD. Newborn temperature during skin-skin breastfeeding in couples having breastfeeding difficulties. *Birth.* 2005;32:115–121.

Christensson K. Fathers can effectively achieve heat conservation in healthy newborn. *Acta Paediatr.* 1996;85(11):1354–1360

Christensson K, Cabrera T, Christensson E, et al. Separation distress call in the human neonate in the absence of maternal body contact. *Acta Paediatr.* 1995;84:468–473.

Cotterman KJ. Reverse pressure softening: a simple tool to prepare areola for easier latching during engorgement. *J Hum Lact.* 2004;20:227–237.

Dashe JS, Rogers BB, McIntire DD, Leveno KJ. Epidural analgesia and intrapartum fever: placental findings. *Obstet Gynecol.* 1999;93:341–344.

FDA Public Health Warning: Need for caution when using vacuum assisted delivery devices. May 21, 1998. Available at: http://www.fda.gov/cdrh/fetal598.html.

Fletcher D, Harris H. The implementation of the HOT [hands off technique) program at the Royal Women's Hospital. *Breastfeed Rev.* 2000;8:19–23.

Gordon NP, Walton D, McAdam E, et al. Effects of providing hospital-based doulas in health maintenance organization hospitals. *Obstetr Gynecol.* 1999;93:422–426.

Gross JB, Cohen AP, Lang JM, et al. Differences in systemic opioid use do not explain increased fever incidence in patients receiving epidural analgesia. *Anesthesiology.* 2002;97:157–161.

Hall RT, Mercer AM, Teasley SL, et al. A breastfeeding assessment score to evaluate the risk for cessation of breastfeeding by 7 to 10 days of age. *J Pediatr.* 2002;141:659–664.

Karl DJ. Using principles of newborn behavioral state organization to facilitate breastfeeding. *Am J Matern Child Nurs.* 2004;29:292–298.

Kennell J, Klaus M, McGrath S, Robertson S. Continuous emotional support during labor in a U.S. hospital. A randomized controlled trial. *JAMA.* 1991;256:2197–2201.

Kennell JH, Klaus MH. Bonding: recent observations that alter perinatal care. *Pediatr Rev.* 1998;19:4–12.

Langer A, Compero L, Garcia C, Reynoso S. Effects of psychosocial support during labor and childbirth on breastfeeding, medical interventions, and mothers' well-being in a Mexican public hospital: a randomized clinical trial. *Br J Obstet Gynaecol.* 1998;105:1056–1063.

Lauwers J, Swisher A. *Counseling the Nursing Mother: A Lactation Consultant's Guide.* 4th ed. Sudbury, MA: Jones and Bartlett Publishers; 2005.

Lawrence RA, Lawrence RM. *Breastfeeding: A Guide for the Medical Profession.* 6th ed. New York: C.V. Mosby; 2005.

Leighton BL, Halpern SH. The effects of epidural analgesia on labor, maternal, and neonatal outcomes: a systematic review. *Am J Obstet Gynecol.* 2002;186(5 Suppl Nature):S69–S77.

Lieberman E, Eichenwald E, Mathur G, et al. Intrapartum fever and unexplained seizures in term infants. *Pediatrics.* 2000a;106:983–988.

Lieberman E, Lang J, Richardson DK, et al. Intrapartum maternal fever and neonatal outcome. *Pediatrics.* 2000b;105:8–13.

Lieberman E, Lang JM, Frigoletto F Jr, et al. Epidural analgesia, intrapartum fever, and neonatal sepsis evaluation. *Pediatrics.* 1997;99:415–419.

Lieberman E, O'Donoghue C. Unintended effects of epidural analgesia during labor: a systemic review. *Am J Obstet Gynecol.* 2002;186(5 Suppl Nature):531–568.

Lindow SW, Hendricks MS, Nugent FA, et al. Morphine suppresses the oxytocin response in breastfeeding women. *Gynecol Obstet Invest.* 1999;48:33–37.

Ludington-Hoe SM, Anderson GC, Simpson S, et al. Birth-related fatigue in 34–36 week preterm neonates: rapid recovery with very early Kangaroo (Skin-to-Skin) Care. *J Obstet Gynecol Neonatal Nurs.*1999;28:94–103.

Marlier L, Schaal B, Soussignan R. Orientation responses to biological odours in the human newborn. Initial pattern and postnatal plasticity. *C R Acad Sci III.* 1997;320: 999–1005.

Mennella JA, Jagnow CP, Beauchamp GK. Prenatal and postnatal flavor learning by human infants. *Pediatrics.* 2001;107:e88 http://pediatrics.aappublications.org/cgi/content/full/107/6/e88.

Merry H, Montgomery A. Do breastfed babies whose mothers have had labor epidurals lose more weight in the first 24 hours of life? Annual Meeting Abstracts. *Academy of Breastfeeding Medicine News and Views.* 2000;6:21.

Michelsson K, Christensesson K, Rothganger H, Winberg J. Crying in separated and nonseparated newborns: sound spectrographic analysis. *Acta Paediatr.* 1996;85: 471–475.

Mikiel-Kostyra K, Mazur J, Boltruszko I. Effect of early skin-to-skin contact after delivery on duration of breastfeeding: a prospective cohort study. *Acta Paediatr.* 2002;91:1301–1306.

Mohrbacher N, Stock J. *The Breastfeeding Answer Book*, revised edition. Schaumburg, IL: La Leche League International; 2003.

Negishi C, Lenhardt R, Ozaki M, et al. Opioids inhibit febrile responses in humans, whereas epidural analgesia does not: an explanation for hyperthermia during epidural analgesia. *Anesthesiology.* 2001;94:218–222.

Newman J, Pitman T. *Dr. Jack Newman's Guide to Breastfeeding.* Toronto: Harper Collins; 2000.

Perlman JM. Maternal fever and neonatal depression: preliminary observations. *Clin Pediatr.* (Phila) 1999;38:287–291.

Perez PG. Labor support to promote vaginal delivery. *Baby Care Forum*. Spring 1998;1:3.

Petrova A, Demissie K, Rhoads GG, et al. Association of maternal fever during labor with neonatal and infant morbidity and mortality. *Obstet Gynecol*. 2001;98:20–27.

Philip J, Alexander JM, Sharma SK, et al. Epidural analgesia during labor and maternal fever. *Anesthesiology*. 1999;90:1271–1275.

Powers O, Slusser W. Breastfeeding update 2: clinical lactation management. *Pediatr Rev*. 1997;18:147–161.

Ransjo-Arvidson A-B, Matthiesen A-S, Lilja G, et al. Maternal analgesia during labor disturbs newborn behavior: effects on breastfeeding, temperature and crying. *Birth*. 2001;28:5–12.

Righard L, Alade MO. Effect of delivery room routines on success of first breastfeed. *Lancet*. 1990;336:1105–1107.

Riordan J, ed. *Breastfeeding and Human Lactation*. 3rd ed. Sudbury, MA: Jones and Bartlett Publishers; 2005.

Rosen P. Supporting women in labor: analysis of different types of caregivers. *J Midwifery Women's Health*. 2004;49:24–31.

Schaal B, Hummel T, Soussignan R. Olfaction in the fetal and premature infant: functional status and clinical implications. *Clin Perinatol*. 2004;31:261–285, vi–vii.

Sepkoski C, Lester BM, Ostheimer GW, Brazelton TB. Neonatal effects of maternal epidurals. *Dev Med Child Neurol*. 1994;36:375–376.

Stainton C, Edwards S, Jones B, Switonski C. The nature of maternal postnatal pain. *J Perinatal Educ*. 1999;8(2):1–10.

Thureen P, Deacon J, O'Neill P, Hernandez J, eds. *Assessment and Care of the Well Newborn*. Philadelphia: W.B. Saunders Company; 1999.

Towner D, Castro MA, Eby-Wilkins E, Hilbert WM. Effect of mode of delivery in nulliparous women on neonatal intracranial injury. *N Engl J Med*. 1999;341:1709–1714.

Varendi H, Christensson K, Winberg J, Porter RH. Soothing effect of amniotic fluid smell in newborn infants. *Early Hum Dev*. 1998;51:47–55.

Varendi H, Porter RH. Breast odor as the only maternal stimulous elicits crawling towards the odour source. *Acta Paediatr*. 2001;90:372–375.

Vestermark V, Hogdall CK, Birch M, et al. Influence of the mode of delivery on initiation of breast-feeding. *Eur J Obstet Gynecol Reprod Biol*. 1991;38:33–38.

Walker M. *Breastfeeding Management for the Clinician: Using the Evidence*. Sudbury, MA: Jones and Bartlett Publishers; 2006.

Walker M. Do labor medications affect breastfeeding? *J Hum Lact*. 1997;13:131–137.

Widstrom AM, Ransjo-Arvidson AB, Christensson K, et al. Gastric suction in healthy newborn infants. Effects on circulation and developing feeding behaviour. *Acta Paediatr Scand*. 1987;76:566–572.

Suggested Readings

Akre J, ed. *Infant Feeding: The Physiological Basis.* Geneva: World Health Organization; 1989.

Crowell M, Hill P, Humenick S. Relationship between obstetrical analgesia and time to effective breastfeeding. *J Nurs Midwifery.* 1994;39:150–155.

DiGirolamo AM, Grummer-Strawn LM, Fein S. Maternity care practices: implications for breastfeeding. *Birth.* 2001;28:94–100.

Ferber S, Makhoul I. The effect of skin-to skin contact (Kangaroo Care) shortly after birth on the neurobehavioral responses of the term newborn: a randomized, controlled trial. *Pediatrics.* 2004;113:858–856.

Klaus M, Kennell J, Klaus P. *Mothering the Mother.* New York: Addison-Wesley; 1993.

Nelson E, Panksepp J. Brain substrates of infant-mother attachment: contributions of opoids, oxytocin, and norepinephrine. *Neurosci Biobehav Rev.* 1998;22:437–452.

Pinelli J. Non-nutritive sucking for promoting physiologic stability and nutrition in preterm infants. Cochrane Rev Abstract (last amendment 7/17/2005). Available at: http://www.nichd.nih.gov/COCHRANE/Pinelli/PINELLI.HTM. Accessed January 3, 2007.

Righard L, Flodmark CE, Lothe L, Jacobsson I. Breastfeeding patterns: comparing the effects on infant behavior and maternal satisfaction of using one or two breasts. *Birth.* 1993;20:182–185.

Righard L. How do newborns find their mother's breast? *Birth.* 1995;22:174–175.

Riordan J, Auerbach KG, eds. *Breastfeeding and Human Lactation.* 2nd ed. Sudbury, MA: Jones and Bartlett Publishers; 1998.

Riordan J, Riordan S. The effect of labor epidurals on breastfeeding. Lactation Consultant Series Two, Unit 4. Schaumburg, IL: La Leche League International; 2000.

Sinusas K, Gagliardi A. Initial management of breastfeeding. *Am Fam Physician.* 2001;64:981–988, 991–992.

Southall DP, Burr S, Smith RD, et al. The Child Friendly Healthcare Initiative (CFHI): Healthcare Provision in Accordance with the UN Convention on the Rights of the Child. *Pediatrics.* 2000;106:1054–1064.

World Health Organization (WHO). *International Code of Marketing of Breastmilk Substitutes.* Geneva: WHO; May 1981.

BREASTFEEDING A PRETERM INFANT

Mary Grace Lanese, RN, BSN, IBCLC
Melissa Cross, RN, IBCLC
Based on original version by
Ruth Worgan, RN, CM, C&FH, IBCLC
Heather Jackson, RGON, RM, MA, IBCLC

OBJECTIVES

- Understanding problems associated with prematurity and their effects on the establishment of breastfeeding.

- Understanding the nutritional needs of the preterm infant and the importance of human milk.

- List the scientific basis for breastfeeding the preterm infant.

- Describe how maturation influences suckling, swallowing, and breathing coordination and the impact on the preterm infant's ability to breastfeed.

- List characteristics of preterm infants that challenge successful breastfeeding.

- Understand importance of Kangaroo Care to parents, infants, and establishing successful breastfeeding.

- Describe the importance of a developmentally sensitive environment in the intensive care nursery.

- Describe the importance of a discharge feeding plan for the preterm infant.

Introduction

Establishing breastfeeding for a preterm infant can be a challenge. Problems include how to provide adequate nutrients the infant can absorb and utilize in amounts that promote optimal growth and development without causing unnecessary stress to the immature infant. Mother's own breast milk is the most appropriate milk to provide adequate nutrition as well as protection from disease and infections. Infants not fed mother's own breast milk have an increased morbidity and mortality rate in all regions of the world.

Support and appropriate management in establishing and maintaining milk production when the infant is unable to initiate breastfeeding are critical to a successful outcome. The lactation consultant must take into consideration the special needs of the preterm infant and incorporate into these her knowledge of the physiological process of breastfeeding the healthy term infant. Ideally, the lactation consultant will be a member of a multidisciplinary collaborative team that, in addition to parents, also may include nurses, physicians, nutritionists, occupational therapists, massage therapists, social workers, developmental specialists, and discharge planners. Lactation support must be a team effort that is research-based and comprehensive. Breastfeeding the preterm infant requires commitment of maternal time and energy, and nurturing support and compassion from the health care team.

An important factor affecting breastfeeding success is maternal morbidity. Many mothers experience a complicated pregnancy, possibly including illness, prolonged bed rest, and cesarean birth. They also may lack breastfeeding knowledge. Social and economic factors of the parents, and gestational age, weight, and morbidity of the infant are other factors that impact successful breastfeeding. Due to improved technology, the age of viability has improved so that infants of gestational age as early as 23 to 24 weeks are surviving. This situation presents a unique set of hurdles in achieving optimal short-term nutrition and long-term physical and cognitive development. Mothers of preterm infants experience challenges that are unique to the preterm situation in addition to the stress that is involved in a life event that has an uncertain outcome.

I. Definition of a Preterm Infant

A. Birth prior to 37th week of gestation.

B. Weight.

1. Less than 2500 grams is referred to as low birth weight.

2. Less than 1500 grams is referred to as very low birth weight (VLBW).

3. Less than 1250 grams is often referred to as extremely low birth weight (ELBW).

C. Gestational age and weight are assessed together to determine if the infant is small for gestational age as a result of intrauterine growth retardation, appropriate for gestational age, or large for gestational age.

D. Each preterm infant is unique in development and required care; a 35-week preterm infant who was born at 24 weeks is developmentally different from a preterm infant born at 35 weeks.

II. Hospital Obstacles to Breastfeeding the Preterm Infant

A. Inconsistent or incorrect information.

1. Information should be based on research and not personal experience or opinion.

2. Mothers can be confused by the same information being said in different ways; scripting can help.

B. Lack of family-centered developmental care philosophy that actively involves parents in the care of their infant (Huppertze et al., 2005).

C. Lack of private space for nursing or pumping.

D. Lack of proper equipment.

E. Lack of acknowledgment of the value of human milk.

F. Pressure for early discharge.

III. Needs of the Preterm Infant to Facilitate Normal Growth and Development

A. Respiratory rate within normal range and stable.

B. Maintain blood sugar above 2.5 mM/L (> 40 mg/dL).

C. Maintain body temperature within normal range.

D. Adequate nutrition unique to each infant.

   1. The metabolized energy requirement varies according to gestational age, weight, and wellness of the preterm; it can vary from 109 to 140 kcal/kg/day.

   2. Feedings for a 2,000 g and more than 32 weeks at birth preterm infant usually vary only in volume and frequency from the full-term infant.

E. Regular kangaroo care skin-to-skin contact with parents, daily, if possible (Anderson, 2003).

IV. Needs of Mother and Father Who Have a Preterm Infant

A. It is common for the mother of the preterm infant to be ill as a result of complications of the pregnancy or labor. The mother may require special medical considerations.

B. Mothers should be provided with information to make an informed decision regarding breastfeeding and/or providing human milk for their infants.

   1. Withholding information in attempts to avoid making mothers feel guilty if they choose not to breastfeed or provide milk denies women the right to make decisions based on factual information (Miracle, Meier, & Bennett, 2004).

C. Support and education on parenting a preterm infant.

D. Facilitating parental infant care in the nursery.

E. Establishment and maintenance of lactation by regular, frequent milk expression.

   1. Milk expression and breastfeeding can be highly significant for the mother.
      a. These two actions are contributions to the infant's care that only the mother can make.
      b. They represent a normalization of an abnormal event.
      c. Breastfeeding is a caregiving behavior that does not have to be forfeited because of the preterm birth.

F. Maintaining equipment and safe storage of milk.

G. Open visiting/accommodations for parents with their infant.

    1. Parents have a need for close physical contact with their infant, such as early and frequent kangaroo care.

H. Skilled health professionals knowledgeable about breastfeeding management are an important element of the support of the mother in her goal to breastfeed.

    1. The mother and health care team should establish a breastfeeding plan.

    2. Mother's breastfeeding plan should be regularly reviewed to ensure it reflects the infant's current state of development.

I. Mothers have identified five positive outcomes or rewards from their preterm breastfeeding experience and have concluded that the rewards outweigh the efforts (Kavanaugh et al., 1997).

    1. The health benefits of breast milk.

    2. Knowing that they gave their infants the best possible start in life.

    3. Enjoyment of the physical closeness and the perception that their infant preferred breastfeeding to bottle-feeding.

    4. Knowing that they made a unique contribution to the infant's care.

    5. Belief and experience that breastfeeding was more convenient.

V. Lactation Consultants Should Be Familiar with Common Conditions Associated with Prematurity and Their Effects on Breastfeeding

A. Respiratory distress syndrome: severe impairment of respiratory function in a preterm newborn, caused by immaturity of the lungs.

B. Necrotizing enterocolitis (NEC): a potentially fatal inflammation with cell death in the lining of the intestines.

    1. Preterm infants who are fed formula demonstrate a six to ten times greater incidence of NEC compared to preterm infants who are fed breast milk (Lucas & Cole, 1990).

C. Hyperbilirubinemia.

D. Intracranial hemorrhage.

E. Hypoglycemia.

F. Bronchopulmonary dysplasia: iatrogenic chronic lung disease that develops in preterm infants after a period of positive pressure ventilation.

G. The optimal growth of preterm infants.

H. All of the conditions above and their treatments usually result in prolonged separation of the preterm infant and the mother resulting in the delay and/or interruption of breastfeeding.

VI. Advantages of Human Milk for Preterm Infants

A. Mother's own milk is the optimal milk for the preterm infant.

1. Morbidity and mortality rates increase significantly when the infant is not fed human milk (Lucas & Cole, 1990; Schanler, 2001).

2. Preterm infants who are fed human milk accrue immune system enhancement, gastrointestinal (GI) maturation, and nutrient availability (Schanler & Hurst, 1994; Schanler, 2001).

3. If mother's own milk is not available, fortified donor human milk or preterm formula are options.

B. Achievement of greater enteral feeding tolerance and more rapid advancement to full enteral feeds.

1. Physiologic amino acids and fatty acid profiles enhance the digestion and absorption of these nutrients.

2. Low renal solute load.

C. Gastric half emptying time in a formula-fed preterm infant can be up to twice the time of a breast milk-fed infant (51 vs. 25 min; Van den Driessche et al., 1999).

D. Contains active enzymes (such as lipase, amylase, and lysozyme) that are lacking in the underdeveloped intestine or intestinal system and provide trophic factors that hasten the maturation of the preterm intestinal system (Lawrence & Lawrence, 2005).

E. Reduced risk of allergy in atopic families (AAP, 2005; Saarinen & Kajosaari, 1995).

F. Weight gain of not only fat and water, but also bone and other tissue.

G. Optimal development of visual acuity and retinal health.

1. Retinopathy of prematurity found to be 2.3 times higher in formula-fed preterm infants (Hylander et al., 2001; Jorgensen et al., 1996).

H. Cognitive and neurodevelopmental outcomes are enhanced, with preterm infants who have been fed breast milk showing higher IQs.

1. Long-chain polyunsaturated fatty acids present in breast milk but not in many formulas are considered to be closely linked to this outcome (Lucas et al., 1992; Vohr et al., 2006).

I. Protection from environmental pathogens.

1. Particularly important in a special care nursery with invasive treatments and many staff members handling the infant.

J. Preterm human milk is optimally suited to the maturation of systems, immunological requirements, and growth of the preterm infant.

VII. Components of Preterm Human Milk

A. According to Gross et al. (1980), differences and changes exist in preterm breast milk compared to full-term breast milk. Preterm milk has higher concentrations of calories, lipids, high nitrogen protein, sodium, chloride, potassium, iron, and magnesium.

B. Calcium and phosphorus are the most commonly lacking macrominerals (Polberger & Lonnerdal, 1993).

C. The addition of extra nutrients, vitamins, and minerals is needed by the VLBW infant.

D. Preterm human milk is optimal for the preterm infant due to his or her limited renal concentration and diluting capacities, a large surface area in relation to weight, and to insensible water loss.

E. The milk of mothers of preterm infants matures to the level of term milk at about four to six weeks.

F. Preterm milk might not meet all nutritional needs of the growing preterm infant, and caloric intake might be inadequate for growth (particularly in preterm infants who are born under 30 weeks gestation and/or are born at less than 2.5 kg), so fortification of mother's milk may be necessary (Schanler, 1996).

VIII. Nutritional Consideration and Optimal Growth of Preterm

A. Optimal growth is typically based on the growth curve that would have been followed if the preterm infant had remained in utero.

1. This target can be achieved more easily in infants who have higher gestational ages.

2. The ELBW infant has a high energy requirement but limited volume tolerance, so intake may be restricted.

B. Early enteral feedings of breast milk before the infant is actually ready to be fed by mouth are sometimes used to prime the gut.

1. These are variously referred to as trickle feeds, trophic feeds, or GI priming feeds: 0.5–1 mL bolus via nasogastric tube every 3 or 6 hours (McClure & Newell, 2000).

2. These are based on the concept that GI hormones are absent in the gut of infants who have never been fed.

3. Trophic feeds facilitate protective gut flora, improve bowel emptying of meconium, and decrease morbidity and mortality from NEC.

4. More mature motor patterns in the gut are seen with these small feeds (Schanler, Schulman et al., 1999a).

5. If infusion pumps are used for feeding, the syringe should be tilted upward at a 25- to 45-degree angle so that the lipids rise to the Leur of the syringe and are infused first.

C. Many guidelines for the progression of preterm infant feeding exist throughout the world.

1. Practices depend on the level and availability of technology within each country and within each individual nursery.

2. Many nurseries are implementing Kangaroo Care, which reduces or changes the need for extensive policies for initiating and maintaining breastfeeding in the preterm infant.

IX. Fortification of Human Milk

A. Human milk can be fortified with commercial fortifiers that include cow's milk-based protein, electrolytes, and a number of vitamins and minerals (Schanler, 1996).

B. Human milk can be fortified with specific nutrients, such as calcium and phosphorus.

C. Fortification is usually begun after full feeding is established and discontinued before discharge from the intensive or special care unit.

D. Using the hindmilk portion of expressed milk (lacto-engineering) as a concentrated source of lipids provides a high calorie, low volume, low osmolaric, readily absorbable supplement (Kirsten & Bradford, 1999).

E. Hindmilk and commercial fortifiers are used for different purposes.

1. Commercial fortifiers are used to supplement essential nutrients.

2. Hindmilk provides a concentrated source of lipids and calories.

F. "Lacto-engineering" can further refine and tailor the milk to a specific infant's needs (Meier & Brown, 1996).

G. The lipid and caloric content of breast milk can be estimated by creamatocrit (Griffin et al., 2000).

1. Creamatocrit is determined by centrifuging a small milk specimen in a capillary tube, separating the lipid portion, and then measuring the content as a percentage of total milk volume (Meier & Brown, 1996).

X. Issues Associated with Fortification of Human Milk

A. Significantly lower gastric emptying times and, therefore, implications for feeding intolerance (Ewer & Yu, 1996).

B. Neutralizing effect of some of the anti-infective (lactoferrin) properties of human milk (Quan et al., 1994).

C. May increase the risk of infection.

D. Incomplete absorption of additives such as medium chain triglyceride oil.

E. Increased osmolarity of fortified milk increasing the morbidity from GI disease.

F. Some nutrient loss can occur through enteral feeding tubes.

   1. Lipids can adhere to the lumen of a feeding tube and not reach the infant; this is more common when giving continuous enteral feeds.

   2. The greatest lipid losses occur with continuous slow infusions; therefore, bolus feedings (intermittent gavage) are recommended when possible.

G. Fortification might influence short-term outcomes (such as weight gain and bone mineralization) but long-term growth and development outcomes have not been shown to be enhanced (Lucas et al., 1999).

   1. Bone mineral content of 8- to 12-year-old children who are born preterm and are fed breast milk is as high or higher than children who are born at term (Lucas et al., 1999).

H. The use of powdered fortifiers is controversial and requires surveillance and additional research (Schanler, 1996).

   1. Powdered fortifiers and preterm formulas are not sterile.

   2. The U.S. Food and Drug Administration and European Food Safety Authority have issued guidelines stating that powdered formulas should not be used in preterm or immunocompromised infants.

   3. There is no evidence that the use of powdered fortifiers in the special or intensive care unit has caused an increased infection rate.

I. An alternative for powdered fortification is the use of liquid fortifiers.

   1. Often used in a 1:1 ratio with human milk, resulting in a reduction of the milk intake.

   2. May be used when the volume of available human milk is inadequate.

J. It has been reported that some centers are using fortified pasteurized donor human milk.

XI. Scientific Basis for Breastfeeding a Preterm Infant

A. No scientific evidence justifies delaying or discouraging the initiation of breastfeeding preterm infants because the infant is unable to bottle-feed.

   1. Strong evidence shows that delaying initiation of direct breastfeeding until after hospital discharge or discouraging it completely leads to premature weaning and/or suboptimal breast milk intake (Buckley & Charles, 2006; Callen et al., 2005).

   2. Until recently, it was widely assumed that breastfeeding was more tiring and bottle-feeding was less work; consequently, preterm infants were required to

demonstrate the ability to consistently bottle-feed before being introduced to breastfeeding.

3. Prolonged bottle-feeding in the absence of breastfeeding frequently leads to feeding patterns that do not transfer well to the breast.

4. Early breastfeeding has been shown to be less stressful to a preterm infant than bottle-feeding (Meier & Anderson, 1987).

5. Bottle-feeding has been shown to produce adverse and undesirable physiologic and biochemical changes in small infants, including: hypoxia, apnea, bradycardia, oxygen desaturation, hypercarbia, reduced minute and tidal volume hypothermia, and irregular breathing frequency (Chen et al., 2000).

6. Bottle-feeding when a mother's goal is to breastfeed undermines her efforts at expressing and supplying her breast milk for her infant.

XII. Maturation and Influences on Sucking, Swallowing, and Breathing Coordination

A. The ability of an infant to breastfeed depends on the suck, swallow, and breathing coordination of the innate reflexes.

1. Esophageal peristalsis and swallowing have been seen in the fetus as early as 11 weeks of gestation.

2. Sucking has been described between 18 and 24 weeks.

3. Lactase, a brush border intestinal enzyme that digests lactose, is present at 24 weeks.

4. Lingual and gastric lipases are detectable at 26 weeks.

5. The gag reflex is seen in preterm infants at 26 to 27 weeks.

6. Rooting is seen around 32 weeks.

7. The coordination of suck, swallow, and breathe actions is seen at 32 to 35 weeks.

8. Some infants as young as 28 weeks are able to lick expressed milk from the mother's nipple.

9. At 28 to 30 weeks, some oral feeding might be possible at the breast.

10. From 32 to 34 weeks, some infants might be able to take a complete breastfeed once or twice a day (Wolf & Glass, 1992).

11. From 35 weeks onward, efficient breastfeeding that maintains adequate growth is possible (Wolf & Glass, 1992).

12. Some characteristics of preterm infants that challenge successful breastfeeding.
    a. Weak, immature, disorganized suck.
    b. A lack of coordination between sucking, swallowing, and breathing.
    c. Diminished stamina.
    d. Low muscle tone.

13. Immature suck pattern.
    a. Three to five sucks per burst.
    b. A pause of equal duration, often detaching from the breast.

14. Transitional suck pattern (Palmer, 1993).
    a. Six to ten sucks per burst.
    b. A pause of equal duration with occasional detaching.
    c. An apneic episode can follow longer suck bursts.

15. Mature suck pattern.
    a. Ten to thirty sucks per burst.
    b. Brief pauses.
    c. Suck/swallow in a 1:1 ratio.

16. Disorganized sucking is a lack of rhythm of the total sucking activity.

17. Dysfunctional sucking is the interruption of the feeding process by abnormal movements of the tongue and jaw.

B. Non-nutritive sucking (sucking without significant intake of milk).

1. Some characteristics.
   a. Can be observed from 18 weeks gestation.
   b. Rate of two sucks per second.
   c. Weak, uncoordinated flutter sucking.
   d. Absence of swallow.

2. Advantages.
   a. Reduces the length of hospital stay (Schanler, Hurst, & Lau, 1999).
   b. When the infant is provided non-nutritive sucking opportunities during gavage feedings, the infant associates the act of sucking with the pleasurable feeling of a full stomach.
   c. Non-nutritive sucking opportunities are sometimes provided by the mother's softened, drained breast or a pacifier.

3. When possible, it is advantageous for non-nutritive sucking to occur at the mother's "empty" breast during gavage feeding.
   a. To avoid imprinting on an artificial nipple.
   b. To begin developing early breastfeeding skills (suck, swallow, and breathe coordination).
   c. To increase maternal milk production.
   d. To increase maternal involvement in infant care.

XIII. Kangaroo Care

A. Can begin when infant is stable, but still intubated (Gale, Franck, & Lund, 1993).

B. Infant and parent maintain skin-to-skin contact.

    1. Infant is naked except for diaper.

    2. Infant is held mostly upright and snuggled between mother's breasts or against father's bare chest.

    3. Infant's back is covered.
        a. Inside parent's shirt.
        b. With parent's hand.
        c. With clothing.
        d. With a blanket.

C. Benefits of kangaroo care to infant (Anderson, 2003; WHO, 2003).

    1. Stable heart rate (de Leeuw et al., 1991; Ludington-Hoe et al., 2004).

    2. More regular breathing.
        a. A 75% decrease in apneic episodes (de Leeuw et al., 1991; Ludington-Hoe et al., 2004).

    3. Improved oxygen saturation levels (Acolet, Sleath, & Whitelaw, 1989).

    4. No cold stress, that is, there are more stable temperatures (Acolet et al., 1989).

    5. Longer periods of sleep (Ludington-Hoe & Kasper, 1995).

    6. More rapid weight gain (Charpak et al., 2001).

    7. Less caloric expenditures (Ludington-Hoe & Kasper, 1995).

    8. More rapid brain development (Feldman et al., 2002).

    9. Reduction of "purposeless" activity (flailing of arms and legs).

    10. Decreased crying (Ludington-Hoe, Cong, & Hashemi, 2002).

    11. Longer periods of alertness.

    12. More successful breastfeeding episodes (Whitlaw et al., 1988).

    13. Increased breastfeeding duration (Hurst et al., 1997; Whitlaw et al., 1988).

    14. Earlier hospital discharge (Charpak et al., 2001).

D. Benefits of kangaroo care to parents (WHO, 2003).

    1. Increased bonding due to increased serum oxytocin levels (Uvnas-Moberg & Eriksonn, 1996).

    2. Promotes confidence in the parents' caregiving (Affonso, Wahlberg, & Persson, 1989).

    3. Parents feel more in control.

    4. Relief of parental stress over having an infant in the intensive care nursery (Boyd, 2004).

    5. Increased maternal milk production (Whitlaw et al., 1988).

    6. Significantly reduced cost due to decreased length of stay (Charpak et al., 2001).

    7. Earlier discharge from hospital.

E. Early breastfeeding practice can be a component of kangaroo care, with skin-to-skin care gradually transitioning to breastfeeding (Anderson, 2003; WHO, 2003).

XIV. Developmental Care

A. Neonatal individualized developmental care can be incorporated into practice in all intensive or special care nurseries.

    1. It is based on the positive development of the five senses: sight, hearing, taste, touch, and smell (Als et al., 2004).

B. Some benefits of a developmentally sensitive environment include:

    1. Greater parental involvement and nurturing care.

    2. More time for adequate rest for infant, which promotes brain development.

    3. Prevention of overstimulation.
       a. Reduced heart rate.
       b. Reduced need for oxygen.

    4. Earlier removal from ventilator.

    5. Earlier initiation of breastfeeding.

    6. Better weight gain (Charpak et al., 2001; Ludington-Hoe & Swinth, 1996).

    7. Reduction in rates of infection (Charpak et al., 2001).

    8. Shorter hospital stays (Charpak et al., 2001).

    9. Improved medical outcomes (Ludington-Hoe et al., 1994).

C. Some examples of an environmentally sensitive special care nursery are:

    1. Lights below 60 foot candles (Committee to Establish Recommended Standards for Newborn ICU Design, 1999).

    2. Blanket-covering isolette low enough to protect eyes.

    3. Day and night rhythmicity (Mirmiran & Arigagno, 2000).

    4. Cluster care across disciplines allowing for longer sleep periods.

    5. Control noise levels.
       a. Less than 50 decibels (AAP, 1997; AAP/ACOG, 2002).
       b. Voices level, particularly at shift change.
       c. Ensure quiet trash removal.
       d. Ensure quiet closing of isolette doors.
       e. Ensure quiet monitor/vent alarms.
       f. Ensure that telephone rings are not disruptive.

6. Positioning infant to promote feelings of security (that is, side and foot rolls to provide borders for infant to lie or push against).

7. Hand containment.
   a. Gentle pressure on infant's back or chest with opened hand helps infant to organize him- or herself.

8. Support infant with blankets and rolls while supine or prone.

9. Midline flexion and containment.

10. Provide boundaries.

11. When infant is lying prone, wet fist with breast milk and position it near nose and mouth (Sullivan & Toubas, 1998).

12. Use of breast milk for oral care helps the infant identify his or her mother's smell and the taste of her milk.

13. Preterm infants have a keen sense of smell and usually respond to human milk by extending the tongue to taste milk and then opening mouth.
   a. Once infant is comfortably positioned at the breast, the mother can express a drop of milk that remains on the tip of her nipple for the infant to smell and then taste.
   b. Preterm infants are slow to respond to stimuli, so the mother should be patient.

14. Sucking pressures are lower in preterm infants, increasing the difficulty in transferring milk.
   a. Goal of early feedings is to allow the infant to gradually increase breastfeeding skill and stamina, which will come with time and patience.
   b. Focusing on weight or milk transfer too early will undermine mother's confidence and put breastfeeding at risk.

15. Breastfeeding is a developmental skill and will happen when an infant is neurobehaviorally ready.

16. Encourage continual skin-to-skin/kangaroo care when mother/parents are present.

17. Appropriate pain management.

18. Massage therapy (Als et al., 2004; Lindrea & Stainton, 2000).

XV. Readiness to Breastfeed

A. Readiness to breastfeed depends on the individual infant's cues.

1. There are no universally agreed-upon criteria for when to initiate feedings at the breast.

2. Traditionally, infants needed to be of a certain weight or gestational age before attempts were made at the breast; these criteria had no scientific basis.

3. The literature supports the observations that infants vary considerably in ability to consume measurable amounts of milk at the breast and require an individualized approach to initial feeding readiness.

4. The transition to the breast can be gradual, with daily kangaroo care advancing to limited periods of sucking on a partially drained breast.

5. There are numerous protocols used to transition the infant to the breast; while some use bottles in the absence of the mother, many protocols currently use gavage feeding or cup feeding in the mother's absence (Kliethermas et al., 1999; Lang, Lawrence, & Orme, 1994; Valentine and Hurst, 1995;).

B. Positions for breastfeeding the preterm infant.

1. The preterm infant's head is heavy in relation to the weak neck musculature that is supposed to support it.
   a. Failure to provide suitable head and jaw stability can result in the infant not effectively latching onto the breast, tiring too quickly, biting the nipple to maintain latch, or frequently slipping off the breast.
   b. The preterm infant usually breastfeeds in positions that provide extra support for the head and torso.

2. Two positions that work well with the preterm are the cross-cradle hold and the football hold.

3. In order to bring the chin into the breast first, the head can be supported by the mother's fingers and the shoulders by the palm of her hand, giving support to the infant's head, neck, and torso, but not bringing the nose in first.
   a. Bringing the chin in first when the infant opens his mouth increases the success of effective latch. The breast is then well supported with the mother's opposite hand in a U hold, being careful to push into the breast, rather than pinch the fingers together (Figure 26-1).
   b. It is helpful to hold the breast throughout the feeding so that there is less stress and weight on the infant's jaw.
   c. The preterm infant might have difficulty opening his or her mouth wide enough to latch properly.

4. The infant's entire head can be encircled by the mother's hand, or she can use the Dancer hand position for jaw stability.
   a. This position may be particularly helpful with larger preterm infants and neurologically impaired infants, but less so when breastfeeding the small preterm (see Chapter 35).

C. Intake of milk while breastfeeding.

1. Intake can be estimated by the use of pre- and post-feed weights (also known as test weights) if accuracy is paramount. Pre- and post-feed weights are helpful in situations where decisions must be made regarding the amounts of

Figure 26-1 Position for breastfeeding the preterm infant. *Source:* Used with permission.

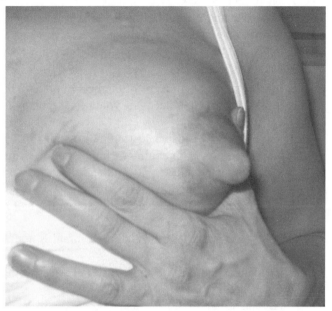

supplement, determination of milk transfer problems, or simple reassurance to the mother or staff (Meier et al., 1996).

2. Mother's milk supply also plays a part in assessing infant intake.
   a. When determining amount of supplement needed, it is helpful to know status of mother's milk supply.
   b. Low milk supply dictates greater amount of supplement.

3. Daily weights or weights every second day are used as the infant begins taking more milk at the breast and the supplement is decreased.

4. Preterm infants often do not demonstrate a predictable, cue-based feeding pattern until close to their corrected term age.

5. Intake-related problems can also be helped by the use of a tube feeding device at the breast that delivers additional milk as the infant suckles at the breast (see Chapter 31).

6. Indications for use of a tube feeding device at the breast.
   a. An infant who latches on to the breast but exerts low sucking pressures.
   b. Lack of sucking rhythm.
   c. Mother's request to supplement at breast.
   d. Mother who has a limited milk supply.
   e. Impaired milk ejection reflex.

7. When limited intake is a result of the infant's inability to draw in enough of the nipple/areola (or if the areola is puffy or the nipple very large in relation to the infant's mouth), a thin nipple shield has been successfully used on a temporary basis until the infant is capable of forming a teat by him- or herself (Meier et al., 2000).

8. One of the major concerns of mothers of preterm infants relates to whether the infant is consuming adequate volumes of milk by breastfeeding (Kavanaugh et al., 1995).
   a. Milk transfer is dependent on milk supply, milk ejection, and infant sucking.
      i. If sucking is immature, then interventions can be targeted toward optimizing milk production and milk ejection in order to compensate for weak or immature sucking patterns.
      ii. The infant should thoroughly soften the first breast before being placed on the other side.
   b. Mothers might perceive that their infant is not taking the majority of the milk available.
   c. Infants might slip off the breast, fall asleep at the breast, or simply stop feeding.
   d. Immature feeding patterns are gradually replaced with more mature patterns as the infant nears his or her term-corrected age.

XVI. Establishing Full Breastfeeding

A. Phase one: Initiate lactation by the expression and collection of breast milk.

1. Lactation should be initiated with a breast pump as early as possible following delivery.

2. Hand expression can be used effectively where mechanical expression is not practical or possible.

3. Mothers should plan to pump, or hand express, 8 to 12 times each 24 hours for the first 7 to 10 days for optimal milk yield. This plan might change to fewer sessions if the level of production is maintained.

4. This plan should yield 800 to 1000 mL of milk daily by day 7 to 10.

5. An abundant milk supply at this point greatly reduces the risk of insufficient milk later (Hill et al., 2005).

6. A 50% breast milk over-supply provides a cushion.
   a. If the milk production drops for any reason, saved milk can be fractionated to provide hindmilk supplements.
   b. An oversupply aids the infant with an easy flow of milk from a full breast.

7. Mothers might find that massaging and compressing each breast during expression contributes to increased milk yields, more thorough draining of the breast, and higher fat content of the expressed milk (Foda et al., 2004).

8. Mothers should plan to use a hospital-grade electric breast pump with double collection kits, if available (see Chapter 30).

9. Simultaneous milk pumping can increase prolactin levels, increase milk yield, and reduce the time spent pumping.

10. Mother's milk should be fed to preterm infants immediately after it is pumped, when possible. Fresh breast milk is preferable for preterm infants (Jones & Tully, 2006).

11. Previously frozen colostrum can be given first before fresh breast milk if the infant cannot be fed enterally for the first few days.
    a. Colostrum coats the immature porous intestine and reduces the absorption of harmful bacteria and food antigens.

12. Fresh breast milk can be refrigerated 24 to 48 hours before use (Jones & Tully, 2006).

13. Breast milk can be frozen for later use; it should be used in the order it was expressed. Frozen milk can be used up to 24 hours after thawing.

14. Low milk volume is a common problem, especially if the infant cannot come to the breast for several weeks or if the infant was born extremely early; a number of possible interventions have proven helpful (Clavey, 1996).
    a. Frequent kangaroo care.
    b. Encourage the infant to suckle at the emptied breast; pump during or right after skin-to-skin contact (Ehrenkranz & Ackerman, 1986).
    c. Pump at the infant's bedside.
    d. Medications may increase milk supply in some mothers.
        i. Metoclopramide (Budd et al., 1993).
        ii. Domperidone (motilium; da Silva et al., 2001).
        iii. The use of oxytocin nasal spray has been used to stimulate the milk ejection reflex (Ruis et al., 1981). However, a recent randomized, controlled trial (Fewtrell et al., 2006) showed no significant difference in milk collection with the use of oxytocin nasal spray.
    e. Acupuncture (Clavey, 1996).
    f. Human growth hormone (Gunn et al., 1996).
        i. Shown to increase breast milk volume with no adverse effects seen in mothers or infants.
        ii. Not widely used due to expense.

B. Phase two: Introduction of the infant to the breast.

1. Will require continued gavage feedings of expressed breast milk in the beginning.

2. Maintenance of milk supply by expression.

3. Scheduled feeds every three hours are typically required until the infant is mature enough to begin cue-based feeding.

4. Cue-based feeding frequency may gradually increase to every two hours (Saunders, Friedman, & Stramoski, 1991).

5. Combination of breastfeeds and supplemental feedings until mature enough to sustain all feeding at the breast.

C. Phase three: Optimizing early feedings.

1. Optimal positioning and attachment of the infant.
   a. Football (clutch) hold, cross-cradle hold, and use of the Dancer hand position with larger preterm infants.

2. Continue frequent kangaroo care.

D. Phase four: Transition to full cue-based breastfeeding.

1. Health care team will assess the readiness to breastfeed.

2. Will occur over time with most infants able to achieve cue-based feeding by the time they are term equivalent.

3. Infant shows signs of demand sucking.

4. Able to sustain full breastfeeding on demand and gain adequate weight.

5. Awake and alert at feeding times.

6. Sucking on fist.

7. Mouthing.

8. Able to sustain a full breastfeed.

9. Stamina to fully breastfeed on demand and gain adequate weight.

E. Several sample feeding protocols have been published.

1. Feeding regimens.
   a. Six-step feeding strategy for preterm infants (Valentine & Hurst, 1995).
      i. Infants begin 10 to 20 mL/kg/day of expressed breast milk (oral-gastric, bolus, or continuous drip by using an automated syringe pump) and are progressed daily at the same rate (if tolerated) to the goal of 150 mL/kg/day of expressed breast milk. During this time period, infants are transitioning off parenteral nutrition.
      ii. Once the infant is receiving 150 mL/kg/day, a powdered human milk fortifier is added at two packets per 100 mL of mother's milk; after 24 hours of tolerance, this amount is increased to four packets per 100 mL of mother's milk.
      iii. If infant growth falters (less than 15 g/kg/day), then the volume of fortified human milk is increased to 160 to 180 mL/kg/day. Other clinical factors associated with slow growth are first ruled out (for example, acidosis or anemia).

iv. If growth remains < 15 g/kg/day, use fortified hindmilk at 180 mL/kg/day and fortify as above.

v. If growth falters, the infants are supplemented with corn oil 0.5 mL every three hours given as a bolus rather than mixed with the milk.

vi. If growth falters, four feedings are replaced with premature formula, and four fortified breast milk feeds are continued.

2. Transition to breastfeeding.

a. Breastfeeding the preterm newborn: a protocol without bottles (Stine, 1990).

i. Gavage feeding until the infant is in stable condition and can tolerate short periods outside the isolette.

ii. Practice sessions at the breast followed by gavage feeding.

iii. When the infant consistently latches on during maternal visits, feeds with swallowing for five minutes, and demonstrates steady weight gain, the amount of supplement should be based on observations of feeding at the breast.

iv. Supplemental milk is given by a nasogastric tube as needed. None is given if the infant breastfed well for five minutes with swallowing.

v. Half the usual volume is given if the infant breastfed for less than five minutes.

vi. The full amount of supplement is given if the infant did not breastfeed.

b. Transitioning preterm infants with nasogastric tube supplementation: increased likelihood of breastfeeding (Kliethermas et al., 1999).

i. Supplementation provided through an indwelling #3.5 French nasogastric tube when the mother was not available to breastfeed or if additional supplemental feedings were required.

ii. Daily weights, with supplements reduced gradually as the infant consistently met or surpassed the expected weight gain of 20 to 30 g/day.

iii. Nasogastric tube removed 24 to 48 hours prior to discharge with supplements given if needed by cup.

iv. Definitions of latch and breastfeeding abilities.
Breastfeeds well.
(1) Good latch-on with a wide-open mouth and lips flanged.
(2) Areola drawn in with sucking.
(3) Tongue is down and cupped; infant retains a vacuum when the forehead is gently pushed away from the breast.
(4) No dimpling of infant's cheeks.
(5) Long draws with rhythmical sucking and audible swallowing.
(6) Mother requires minimal help with positioning and latch-on.
(7) Breastfeeding is greater than or equal to five to eight minutes.
Breastfeeds fairly.
(1) Occasional latch-on.

(2) Short sucks, fewer long draws, infrequent audible swallowing, mother requires help with positioning.

(3) Time of active suckling is less than five minutes.

Breastfeeds poorly

(1) Some rooting or licking movements.

(2) No latch-on.

(3) Mother requires assistance with positioning.

XVII. Discharge Planning

A. Parents require a detailed plan of caring/parenting their preterm infant after discharge with support and encouragement for ongoing care and information should include the following (Academy of Breastfeeding Medicine Protocol No. 12):

1. Signs that the infant is getting enough breast milk; weight checks; pre- and post-feed weights if necessary; diaper counts of wet diapers and bowel movements.

2. Expected feeding patterns; at least eight feeds per 24 hours with only one prolonged sleep period of up to five hours, maximum; cues that indicate the infant is ready to feed.

3. Continued use of a breast pump until the infant is fully established at the breast, with adequate weight gain and no need for supplemental feedings.
   a. Mothers usually need to continue using the breast pump after the infant has been discharged; pumping might be needed after each feeding or only a few times each day, depending on the number of supplemental feedings.
   b. Experts recommend that the mother produce about 50% more milk than the infant needs at discharge because the increased volume helps the milk flow freely in the presence of a weaker suck.

4. Proper use of supplemental feeding devices, when appropriate.
   a. Cup.
   b. Feeding tube at breast.
   c. Supervision of the use of a nipple shield.
   d. Close follow-up should continue as progress is made toward full breastfeeding.

5. If parents choose to bottle-feed human milk during the infant's hospitalization, the lactation consultant can help transition the infant to the breast before or after discharge.

6. The lactation consultant should conduct post discharge telephone follow-up (Elliott & Reimer, 1998).

B. Parents should be provided information about the availability of support services.

1. Primary health care provider.

2. International Board Certified Lactation Consultant.

3. Health professional who has expertise in breastfeeding preterm infants (that is, specially trained midwives, doulas and peer counselors; Elliott & Reimer, 1998).

4. Community support groups.

5. Social services.

6. La Leche League.

7. Women, Infants, and Children Program (in the United States).

References

Academy of Breastfeeding Medicine: Clinical Protocol No 12: Transitioning the breastfeeding/breast milk-fed premature infant from neonatal intensive care unit to home. Available (under "Protocols") at: http://www.bfmed.org. Accessed January 5, 2007.

Acolet D, Sleath K, Whitelaw A. Oxygenation, heart rate and temperature in very low birthweight infants during skin-to-skin contact with their mothers. *Acta Paediatr Scand.* 1989;78:189–193.

Affonso D, Wahlberg V, Persson V. Exploration of mother's reactions to the kangaroo method of prematurity care. *Neonatal Netw.* 1989;7:43–51.

Als H, Duffy FH, McAnulty GB, et al. Early experience alters brain function and structure. *Pediatrics.* 2004;114:1738–1739.

American Academy of Pediatrics (AAP). Noise: a hazard for the fetus and newborn. *Pediatrics.* 1997;100:724–727.

American Academy of Pediatrics (AAP). Policy Statement, Breast feeding and the use of human milk. *Pediatrics.* 2005;115;496–506.

American Academy of Pediatrics and American College of Obstetricians and Gynecologists. *Guidelines for Perinatal Care.* 5th ed. Elk Grove Village, IL; AAP, ACOG; 2002.

Anderson GC. Mother-newborn contact in a randomized trial of kangaroo (skin-to-skin) care. *J Obstet Gynecol Neonatal Nurs.* 2003;2:604–611.

Boyd S. Within these walls: moderating parental stress in the neonatal intensive care unit. *J Neonatal Nurs.* 2004;10:80–84.

Buckley K, Charles GE. Benefits and challenges to transitioning preterm infants to at-breast feeding. *Int Breastfeed J.* 2006;1:13.

Budd SC, Erdman SH, Long DM, Trombley SK, Udall JN Jr. Improved lactation with Metoclopramide, as case report. *Clin Pediatr.* (Phila) 1993;32:53–57.

Callen J, Pinelli J, Atkinson S, Saigal S. Qualitative analysis of barriers to breastfeeding in very low birth weight infants in the hospital and post discharge. *Adv Neonatal Care.* 2005;5:93–103.

Charpak N, Ruiz-Pelaez JG, Figueroa de CZ, Charpak Y. A randomized, controlled trial of kangaroo mother care: results of a follow-up at one year of corrected age. *Pediatrics.* 2001;108:1072–1079.

Chen C-H, Wang T-M, Chang H-M, Chi C-S. The effect of breast- and bottle-feeding on oxygen saturation and body temperature in preterm infants. *J Hum Lact.* 2000;16: 21–27.

Clavey S. The use of acupuncture for the treatment of insufficient lactation. *Am J Acupunct.* 1996;24:35–46.

Committee to Establish Recommended Standards for Newborn ICU Design. Recommended standards for newborn ICU design small. *J Perinatol.* 1999;19: S1–S12.

da Silva OP, Knopport DC, Angelini MM, Forret PA. Effect of domperidone on milk production in mothers of premature newborns; a randomized, double-blind, placebo-controlled trial. *CMAJ.* 2001;164:17–21.

De Leeuw R, Collin EM, Dunnebbier EA, Mirmiran M. Physiologic effects of kangaroo care in very small preterm infants. *Biol Neonate.* 1991;59:149–155.

Ehrenkranz RA, Ackerman BA. Metoclopramide effect on faltering milk production by mothers of premature infants. *Pediatrics.* 1986;78:614–620.

Elliott S, Reimer C. Postdischarge telephone follow-up program for breastfeeding preterm infants discharged from a special care nursery. *Neonatal Netw.* 1998;17: 41–45.

Ewer AK, Yu VYH. Gastric emptying in preterm infants: the effect of breast milk fortifier. *Acta Paediatr.* 1996;85:1112–1115.

Feldman R, Eidelman A, Sirota L, Weller A. Comparison of skin-to-skin (Kangaroo) and traditional care: parenting outcomes and preterm infant development. *Pediatrics.* 2002;110:16–26.

Fewtrell MS, Loh KL, Blake A, et al. Randomised, double blind trial of oxytocin nasal spray in mothers expressing breast milk for preterm infants. *Arch Dis Child Fetal Neonatal Ed.* 2006;91:F169–F174.

Foda, MI, Kawashima T, Nakamura S, et al. Composition of milk obtained from unmassaged versus massaged breasts of lactating mothers. *J Pediatr Gastroenterol Nutr.* 2004;38:477–478.

Gale G, Franck L, Lund C. Skin-to-skin (Kangaroo) holding of the intubated premature infant. *Neonatal Netw.* 1993;12:49–57.

Griffin TL, Meier PP, Bradford LP, et al. Mother's performing creamatocrit measures in the NICU: Accuracy, reactions, and cost. *J Obstet Gynecol Neonatal Nurs.* 2000;29: 249–257.

Gross SJ, David RJ, Bauman L, et al. Nutritional composition of milk from mothers delivering preterm and at term. *J Pediatr.* 1980;96:641–644.

Gunn AJ, Gunn TR, Rabone DL, et al. Growth hormone increases breast milk volumes in mothers of preterm infants. *Pediatrics.* 1996;98:279–282.

Hill PD, Aldag JC, Chatterton RT, Zinamann M. Primary and secondary mediators' influence on milk output in lactating mothers and preterm infants. *J Hum Lact.* 2005;21:138–150.

Huppertze C, Gharavi B, Schott C, Linderkamp O. Individual development care based on Newborn Individualized Developmental Care and Assessment Program (NIDCAP). *Kinderkrankenschwester.* 2005;9:359–364.

Hurst NM, Valentine CJ, Renfro L, et al. Skin-to-skin holding in the neonatal intensive care unit influences maternal milk volume. *J Perinatol.* 1997;17:213–217.

Hylander MA, Strabino DM, Pezzullo JC, Dhaniraddy R. Association of human milk feeding with a reduction in retinopathy of prematurity among very low birth weight infants. *J Perinatol.* 2001;21:356–362.

Jones F, Tully MR. Best practices for expressing, storing and handling human milk in hospital, homes and child care settings. Raleigh, NC: Human Milk Bank Association of North America (HMBANA); 2006.

Jorgensen MH, Hernell O, Lund P, et al. Visual acuity and erythrocyte docosahexaenoic acid status in breast-fed and formula-fed term infants in first four months of life. *Lipids.* 1996;31:99–105.

Kavanaugh K, Mead L, Meier P, Mangurten HH. Getting enough: mothers' concerns about breastfeeding a preterm infant after discharge. *J Obstet Gynecol Neonatal Nurs.* 1995;24:23–32.

Kavanaugh K, Meier P, Zimmerman B, Mead L. The rewards outweigh the efforts: breastfeeding outcomes for mothers of preterm infants. *J Hum Lact.* 1997;13:15–21.

Kirsten D, Bradford L. Hindmilk feedings. *Neonatal Netw.* 1999;18:68–70.

Kliethermas P, Cross ML, Lanese MG, et al. Transitioning preterm infants with nasogastric tube supplementation: Increased likelihood of breastfeeding. *J Obstet Gynecol Neonatal Nurs.* 1999;28:264–273.

Lang S, Lawrence CJ, Orme RL. Cup feeding: An alternative method of infant feeding. *Arch Dis Child.* 1994;71:365–369.

Lawrence RA, Lawrence RM. *Breastfeeding, A Guide for the Medical Profession.* 6th ed. Philadelphia: Mosby-Elsevier; 2005.

Lindrea KB, Stainton MC. A case study of infant massage outcomes. MCN *Am J Matern Child Nurs.* 2000:25:95–99.

Lucas A, Cole TJ. Breast milk and necrotising enterocolitis. *Lancet.* 1990;336: 1519–1523.

Lucas A, Fewtrell MS, Morley R, et al. Randomized outcome trial of human milk fortification and developmental outcome in preterm infants. *Am J Clin Nutr.* 1999; 64:142–151.

Lucas A, Morley R, Cole TJ, et al. Breast milk and subsequent intelligence quotient in children born preterm. *Lancet.* 1992;339:261–264.

Ludington-Hoe SM, Thompson C, Swinth J, et al. Kangaroo care: research results, and practice implications and guidelines. *Neonatal Netw.* 1994;13:19–27.

Ludington-Hoe SM, Kasper CE. A physiologic method of monitoring preterm infants during kangaroo care. *J Nurs Manag.* 1995;3:13–29.

Ludington-Hoe SM, Swinth JY. Developmental aspects of kangaroo care. *J Obstet Gynecol Neonatal Nurs.* 1996;25:691–703.

Ludington-Hoe SM, Cong X, Hashemi F. Infant crying: nature, physiologic consequences, and select intervention. *Neonatal Netw.* 2002;21:29–36.

Ludington-Hoe SM, Swinth JV, Thompson C, Hadeed AJ. Randomized controlled trial of kangaroo care: cardiorespiratory and thermal effects on healthy preterm infants. *Neonatal Network.* 2004;23:39–48.

McClure RJ, Newell SJ. Randomized control study of clinical outcome following trophic feeding. *Arch Dis Child Fetal Neonatal E.* 2000;82:F29–F33.

Meier P, Anderson GC. Responses of small preterm infants to bottle- and breast-feeding. *MCN Am J Matern Child Nurs.* 1987;12:97–105.

Meier PP, Brown LP. State of the science: Breastfeeding for mothers and low birth weight infants. *Nurs Clin N Am.* 1996;31:351–365.

Meier PP, Brown LP, Hurst NM, et al. Nipple shields for preterm infants: effect on milk transfer and duration of breastfeeding. *J Hum Lact.* 2000;16:106–114.

Meier PP, Engstrom JL, Fleming BA, et al. Estimating intake of hospitalized preterm infants who breastfeed. *J Hum Lact.* 1996;12:21–26.

Miracle DJ, Meier PP, Bennett PA. Mother's decision to change from formula to mothers' milk for very-low-birth-weight infants. *J Obstet Gynecol Neonatal Nurs.* 2004;33: 692–703.

Mirmiran M, Arigagno A. Influence of light in the NICU on the development of circadian rhythms in preterm infants. *Semin Perinatol.* 2000;24:247–257.

Palmer MM. Identification and management of the transitional suck pattern in premature infants. *J Perinat Neonatal Nurs.* 1993;7:66–75.

Polberger S, Lonnerdal B. Simple and rapid macronutrient analysis of human milk for individualized fortification: basis for improved nutritional management of very-low-birth-weight infants? *J Pediatr Gastroenterol Nutr.* 1993;17:283–290.

Quan R, Yang C, Rubinstein S, et al. The effect of nutritional additives on anti-infective factors in human milk. *Clin Pediatr.* June 1994;325–328.

Ruis H, Rolland R, Doesburg W, et al. Oxytocin enhances onset of lactation among mothers delivering prematurely. *BMJ.* 1981;283:340–342.

Saarinen UM, Kajosaari M. Breastfeeding as prophylaxis against atopic disease: prospective follow-up study until seventeen years old. *Lancet.* 1995;346:1065–1069.

Saunders RB, Friedman CB, Stramoski PR. Feeding preterm infants: schedule or demand? *J Obstet Gynecol Neonatal Nurs.* 1991;20:212–218.

Schanler RJ. Human milk fortification for premature infants. *Am J Clin Nutr.* 1996; 64:249–250.

Schanler RJ. Human milk for premature infants. *Pediatr Clin North Am.* 2001;48:207–219.

Schanler RJ, Hurst NM. Human milk for the hospitalized preterm infant. *Semin Perinatol.* 1994;18:476–484.

Schanler RJ, Hurst NM, Lau C. The use of human milk and breastfeeding in premature infants. *Clin Perinatol.* 1999;26:379–398.

Schanler RJ, Shulman RJ, Lau C, et al. Feeding strategies for premature infants: randomized trial of gastrointestinal priming and tube feeding method. *Pediatrics.* 1999a;103:434–439.

Stine MJ. Breastfeeding the premature newborn: a protocol without bottles. *J Hum Lact.* 1990;6:167–170.

Sullivan RM, Toubas P. Clinical usefulness of maternal odor in newborns: Mouthing and feeding preparatory responses. *Biol Neonate.* 1998;74:402–408.

Uvnas-Moberg K, Eriksonn M. Breastfeeding: physiological endocrine and behavioral adaptation caused by oxytocin and local neurogenic activity in the nipple and mammary gland. *Acta Pardiatr Scand.* 1996;85:523–530.

Valentine CJ, Hurst NM. A six-step feeding strategy for preterm infants. *J Hum Lact.* 1995;11:7–8.

Van den Driessche M, Peeters K, Marien P, et al. Gastric emptying in formula-fed and breast-fed infants measured with the 13C-octanoic acid breath test. *J Pediatr Gastroenterol Nutr.* 1999;29:46–51.

Vohr B, Poindexter, et al. Beneficial effects of breast milk in the neonatal intensive care unit on development outcome of extremely low birth weight infants at eighteen months of age. *Pediatrics.* 2006;118E:115–123.

Whitlaw A, Heisterkanp G, Sleath K, et al. Skin-to-skin contact for very low birthweight infants and their mothers. *Arch Dis Child.* 1988;63:1377–1381.

Wolf LS, Glass RP. *Feeding and Swallowing Disorders in Infancy: Assessment and Management.* Tucson, AZ: Therapy Skill Builders; 1992.

World Health Organization (WHO). *Kangaroo Mother Care: A Practical Guide.* Geneva: WHO; 2003.

Suggested Readings

Affonso D, Bosque E, Wahlberg V, Brady JP. Reconciliation and healing for mothers through skin-to-skin contact provided in an American tertiary-level intensive care nursery. *Neonatal Netw.* 1993;12:25–32.

Als H, Gilkerson L. Developmentally supportive care in the neonatal intensive care unit. *Zero to Three.* 1995;15:2–10.

Anderson GC. Current knowledge about skin-to-skin (Kangaroo) care for preterm infants. *J Perinatol.* 1991;11:216–226.

Arenson J. Discharge teaching in the NICU: The changing needs of NICU graduates and their families. *Neonatal Netw.* 1988;7:29–30, 47–52.

Armstrong HC. Breastfeeding low birthweight infants: advances in Kenya. *J Hum Lact.* 1987;3:34–37.

Barnes LP. Lactation consultation in the neonatal intensive care unit. *MCN Am J Matern Child Nurs.* 1991;16:167.

Becker PT, Grunwald PC, Moorman J, Stuhr S. Effects of developmental care on behavioral organization in very-low-birth-weight infants. *Nurs Res.* 1993;42:214–220.

Bell RP, McGrath JM. Implementing a research-based kangaroo care program in the NICU. *Nurs Clin N Am.* 1996;31:387–403.

Bell EH, Geyer J, Jones L. A structured intervention improves breastfeeding success for ill or preterm infants. *Am J Matern Child Nurs.* 1995;20:309–314.

Bier JB, Ferguson A, Anderson L, et al. Breast-feeding of very low birth weight infants. *J Pediatr.* 1993;123:773–779.

Bier JB, Ferguson A, Cho C, et al. The oral motor development of low-birth-weight infants who underwent orotracheal intubation during the neonatal period. *Am J Dis Child.* 1993;147:858–862.

Bier JB, Ferguson AE, Morales Y, et al. Comparison of skin-to-skin contact with standard contact in low birth weight infants who are breastfed. *Arch Pediatr Adolesc Med.* 1996;150:1265–1269.

Bishop NJ, Dahlenburg SL, Fewtrell MS, et al. Early diet of preterm infants and bone mineralization at age five years. *Acta Paediatr.* 1996;85:230–236.

Bosque EM, Brady JP, Affonso DD, Wahlberg V. Physiologic measures of kangaroo versus incubator care in a tertiary-level nursery. *J Obstet Gynecol Neonatal Nurs.* 1995;24:219–226.

Bowles BC, Stutte PC, Hensley JH. Alternate massage in breastfeeding. *Genesis.* 1988;9:5–9, 17.

Charpak N, Ruiz-Pelaez JG, Charpak Y, Rey-Martinez. Kangaroo mother program: an alternative way of caring for low birth weight infants? One year mortality in a two cohort study. *Pediatrics.* 1994;94:804–810.

Costello A, Chapman J. Mothers' perceptions of the care-by-parent program prior to hospital discharge of their preterm infants. *Neonatal Netw.* 1998;17:37–42.

D'Appolito K. What is an organized infant? *Neonatal Netw.* 1991;10:23–29.

Drosten-Brooks F. Kangaroo care: skin-to-skin contact in the NICU. *Am J Matern Child Nurs.* 1993;18:250–253.

Durand R, Hodges S, LaRock S, et al. The effect of skin-to-skin breastfeeding in the immediate recovery period on newborn thermoregulation and blood glucose values. *Neonatal Intensive Care.* 1997; March/April:23–27.

El-Mohandes, Schatz V, Keiser JF, Jackson BJ. Bacterial contaminants of collected and frozen human milk used in an intensive care nursery. *Am J Infect Control.* 1993;21:226–230.

Evanochko CM. Bacterial growth in expressed breast milk in continuous feeding setups in the NICU. *Neonatal Netw.* 1995;14:52.

Feher SDK, Berger LR, Johnson JD, Wilde JB. Increasing breast milk production for premature infants with a relaxation/imagery audiotape. *Pediatrics.* 1989;83:57–60.

Fewtrell MS, Prentice A, Jones SC, et al. Bone mineralization and turnover in preterm infants at 8–12 years of age: the effect of early diet. *J Bone Miner Res.* 1999;14:810–820.

Forsyth TJ, Maney LA, Ramirez A, et al. Nursing case management in the NICU: enhanced coordination for discharge planning. *Neonatal Netw.* 1998;17:23–34.

Gennaro S, Brooten D, Bakewell-Sachs S. Postdischarge services for low-birth-weight infants. *J Obstet Gynecol Neonatal Nurs.* 1991;20:29–36.

Glass RP, Wolf LS. A global perspective on feeding assessment in the neonatal intensive care unit. *Am J Occup Ther.* 1994;48:514–526.

Goldman AS, Chheda S, Keeney SE, et al. Immunologic protection of the premature newborn by human milk. *Semin Perinatol.* 1994;18:495–501.

Groh-Wargo S, Toth A, Mahoney K, et al. The utility of a bilateral breast pumping system for mothers of premature infants. *Neonatal Netw.* 1995;14:31–36.

Gupta A, Khanna K, Chattree S. Cup feeding: An alternative to bottle feeding in a neonatal intensive care unit. *J Trop Pediatr.* 1999;45:108–110.

Hamosh M. Digestion in the premature infant: the effects of human milk. *Semin Perinatol.* 1994;18:485–494.

Hamosh M, Ellis LA, Pollock DR, et al. Breastfeeding and the working mother: effect of time and temperature of short-term storage on proteolysis, lipolysis, and bacterial growth in milk. *Pediatrics.* 1996;97:492–498.

Harrison H. The principles for family-centered neonatal care. *Pediatrics.* 1993;92:643–650.

Hill AS, Rath L. The care and feeding of the low-birth-weight infant. *J Perinat Neonatal Nurs.* 1993;6:56–68.

Hill PD, Hanson KS, Mefford AL. Mothers of low birthweight infants: breastfeeding patterns and problems. *J Hum Lact.* 1994;10:169–176.

Hill PD, Andersen JL, Ledbetter RJ. Delayed initiation of breast-feeding the preterm infant. *J Perinat Neonatal Nurs.* 1995;9:10–20.

Hill PD, Brown LP, Harker TL. Initiation and frequency of breast expression in breastfeeding mothers of LBW and VLBW infants. *Nurs Res.* 1995;44:352–355.

Hill PD, Aldag JC. Milk volume on day 4, and income predictive of lactation adequacy at 6 weeks of mothers of preterm infants. *J Perinat Neonatal Nurs.* 2006;19:273–282.

Hill PD, Aldag JC, Chatterton RT. The effect of sequential and simultaneous breast pumping on milk volume and prolactin levels: a pilot study. *J Hum Lact.* 1996;12:193–199.

Hill PD, Aldag JC, Chatterton RT Jr. Breastfeeding experience and milk weight in lactating mothers pumping for preterm infants. *Birth.* 1999;26:233–238.

Hill PD, Aldag JC, Chatterton RT. Effects of pumping style on milk production in mothers of non-nursing preterm infants. *J Hum Lact.* 1999;15:209–216.

Hill PD, Ledbetter RJ, Kavanaugh KL. Breastfeeding patterns of low birth weight infants after hospital discharge. *J Obstet Gynecol Neonatal Nurs.* 1997;26:189–197.

Hopkinson JM, Schanler RJ, Garza C. Milk production by mothers of premature infants. *Pediatrics.* 1988;81:815–820.

Hopkinson JM, Schanler RJ, Fraley JK, Garza C. Milk production by mothers of premature infants: influence of cigarette smoking. *Pediatrics.* 1992;90:934–938.

Hurst NM, Myatt A, Schanler RJ. Growth and development of a hospital-based lactation program and mother's own milk bank. *J Obstet Gynecol Neonatal Nurs.* 1998;27:503–510.

Inoue N, Sakashita R, Kamegai T. Reduction of masseter muscle activity in bottle-fed infants. *Early Hum Dev.* 1995;42:185–193.

Jocson ML, Mason EO, Schanler RJ. The effects of nutrient fortification and varying storage conditions on host defense properties of human milk. *Pediatrics.* 1997;100: 240–243.

Jones E. Breastfeeding in the preterm infant. *Mod Midwife.* 1994;4:22–26.

Koenig JS, Davies AM, Thach BT. Coordination of breathing, sucking, and swallowing during bottle feedings in human infants. *J Appl Physiol.* 1990;69:1623–1629.

Lang S. *Breastfeeding Special Care Infants.* Philadelphia: W.B. Saunders Company; 1997.

Law H. The use of comforting touch and massage to reduce stress for preterm infants in the neonatal intensive care unit. *Newborn Infant Nurs.* 2001;1:235–241.

Lawhon G, Melzar A. Developmental care of the very low birth weight infant. *J Perinat Neonatal Nurs.* 1988;2:56–65.

Ludington SM. Energy conversion during skin-to-skin contact between premature infants and their mothers. *Heart Lung.* 1990;19:445–451.

Ludington S. *Kangaroo Care: The Best You Can Do for Your Preterm Infant.* New York: Bantam Books; 1993.

Luukkainen P, Salo MK, Nikkari T. The fatty acid composition of banked human milk and infant formulas: the choices of milk for feeding preterm infants. *Eur J Pediatr.* 1995;154:316–319.

Makrides M, Neumann MA, Gibson RA. Effect of maternal docosahexaenoic acid (DHA) supplementation on breast milk composition. *Eur J Clin Nutr.* 1996;50:352–357.

Malhotra N, Vishwambaran L, Sundaram KR, Narayanan I. A controlled trial of alternative methods of oral feeding in neonates. *Early Hum Dev.* 1999;54:29–38.

Martell M, Martinez G, Gonzalez M, et al. Suction patterns in preterm infants. *J Perinat Med.* 1993;21:363–369.

Matthew OP. Respiratory control during nipple feeding in preterm infants. *Pediatr Pulmonol.* 1988;5:220–224.

Matthew OP. Science of bottle feeding. *J Pediatr.* 1991a;119:511–519.

Matthew OP. Breathing patterns of preterm infants during bottle feeding: role of milk flow. *J Pediatr.* 1991b;119:960–965.

McCoy R, Kadowaki C, Wilks S, et al. Nursing management of breast feeding for preterm infants. *J Perinat Neonatal Nurs.* 1988;2:42–55.

Medoff-Cooper B, Verklan T, Carlson S. The development of sucking patterns and physiologic correlates in very-low-birth-weight infants. *Nurs Res.* 1993;42:100–105.

Meier P. Bottle- and breast-feeding: effects on transcutaneous oxygen pressure and temperature in preterm infants. *Nurs Res.* 1988;37:36–41.

Meier P, Pugh EJ. Breast-feeding behavior of small preterm infants. *Am J Matern Child Nurs.* 1985;10:396–401.

Meier P, Wilks S. The bacteria in expressed mothers' milk. *Am J Matern Child Nurs.* 1987;12:420–423.

Meier PP, Engstrom JL, Mangurten HH, et al. Breastfeeding support services in the neonatal intensive-care unit. *J Obstet Gynecol Neonatal Nurs.* 1993;22:338–347.

Meier PP, Engstrom JL, Crichton CL, et al. A new scale for in-home test-weighing for mothers of preterm and high risk infants. *J Hum Lact.* 1994;10:163–168.

Meier PP, Brown LP. Breastfeeding a preterm infant after NICU discharge: reflections on Ryan's story. *Breastfeeding Abstracts.* 1997;17:3–4.

Mennella JA, Beauchamp GK. The human infants' response to vanilla flavors in mother's milk and formula. *Infant Behav Dev.* 1996;19:13–19.

Milsom SR, Breier BH, Gallaher BW, et al. Growth hormone stimulates galactopoiesis in healthy lactating women. *Acta Endocrinol.* 1992;127:337–343.

Moran M, Radzyminski SG, Higgins K, et al. Maternal Kangaroo (skin-to-skin) care in the NICU beginning 4 hours postbirth. *Am J Matern Child Nurs.* 1999;24:74–79.

Moro GE, Minoli I, Ostrom M, et al. Fortification of human milk: evaluation of a novel fortification scheme and of a new fortifier. *J Pediatr Gastroenterol Nutr.* 1995;20: 162–172.

Narayanan I. Human milk for low birthweight infants: Immunology, nutrition and newer practical technologies. *Acta Paediatr.* Jpn. 1989;31:455–461.

Newell SJ, Chapman S, Booth IW. Ultrasonic assessment of gastric emptying time in the preterm infant. *Arch Dis Child.* 1993;69:32–36.

Nyqvist KH, Sjoden PO, Ewald U. Mothers' advice about facilitating breastfeeding in a neonatal intensive care unit. *J Hum Lact.* 1994;10:237–243.

Nyqvist KH, Rubertsson C, Ewald U, et al. Development of the preterm infant breastfeeding behavior scale (PIBBS): A study of nurse-mother agreement. *J Hum Lact.* 1996;12:207–219.

Nyqvist KH, Ewald U, Sjoden PO. Supporting a preterm infant's behavior during breastfeeding: a case report. *J Hum Lact.* 1996;12:221–228.

Nyqvist KH, Sjoden P-O, Ewald U. The development of preterm infants' breastfeeding behavior. *Early Hum Dev.* 1999;55:247–264.

Orlando S. The immunologic significance of breast milk. *J Obstet Gynecol Neonatal Nurs.* 1995;24:678–683.

Pardou A, Serruys E, Mascart-Lemone F, et al. Human milk banking: influence of storage processes and of bacterial contamination on some milk constituents. *Biol Neonate.* 1994;65:302–309.

Schanler RJ, Shulman RJ, Lau C. Feeding strategies for premature infants: beneficial outcomes of feeding fortified human milk versus preterm formula. *Pediatrics.* 1999b; 103:1150–1157.

Siddell EP, Froman RD. A national survey of neonatal intensive care units: criteria used to determine readiness for oral feedings. *J Obstet Gynecol Neonatal Nurs.* 1994;23:783–789.

Stutte PC, Bowles BC, Morman GY. The effects of breast massage on volume and fat content of human milk. *Genesis.* 1988;10:22–25.

Thompson DG. Critical pathways in the intensive care and intermediate care nurseries. *Am J Matern Child Nurs.* 1994;19:29–32.

Valentine CJ, Hurst NM, Schanler RJ. Hindmilk improves weight gain in low-birth-weight infants fed human milk. *J Pediatr Gastroenterol Nutr.* 1994;18:474–477.

Walker M. *Breastfeeding Premature Infants.* Lactation Consultant Series Unit 14. New York: Avery; 1990.

Walker M. Management guidelines for breastfeeding mothers with LBW infants. *J Perinat Educ.* 1992a;1:25–30.

Walker M. Breastfeeding the premature infant. *Women's Health Nurs.* 1992b;3:620–633.

Walker M. *Breastfeeding Your Premature or Special Care Infant: A Practical Guide for Nursing the Tiny Infant.* Weston, MA: Lactation Associates; 1998.

Wang CD, Chu PS, Mellen BG, Shenai JP. Creamatocrit and the nutrient composition of human milk. *J Perinatol.* 1999;19:343–346.

Wight N. Donor milk: down but not out. (letter) *Pediatrics.* 2005;116:1610–1611.

Williamson MT, Murti PK. Effects of storage, time, temperature, and composition of containers on biologic components of human milk. *J Hum Lact.* 1996;12:231–235.

Breastfeeding Multiples

Karen Kerkhoff Gromada, MSN, RN, IBCLC

OBJECTIVES

- Discuss the ways that antenatal, intrapartum, and postnatal conditions and events often affect the initiation of breastfeeding and lactation after multiple births.

- Describe strategies for initiating and coordinating breastfeeding with multiple-birth neonates.

- Identify physiologic and psychosocial factors that often affect breastfeeding multiple-birth infants/children.

Introduction

A number of assumptions are associated with breastfeeding twins or higher-order multiples (HOMs). When providing breastfeeding/lactation care to women who have multiple-birth children, the lactation consultant may assume the following:

- Single-infant pregnancy and birth are the species norms for Homo sapiens. As such, multiple-birth infants/children strain maternal physical and emotional reserves. This strain extends to the breastfeeding relationship(s).

- Breastfeeding initiation and duration with multiples is affected by more than an ability to replicate appropriate breastfeeding mechanics or typical lactation management strategies with two or more infants/children.

- Infant and maternal complications present at birth affect breastfeeding initiation and may have long-lasting effects on breastfeeding duration or the feeding pattern of one or more of the multiple infants.

- Coordinating the breastfeeding of two or more infants who have differing but normal suckling abilities, feeding patterns, and feeding styles may be perceived by a mother as breastfeeding problems as opposed to being part of the reality of having multiple infants/children.

• Older infant and toddler multiples engage in interactive behaviors between themselves during breastfeeding that may affect each maternal-child breastfeeding relationship.

I. Factors Associated with Multiple Pregnancy That Affect the Initiation of Breastfeeding

A. Increased incidence of twin and HOM births in Western cultures (Statistics cited are for the United States, but most industrial nations report a similar percent of increase in multiple births; Denton & Bryan, 2002; Martin et al., 2003).

1. Twins: More than 65% increase between 1980 and 2002 (Figure 27-1).
   a. In 2002, 3.15 per 100 births were twins.

2. HOM: More than 340% increase between 1980 and 2002 (see Figure 27-2).
   a. Prior to 1980, 37 per 100,000 births were HOM.
   b. In 2002, 184 per 100,000 births were HOM.

3. Most of the increased incidence of multiple births is related to factors associated with a higher incidence of dizygotic (fraternal) multiples, that is, fertilization of two or more separate ova by separate sperm (Martin et al., 2003).

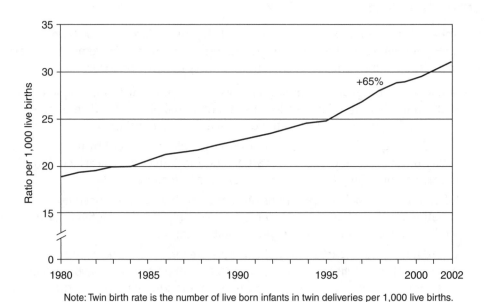

Note: Twin birth rate is the number of live born infants in twin deliveries per 1,000 live births.

Figure 27-1   Twin birth rate: U.S., 1980–2002. *Source:* Retrieved from http://www.cdc.gov/.

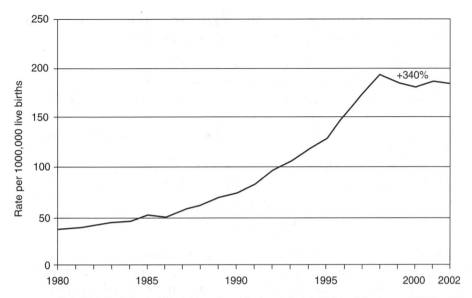

Note: Triplet/ + birth rate is the total number of live born infants in triplet + deliveries per 1,000 live births.
Triplet/ + includes births in greater than twin deliveries.

Figure 27-2   Triplet/+birth rate: U.S., 1980–2002. *Source:* Retrieved from
http://www.cdc.gov/.

 4. Factors that have affected the incidence of dizygotic twinning since 1980.
     a. Ovarian stimulation medications or ovulatory induction medications.
     b. Assisted reproductive technologies (ART) such as in vitro fertilization,
        intrauterine insemination, and gamete or zygote intrafallopian tube transfer.
 B. Effect of increased incidence of multiple births on breastfeeding and lactation.

 1. Increased numbers of mothers of multiples (MOM) initiating breastfeeding/
    lactation (Boyle and Collopy, 2000; Damato et al., 2005; Geraghty et al., 2004a;
    MOST, 2005).
    a. Twin breastfeeding initiation rates: reports range from 64% to 89.4%.
    b. HOM breastfeeding initiation rates: reports range from 55% to 86%.

 2. The demographics of women who are using ART to achieve pregnancy are
    often the same mothers or the same population who are experiencing increased
    rates of breastfeeding initiation and duration (Gromada & Bowers, 2005).

II. Risk Factors of Multiple Pregnancy/Birth (Bowers & Gromada, 2006; Boyle & Collopy, 2000; Martin et al., 2003)

A. Infants have an increased incidence of the following:

1. Preterm labor and birth (preterm is < 37 weeks gestation; very preterm < 32 weeks). The average duration of gestation (Figure 27-3) is as follows:
   a. Single infant, 38.8 weeks (10% < 37 weeks/2% < 32 weeks).
   b. Twins, 35 to 36 weeks (58.2% < 37 weeks/11.9% < 32 weeks); < 14% born full-term.
   c. Triplets, 33 weeks (92.4% < 37 weeks/36.1% < 32 weeks).
   d. Quadruplets, 29 weeks (96.8% < 37 weeks/59.9% < 32 weeks).

2. Intrauterine growth restriction (IUGR)/fetal growth restriction.
   a. Decreasing fetal growth curves beginning at approximately 27 weeks for HOM and 30 weeks for twins.
   b. Discordant growth related to placental or cord anomalies.
   c. Twin-to-twin transfusion syndrome (TTTS) related to vascular connections when monozygotes (identical/single ovum-sperm) share a single placenta.

3. Low birth weight (LBW; defined as ≤ 5 lb, 8 oz or 2,500 g) and very, or extremely, low birth weight (VLBW; ≦ 3 lb, 3 oz or 1,500 g; ELBW < 1,250 g) [Figure 27-4].
   a. Single infant: 6.1% LBW/1.1% V/ELBW; average birth weight (ABW) 7 lb, 1 oz (3332 g).
   b. Twins: 55.4% LBW/10.2% V/ELBW; ABW 5 lb, 2.7 oz (2347 g).

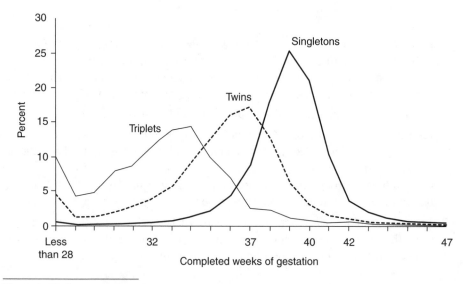

Figure 27-3   Gestational age distribution by plurality: U.S., 2002. *Source:* Retrieved from http://www.cdc.gov/.

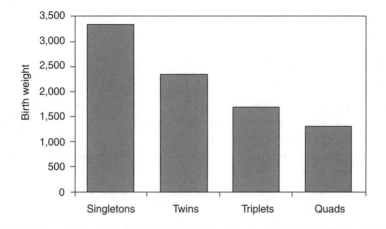

Figure 27-4   Mean birth weight by plurality: U.S., 2002. *Source:* Retrieved from http://www.cdc.gov/.

    c. Triplets: 94.4% LBW/34.5% V/ELBW; ABW 3 lb, 11.5 oz (1687 g).
    d. Quadruplets: 98.8% LBW/61.1% V/ELBW; ABW 2 lb, 14.25 oz (1309 g).
    e. 2003 Multiples = < 3.2% of all births but >1 of 4 overall VLBW infants.

4. Increased incidence of congenital or pregnancy-related anomalies, such as cardiac, club foot, hip dislocation, developmental delays, cerebral palsy, Down syndrome, and so on.
    a. Singletons 2.4%; twins 8.3%; monozygotic twins 12% to 15%.

5. Infant mortality per 1,000 live births by plurality for 1999 through 2001 (Martin et al., 2004; Figure 27-5).

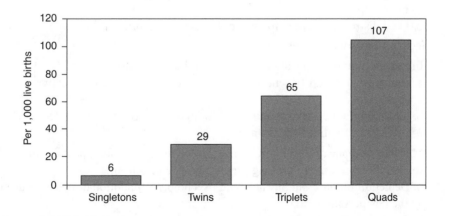

Figure 27-5   Infant mortality rates by plurality: U.S. combined years 1999–2001. *Source:* Retrieved from http://www.cdc.gov.

  a. Singleton 6 per 1000

  b. Twin 29 per 1000

  c. Triplet 65 per 1000

  d. Quadruplet 107 per 1000.

B. Maternal.

 1. Pregnancy-induced hypertension; may be referred to as preeclampsia or toxemia.

  a. Incidence: singleton pregnancies 7%; twins 14%; triplets 21%; quadruplets 40% (Bowers & Gromada, 2006).

  b. Symptoms often more severe or initially present with more advanced symptoms in multiple pregnancy.

  c. Progression to HELLP syndrome (see Chapter 34) more common with multiple pregnancy.

 2. Anemia found in 21% to 36% of multiple pregnancies, 2 to 3 times higher than for singleton pregnancy.

 3. Gestational diabetes mellitus prevalence varies.

  a. Singleton pregnancy, 4%.

  b. Twin pregnancy, 7%.

  c. Triplet pregnancy, 9%.

  d. Quadruplet pregnancy, 11%.

 4. Perinatal hemorrhage.

  a. Antenatal or intrapartum bleeding related to placental conditions; for example, increased incidence of placenta previa, abruption.

  b. Postnatal hemorrhage related to increased implantation site(s) and increased uterine atony.

 5. Surgical delivery (~50% both twins, 7%–10% second twin only; 95% HOM).

  a. Malpresentation of fetal presenting part (increased for second/subsequent multiple).

  b. Fetal distress (increased for second/subsequent multiple).

C. Effects on breastfeeding initiation.

 1. Increased infant complications result in an increase of:

  a. Immature or insult to central nervous system and decreased effective suckling.

  b. Mother–infant(s) separation related to increased need for infant neonatal intensive care unit (NICU) stays.

 2. Maternal complications or conditions (preconception through postpartum) and related interventions to prolong pregnancy often result in:

  a. Depletion of maternal physical and psychological/emotional reserves during the postpartum period.

  b. Delayed initiation of breastfeeding or compensatory milk expression.

  c. Delayed or lower milk production.

D. Prenatal preparation (Gromada, in press; Leonard, 2003).

1. Infant-feeding decision; advantages and disadvantages pertinent to the breastfeeding of two or more newborns/infants.

2. Milk production adaptation for multiple infants (Mead et al., 1992; Saint, Maggiore, & Hartmann, 1986).

3. Anticipatory guidance related to:
   a. Improving infant outcomes associated with a pregnancy weight gain of 38 to 54 lb (17.3–24.5 kg) for twins, 50 to 60 lb (22.7–27.2 kg) for triplets (Bowers & Gromada, 2006), means improved effective breastfeeding/suckling in the early postpartum period.
   b. Initiation related to potential infant or maternal complications means maternal flexibility and perspective.
   c. Short- and long-term breastfeeding goals and possible adaptations related to the reality of multiple infants.

III. Initiating Breastfeeding (Gromada, in press; Gromada & Spangler, 1998; Leonard, 2003)

A. Healthy, full/near-term twins and triplets.

1. Early, frequent, "cued" breastfeeding for each.

2. Individual versus simultaneous feedings until at least one is assessed for consistent, effective breastfeeding.

3. Discharge planning.
   a. Coordinating breastfeeding (see below) and other infant care.
   b. Distinguishing breastfeeding issues versus "two or more infants" issues.
   c. Reviewing support systems, including physical (such as household help) and emotional support.

B. Maternal complications.

1. Direct breastfeeding.
   a. Round-the-clock, supportive assistant (partner, relative, friend, etc.) to help with infants' care and breastfeeding, such as for positioning infants, holding infant in place if needed, etc.

2. Compensatory milk expression per self or caregiver (at least 8 times or >100 min/24 h).

C. Preterm or sick twins/HOMs.

1. Establishing a realistic plan for lactation via milk expression for two or more newborns.
   a. Initiate milk expression as soon as possible following birth for at least eight times or 100 minutes/24 hours.

  b. Increase the number of pumping sessions or the total number of minutes pumped as needed.

  c. Increased need for rental, hospital-grade, electric pump with a double collection kit and properly-sized breast shields/flanges UNTIL all multiples effectively breastfeed.

 2. If milk volume obtained is inadequate for all babies.

  a. Review milk expression/breast pumping management routine and breast pump equipment being used by mother, revising as needed.

  b. Review maternal health history for preconception, including lowered fertility, and pregnancy issues associated with a delayed or lower milk production.

  c. Consider use of one/more galactogogues as needed based on individual situation; postpartum depression (PPD) is more common for MOM (Leonard, 1998), which should be kept in mind when suggesting galactogogue agents associated with feelings of depression as a side effect, such as metoclopramide.

  d. Discuss with mother (and other parent) and the neonatologist to determine if babies should get equal amounts of available mother's milk or whether one (or more) sicker babies would benefit from greater amounts of available milk.

  e. Provide possible options regarding banked donor human milk.

 3. Transitioning two or more preterm or sick neonates to breastfeeding.

  a. Assess and intervene based on individual infant ability.

  b. Expect a learning curve for breastfeeding, including the necessity of maternal patience and persistence in situations of two or more preterm or sick newborns (of differing abilities) learning to breastfeed effectively.

 4. Discharge planning.

  a. Staggered discharge is common; one baby discharged to the home and one baby is in the NICU.

  b. Parental anxiety related to the growth and development of preterm or sick newborns.

  c. Differing breastfeeding "learning" curves for individual infants.

IV. Maternal Postpartum Biopsychosocial Issues Affecting Breastfeeding and Lactation (Auer & Gromada, 1998; Gromada & Bowers, 2005; Leonard, 2003).

 A. Physiologic conditions related to depleted reserves or a decreased resistance to illness.

  1. Some physiologic condition(s) contributing to infertility may affect milk production to varying degrees, such as polycystic ovary syndrome, thyroid conditions, chronic hypertension, etc.

2. Sequelae related to the stress of a multiple pregnancy; complications or interventions to prolong the pregnancy, such as pregnancy-induced hypertension, preterm labor or birth, postpartum hemorrhage, strict bed rest, etc.

3. Recovery from surgical birth.

4. Profound sleep deprivation related to frequent interruptions for multiples' care/feeding.

B. Emotional; chronic feeling of being overwhelmed (Beck, 2002a, 2002b; Geraghty, Khoury, & Kalkwarf, 2004b; Gromada, in press; Leonard, 2000).

1. Incidence of PPD 2 to 3 times higher in mothers of multiples.

2. Unrealistic expectations for the maternal role with multiple infants.

3. Lack of support systems.

C. Mother-infant(s) attachment is a different process than with a single infant.

1. Common variations (Gromada, in press).
   a. Unit attachment: initial feelings of attachment are for the set of babies as a whole.
   b. Flip-flop attachment: alternating focus of attention on one infant at a time.
   c. Preferential attachment: a persistent, deeper attachment for one baby; harmful to all.

2. Differentiation. Parental comparisons of multiples' physical and behavioral traits.
   a. Desire to treat infants as separate yet also treat all equally.
   b. "Equal" treatment results in ignoring infants' individual feeding cues.

V. Maintaining Breastfeeding (Gromada, in press; Gromada & Bowers, 2005)

A. Coordinating breastfeeding related to multiple infant feeding patterns.

1. Individual variations related to normal variations in breastfeeding patterns (for example, the typical number of feedings per 24 hours) or breastfeeding styles (for example, the typical length of feedings).

2. Affected by zygosity (genetically-based patterns) and the maternal perception of the infants as per the differentiation process.
   a. Monozygotes: more likely to have similar behavioral approaches/patterns related to breastfeeding. For example, similar number of breastfeedings in 24 hours and cues to feed at approximately the same times.
   b. Dizygotes: more genetic variation results in more varied feeding approaches and pattern; may be similar (each cueing 10 times in 24 h) or quite different (one cueing 8 times, one cueing 14 times, and one cueing 10 times in 24 h).

3. MOM face a competing desire to treat multiples as individuals but also as equals (Beck, 2002b).
   a. Influences maternal response to individual cues, including feeding cues.
   b. Potential for adverse impact on individual multiples' growth and development.

4. Individual outcome measures related to within normal limits outputs and weight gains.
   a. Coordinate 24-hour feeding charts by clearly marking for each infant or using a different color paper for each infant's chart.
   b. Outcomes might reflect individual breastfeeding ability/effectiveness of the milk transfer.

B. Feeding rotation (assuming effective breastfeeding for each multiple); anything works if based on the individual infants' cues.

1. Alternate breasts each feeding.

2. Alternate breasts every 24 hours (more often if you have an odd number of multiples).
   a. Today, baby A feeds using the right breast and B using the left breast; tomorrow A at left and B at right breast.
   b. Appears strategy favored by most mothers due to ease of remembering rotation; provides benefits of alternating breasts.

3. Assign each multiple to a specific breast.
   a. Benefits.
      i. Breast self-regulation by two individual infants may (1) enhance one/both ability to suckle effectively; (2) decrease consequences of overactive milk ejection reflex or gastroesophageal reflux.
      ii. Minimize cross contamination with certain infective conditions, for example, thrush.
   b. Risks.
      i. Infant refusal to feed on the opposite breast if one breast cannot be suckled for any reason; problematic due to more nursing strikes with multiples.
      ii. Significant difference in maternal breast size.
      iii. Less infant eye and side-to-side stimulation; counteractive positional changes less likely to occur with simultaneous breastfeeding and caring for multiples.

C. Individual versus simultaneous feeding.

1. Affected by infants' suckling abilities and maternal choice.

2. Rationale for simultaneous feeding.
   a. Saves maternal time and facilitates the development of a routine.
   b. Theoretical increase in milk production (based on breast pumping research).
      i. Many mothers have had no milk production issue when multiples generally breastfeed separately if cue-based breastfeeding occurs.

    c. Effective breastfeeding of one infant might stimulate improved breastfeeding in another by triggering the milk ejection reflex.

  3. Most MOM combine simultaneous with separate feeding.

  4. For simultaneous feedings, household pillows or a larger, deeper nursing pillow designed for feeding two babies at once can provide support/"extra arms."

  5. Positions for simultaneous feeding (Gromada, in press).
    a. Double clutch/double football (variation, double perpendicular).
    b. Double cradle or criss-cross cradle (variation, V-hold).
    c. Cradle/clutch combination (variation, layered/parallel).
    d. Double straddle with babies seated, facing mother's breasts (variation, double upright with one/both babies in kneeling or standing position).
    e. Positions with mother in reclining or supine position.
      i. Double prone with both babies prone or slightly sidelying on mother's body.
      ii. Double "alongside," with one baby cradled in each of mother's arms, alongside her body, breast to hip.
      iii. Kneeling/standing, a modification of double clutch with an infant "standing" or kneeling on the surface next to mother, their bodies draped or supported along the rib area of mother's supine body.

D. Maternal comfort (Gromada, in press).

  1. Because of the increased time spent breastfeeding multiple infants, many mothers create a nursing station consisting of:
    a. A wide, padded chair or sofa; for example, an upholstered recliner.
    b. A nearby table for snacks, beverages, portable telephone, remote controls, and so on.
    c. Convenient location, such as a room where the mother spends the most time.

  2. Nutrition. Effective breastfeeding/lactation for multiples should result in a natural increase in maternal hunger and thirst.
    a. Strategies for eating while breastfeeding; for example, one-handed snacks, a large sports mug (optional built-in straw).
    b. Hydration needs vary, so mother should drink to thirst and produce pale, yellow urine.
      i. Involvement with infants' care may result in ignoring personal thirst cues.
    c. A suppressed/minimal appetite in breastfeeding MOM may be a symptom of a postpartum mood disorder.

E. Role of routine or "scheduling" feeds.

  1. Maternal need for control (in a situation associated with increased feelings of loss of control [Beck, 2002a]).

  2. Related to profound sleep deprivation/recovery from multiple pregnancy and birth.

  3. Ability to "schedule" or anticipate infants' care/feeding needs appears to increase with HOMs.

4. Strategies.
  a. Discuss realistic expectations for the individual infant temperaments/behavioral patterns.
  b. Wake a second infant to feed with or immediately after another; day and/or night.
    i. Risks of strategy include inadequate feeding of one or more babies or ignoring an infant's higher need for attention.
  c. Co-sleeping options to increase maternal sleep.
    i. If bedsharing with parent(s), the research is less clear for preterm/near-term infants or when more than one baby bedshares. See Chapter 4 for information on safe sleep environments.
    ii. Co-bedding of twins in a single crib appears to improve synchronous sleep for babies and assist in sleep near parents without increasing sleep-related situational risks (Ball, 2006).

VI. Ongoing Breastfeeding Difficulties (see related chapters; Auer & Gromada, 1998; Gromada, in press)

A. Infant-related (cited as most commonly associated with early weaning by mothers of multiples).
  1. An ongoing latch-on or suckling difficulty of one may affect breastfeeding for all.
    a. Limited maternal time/effort available to work with affected multiple(s).
    b. Limited time for compensatory milk expression related to decreased milk removal by the affected infant(s).
    c. Lack of effective milk removal results in down-regulation of/decreased milk production.
  2. Inadequate weight gain of one or more multiples.
    a. Real: inadequate outputs or consistent poor gain: < 2/3 oz (20 g)/day or < 4 oz (120 g)/week.
    b. Perceived: genetic or prenatal-related, slower, but within normal limits growth/gain of one; slow, steady gain of 1/2 to 2/3 oz (15–20 g)/day or 3 to 4 oz (90–120 g)/week for one or more.
      i. Postnatal growth and development for multiple infants may be associated with prenatal growth (Monset-Couchard, Bethmann, & Relier, 2004).
      ii. Caution mother that the tracking of growth curves may be inappropriate if using formula-fed infant-based charts, so refer her to the appropriate growth charts (WHO growth charts, 2006).

B. Maternal
  1. Milk sufficiency, cited as most commonly associated with early weaning by MOM (Damato et al., 2005).

    a. Real: related to sequelae of pregnancy/birth complications, underlying maternal condition, or as result of delayed, infrequent, or insufficient milk emptying due to "scheduled" or ineffective breastfeeding or inadequate compensatory milk expression.

    b. Perceived: related to confusion resulting from an increase in the total number of daily breastfeedings or confusion from variations in the infants' breastfeeding patterns; difficulty differentiating one infant from another.

    c. Intervention: establish/increase/maintain milk production via increased compensatory milk expression by temporarily decreasing time at breast for any multiple affected by ineffective breastfeeding.

      i. A mother is more likely to feel confident and continue breastfeeding efforts when milk production is less of a concern.

      ii. Addition of galactogogues as needed and under the guidance of medical personnel, as an adjunct to increased milk removal (per III, C, 2, c above).

      iii. The infant's ability at the breast often improves with time/maturity; milk production can improve or be maintained only if milk is removed with adequate frequency.

2. Nipple or breast pain.

    a. Nipple pain or damage may occur more often due to the increased likelihood of ineffective breastfeeding related to the increase of preterm and near-term birth for multiples with related immature suck-swallow-breathe coordination.

      i. Infant-related complications and maternal surgical birth are more likely to result in antibiotic use and development of fungal infection that may spread to a mother's nipples and areola.

      ii. There is less time to consistently implement suggested interventions for sore/damaged nipples related to the number of infants requiring care.

    b. Delayed or missed feedings combined with increased milk production and/or decreased maternal resistance for illness may have a greater impact on the maternal system; for example, milk stasis may lead more quickly to engorgement, a plugged duct, or mastitis if a breastfeeding is postponed or missed.

3. Issues associated with long-term pumping and a mother's return to work are related to weaning at 6 months for MOM (Damato et al., 2005).

VII. Full/Exclusive or Partial Breastfeeding and Breast-Milk-Feeding Options (Gromada, in press)

A. Definitions.

1. Full/exclusive breastfeeding: achieved for weeks to months with two to four multiples.

2. Partial breastfeeding: from occasional "topping off" of/complementary feedings to scheduled supplementary feedings that replace one or more breastfeedings.

3. Full/exclusive or partial breast-milk-feeding: feeding of expressed breast milk via an alternative feeding method for some/all feedings.
   a. Appears to be associated with preterm birth or for one affected by an ongoing health issue or congenital anomaly affecting ability to transition to direct breastfeeding.
   b. Breastmilk feeding of multiples, in the absence of any direct breastfeeding, has been associated with an earlier end to lactation (Geraghty, Khoury, & Kalkwarf, 2005).

B. Implementation of full/exclusive versus partial breastfeeding or breast milk-feeding options.

1. Any option may be used with one/more/all multiple(s) at any time during lactation.

2. Any option may be used short or long term for feeding.
   a. MOM have moved from breast-milk-feeding to partial or full/exclusive direct breastfeeding.
   b. MOM have moved from full/exclusive to partial breastfeeding and the reverse, that is, from partial to full/exclusive breastfeeding.
   c. Movement within feeding options generally depends on complex interaction between/among maternal personal, infant-related, and environmental factors.

3. Partial breastfeeding can include the use of expressed breast milk (EBM) or artificial baby milk (ABM).

4. Factors involved in maternal decision-making often include:
   a. Effect of ongoing infant or maternal physical conditions affecting breastfeeding or lactation.
   b. Psychosocial issues related to the care of two or more newborns/infants.
   c. A choice for continuing to breastfeed (or pumping for) all versus total weaning.

C. Factors associated with partial breastfeeding.

1. Benefits (actual or perceived).
   a. Adequate infant nutrition (when intake is of concern for one or more infants).
   b. Help with infant feedings.
   c. Some breastfeeding/breast milk is better than no breastfeeding/breast milk related to milk properties and the maternal-infant(s) attachment.

2. Risks (actual).
   a. Decreased milk production with less time and, therefore, increased difficulty improving milk production for multiple infants.
   b. Increased infant illnesses related to a decreased human milk intake.
   c. Increased infant "preference" for an alternative feeding method yet less time to work with/help any infant at breast due to caring for two or more infants.

3. Maintaining milk production when implementing partial breastfeeding.
   a. Limit use of other feeding alternatives.
     i. "Top off" or complement a breastfeeding rather than supplement, which replaces an entire feeding.
     ii. Minimize amount of EBM or ABM offered as complement or supplement to encourage more frequent direct breastfeeding to any multiple able to breastfeed effectively.
   b. Supplement one or more on an as-needed basis only; for example, a need for several hours of uninterrupted sleep.
   c. Avoid alternating feeding methods every other feeding; equals all the work (time and energy) needed for both breastfeeding and the chosen alternative method; may work if full-time help handles alternative feedings.
   d. Maintain effective/thorough milk removal *at least* 8 times/24 hours.

VIII. Breastfeeding Older Infant and Toddler Multiples

A. Supplementary vitamins or iron: factors affecting multiples.

   1. Collective (preterm birth of all) versus individual (IUGR of one) multiple's situation/(blood count) outcomes.

   2. Preterm birth or other intrauterine conditions, such as TTTS in which "donor" is affected.

B. Introducing solid foods.

   1. MOM may be encouraged to introduce solid foods earlier.
     a. The perception that solid feedings lengthen the time between feedings (despite research evidence to the contrary).
     b. Preterm multiples' gastrointestinal tracts are less mature and usually less ready for early solids introduction.

   2. Individual multiples are likely to demonstrate readiness at different times, especially dizygotic multiples.
     a. Parental tendency to treat multiples as "equal" is likely to result in the introduction of solid food to both/all at once.

C. Strategies to assist parents with introducing other foods; anticipatory guidance.

   1. Address common misconceptions, such as using cereal to prolong infant sleep.

   2. Blood testing, such as hematocrit testing, to obtain quantitative information regarding possible need for supplementary iron.

   3. Signs of "readiness" for other foods, stressing sensitivity to multiples' individual differences.

D. Weaning (Gromada, in press).

   1. Individual baby-led/child-led weaning.
     a. May occur weeks, months, or years apart.

    b. Early (10–12 months), abrupt baby-led weaning is slightly more common with multiples, even in the absence of regular, supplementary bottle-feedings; may affect one or more.

  2. Mother-encouraged, baby-led weaning is an imposition of some type of limits on breastfeeding, such as when or where breastfeeding may occur.
    a. Often related to the effect of multiples' interactions while at the breast.

  3. Mother-led weaning is a purposeful decrease in the number of breastfeedings by the mother; often related to maternal feelings of being overwhelmed by multiple infants/toddlers.
    a. Gradual: a purposeful decrease in breastfeeding yet accommodates multiples' responses to decrease.
    b. Abrupt: a sudden, complete weaning.
      i. A plan for gradual weaning may become acceptable if the mother understands implications of abrupt weaning for self as well as infants related to greater milk production with two or more infants/toddlers.

E. How multiples differ from singletons.

  1. Increased nursing strikes in older infancy (etiology unknown).
    a. Possible contributing factors are inadvertent delays or purposeful "scheduling" of breastfeeding due to increased infant care needs.

  2. Increased biting (of maternal nipple/areola) during breastfeeding possibly related to simultaneous feeding and less ability to monitor for signs that one baby is on verge of biting.

  3. Increased interaction between multiples during breastfeeding.
    a. Playful to punching behaviors; often builds up from being playful to pushing to punching.
    b. "Jealous" breastfeeding, a demand by one to breastfeed unrelated to apparent need; request appears to be associated with sibling's breastfeeding.

References

Auer C, Gromada K. A case report of breastfeeding quadruplets: factors perceived as affecting breastfeeding. *J Hum Lact.* 1998:14:135–141.

Ball HL. Sleep arrangements of twin infants. Durham University, Department of Anthropology Parent-Infant Sleep Lab 2006. Available at: http://www.dur.ac.uk/sleep.lab/projects/twins/. Accessed January 23, 2007.

Beck CT. Releasing the pause button: mothering twins during the first year of life. *Qual Health Res.* 2002a;12:593–608.

Beck CT. Mothering multiples: a meta-synthesis of qualitative research. *The Am J Matern Child Nurs.* 2002b;27:214–221.

Bowers N, Gromada KK. *Care of the Multiple-Birth Family: Pregnancy and Birth*, rev. ed., nursing module. White Plains, NY: March of Dimes; 2006.

Boyle M, Collopy K. *Membership Report 2000: An Analysis of Pregnancy, Birth, and Neonatal Data from Over 1,000 Higher Order Multiple Pregnancies*. Brentwood, NY: Mothers of Supertwins (MOST); 2000.

Damato EG, Dowling DA, Standing TS, Schuster SD. Explanation for the cessation of breastfeeding in mothers of twins. *J Hum Lact*. 2005;21:296–304.

Denton J, Bryan E. Multiple birth children and their families following ART. In: E Vayena, PJ Rowe, PD Griffen, eds. Current Practices and Controversies in Assisted Reproduction: Report of a Meeting on Medical, Ethical and Social Aspects of Assisted Reproduction. Geneva: World Health Organization (WHO); 2002. Available at: http://www.who.int/reproductive-health/infertility/24.pdf. Accessed January 18, 2007.

Geraghty SR, Khoury JC, Kalkwarf HJ. Human milk pumping rates of mothers of singletons and mothers of multiples. *J Hum Lact*. 2005;21:413–420.

Geraghty SR, Pinney SM, Sethurman G, et al. Breast milk feeding rates of mothers of multiples compared to mothers of singletons. *Ambul Pediatr*. 2004a;4:226–231.

Geraghty SR, Khoury JC, Kalkwarf HJ. Comparison of feeding among multiple birth infants. *Twin Res*. 2004b;7:542–547.

Gromada KK. *Mothering Multiples: Breastfeeding and Caring for Twins or More*, revised edition. Schaumburg, IL: La Leche League International; in press.

Gromada KK, Bowers N. *Care of the Multiple-Birth Family: Birth Through Early Infancy*, revised edition, nursing module. White Plains, NY: March of Dimes; 2005.

Gromada KK, Spangler A. Breastfeeding twins and higher-order multiples. *J Obstet Gynecol Neonatal Nurs*. 1998;27:441–449.

Leonard LG. Breastfeeding rights of multiple birth families and guidelines for health professionals. *Twin Res*. 2003;6:34–45.

Leonard LG. Breastfeeding triplets: the at-home experience. *Public Health Nurs*. 2000;17:211–221.

Leonard LG. Depression and anxiety disorders during multiple pregnancy and parenthood. *J Obstet Gynecol Neonatal Nurs*. 1998;27:329–337.

Martin JA, Hamilton BE, Cosgrove CM, Munson ML. The New Matched Multiple Birth File, 1995–2000. Atlanta, GA: Center for Disease Control and Prevention (CDC)/National Center for Health Statistics (NCHS); 2004. Available at: http://www.cdc.gov/nchs/ppt/duc2004/martin_plus.pps. Accessed January 18, 2007.

Martin JA, Hamilton BF, Sutton PD, et al. Births: Final Data for 2002. *National Vital Statistics Report*. 52(12). Hyattsville, MD: National Center for Health Statistics; 2003.

Mead L, Chuffo R, Lawlor-Klean P, Meier P. Breastfeeding success with preterm quadruplets. *J Obstet Gynecol Neonatal Nurs*. 1992;21:221–227.

Monset-Couchard M, de Bethmann O, Relier JP. Long term outcome of small versus appropriate size for gestational age co-twins/triplets. *Arch Dis Child Fetal Neonatal Ed*. 2004;89:F310–F314.

Mothers of Supertwins (MOST). Most comprehensive study to date of 1300 multiple birth mothers develops first-ever profile of average multiple birth mother and baby.

Research on Multiples (web site press release); 2005. East Islip, NY: Author. Available at: http://www.preemiecare.org/newsletter_05.htm. Accessed January 20, 2007.

Saint L, Maggiore P, Hartmann P. Yield and nutrient content of milk in eight women breast-feeding twins and one woman breast-feeding triplets. *Br J Nutr.* 1986;56:49–58.

Breastfeeding and Growth: Birth Through Weaning

Nancy Mohrbacher, IBCLC

OBJECTIVES

- Discuss normal growth in the full-term breastfeeding baby and compare differences in growth when babies are not breastfed.
- Explain how culture, infant stomach size, and mothers' breast storage capacity can affect breastfeeding patterns.
- Recognize how breastfeeding behaviors change during the first 12 months and beyond as a result of normal growth and development.
- Identify recommendations for breastfeeding duration and compare them to the natural age of weaning.
- Describe safe and gentle weaning strategies for families who choose to end breastfeeding prior to their child's natural readiness to wean.

Introduction

Expectations of breastfeeding behavior are influenced by culture, and a wide range of breastfeeding behaviors and weaning ages are considered normal in different times and places. At one end of the spectrum, it is culturally normal to breastfeed four times per hour round the clock for the first two years of life among the !Kung of Africa, one of the world's last hunter-gatherer societies (Stuart-Macadam, 1995). This culture also expects frequent and intense breastfeeding for the first three to four years of life. At the other end of the spectrum is the modern-day United States, where cultural beliefs about breastfeeding are influenced by bottle-feeding norms. During the first few months of life, babies in the United States are generally expected to breastfeed at regular intervals of no less than two to three hours. In this culture, as babies age, the intervals between breastfeedings are expected to increase. When babies indicate they want to breastfeed more often than these cultural expectations, mothers are often encouraged to supplement with formula. Complete weaning is generally expected by about one year of age.

I. Human Babies Are Born with Instinctive Breastfeeding Behaviors

A. Mammalian biology suggests that frequent feedings and continuous contact are normative for human babies.

B. If kept skin-to-skin with mother after birth, healthy newborns instinctively move to the breast and breastfeed.

1. After birth, healthy newborns follow a predictable series of behaviors that move them to the breast, stimulate oxytocin release in the mother (Matthiesen et al., 2001), and lead to breastfeeding, usually about an hour after birth (Table 28-1).

2. If a mother receives certain pain medications during labor or mother and baby are separated before the first breastfeeding, these instinctive behaviors are temporarily suppressed in some newborns (Righard & Alade, 1990).

C. If human infants are separated from their mothers during the newborn period, they are at risk for unstable body functions and feeding problems.

1. Human newborns separated from their mother exhibit the "protest-despair" response that also occurs in other mammals.

a. The baby uses a distinctive "separation distress" cry to alert the mother of his or her need to be reunited (Christensson et al., 1995).

b. Levels of stress hormones rise and body functions such as temperature, blood sugar, breathing, and heart rate become unstable (Christensson et al., 1992).

c. If the cry is not responded to, the newborn's physiology changes to "despair mode," slowing digestion and growth to increase odds of survival.

Table 28-1 Newborn Instinctive Behaviors After Birth

Median	Behavior
Time *minutes*	
6	Opens eyes
11	Massages the breast
12	Hand to mouth
21	Rooting
25	Moistened hand to breast
27	Tongue stretches and licks nipple
80	Breastfeeding

Source: Adapted from Matthieson A, Ransjo-Arvidson A, Nissen E, Uvnäs-Moberg K. Postpartum maternal oxytocin release by newborns: effects of infant hand massage and sucking. *Birth.* 2001; 28:13–19.

2. Continuous contact between mother and baby is associated with fewer feeding problems, less crying, and more stable body functions (Christensson et al., 1992).

D. Mammalian species fall into four broad categories, with maturity at birth and milk composition (especially fat and protein content) determining normative feeding frequency (Bergman, 2001).

1. Cache mammals (such as deer, rabbit) are born most mature; mothers are able to leave the newborns for up to 12 hours before returning to feed because their milks are highest in fat and protein.

2. Follow mammals (such as giraffe, cow) are less mature at birth; newborns must follow the mothers to feed at shorter intervals because their milks are lower in fat and protein than the milks of cache mammals.

3. Nest mammals (such as dog, cat) are less mature still at birth; mothers must return to their litter to feed more often because their milks are lower than follow mammals' milks in fat and protein.

4. Carry mammals (such as marsupials, primates, humans) are the least mature at birth; the young must maintain continuous contact with the mother's body throughout infancy and feed round-the-clock, because their mothers' milks are lowest in fat and protein (human milk is among the lowest).

II. Growth Curves for Breastfed Babies Differ from Babies Fed Nonhuman Milks

A. In 2006, the World Health Organization (WHO) published its child growth standards, based on primary growth data from 8500 children from six ethnically and culturally diverse countries, using breastfed children as the normative model for growth and development (WHO Multicentre Study Group, 2006a).

1. Previous growth charts did not control for differences in feeding method and provided a basis for comparison only.

2. The current standards set international benchmarks and serve as guidelines for how all children should grow.

3. Mothers who participated in the study that led to these standards optimally, did not smoke and added healthy complementary foods to their baby's diet between four and six months, the recommended age at the time of the study.

B. Breastfed babies are leaner than babies fed nonhuman milks from four to twelve months, and boys gain weight slightly faster than girls (Figures 28-1 and 28-2).

1. Using the 2006 growth standards, more children will be considered overweight than with previous charts.

2. In comparison to the previous growth references, when the 2006 growth standards are used, from birth to six months more children will be considered underweight, and from six and twelve months fewer children will be considered underweight.

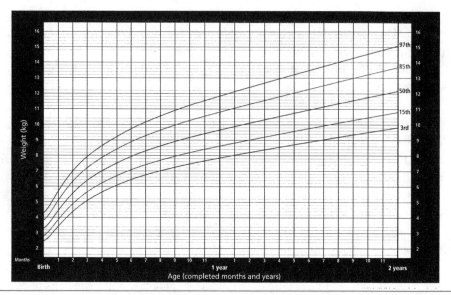

Figure 28-1   WHO Weight-for-age Boys, Birth to 2 years (percentiles). *Source:* WHO Multicentre Growth Reference Study Group. *WHO Child Growth Standards.* Geneva, Switzerland: World Health Organization, 2006. Web site: http://www.who.int/childgrowth/en.

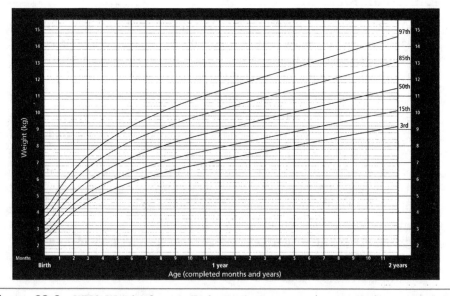

Figure 28-2   WHO Weight-for-age Girls, Birth to 2 years (percentiles). *Source:* WHO Multicentre Growth Reference Study Group. *WHO Child Growth Standards.* Geneva, Switzerland: World Health Organization, 2006.

C. Growth in length varies by sex, with boys growing slightly faster than girls (Figures 28-3 and 28-4), and occurs in spurts rather than continuously (Lampl, Velduis, & Johnson, 1992).

D. Included in these data are internationally valid windows of achievement for gross motor milestones (Figure 28-5).

III. Breastfeeding Patterns During Infancy Vary by Cultural Expectations, Infant Stomach Size, and Time of Day

A. Cultural expectations influence breastfeeding patterns.

1. In some traditional cultures, babies breastfeed intensely—as often as several times each hour—day and night for three to four years (Stuart-Macadam, 1995).
   a. In these cultures, mothers keep their babies against their bodies as they work, and babies have ready access to the breast at all times.
   b. Intense breastfeeding is considered normal and desirable.

2. In many Western cultures, mothers are expected to regulate breastfeeding by the clock.
   a. Mothers are told to encourage babies—even newborns—to breastfeed at set intervals of no less than two to three hours.
   b. The use of breast substitutes, such as pacifiers/dummies and bottles, is common and encouraged.

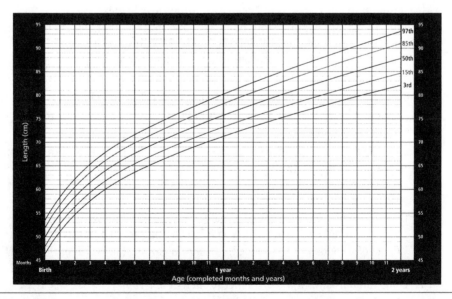

Figure 28-3   WHO Length-for-age Boys, Birth to 2 years (percentiles). *Source:* WHO Multicentre Growth Reference Study Group. *WHO Child Growth Standards.* Geneva, Switzerland: World Health Organization, 2006.

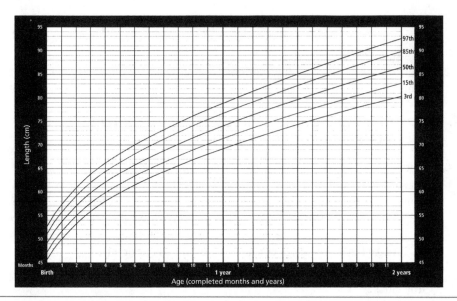

Figure 28-4   WHO Length-for-age Girls, Birth to 2 years (percentiles). *Source:* WHO Multicentre Growth Reference Study Group. *WHO Child Growth Standards.* Geneva, Switzerland: World Health Organization, 2006.

    c. Separation of mothers and babies is considered normal and desirable, and mothers are encouraged to "get away" from their babies.
    d. Work is usually distinct from home life, and most mothers leave their babies with a caregiver to do their work in another location.
    e. Babies are expected to self-soothe, sleep alone, and be weaned at an early age.
  B. A baby's age and stomach size will determine in part how much milk is taken at each feeding, which affects how many times per day a baby needs to breastfeed to thrive (Kent et al., 2006).
    1. A baby needs a certain amount of milk per day to thrive, which varies by age until about one month (Butte et al., 2000; Kent et al., 2006).
    a. On the first day, a breastfed baby needs about 30 mL/day.
    b. At about one week, this has increased to about 300 to 450 mL/day.
    c. By about one month, a breastfed baby needs about 750 to 1050 mL/day.
    d. Daily milk intake stays relatively stable from one to six months.
    e. When solid foods are introduced, ideally no earlier than six months (WHO, 2001), the amount of human milk needed will decrease, as solid food replaces some human milk in a baby's diet (Cohen et al., 1994).
    2. A baby is born with a tiny stomach that stretches little to none during the first 24 hours (Silverman, 1961; Zangen et al., 2001).

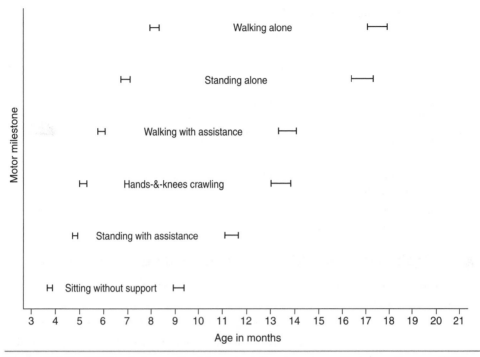

Figure 28-5   WHO windows of achievement for six gross milestones. *Source:* WHO Multicentre Growth Reference Study Group. *WHO Child Growth Standards.* Geneva, Switzerland: World Health Organization, 2006. Web site: http://www.wo.int/childgrowth/en/.

   a. During the first day, a newborn's stomach can hold on average 5 to 7 mL/feeding.
   b. By day three, an infant's stomach can hold on average 22 to 27 mL.
   c. By day ten, it can hold on average 60 to 81 mL.
   d. By one month, a breastfed baby averages 60 to 120 mL per feeding (Kent et al., 2006).

C. Mother's breast storage capacity (how much milk the glandular tissue in her breasts can comfortably hold) affects the amount of milk a baby has access to at a feeding (Daly & Hartmann, 1995; Daly, Owens, & Hartmann, 1993; Kent et al., 2006).

   1. A mother with a large breast storage capacity has more milk available at each feeding, which in some cultures may have a profound effect on breastfeeding patterns.
   a. The baby may always be satisfied with one breast per feeding.
   b. The baby may feed fewer times per day than average but gain weight at an average or above-average rate.

c. The baby may feed less often at night at an earlier age than an average baby.

2. The mother with a small breast storage capacity can produce plenty of milk overall, but her baby will likely have a very different breastfeeding pattern.
   a. The baby will need to breastfeed more times per day to get the same amount of milk.
   b. The baby may always want both breasts at a feeding.
   c. The baby may need to feed often at night throughout infancy and beyond.

D. Time of day also can influence breastfeeding patterns, especially in Western cultures where babies are expected to feed at regular intervals (Kent et al., 2006).

1. It is common for babies in Western cultures to breastfeed less often during morning hours.

2. It is common for babies in Western cultures to breastfeed more often or even continuously during the evening.

IV. As Babies Grow and Mature, Breastfeeding Behaviors Change

A. Irrespective of cultural expectations, babies tend to breastfeed long and often during the first 40 days postpartum.

1. Newborns in Western cultures breastfeed on average 20 to 40 minutes per feeding, with their feeding times tending to shorten with practice and maturity.

2. During the first six weeks or so, breastfed babies typically breastfeed at least 8 to 12 times per day and "cluster" their feedings together, especially during the evening.

B. After six weeks, the breastfed baby in a Western culture tends to spend much less time breastfeeding.

1. Feeding length tends to shorten from about 20 to 40 minutes on average during the newborn period to about 15 to 20 minutes later.

2. Number of feedings decreases as a baby's stomach size increases and he or she can hold more milk (WHO Multicentre Study Group, 2006b).

C. Older babies may return to intense breastfeeding to adjust their mothers' milk supply as needed, which is sometimes referred to as *growth spurts* that typically occur around two to three weeks, six weeks, and again at three months (Mohrbacher & Stock, 2003).

D. Beginning at around three months, babies who were previously content to breastfeed without interruption now become easily distracted from the breast by activities going on around them (Mohrbacher & Stock, 2003).

1. Mothers are sometimes concerned about this change in breastfeeding and worry about whether their babies are getting enough milk.
   a. During this developmental phase, many babies breastfeed better at night.

    b. If a mother wants to encourage more consistent breastfeeding during the day, she can try breastfeeding in a darkened room with fewer distractions. Usually babies outgrow this distraction phase, so this will be a temporary situation.

    c. If a mother has other children, avoiding distractions during the day may be difficult.

  2. Even with distractions during breastfeeding, as long as a mother allows baby ready access to the breast, a baby can get the milk needed by breastfeeding more often or longer at other times.

E. As babies begin to teethe and teeth appear, they may bear down on the breast during feedings to help relieve gum soreness, causing nipple pain or trauma.

  1. To prevent this, suggest the mother give her baby something cold to chew on to numb the gums before breastfeeding, like a cold wet cloth.

  2. If the baby is taking other foods, the mother may choose to provide cold or frozen foods before breastfeeding.

  3. If the baby persists in biting, the mother can pull baby in close enough to block his or her airway with the breast.

    a. This will cause the baby to open his or her mouth to breathe, avoiding further skin damage as baby comes off the breast.

    b. It also discourages future biting.

F. As a baby learns to crawl and then walk, he or she may become even more distracted during breastfeeding, especially during daylight hours, and may begin to take more milk at night.

V. A Minimum of One Year (AAP, 2005) to Two Years (WHO, 2001) of Breastfeeding Is Recommended, with Solid Foods Added at About Six Months of Age

A. These recommendations are based on a large body of research linking shorter duration of breastfeeding to increased incidence of many health problems later in life, including obesity, childhood cancers, Crohn's disease, Hodgkin's disease, allergies, inflammatory bowel diseases, and others (AAP, 2005).

B. Women who have not breastfed or those with shorter breastfeeding durations are at increased risk for premenopausal breast cancer, ovarian cancer, osteoporosis, and diabetes (AAP, 2005).

VI. When Weaning Age Is Considered Independent of Culture, the Human Norm Is Between Three and Seven Years (Dettwyler, 1995; Figure 28-6)

A. Weaning before age three years is associated with a higher risk of morbidity and mortality (Molbak et al., 1994).

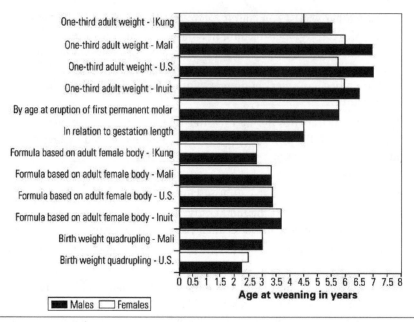

Figure 28-6 Natural age at weaning according to technique used. *Source:* Dettwyler, K. A time to wean: The hominid blueprint for the natural age of weaning in modern human populations. In *Breastfeeding: Biocultural Perspectives,* edited by P. Stuart-Macadam and K. Dettwyler. New York: Aldine de Gryter, 1995.

B. Breastfeeding is the natural outlet for a child's sucking urge until this urge is outgrown.

1. In some cultures, this desire to suck is satisfied with breast substitutes, such as pacifiers/dummies or bottles, which increase the risk of abnormal mouth and dental formation.

2. Early weaning is associated with an increased need for orthodontia (Labbok & Hendershot, 1987) and speech and reading problems, especially in boys (Broad & Dungazich, 1983).

C. No matter what the child's age, the sucking and skin-to-skin of breastfeeding release oxytocin in mother and child (Uvnäs-Moberg, 1998), which is associated with:

1. Enhanced maternal/infant attachment.

2. Easier transition to sleep for both mother and child.

3. Greater calm during times of crisis or upset.

VII. Clinical Breastfeeding Challenges from Six to Twelve Months and Beyond

A. Candidiasis and mastitis (breast inflammation sometimes referred to as *plugged ducts* or *breast infections*) can occur any time during the course of breastfeeding.

B. Some situations are unique to the mother of an older breastfeeding baby and child.

   1. Return of menstruation.

     a. Most women who exclusively breastfeed for the first six months, add solid foods gradually, and continue to breastfeed at night, on average resume menstruation at about one year postpartum (Lewis et al, 1991).

     b. Some mothers report that their baby is reluctant to breastfeed or refuses the breast right before their period or during the first day or two.

     c. Some women report a diminishing milk supply around their period, with supply increasing after a day or two of frequent breastfeeding.

     d. Some women feel nipple pain or tenderness during this time each month.

   2. New pregnancy.

     a. Research indicates that 74% of breastfeeding women experience nipple pain during pregnancy (Mead & Newton, 1967).

     b. Mature milk reverts to colostral fluid at about four to five months of pregnancy.

     c. About two thirds of babies wean during pregnancy (Newton & Theotokatos, 1979), which may be due to diminished milk volumes or a change in the taste of the milk.

     d. Abrupt weaning by the baby or child is possible, as is the desire to continue breastfeeding.

     e. Some children wean during the pregnancy but resume breastfeeding after the birth of the baby.

   3. Nursing strikes (Mohrbacher & Stock, 2003).

     a. Sudden refusal to breastfeed can occur after a period of uneventful breastfeeding.

     b. Common causes include otitis media, nasal congestion, unusual separation of mother and baby, a negative emotional encounter (often associated with a bite), frequent use of bottles and/or pacifiers, low milk supply, and sometimes the cause is unknown.

     c. This problem is almost always temporary and can be resolved with frequent skin-to-skin contact without pressure to breastfeed, attempting breastfeeding while baby is asleep or half asleep, and elimination of artificial nipples.

     d. Illness should always be ruled out as a cause.

     e. Mothers may feel this as a personal rejection.

     f. Suggest the mother express her milk as often as her baby was breastfeeding to preserve her milk supply until the baby accepts the breast again.

VIII. The Lactation Consultant Should Be Prepared to Offer Help to a Family Who Chooses to Wean Before the Child Is Developmentally Ready

A. Examine own beliefs regarding appropriate age of weaning.

B. Assist the family in viewing breastfeeding within the context of the child's normal development.

C. Discuss their feelings and reasons for wanting to wean.

1. In cultures or families where breastfeeding an older baby or child is viewed with disapproval, social pressure can influence parents' decision to wean.

2. If their goals for weaning are unlikely to be met (that is, the child will become more independent or start sleeping more at night), be sure to inform them that weaning may not accomplish this goal.

3. Depending on the reason for weaning (that is, the mother feels "touched out"), it may be appropriate to suggest a partial rather than a full weaning.

4. If a medical issue is involved, encourage the parents to get a second opinion.

D. Provide specific strategies for gradual weaning that are consistent with the age of the child and the parents' cultural beliefs.

1. If possible, abrupt or sudden weaning should be avoided, because it increases the mother's risk of severe pain, mastitis, and breast abscess.

2. When weaning a baby younger than 12 months, discuss weaning issues specific to this age range.
   a. An appropriate substitute for human milk needs to be chosen, which should be done in consultation with the baby's health care provider.
   b. Discuss feeding method; in countries where bottles are not safe, a young baby may need to be fed the substitute milk by cup or spoon.
   c. Babies older than six to eight months may be able to take all their liquid from a cup.
   d. To allow her milk supply to decrease gradually and comfortably, suggest the mother substitute one daily breastfeeding with a feeding of the substitute milk and then wait two to three days before eliminating another breastfeeding.
   e. Repeat this process until the mother has weaned from all feedings at the breast.
   f. If at any time during weaning a mother's breasts feel uncomfortably full, suggest she express just enough milk to make herself comfortable, which will prevent pain and health risk.

3. When weaning a baby older than 12 months, discuss issues specific to the older child (Mohrbacher & Stock, 2003).
   a. A child will need more food to offset the loss of human milk in the diet, but these can be foods from the family table.

    b. For weaning to be a positive transition, explain that the older baby or child considers breastfeeding to be more than a feeding method; it is also a way to be close and receive comfort, and to have more "mommy time."

    c. There are many time-tested strategies for helping the older baby or child make this a gentle transition (Mohrbacher & Kendall-Tackett, 2005).

       i. Don't offer the breast but don't refuse if the child asks.

      ii. Change daily routines so that the child asks to breastfeed less, which (depending on the child) may mean getting away from home more or staying home more.

     iii. Have the mother's partner take a more active role by getting up with the child at night and getting up with the child in the morning and providing breakfast.

     iv. Offer other foods and drinks before the child usually asks to breastfeed to decrease hunger and thirst.

      v. Avoid the place where breastfeeding normally occurs.

     vi. Breastfeed when asked, but for a shorter time than usual.

    vii. Postpone breastfeeding.

   viii. Bargaining can sometimes be used with an older child, but only with a child old enough to understand the meaning of a promise.

    d. Encourage the family to use those strategies that work well for their child and avoid those that don't.

References

American Academy of Pediatrics Work Group on Breastfeeding (AAP). Breastfeeding and the use of human milk. *Pediatrics.* 2005;115:496–506.

Bergman N. Kangaroo mother care: restoring the original paradigm for infant care and breastfeeding. Video 2001. Cape Town, South Africa: Kangaroo Mother Care. Available at: http://www.kangaroomothercare.com. Accessed January 19, 2007.

Broad F, Duganzich D. The effects of infant feeding, birth order, occupation and socio-economic status on speech in six-year-old children. *NZ Med J.* 1983:483–486.

Butte N, Wong WW, Hopkinson JM, et al. Infant feeding mode affects early growth and body composition. *Pediatrics.* 2000;106:1355–1366.

Christensson K, Cabrera T, Christensson E, et al. Separation distress call in the human neonate in the absence of maternal body contact. *Acta Paediatr.* 1995;84:468–473.

Christensson K, Siles C, Moreno L, et al. 1992. Temperature, metabolic adaptation and crying in healthy full term newborns cared for skin to skin or in a cot. *Acta Paediatr.* 1992;81:488–493.

Cohen R, Brown KH, Canahuati J, et al. Effects of age of introduction of complementary foods on infant breast milk intake, total energy intake, and growth: a randomised intervention in Honduras. *Lancet.* 1994;344:288–293.

Daly S, Hartmann P. Infant demand and milk supply. Part 2: The short-term control of milk synthesis in lactating women. *J Hum Lact.* 1995;11:27–31.

Daly S, Owens RA, Hartmann PE. The short-term synthesis and infant-regulated removal of milk in lactating women. *Exp Physiol.* 1993;78:209–220.

Dettwyler K. A time to wean: the hominid blueprint for the natural age of weaning in modern human populations. In: Stuart-Macadam P, Dettwyler K, eds. *Breastfeeding: Biocultural Perspectives.* New York: Aldine de Gryter; 1995.

Kent J, Mitoulas L, Cregan M, et al. Volume and frequency of breastfeedings and fat content of breast milk throughout the day. *Pediatrics.* 2006;117:387–395.

Labbok M, Hendershot G. Does breast-feeding protect against malocclusion? *Am J Prev Med.* 1987;3:227–332.

Lampl M, Velduis J, Johnson M. Saltation and stasis: a model of human growth. *Science.* 1992;258:801–803.

Lewis P, Brown JB, Renfree MB, Short RV. The resumption of ovulation and menstruation in a well-nourished population of women breastfeeding for an extended period of time. *Fertil Steril.* 1991;55:529–536.

Matthieson A, Ransjo-Arvidson A, Nissen E, Uvnäs-Moberg K. Postpartum maternal oxytocin release by newborns: Effects of infant hand massage and sucking. *Birth.* 2001;28:13–19.

Mead M, Newton N. Cultural patterns of perinatal behavior. In: Richardson S, Guttmacher A. *Childbearing: Its Social and Psychological Aspects.* Baltimore: Williams & Wilkins Company; 1967.

Mohrbacher N, Kendall-Tackett K. *Breastfeeding Made Simple: Seven Natural Laws for Nursing Mothers.* Oakland, CA: New Harbinger Publications; 2005.

Mohrbacher N, Stock J. *The Breastfeeding Answer Book.* 3rd ed. Schaumburg, IL: La Leche League International; 2003.

Molbak K, Gottschau A, Aaby P, et al. Prolonged breastfeeding, diarrhoeal disease, and survival of children in Guinea-Bissau. *BMJ.* 1994;308:1403–1406.

Newton N, Theotokatos M. Breastfeeding during pregnancy in 503 women: does a psychobiological weaning mechanism exist in humans? *Emotion Reprod.* 1979; 20B:845–849.

Righard L, Alade M. Effects of delivery room routines on success of first breast-feed. *Lancet.* 1990;336:1105–1107.

Silverman MA, ed. *Dunman's Premature Infants.* 3rd ed. New York: Paul B. Hoeber, Inc., Medical Division of Harper and Brothers; 1961:143–144.

Stuart-Macadam P. Breastfeeding in prehistory. In: Stuart-Macadam P, Dettwyler K. *Breastfeeding: Biocultural Perspectives.* New York: Aldine de Gryter; 1995.

Uvnäs-Moberg K. Oxytocin may mediate the benefits of positive social interaction and emotions. *Psychoneuroendocrinology.* 1998;23:819–835.

World Health Organization (WHO) Multicentre Growth Reference Study Group. WHO Child Growth Standards. Geneva: World Health Organization; 2006a. Available at: http://www.who.int/childgrowth/en/. Accessed January 19, 2007.

World Health Organization (WHO) Multicentre Growth Reference Study Group. Breastfeeding in the WHO Multicentre Growth Reference Study. *Acta Paediatr.* 2006b;95(suppl 450):16–26.

World Health Organization (WHO). The optimal duration of exclusive breastfeeding: report of an expert consultation. Geneva: World Health Organization; 2001.

Zangen S, Di Lorenzo C, Zangen T, et al. Rapid maturation of gastric relaxation in newborn infants. *Pediatr Res.* 2001;50:629–632.

Breastfeeding with Maternal Physical Impairments

Noreen Siebenaler, MSN, RN, IBCLC
Judi Rogers, OTR/L

OBJECTIVES

- List five maternal disabilities that may create barriers to successful breastfeeding.
- State one to two methods of assisting or adaptations that are most appropriate for each disability listed in objective one.
- Discuss four reasons why women with physical, sight, or hearing disabilities often find breastfeeding easier than bottle-feeding.
- List three community services for breastfeeding mothers with physical, sight, or hearing disabilities.

Introduction

An increasing number of women with physical and sensory disabilities are choosing to become mothers. Disabled women have the same desires as other women to have children. Lactation consultants will hopefully have increasing opportunities to work with them. Many professionals have not seen anyone with a disability take care of and breastfeed a baby, and it can be difficult to imagine how they might manage. Some mothers with disabilities have been able to successfully breastfeed as well as take care of their babies even without proper equipment and support. Having appropriate equipment and support can make breastfeeding and baby care more successful. Many people with and without disabilities have learning difficulties. When working with a disabled mother who seems to have difficulty grasping information, try to give small pieces of information separately and check for understanding before giving more information. A small percentage of people with cerebral palsy (CP) have some learning difficulties. Do not confuse people who have speech involvement with people who have learning difficulties. People who have speech involvement have their tongue and mouth muscles affected by their disability. Multiple sclerosis (MS) may cause some learning difficulties such as short-term memory loss or slowed processing of information. A part of developing skills as a professional is to expand the perception you have of women breastfeeding to include women with disabilities. When working with mothers who have disabilities, it is important to remember that they are mothers first. Be respectful when asking questions; explain exactly what you need to know and why.

Women with disabilities who want to breastfeed do not always have support from their families and friends. Family members may think breastfeeding will drain the mother of her limited energy, or that it will be too physically demanding. One mother, who had a neuromuscular disability, when expressing why breastfeeding was so important to her said, "This is the only thing I can do for my baby that no one else can do" (Rogers, 2005).

Mothers with sensory disabilities care for and bond with their infants in the same ways as nondisabled mothers do, through their senses of touch, smell, and intuitive sensitivity (Martin, 1992). There is no physiological reason why mothers who are blind or deaf should not breastfeed.

Women with muscular dystrophy, CP, MS, and other physical disabilities may be unable to hold and position their babies for breastfeeding without proper equipment. They often have difficulty breastfeeding outside of their homes.

Breastfeeding a baby without appropriate aids and techniques can increase pain for women who have repetitive stress disorders such as carpel tunnel, tendonitis, or thoracic outlet syndrome (TOS). Partial breastfeeding may be most appropriate for women with specific disabilities and situations (Carthy, Conine, & Hall, 1990).

The following are guidelines for lactation consultants to use in their practice:

1. Women who have been physically disabled for a long time are usually very knowledgeable about their abilities and limitations. Involve them in decision-making. Ask for their opinions (Mohrbacher & Stock, 2003).

2. Help mothers find comfortable positions and appropriate, supportive breastfeeding pillows.

3. Assist the mother in locating other types of supportive equipment such as adaptable pumps and bras that will make breastfeeding easier.

4. Use creativity in problem solving, involve supportive family members, promote coordination of services that enhance the mother's abilities, and locate appropriate community and Internet resources.

5. Be aware that this may be the first time the mother has handled a baby.

I. Carpel Tunnel Syndrome (repetitive stress disorder)

A. Etiology and symptoms.

1. A painful disorder of the wrist and hand where the median nerve is compressed causing part of the wrist and hand to have parasthesia (numbness, tingling, and weakness).

    2. Swelling from irritated tendons narrows the carpel tunnel and causes the median nerve to be compressed.

    3. More common in women, especially during pregnancy.

    4. During pregnancy, the hormone relaxin loosens connections between tendons, which may result in pressure on the median nerve.

    5. Compression of the median nerve causes weakness, pain with opposition of the thumb as well as burning, tingling, or aching that radiates to the forearm and shoulder joint. Pain is intermittent or constant and often is most intense at night.

    6. Diagnosis is by physical exam, electromyography (EMG), and magnetic resonance imaging (MRI).

  B. Treatment.

    1. See De Quervain's tendonitis treatment (section II).

    2. Methods of assisting are similar to those for TOS (section III) and De Quervain's tendonitis (section II).

II. De Quervain's Tendonitis (repetitive stress disorder)

  A. Etiology and symptoms.

    1. Also called *new mother's tendonitis*. Pain and inflammation is caused by an irritation of two tendons at a point where they run through a very tight channel on the thumb side of the wrist.

    2. The irritation at the base of the thumb can cause difficulty in turning the wrist and gripping.

    3. Repetitive stress disorder may be present as a work-related injury prior to childbirth.

    4. Can be caused by repetitive wrist motions new mothers use as they care for their infants and the repetitive wrist-bending movements a mother may use to attach a baby to breastfeed (Wagman, 1993).

    5. Diagnosed by a physical examination, EMG, and MRI.

  B. Treatment (carpel tunnel and De Quervain's tendonitis).

    1. Anti-inflammatory medications, oral analgesics, ice or cool packs to relieve symptoms.

    2. Injections of cortisone often bring dramatic relief of pain.

    3. Wrist splint can minimize pressure on the nerves; keeps the wrist straight at night to minimize pain; also forearm splint for carpel tunnel.

    4. Change repetitive work activities, resting affected area for two weeks if possible.

    5. Physical therapy exercise and ultrasound over affected areas to strengthen and reduce swelling.

    6. Surgical intervention is occasionally needed to relieve symptoms.

C. Methods of assisting are similar to and can be combined with TOS and carpel tunnel syndrome.

III. Thoracic Outlet Syndrome (TOS; a repetitive stress disorder)

A. Etiology and symptoms.

1. A group of distinct disorders that result in compressions of nerves and blood vessels in the brachial plexus, a network of nerves that extends from the base of the neck to the axilla and conducts signals from the shoulder, arm, and hand.

2. Many physical and occupational therapists believe TOS is caused by injury to the nerves in the brachial plexus.

3. The main symptom of this disorder is pain. Shoulder and elbow pain can radiate to the little finger and ring finger.

4. Abnormal burning or prickling sensations may be felt in the arms or hands.

5. TOS is often caused by repetitive activities or by a hyperextension injury.

6. Diagnosed by physical exam, EMG, and MRI.

B. Treatment.

1. Physical therapy.
   a. Can strengthen surrounding muscles of the shoulder.
   b. Can stretch muscles in the arm and shoulder as well as the scalenes in the neck.

2. Postural exercises help with standing and sitting straighter, which reduces pressure on nerves and blood vessels, relieving pain.

3. Ergonomic assessment of work environment to avoid strenuous activities.

4. Anti-inflammatory medications and oral analgesics.

C. Possible effect on breastfeeding (carpel tunnel, De Quervain's tendonitis, TOS).

1. Difficulties with picking up the baby, positioning baby, moving the baby at the breast or between breasts, and burping the baby, due to pain that impacts wrist and hand movements.

2. Limited ability to use two hands to assist baby with latch-on.

3. Reduced finger dexterity to open and close bra.

D. Methods of assisting (carpel tunnel, De Quervain's tendonitis, TOS).

1. Firm breastfeeding pillows that go around mother's waist and bring baby up to breast level, thus keeping the baby's weight off mother's arms, wrists, and hands.

2. Football or clutch positions using pillows to hold baby so mother does not have to use arms, wrists, and hands when breastfeeding.

3. Breastfeed one breast per feeding.

4. Latch on using one hand and without bending wrists (Figure 29-1).

5. Velcro bra attachments for opening and closing bra.

6. Mothers with TOS often find a side lying position too painful, due to compression of thoracic nerves. A 45-degree supine position may be the most effective and least painful for nighttime feedings.

7. Slings may make breastfeeding easier for mothers with carpel tunnel and tendonitis because babies can breastfeed in slings with less wrist and hand movement.

8. Women with TOS will have increasing pain and related symptoms if they use small electric breast pumps that vibrate. Hospital-grade automatic cycling pumps or other higher level non-vibrating pumps would be most appropriate.

9. Hands-free pumping bras and devices that hold pump pieces in place during pumping without using hands prevent symptoms of repetitive stress and are available over Internet sites (see Internet Resources).

IV. Multiple Sclerosis

A. Etiology and symptoms.

   1. MS usually appears between the ages of 20 and 40.
     a. It has a variety of symptoms that vary over time.
     b. It may not be diagnosed until years after the first symptoms occur because the symptoms are variable and confusing.
     c. There are four subtypes.

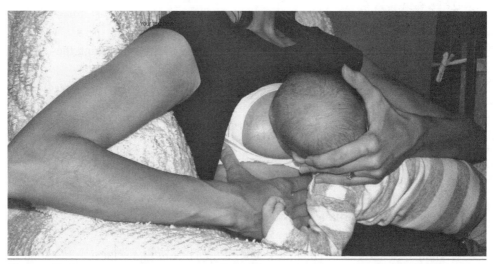

Figure 29-1   Latch on without bending wrists. Used with permission.

2. Symptoms are caused by demyelinization (reduction of the myelin sheaths covering nerves).
    a. Myelin sheaths help with nerve conduction.
    b. Remission of symptoms will result when the glial scar forms over the myelin sheath repairing the sheath.
3. Symptoms of MS can be sensory (visual problems, numbness and/or tingling in hands and feet).
4. There can be limitations in movement to one or all four extremities as well as limitations to fine motor skills, speech, and central body movement.
5. Causes of MS are not completely understood. It is an autoimmune disorder in which a person's antibodies attack the myelin sheath covering the nerves.
6. Depression is often associated with MS.

B. Diagnosis.
1. Physical exam, symptom history, MRI, and spinal tap.
    a. A greater than normal amount of protein in cerebrospinal fluid is characteristic of MS.
    b. The diagnosis is difficult to make because many other conditions affect the nervous system and produce similar symptoms.

C. Treatment.
1. Corticosteroids and other medications are used both to treat symptoms such as bladder, bowel, and visual disturbances, and to slow the progression.
2. Treatment goals include maintaining mobility and providing adaptations needed during exacerbations.

D. Possible effects on breastfeeding.
1. All medications should be evaluated for their passage into breast milk and any effect they may have on the baby (Hale, 2006).
2. Symptoms (exacerbations) of MS are more likely to increase during the postpartum period (Lorenzi & Ford, 2002).
3. A preliminary study showed an association between increased breastfeeding and decreased postpartum exacerbations (Gulick & Halper, 2002).
4. Upper extremities can be affected causing difficulty with picking up, holding, and latching on (see Figure 29-2).
5. If the baby breastfeeds easily, a mother may find breastfeeding easier than bottle-feeding (Adelson, 2003).
6. Some mothers may find the first weeks of breastfeeding stressful and tiring and may choose to partially breastfeed (Eggum, 2001).

E. Methods of assisting for MS.
1. Similar to and can be combined with CP, spinal cord injury (SCI), rheumatoid arthritis (RA), and myasthenia gravis (MG).

Figure 29-2 Supportive position for mothers with MS.

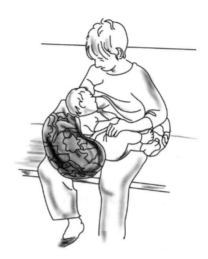

V. Cerebral Palsy

A. Etiology and symptoms.

1. CP involves damage to the motor area of the brain. Damage may occur prenatally, during birth or the postpartum period, or in infancy/childhood.

2. Limitations involve one to four limbs, trunk, and speech. When one side is affected, it is called *hemiplegia*; both legs affected is *diplegia*, three limbs affected is *triplegia*, four limbs affected is *quadriplegia (or tetraplegia)*.

3. Classifications of cerebral palsy (CP).
   a. Athetoid CP is characterized by involuntary, irregular, slow movements of the affected body part.
   b. Spastic CP is characterized by increased muscle tone that results in the affected limb being stiffly held, making it hard to move the limb.
   c. Ataxic CP is characterized by a wide-based, unsteady gait and often reduced manual dexterity.
   d. Types of CP are distinguished by muscle tone and pattern of movement.

B. Diagnosis.

1. Usually occurs during infancy.

2. Based upon symptoms, delays in developmental milestones, and MRI.

C. Treatment.

1. Physical therapists and occupational therapists can help with increasing and maintaining ability to function.

D. Possible effects on breastfeeding.

1. Limited upper extremity functioning if there is hemiplegia, triplegia, or quadriplegia. This results in difficulty with positioning on nonaffected side, plus difficulty switching baby from the nonaffected side to the affected side.

2. Upper extremities can be affected, causing difficulty with picking up or holding the baby as well as latching on and burping.

E. Methods of assisting for CP are similar to and can be combined with those for MS, SCI, MG, and RA.

VI. Spinal Cord Injury

A. Etiology and symptoms.

1. SCI refers to irreversible damage to the spinal cord caused by trauma or tumor.
   a. The spinal cord is a bundle of nerves inside the vertebral column that carries messages between the brain and the rest of the body.
   b. Nerves from the cord come out at each vertebrae, and it is at the vertebral level where the extent of injury is determined.
   c. Neck vertebrae are C1 to C7; injuries at this level will affect all four limbs (quadriplegia).

2. Injury to the spinal cord usually causes both loss of movement (paralysis) and loss of sensation. There can also be movement with loss of sensation or sensation with loss of movement.

3. Thoracic vertebrae are located on the upper and mid back.
   a. Vertebrae are numbered T1 to T12. Injury between T1 and T8 causes high paraplegia in which trunk control is affected.

4. Injury to the lumbar level vertebrae affects leg movement and sensation; injury to the sacral level affect groin, leg, and toe movement.

5. The level of injury determines the level of function lost.
   a. The higher the injury, the more functions are lost.
   b. Breathing is affected if the injury is above C4.

6. An SCI at T6 or above places people at risk for autonomic dysreflexia, a condition caused by noxious or painful stimuli below the level of the injury.
   a. A noxious stimulus can include an extended bladder, labor and delivery, nipple pain, or breast pain.
   b. Some symptoms of dysreflexia, such as headaches, sweating, goose bumps, and fluctuations of blood pressure, if unresolved can result in stroke (Walker, 2006).

B. Treatment.

1. Treatment involves working with physical therapy and occupational therapy to increase functional abilities (Herman, 2002).

C. Possible effects on breastfeeding.

1. A reduction in milk production may be seen as soon as three to five days after the birth and as late as six weeks postpartum in a mother with an injury at T4 (Rogers, 2005).
   a. Colostrum does not seem to be affected.
   b. Reduced milk production may be due to the lack of sensation at the nipples and the decreased sympathetic nervous system feedback to the pituitary, resulting in decreased prolactin secretion (Halbert, 1998; Walker, 2006).

2. In a woman who has an SCI below the T6 level, milk production is not affected (Rogers, 2005).

3. Pain associated with breastfeeding can cause dysreflexia. Nausea, anxiety, sweating, and goose bumps below the level of the SCI are the first symptoms of dysreflexia (see section VI, Etiology and symptoms).

4. Possible limited ability to hold, position for breastfeeding, lift, or burp the baby.

D. Methods of assisting for SCI are similar to and can be combined with those for MS, CP, RA, and MG.

VII. Rheumatoid Arthritis (RA)

A. Etiology and symptoms.

1. Defined as an inflammatory condition of the joints, characterized by pain and swelling (Andersen, Anderson, & Glanze, 1994).
   a. A chronic, destructive, sometimes deforming, autoimmune collagen disease most commonly beginning in the joints of the hands and wrists.
   b. Results in a symmetric inflammation of the synovium (fluid surrounding joints) and swelling of joints.
   c. Joint involvement is usually symmetrical, meaning that if a joint hurts on the left hand, the same joint will hurt on the right hand.
   d. Effects of RA can vary from person to person. There is growing evidence that RA is not one disease but may be several different diseases with the same symptoms (Brennan & Silman, 1994; see Figure 29-3).

2. Common physical symptoms include: fatigue, stiffness especially in the morning, pain associated with prolonged sitting, weakness, flu-like symptoms and muscle pain, including a low-grade fever (Brun, Nilssen, & Kvale, 1995).
   a. Loss of appetite may be present as well as depression, weight loss, anemia, cold and/or sweaty hands and feet.

3. Exacerbations and remissions are common.
   a. Remission often occurs during pregnancy (Jacobsen, Askling, & Knowler, 2003).
   b. Exacerbations are likely to occur during the postpartum period.
   c. Research suggests that exposure to high levels of prolactin could stimulate the development of RA in susceptible women (Barrett et al, 2000; Brennan et al., 1996).

Figure 29-3 This jacket for arthritis sufferers has a Velcro™ closure for easy access, and the jacket helps keep the mother's stiff shoulders warm.

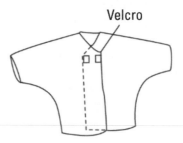

d. Karlson showed that women who breastfed for 13–24 months had a 20% reduction in risk for development of RA while those breastfeeding for at least 24 months during their childbearing years increased their risk reduction to 50% (Karlson et al, 2004).

4. Stress aggravates RA and increases symptoms.

B. Treatment.

1. In severe pain, intra-articular injections of corticosteroids may give relief.

2. Patients are advised to avoid situations known to cause anxiety, worry, fatigue, and other stressors.

3. Treatment includes sufficient rest, exercise to maintain joint function, medications for the relief of pain and to reduce inflammation, orthopedic interventions to prevent deformities, and dietitian-guided weight loss if needed.

4. Medications used to decrease pain and inflammation are usually compatible with breastfeeding.
   a. Steroids are commonly given.
   b. One possible serious side effect of steroids that may occur is psychosis.

5. Hale (2006) recommends pumping and discarding mother's milk for a minimum of four days when methotrexate therapy is indicated.

C. Diagnosis.

1. Lab tests can verify and differentiate between arthritis and other diseases.

D. Possible effects on breastfeeding.

1. Mothers will need additional rest due to the sometimes overwhelming fatigue, stiffness, and pain that occur postpartum.

2. Worsening of symptoms often impacts baby care activities such as breastfeeding and diapering.

E. Methods of assisting for RA are similar to and can be combined with those for MS, CP, SCI, and MG.

VIII. Myasthenia Gravis (MG)

A. Etiology and symptoms.

   1. Chronic autoimmune disease causing weakness in voluntary muscles throughout the body.

   2. Antibodies interfere with messages sent from nerve endings to muscles.

   3. There are three types: a hereditary type that may cause the baby to have a weakened suck, one type with ocular involvement, and one type with generalized involvement.

   4. Those with generalized involvement comprise 85% to 90% of MG patients.
     a. This type also involves voluntary muscles that control movement, eyelids, chewing, swallowing, coughing, and facial expression.
     b. Involuntary muscles that can be affected are those that control eye movement, eyelids, chewing, swallowing, coughing, and facial expressions.

   5. There is usually no pain experienced with this form of autoimmune disease.

   6. When breathing muscles are affected, *myasthenic crisis* may occur and respiratory support may be needed. Usually there are progressive warning signs before a crisis, and it is more likely to occur when difficulty with swallowing and talking have been present.

   7. Remission of symptoms is common and can last for long periods of time.

B. Diagnosis.

   1. Medical history, physical and neurological exam.

   2. Assessment for impairment of eye movements or muscle weakness without any changes in ability to feel things.

   3. Tests for muscle responsiveness and blood tests for the presence of immune molecules or acetylcholine receptors.

   4. Nerve conduction tests.
     a. The most current information can be found on the National Institutes of Health Web site (see Internet Resources).

C. Treatment.

   1. Medications used to treat MG help improve neuromuscular transmission and increase muscle strength.

   2. Immunosuppressive drugs may also be used to improve muscle strength by suppressing the production of abnormal antibodies.

   3. Thymectomy, surgical removal of the thymus gland, helps reduce symptoms in more than 70% of affected persons and may provide a cure in some cases.

D. Possible effects on breastfeeding.

1. Weakness and fatigue of arm and neck muscles can result in difficulty with positioning and attachment.
2. Fatigue associated with specific muscle groups increases the need for rest periods.

E. Methods of assisting MS, CP, SCI, RA, and MG.

1. MS and CP may affect upper extremity function.
2. Depending on what is needed, demonstrate and provide one-to-one help as follows.
   a. Women with these disabilities may be prescribed medications.
   b. All medications should be evaluated for their passage into breast milk and any effect they may have on the baby.
   c. Refer to physician, text references, and Internet resources to determine the compatibility of these medications with breastfeeding.
3. Partial breastfeeding may be indicated due to the mother's exacerbations, and/or fatigue, stress, etc. If it is indicated, provide information on maintaining adequate milk production (Wade et al., 1999).
4. Trying out different breastfeeding pillows allows a mother to determine which one works best for her.
   a. The pillow should hold the baby at breast level and keep the weight of the baby on the pillow and off the mother's arms.
   b. A pillow that attaches around the waist will ensure stability.
5. Increase the mother's knowledge of different breastfeeding positions so she can find which positions are easiest and most comfortable for her.
6. Encourage and assist the mother to try different positions while lying down. This can help fatigue issues and nighttime feedings.
   a. Lying on the affected side is helpful so the mother can use her unaffected arm.
   b. A 45-degree angle supine position also may be helpful for breastfeeding the baby.
   c. When it is difficult to hold a baby, a baby sling might help with holding and positioning the infant for breastfeeding (Figure 29-4).
7. Use of a lifting harness, after the baby is a month old also may help with changing baby's position and burping (see Internet Resources).
8. Breastfeeding on one side per feeding may be easier.
9. Mothers with limited hand and wrist can use the latch-on and positioning suggestions listed for repetitive stress disabilities.
10. Place a rolled cloth diaper or small cloth towel under the mother's breast so she does not have to use her hand to hold her breast while feeding.
11. Holes can be cut in a bra to expose the areola and nipple.

Figure 29-4 A support
suggestion for mothers with
muscular weakness.

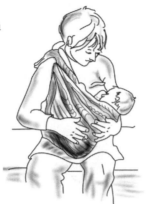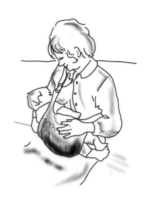

a. This provides breast support while feeding and helps to position the breast
for easier latch-on.

b. Hands-free pumping bras may vary from extremely effective to minimally
effective.

c. For some women with hand and wrist limitations, this may be the only way
they can pump independently or without pain.

12. Prevent nipple pain by teaching the mother how to position and latch her
baby correctly, express milk onto the nipple after feedings, and air dry her
nipples.

13. Women need to be aware of possible pain associated with breastfeeding, such
as the pain of engorgement, mastitis, and nipple pain, so they can minimize
the pain or prevent it by learning different techniques.

a. Breastfeeding pain can trigger increased spasticity in women with a variety
of disabilities.

b. In women with SCI at T6 and above, pain can cause dysreflexia that could
become dangerous (see section VI. Spinal Cord Injury).

14. Support team.

a. If the mother has a personal care attendant (PCA), the mother may choose to
ask the PCA to help her with breastfeeding.

b. Family or friends also may help with positioning, latch-on, and burping.

c. The lactation consultant should show the support team how to assist with
positioning and attachment.

15. Discuss with the mother and determine which baby care activities are most
important to her.

a. Her choice may be determined by her need to conserve energy for the more
enjoyable tasks such as feeding and playing with her baby as well as a

desire for her spouse or partner to do some of the baby care tasks (Rogers, Tuleja, & Vensand, 2004).

16. Adaptive baby care equipment and advice are available to mothers (see Internet Resource list).

17. Help the mother articulate her needs and what type of help she would like.
    a. It is important to take her family dynamics into consideration.
    b. If there is difficulty in matching the mother's needs with the family's desire to help, recommend a consult with a family therapist.

18. Discuss with the mother any adjustments that are necessary to adapt her environment to facilitate breastfeeding, such as breastfeeding in a wheelchair or wheelchair access to the baby's crib (Riordan, 2005).

IX. Sensory Disabilities: Visual Impairment, Deafness, and Hard of Hearing

A. Overview.

1. Mothers who cannot see or hear their infants do care for and bond with them in the same ways as nondisabled mothers, through their senses of touch, smell, and intuitive sensitivity (Martin, 1992).

2. There is no physiological reason why mothers who are blind or deaf should not breastfeed.

B. Etiology and symptoms of visual impairment.

1. Blindness or partial sight can be caused by hereditary conditions and many other medical conditions, including premature birth, or congenital conditions.

2. Blindness can occur at any age, beginning with birth.

3. Total blindness, no light perception, occurs in approximately 3% of the U.S. population (Good Mojab, 1999).

4. Definition: for every 200 feet of normal vision, a legally blind person will see approximately 20 feet (Good Mojab, 1999).

5. Some partially blind individuals will see only shadows or have fluctuating vision. They may see better during the day and be totally blind at night or may be very light sensitive.

C. Etiology and symptoms: deafness and hard of hearing.

1. Deafness may result from prenatal exposure to various conditions such as rubella, cytomegalovirus, hereditary conditions, premature birth, congenital conditions, or medical conditions.

2. Total deafness occurs in approximately 1% of the U.S. population.

D. Diagnoses.

1. Diagnosis of visual impairment occurs through an eye exam by an optometrist.
    a. A more thorough visual evaluation by an ophthalmologist follows, which will include a functional vision assessment.
2. Diagnosis of deafness occurs through audiological screening at a hospital or doctor's office or through newborn hearing screenings.

E. Methods of assisting a mother with visual impairment.

1. Breastfeeding may be easier because there are no bottles to prepare and clean.
2. Ask the mother what she can see, because many mothers have partial vision.
3. Turn visual demonstrations into verbal descriptions.
4. A football hold allows easy access to the baby's face so a mother can feel how the baby's jaw is moving during sucking.
5. A baby sling gives a mother the ability to use both hands for latch by using the index finger (braille finger) to locate the baby's nose and lips.
6. Cradle or cross-cradle hold may give better "tummy to tummy" orientation with the baby's body.
7. Refer to experienced breastfeeding mothers who are partially sighted or blind.
8. Resources for blind mothers: Braille communications and audio tapes for partially sighted or blind mothers are available from La Leche League International (Martin, 1992).

F. Methods of assisting deaf or hard of hearing mothers.

1. Sign language as a communication method to accompany one-to-one breastfeeding assistance for deaf mothers may be available with the mother's clinic, hospital, or community (Bowles, 1991).
2. Deaf mothers communicate in a variety of ways. Ask what they prefer: speaking, writing, signing, or e-mail (Bykowski, 1994).
3. Vibration pagers for deaf mothers have different vibrations for different sounds, so a pager can vibrate a certain way when a baby cries (see Internet Resources).
4. The most effective teaching methods for deaf mothers may be video, written materials, and recommended Web sites.
5. Telephone systems specifically designed for deaf individuals are easily available for home use. Mothers can use these systems to call lactation consultants when questions or problems arise.

"Some of the material in this chapter was developed under Through the Looking Glass' funding from the U.S. Department of Education, National Institute on Disability and Rehabilitation Research (#H133A04001). The content and opinions do not necessarily represent the policy of NIDRR, nor should anyone assume endorsement by the Federal Government."

References

Adelson R. MS and pregnancy: the main event. *Inside MS.* 2003;21: Issue 2.

Anderson K, Anderson L, Glanze W. *Mosby's Medical, Nursing, and Allied Health Dictionary*, 4th ed. St. Louis: Mosby Yearbook; 1994:124–125.

Barrett JH, Brennan P, Fiddler M, Silman A. Breastfeeding and postpartum relapse in women with rheumatoid and inflammatory arthritis. *Arthritis Rheum.* 2000;43: 1010–1015.

Bowles BC. Breastfeeding consultation in sign language. *J Hum Lact.*1991;7(1):21.

Brennan P, Ollier B, Worthington J, et al. Are both genetic and reproductive associations with rheumatoid arthritis linked to prolactin? *Lancet.* 1996;348:106–109.

Brennan P, Silman A. Breastfeeding and the onset of rheumatoid arthritis. *Arthritis Rheum.* 1994;37:808–813.

Brun JF, Nilssen S, Kvale G. Breastfeeding and other reproductive factors and rheumatoid arthritis: a prospective study. *Br J Rheumatol.* 1995;34:542–546.

Bykowski N. Helping mothers who are deaf or hard of hearing. *Leaven.* 1994; May–June:45–46.

Carthy E, Conine TA, Hall L. Comprehensive health promotion for the pregnant woman who is disabled. *J Nurse Midwif.* 1990;35:133–142.

Eggum M. Breastfeeding with multiple sclerosis. Association of Women's Health, Obstetric and Neonatal Nursing (AWHONN) *Lifelines.* 2001; February/March:37–40.

Good Mojab C. Helping the visually impaired or blind mother breastfeed. *Leaven.* 1999;35:51–56.

Gulick E, Halper J. Influence of feeding method on postpartum relapse of mothers with MS. *Int J MS Care.* 2002;4:183–191.

Halbert L. Breastfeeding in the woman with a compromised nervous system. *J Hum Lact.* 1998;14:327–331.

Hale T. *Medications and Mother's Milk.* 12th ed. Amarillo, TX: Hale Publishing; 2006.

Herman A. Challenges and solutions for parents with disabilities. In: *Spinal Network.* 3rd ed. Horsham, PA: Leonard Media Group; 2002:365–368.

Jacobson ME, Askling J, Knowler WC. Perinatal characteristics and risk of rheumatoid arthritis. *BMJ.* 2003;326:1068–1069.

Karlson EW, Mandl LA, Hankinson SE, Grodstein F. Do breastfeeding and other reproductive factors influence future risk of rheumatoid arthritis? Results from the Nurses Health Study. *Arthritis Rheum.* 2004;50:3458–3467.

Lorenzi A, Ford H. Multiple sclerosis and pregnancy. *Postgrad Med J.* 2002:78:460–464.

Martin CD. La Leche League and the mother who is blind. *Leaven.* 1992;5:67–68.

Mohrbacher N, Stock J. Chronic illness or physical limitations. *The Breastfeeding Answer Book.* Shaumberg, IL: La Leche League International; 2003:557–569.

Riordan J. Baby guidelines for physically disabled breastfeeding mothers. *Breastfeeding and Human Lactation.* 3rd ed. Sudbury, MA: Jones and Bartlett Publishers; 2005: 472–475.

Rogers J. *The Disabled Woman's Guide to Pregnancy and Birth.* New York: Demos Medical Publishing; 2005.

Rogers J, Tuleja C, Vensand K. Baby care preparation. In: Welner S, Haselstine F, eds. *Welner's Guide to the Care of Women with Disabilities.* Philadelphia: Lippincott Williams & Wilkins; 2004:171.

Wade M, Foster N, Cullen L, et al. Breast and bottle-feeding for mothers with arthritis and other physical disabilities. *Prof Care Mother Child.* 1999;9:35–38.

Wagman R. *Preventing Repetitive Stress Syndrome for the New Mother.* Englewood, NJ: Hand Rehabilitation Center of Englewood; 1993.

Walker M. *Breastfeeding Management for the Clinician: Using the Evidence.* Sudbury, MA: Jones and Bartlett Publishers; 2006: 411–443.

Internet Resources

Through The Looking Glass (TLG). A community nonprofit organization formed in 1982 as a resource center for families in which one or more members has a disability. TLG's mission is to create, demonstrate, and encourage resources, and model early intervention services that are health promoting and empowering. TLG consults with parents and professionals nationally and internationally. Adaptive baby care equipment including lifting harnesses and advice for mothers is available. Available at: http://www.lookingglass.org. Accessed January 20, 2007.

Arthritis

Arthritis Foundation. Search diseases center. Atlanta, GA. Available at: http://www.arthritis.org. Accessed January 20, 2007.

CBS News. Healthwatch. Breastfeeding Fights Arthritis. Available at: www.cbsnews.com/stories/2004/11/04/health/webmd/main653734.shtml. Accessed January 20, 2007.

Web MD. Search rheumatoid arthritis. Available at: http://www.webmd.com. Accessed January 20, 2007.

Carpel Tunnel

National Institute of Neurological Disorders and Stroke. Bethesda, MD: National Institutes of Health. Search carpel tunnel syndrome. Available at: http://www.ninds.nih.gov. Accessed January 20, 2007.

Thoracic Outlet Syndrome

National Institute of Neurological Disorders and Stroke. Bethesda, MD: National Institutes of Health. Search thoracid outlet syndrome. Available at: http://www.ninds.nih.gov. Accessed January 20, 2007.

Multiple Sclerosis

International Multiple Sclerosis Support Foundation, Jean Sumption. A Web site of physicians with MS. Available at: http://www.msnews.org. Accessed January 20, 2007.

Multiple Sclerosis Association of America, Cherry Hill, NJ. Available at: http://www.msaa.com. Accessed January 20, 2007.

Multiple Sclerosis Foundation, Ft. Lauderdale, FL. Available at: http://www.msfacts.org. Accessed January 20, 2007.

Multiple Sclerosis and Breastfeeding: Personal Stories. Available at: http://www.nationalmssociety.org/pregnancy_letters.asp.

Multiple Sclerosis Medications and Breastfeeding. Available at: www.nationalmssociety.org/clinup_breastfeeding.asp. Accessed January 20, 2007.

National Multiple Sclerosis Society, New York. Available at: http://www.nmss.org.

New Mobility. The Total Wheelchair Resource Book. Horsham, PA. Available at: http://www.spinalnetwork.net. Accessed January 20, 2007.

Spinal Cord Injury

Medline Plus, Bethesda, MD. Available at: http://www.nlm.nih.gov/medlineplus/spinalcordinjuries.html. Accessed January 20, 2007.

National Spinal Cord Injury Association. Common Questions about Spinal Chord Injury. Available at: http://www.Spinalcord.org/html/factsheets/spin.php. Accessed January 20, 2007.

Regional Spinal Cord Injury Center of Delaware Valley, Jefferson Health Care System. Spinal Cord Injury Manual. Available at: http://www.Spinalcordcenter.org/manual/pdf-files/scibook-chp08.pdf. Accessed January 20, 2007.

Spine Universe, Wheaton, IL. Benzel EC. Spinal chord injury (SCI): aftermath and diagnosis. Available at: http://www.Spineuniverse.com/displayarticle.php/article1445.html. Accessed January 20, 2007.

Myasthenia Gravis

Howard JF Jr. Myasthenia gravis—a summary. [monograph on the Web]. Available at: http://www.myasthenia.org/information/summary.htm. Accessed January 20, 2007.

National Institute of Neurological Disorders and Stroke. Bethesda, MD: National Institutes of Health. Myasthenia gravis fact sheet. Available at: http://www.ninds.nih.gov/disorders/myasthenia_gravis/detail_myasthenia_gravis.htm#545531. Accessed January 20, 2007.

Neurology Channel. Health Communities.com. Myasthenia gravis. Available at: http://www.neurologychannel.com/myastheniagravis/. Accessed January 20, 2007.

Deafness

Deaf Counseling, Advocacy, and Referral Agency, San Leandro, CA. Available at http://www.dcara.org. Accessed January 20, 2007.

National Association of the Deaf (NAD), Silver Spring, MD. Available at: http://www.nad.org. Accessed January 20, 2007.

Blindness

American Council of the Blind, Washington, DC. Available at: http://www.acb.org. Accessed January 20, 2007.

American Foundation for the Blind, New York. Available at: http://www.igc.apc.org/afb/. Accessed January 20, 2007.

HEAR-MORE Co., Farmingdale, New York. Sonic Alert Bed Vibrator D/C Auxilliary Jack. Available at: www.hearmore.com/store/prodList.asp?idstore=1. Accessed January 20, 2007.

La Leche League International, Schaumberg, IL. Audiotapes and Braille. Available at: http://www.lalecheleague.org. Accessed January 20, 2007.

Breastfeeding Technology

Milk Expression, Storage, and Handling

Rebecca Mannel, BS, IBCLC
with contributions from Ruth Worgan, RN, CM, IBCLC

OBJECTIVES

- Describe indications and methods for expression of human milk.
- Discuss the types and action of available mechanical pumps.
- Describe the techniques of hand and mechanical expression.
- Discuss current guidelines for storage and handling of human milk.

Introduction

At some time during the course of lactation, many women may choose or need to express their milk. Whether to initiate, maintain, or increase milk production, the removal of a mother's milk from her breasts either by hand or mechanical breast pump is a learned technique. Women benefit from clear instructions and guidelines on how to express milk in an efficient manner and of a sufficient quantity to meet their individual needs.

I. Mothers May Choose or Need to Express Milk for a Number of Reasons

A. To increase the milk supply.

B. To stimulate lactogenesis II when breastfeeding initiation is delayed due to separation of baby and mother.

C. To supply milk if her baby is ill or hospitalized and cannot breastfeed directly.

D. To prevent or relieve breast engorgement.

E. To have milk available if she leaves the baby with another caregiver.

F. To provide her baby with milk while she is at work or at school.

G. To maintain or increase milk production when:

1. Breastfeeding is interrupted due to travel, maternal hospitalization, or maternal use of medications contraindicated during lactation.

2. Milk production has decreased due to infrequent feedings or inadequate milk removal.

3. A mother chooses to provide only expressed milk to her baby rather than directly breastfeed.

H. To contribute to a milk bank.

II. Hand-Expression of Human Milk

A. The most common form of milk expression throughout the world.

1. No equipment or electricity is required.

2. Hands are always available.

3. No cost to mother.

4. Every mother should learn how to hand express her milk (Lawrence, 2005).

B. Reasons to express milk by hand (in addition to I. above).

1. To soften the areola.
   a. Drains overfull milk ducts to make it easier for baby to latch on.

2. To elicit the milk ejection reflex prior to breastfeeding or pumping.

3. If the nipples are sore or macerated and the use of a pump will exacerbate the tissue damage.

III. Mechanical Expression of Human Milk

A. Mechanical devices for expressing milk have been used for centuries (Walker, 2005).

1. Some cost involved to purchase.

2. May require electricity.

3. Replacement parts may be needed at times.

4. Minimal to no regulations for breast pumps exist in most countries.
   a. In the United States, pumps are regulated by the Food and Drug Administration (FDA) for safety. Adverse events are reported to the FDA (http://www.accessdata.fda.gov/scripts/cdrh/cfdocs/cfMAUDE/Search.cfm).

B. Reasons to express milk with a breast pump.

1. See section I.

2. Can be easier, less tiring than hand expression.
   a. Mothers with physical impairments may be unable to hand express.

3. Can be faster than hand expression.
   a. Several types allow for simultaneous pumping of both breasts.

4. Can collect more milk.

   a. Mothers often collect more milk with mechanical expression than with hand expression (Paul et al., 1996; Slusher et al., 2004).

   b. Mothers collect more milk with simultaneous pumping (Auerbach, 1990; Jones, Dimmock, & Spencer, 2001).

5. Can be more comfortable.

   a. Mothers with severely engorged breasts may find hand expression too painful.

6. Some sexual abuse survivors may tolerate mechanical pumping over hand expression or direct breastfeeding (Lauwers & Swisher, 2005; Riordan, 2005).

IV. Factors to Consider in Choosing Type of Pump

A. Age of baby.

B. Condition of the baby.

C. Condition of the mother.

D. Reason/need for pumping.

E. Availability and affordability.

F. Efficacy and comfort.

G. Ease of use and cleaning.

H. Availability of replacement parts/service.

I. Safety.

1. The rubber bulb or "bicycle horn" type manual pumps should be avoided because of the great potential for bacterial contamination of milk as well as nipple pain and damage (Foxman et al., 2002; Lawrence, 2005).

2. Electric or battery-operated pumps that maintain constant negative pressure are more likely to cause nipple/breast trauma (Egnell, 1956; Lawrence, 2005).

V. Action: How Milk Is Removed from the Breast

A. Infants use suction and a compressive, peristaltic tongue motion to remove milk from the breast. Pumps use suction only in a cyclic pattern (Zoppou, Barry, & Mercer, 1997a).

B. When milk flow is low, infants suckle faster. When milk flow is high, infants suckle slower. Average suckling rate is 74 cycles/minute with a range of 36 to 126 cycles/minute (Bowen-Jones, Thompson, & Drewett, 1982).

C. Negative pressure generated by infant suckling averages 50 to 155 mm Hg with a maximum of 241 mm Hg (Prieto et al., 1996).

D. Effective pumps create a vacuum that forms a pressure gradient. Under the higher pressure of the milk ejection reflex, milk flows or is "pushed out" to the lower pressure of the milk collection container.

E. Effective pumps do not suck, pull, or pump milk out of the breast.

F. Effectively nursing infants can transfer more milk from the breast than the mother who is pumping (Chapman et al., 2001; Zoppou, Barry, & Mercer, 1997b).

G. A few pumps also use compression.

VI. Manual or Hand Pumps

A. Advantages.

1. Affordable; least expensive type of pump.

2. Available; easily found in most communities.

3. Portable; no electricity or batteries required.

4. Most are easy to use and easy to clean.

5. Some can be adapted for use on electric pumps.

B. Disadvantages.

1. Inconsistent or inadequate suction levels.

2. Most require sequential pumping rather than simultaneous.

3. Longer pumping sessions (15–20 minutes/breast).

4. User fatigue.

5. Not recommended for frequent, full-time use (such as working mother or mother of preterm, hospitalized infant (ABM #7, 2004).

C. Types/action.

1. Two main types available.

a. Cylinder pumps.

i. Made up of two cylinders, one inside the other. A gasket at the end of the inner cylinder forms a seal with the outer cylinder.

ii. Vacuum is generated when the outer cylinder is pulled while the inner one remains over the areola.

iii. Some have adjustable vacuum and/or mechanism that automatically interrupts the vacuum at the end of the outward pull on the cylinder.

iv. Higher vacuum is generated as the outer cylinder fills with milk. This may become painful.

v. The outer cylinder may come off during pumping, spilling all the expressed milk.

vi. Gaskets need to be removed for cleaning to prevent bacterial contamination.

vii. Gaskets need to be replaced because they can dry out, shrink, or lose ability to create a seal.

b. Squeeze-handle pumps.

i. Vacuum is generated when the mother squeezes and releases a handle.

ii. Some have adjustable vacuum.

iii. Some have adjustable cycling.

iv. Some have several parts that need to be disassembled for adequate cleaning.

v. Gaskets need to be removed for cleaning to prevent bacterial contamination.

vi. Gaskets need to be replaced because they can dry out, shrink, or lose ability to create a seal.

VII. Battery-Operated Pumps

A. Advantages.

1. Portable.
   a. No electricity required.
   b. Batteries are available in most communities.
   c. Rechargeable batteries are an option.

2. Easy to use.
   a. Requires only one hand; one brand is hands-free.
   b. No user fatigue.

3. Some can be adapted for use on larger, electric pumps.

4. Some mothers buy two and use for simultaneous pumping.

5. Some are designed for simultaneous pumping.

6. Most have adjustable vacuum.

7. Most accept an A/C adapter and can be plugged into an electrical outlet when desired.

B. Disadvantages.

1. Require replacement of batteries, which can be frequent depending on how much the mother is pumping.

2. Several types require manual release of the vacuum during the pumping cycle; nipple trauma can occur with prolonged vacuum (Egnell, 1956).

3. Vacuum in some pumps takes up to 30 seconds to reach appropriate level. Time for recovery of the vacuum following release varies from brand to brand and can limit the number of cycles to < 6/minute, which is below acceptable ranges (Riordan, 2005).

4. As batteries deteriorate, the vacuum recovery time lengthens. Some types of batteries are not as effective as others.

5. Maximum vacuum can continue decreasing after each release during the pumping session.

6. Not recommended for mothers pumping for preterm/hospitalized infants (ABM #7, 2004).

C. Types/action.

1. The batteries/electricity power a small motor that generates a vacuum.

2. One type is worn under the bra so the mother can pump hands-free.

3. A/C adapters save on battery life and allow motor to achieve maximum cycling of vacuum.

VIII. Electric Pumps

A. Advantages.
   1. Often available in hospitals for mothers of preterm or sick infants.
      a. Some communities have these pumps available for rental.
      b. Some insurance companies cover the cost of rental for mothers of hospitalized infants.
      c. A prescription for breast milk from the baby's physician might be required to secure the rental and to extend it for use after the baby is discharged.
   2. Some employers make these pumps available to their employees who return to work and continue breastfeeding.
   3. Most allow for simultaneous pumping of both breasts.
   4. No user fatigue.
   5. Shorter pumping sessions (10–15 minutes total for simultaneous pumping).
   6. Most have adjustable vacuum.
   7. Some have automatic cycling that approaches physiological suckling (Mitoulas et al., 2002a).
   8. Recommended for mothers who are pumping for preterm/hospitalized infants (that is, daily use).

B. Disadvantages.
   1. Least affordable type of pump.
   2. May not be readily available in some communities.
   3. Electricity is required. Some have accessory adapter for use in automobiles; some can operate with batteries.
   4. Several types require manual release of the vacuum during the pumping cycle (semi-automatic cycling); nipple trauma can occur with prolonged vacuum (Egnell, 1956).

C. Types/action.
   1. Semiautomatic pumps.
      a. Require manual release of the vacuum during the pumping cycle.
         i. The mother typically has to cover a hole in the flange base to create the vacuum.
      b. Most mothers need practice to find the technique of vacuum release/cycling that facilitates effective milk removal.
      c. Smallest and least expensive of the electric pumps.
   2. Automatic pumps.

    a. Hospital-grade.
      i. Designed for use by many mothers; each mother has a personal collection kit to prevent cross-contamination.
      ii. Some have automatic cycling that approaches physiological suckling (Mitoulas et al., 2002a).
      iii. Mothers of preterm infants more likely to achieve full milk supply (Hill et al., 2005a; 2006).
    b. Personal use.
      i. Designed for daily use by one mother for one or more infants.
      ii. Some have automatic cycling that approaches physiological suckling (Mitoulas et al., 2002a).
      iii. Bacterial contamination may occur when loaned/given to other mothers.
      iv. Motor may wear out when loaned/given to other mothers.

IX. Techniques of Milk Expression: General Guidelines

A. Milk can be expressed into any type of container, such as a bottle, cup, glass, jar, or bowl. It helps if the container has a wide opening.

B. Frequency of milk expression depends upon the reason for expression.

   1. For occasional expressing, pump during, after, or between feedings, whichever gives the best results.

   2. Express as many times as required to obtain the amount of milk needed to use or store.

   3. Many mothers tend to express more milk first thing in the morning due to higher residual volumes of milk (Riordan, 2005).

   4. For employed mothers, expressing may be needed on a regular basis for at least the number of breastfeeds that are missed (ABM #3, 2002).

   5. To increase a low milk supply, she can express after each feeding. Mothers who are supplementing with expressed human milk and/or formula should express at least each time baby receives a supplemental feeding (ABM #3, 2002).

   6. For preterm or ill babies, the mother should begin expressing milk as early as possible within the first 24 hours and 8 to 10 times each 24 hours thereafter (Hill et al., 1999a, 2001, 2005b).

   7. For engorgement, she can express for a few minutes to soften the breasts before she breastfeeds, and express after she breastfeeds if she still feels full or uncomfortable (ILCA, 2005).

C. Eliciting milk ejection reflex (milk release).

   1. An infant on average takes 54 seconds to elicit the milk ejection reflex while a breast pump can take up to 4 minutes (Kent et al., 2003; Mitoulas et al., 2002b).

   2. Some women have difficulty with their milk release when trying to express their milk. "Embarrassment, tension, fear of failure, pain, fatigue, and anxiety

may block the neurochemical pathways required for milk-ejection" (Walker, 2005:348).

3. Some women are successful having their baby nurse and stimulate the milk release before pumping or hand expressing.

4. Applying warm compresses, taking a warm shower, thinking about baby, looking at a picture of baby, and/or relaxation techniques help some women elicit the milk ejection reflex.

5. Gentle nipple stimulation (avoid pulling or squeezing) can stimulate oxytocin release (Rojansky et al., 2001; Summers, 1997).

6. Breast massage is widely recognized to stimulate milk release (see section IX. D).

7. Holding baby skin-to-skin (including during hospitalization) can stimulate oxytocin release (Uvnäs-Moberg & Petersson, 2005).

8. A recent randomized, controlled trial showed no significant difference in milk collection with the use of oxytocin nasal spray (Fewtrell et al., 2006).

D. Breast massage.

1. Stimulates oxytocin release which controls milk ejection reflex (Matthiesen et al., 2001).

2. Increases milk collection and thus milk production (Jones et al., 2001).

3. Improves composition of human milk by increasing gross energy and lipid content (Foda et al., 2004).

4. Various methods (Okeya, Oketani) are widely promoted in Japan (Foda et al., 2004; Kyo, 1982).

5. Adds external pressure, which increases pressure gradient in the breast, facilitating milk flow to negative pressure area of the pump or milk collection container (Walker, 2005).

6. Can be done in different ways, with the mother deciding which method works best for her.
   a. Hold the breast with one or both hands (depending on the size of the breast) so that the thumbs are on top of the breast and the fingers beneath it. Gently compress the breast between the fingers and thumbs, rotating fingers and thumbs around the breast.
   b. Use fingertips to massage in small circles all around the breast. This circular motion can cover some of the harder to reach areas on the underside of the breast and under the arms.

X. Hand Expression

A. Always wash hands before expressing milk.

B. Cup the breast with the thumb and forefingers directly opposite each other without touching the nipple or areola (depending on the extent of the areola). Push back into the chest wall and then forward in a rhythmical movement to 'massage' the breast. Repeat this action, rotating around the breast, being careful to massage forward and not pinch or squeeze (Glynn & Goosen, 2005).

C. Another method that some mothers find helpful is to hold the breast so that the thumb is on the top margin of the areola and the other four fingers are cupping the breast from underneath, with the little finger touching the rib.

   1. To express milk, she will start a wave-like motion from her little finger, pushing gently into the breast followed by the fourth finger, then the third, then the index finger while the thumb compresses from above.

   2. She can perform this action a few times and rotate the hand position so that all areas of the breast are reached.

   3. When she is finished on the first breast, she will continue on the second one.

   4. To obtain more milk, she can return to the first breast again, alternating back and forth to take advantage of the several milk ejection reflexes.

D. Avoid squeezing, rubbing, or pulling breast tissue.

E. Thorough milk removal and softening of the breast may take 20 to 30 minutes (Lawrence, 2005).

XI. Mechanical Expression

A. Follow manufacturer's instructions on use and cleaning for specific types of pumps.

   1. Ensure mother understands mechanism for vacuum release.

B. Wash hands before any milk expression.

C. Assemble collection equipment; ensure cleanliness.

   1. Washing equipment in the dishwasher or with hot soapy water is usually sufficient to keep it clean.

   2. All parts that come in contact with the milk should be washed after each use.

D. Some pumps come with various types of inserts that can be placed inside the flange (cone-shaped part that is placed over the nipple/areola) for a better fit.

E. Many pumps come with variable-sized flanges to accommodate larger nipples.

   1. The mother should use a flange that "fits" her nipple: the nipple should move freely back and forth in the "tunnel" or straight shaft of the flange and should not pinch, chafe, or rub during pumping. Flange diameters range from 21 mm to 40 mm.

   2. Pumping can cause areolar edema (Wilson-Clay & Hoover, 2005).

   3. Continued pumping with a flange that is too tight will cause nipple pain/trauma and reduction of milk supply (Meier, Motykowski, & Zuleger, 2004).

4. More than half of mothers who are pumping for preterm/hospitalized infants may require flanges with diameters > 24 mm (Meier et al., 2004).

F. The flange should be centered over the nipple and areola during pumping.

G. Some mothers massage breasts before and during pumping for optimal milk collection.

    1. If using a double collection kit, the flanges can be held in place with the forearm to free the other hand for breast massage.

    2. Some women secure the flanges to their bra to free one or both hands for breast massage.

    3. Some women express both breasts twice following breast massage.

H. Set the pump on the lowest suction setting, increasing it as needed. The mother should feel firm, non-painful tugging.

    1. Pumps that allow the mother to adjust the suction and cycling should initially be set on lower suction with faster cycling. Once milk release has occurred, the suction can be increased and cycling decreased to more closely mimic physiological suckling (Mitoulas et al., 2002b).

I. Duration of pumping session.

    1. Mothers who are pumping occasionally may pump until they have collected the desired quantity of milk.

    2. Mothers who are pumping for preterm/hospitalized infants or to increase milk production should pump until the milk stops flowing.

J. Mothers who are using a manual pump may choose to prop their arm on a pillow, table, or wide chair arm if their arm gets tired.

XII. Expected Milk Volumes (Hill et al., 2005a)

A. Refer to Table 30-1 for data on expected milk output.

B. Mothers produce 30 to 100 mL of milk in the first 24 hours (ILCA, 2005).

C. The average of milk output at postpartum days 6 and 7 is predictive of milk output at postpartum week 6.

D. Adequate milk volume is defined as ≥ 500 mL/day at postpartum week 6.

    1. Preterm mothers are encouraged to produce more than average (750–1000 mL/day) by postpartum day 14 in order to ensure adequate milk production and facilitate infant transition to direct breastfeeding before hospital discharge (see Chapter 26, Breastfeeding a Preterm Infant).

    2. Milk production < 500 mL/day by postpartum day 14 is a marker for inadequate long-term milk production (Hill et al., 1999a).

E. Preterm mothers are 2.8 times more at risk of producing an inadequate milk supply than term mothers (Table 30-1).

Table 30-1   Expected Milk Output (mL/day)

	Week 1 (days 6 and 7 average)	Week 6
Term, Breastfeeding	511 ± 209	663 ± 218
Preterm, Expressing	463 ± 388	541 ± 461

Source: Data are from Hill et al., 2005a.

XIII. Common Problems

   A. Pain with pumping.

      1. Check flange fit.

         a. Change to wider diameter flange if chafing/pinching nipple (Figure 30-1).

         b. Nipples swell during pumping (Wilson-Clay & Hoover, 2005).

      2. Check vacuum/suction levels of pump.

         a. Reduce suction level (see section XI. H).

      3. Check cycling of pump.

         a. Instruct mother how to release suction consistently during milk expression if her pump does not automatically cycle.

Figure 30-1   Poor flange fit. *Source:* Wilson-Clay, B., Hoover K. *The Breastfeeding Atlas.* Austin, TX: Lactnews Press, 2005.

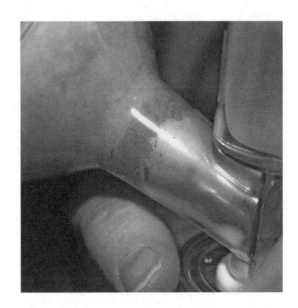

4. Check duration of pumping sessions.
   a. "Marathon" sessions (45–60 minutes) do not increase milk production.
   b. Instruct mother to pump until the milk stops flowing.
5. Consider possible infection of the breast or nipple.
   a. Inadequate breast draining leads to milk stasis, a risk factor for mastitis (ABM #4, 2002).
   b. Nipple trauma is a risk factor for candidiasis and mastitis (ABM #4, 2002; Foxman et al., 2002).
6. Consider changing to a different brand/type of pump.
   a. Breast pump adverse events are likely underreported to the FDA in the United States (Brown et al., 2005).
      i. Most commonly reported adverse events for electric breast pumps were pain/soreness, need for medical intervention, and breast tissue damage.
      ii. Most frequently reported adverse events for manual breast pumps were breast tissue damage and infection.
B. Dwindling or decreasing milk collection.
   1. Preterm mothers who are expressing milk are 2.8 times more at risk of producing an inadequate milk supply than term mothers who are breastfeeding (Hill et al., 2005a).
   2. Many mothers who return to work struggle to maintain an adequate milk supply (Chezem et al., 1998; Hills-Bonczyk et al., 1993).
   3. Table 30-2 lists strategies to increase milk production when expressing milk.
   4. For more information on specific situations related to low milk production, refer to the following chapters:
      a. Insufficient milk production, Chapter 39.
      b. Induced lactation/relactation, Chapter 32.
      c. Preterm/hospitalized infants, Chapter 26.

XIV. Guidelines for Storage and Handling of Human Milk

A. Storage of human milk for the hospitalized infant (HMBANA, 2006).
   1. Milk should be stored in clean, hard-sided containers that are food-grade clean.
      a. Polypropylene or polybutylene plastic or glass with leak-proof lids.
      b. Fill containers ¾ full.
      c. Label with child/mother's name; hospital ID number; date/time of expression.
      d. Milk from each breast at a pumping session can be put in the same container; avoid combining milk from different pumping sessions to minimize contamination.
      e. Human milk does not require biohazard labeling (CDC, 1994).
   2. Table 30-3 shows a list of milk storage guidelines.
      a. While HMBANA guidelines state that fresh, expressed human milk can be

Table 30-2   Dwindling Milk Supply

Assess Expression Technique for Possible Causes of Faltering Milk Supply	Additional Strategies If Pumping Regularly with Effective Pump
Duration of expression/pumping	Expressing while holding/touching baby (skin-to-skin) at least once a day
Adequacy of breast emptying	Breast massage with expression
Frequency of expression/pumping	Conscious relaxation or visualization
Type of pump	Pumping for 2 minutes beyond milk flow
Maternal medication use	Medication/herbs prescribed by physician to increase prolactin levels

Source: Data are from HMBANA, 2006.

stored for less than eight days in the refrigerator, many hospital policies recommend < 48 hours for the hospitalized infant.

B. Storage of human milk for the healthy infant at home or in childcare settings (HMBANA, 2006).

1. Refer to Table 30-4 for milk storage guidelines for the healthy infant.

2. Expressed milk can be stored in glass or plastic baby bottles; clean food storage containers with tight-fitting, solid lids; disposable feeding bottle liners and mother's milk bags.

 a. Double bagging is recommended to protect the milk because some plastic bags/bottle liners can tear easily.

 b. Fill containers ¾ full.

 c. Label with child/mother's name; date/time of expression.

 d. Chill freshly expressed milk before adding it to already refrigerated or frozen milk.

 e. Freeze milk in small amounts of 2 to 4 oz (60–120 mL) to avoid waste and speed thawing.

 f. Human milk does not require biohazard labeling (CDC, 1994).

C. Handling expressed human milk (HMBANA, 2006).

1. Hospitalized infants.

 a. Sample hospital policy: HCA Healthcare (http://www.ilca.org).

2. Healthy infants.

 a. Use any freshly pumped milk if available. Otherwise, use milk with oldest storage date first.

Table 30-3   Milk Storage Guidelines for the Hospitalized Infant

Method	Hospitalized Infant
Room Temperature [77°F or 25°C] (best to refrigerate immediately)	< 4 hours
Refrigerator [39°F or 4°C] (fresh expressed)	< 8 days
Insulated cooler with frozen gel packs [59°F or 15°C] (transported milk)	< 24 hours
Completely thawed and placed in refrigerator [39°F or 4°C]	< 24 hours
Previously frozen, brought to room temperature [77°F or 25°C]	< 4 hours
Freezer Compartment (1 door refrigerator)	Not Recommended
Freezer Compartment [23°F or −5°C] (2 door refrigerator) *not in door	< 3 months
Deep Freezer [−4°F or −20°C]	< 6 months

Source: Data are from HMBANA, 2006.

    b. Milk can be thawed quickly in a container of warm water (not to exceed 37°C or 98°F); ensure water does not touch lid.

    c. Milk can be thawed slowly in the refrigerator or at room temperature. If thawing at room temperature, monitor milk and refrigerate before it is completely thawed, while ice crystals are still present.

    d. Warm milk for feeding by putting container in warm water or holding under running water.

    e. Never microwave human milk, either to defrost it or to warm it.

       i. Microwaving liquids creates hot spots that might burn the baby.

       ii. Microwaving human milk destroys sIgA and other immune components.

    f. If thawed milk has a soapy odor/taste that bothers the baby, the milk can be scalded prior to storing.

       i. Heat milk to ~180°F (82°C) or until small bubbles form around edge of pan; chill quickly and store until use.

       ii. Some mothers have high lipase levels; scalding the milk will inactivate the lipase.

       iii. Milk with soapy odor/taste is not harmful to the baby.

Table 30-4 Milk Storage Guidelines for the Healthy Infant

Method	Healthy Infant
Room Temperature [77°F or 25°C]	< 6 hours
Refrigerator [39°F or 4°C] (fresh expressed)	< 8 days
Insulated cooler with frozen gel packs [59°F or 15°C] (transported milk)	< 24 hours
Completely thawed and placed in refrigerator) [39°F or 4°C]	< 24 hours
Freezer Compartment (1 door refrigerator)	2 weeks
Freezer Compartment [23°F or −5°C] (2 door refrigerator) *not in door	< 6 months
Deep Freezer [−4°F or −20°C]	< 12 months

Source: Data are from HMBANA, 2006; Williams-Arnold, 2000.

References

Academy of Breastfeeding Medicine (ABM). Clinical Protocol Number 3. Hospital guidelines for the use of supplementary feedings in the healthy term breastfed neonate. 2002. Available at: http://www.bfmed.org. Accessed January 20, 2007.

Academy of Breastfeeding Medicine (ABM). Clinical Protocol Number 4. Mastitis. 2002. Available at: http://www.bfmed.org. Accessed January 20, 2007.

Academy of Breastfeeding Medicine (ABM). Clinical Protocol Number 8. Human milk storage information for home use for healthy full term infants. 2004. Available at: http://www.bfmed.org. Accessed January 20, 2007.

Auerbach KG. Sequential and simultaneous breast pumping: a comparison. *Int J Nurs Stud.*1990;27:257–265.

Bowen-Jones A, Thompson C, Drewett RF. Milk flow and sucking rates during breast-feeding. *Dev Med Child Neurol.* 1982;24:626–633.

Brown SL, Bright RA, Dwyer DE, Foxman B. Breast pump adverse events: reports to the food and drug administration. *J Hum Lact.* 2005;21:169–174.

Centers for Disease Control and Prevention. Guidelines for Preventing Transmission of Human Immunodeficiency Virus through Transplantation of Human Tissue and Organs. 1994.

Chapman DJ, Young S, Ferris AM, Perez-Escamilla R. Impact of breast pumping on lactogenesis stage II after cesarean delivery: a randomized clinical trial. *Pediatrics.* 2001;107:E94.

Chezem J, Friesen C, Montgomery P, et al. Lactation duration: influences of human milk replacements and formula samples on women planning postpartum employment. *J Obstet Gynecol Neonatal Nurs.* 1998;27:646–651.

Egnell E. The mechanics of different methods of emptying the female breast. *J Swed Med Assoc.* 1956;40:1–8.

Fewtrell MS, Loh KL, Blake A, et al. Randomised, double blind trial of oxytocin nasal spray in mothers expressing breast milk for preterm infants. *Arch Dis Child Fetal Neonatal Ed.* 2006;91:F169–F174.

Foda MI, Kawashima T, Nakamura S, et al. Composition of milk obtained from unmassaged versus massaged breasts of lactating mothers. *J Pediatr Gastroenterol Nutr.* 2004;38:484–487.

Foxman B, D'Arcy H, Gillespie B, et al. Lactation mastitis: occurrence and medical management among 946 breastfeeding women in the United States. *Am J Epidemiol.* 2002;155:103–114.

Glynn L, Goosen L. Manual expression of breast milk. *J Hum Lact.* 2005;21:184–185.

Hill PD, Aldag JC, Chatterton RT. Effects of pumping style on milk production in mothers of non-nursing preterm infants. *J Hum Lact.* 1999a;15:209–216.

Hill PD, Aldag JC, Chatterton RT. Initiation and frequency of pumping and milk production in mothers of non-nursing preterm infants. *J Hum Lact.* 2001;17:9–13.

Hill PD, Aldag JC, Chatterton RT, Zinaman M. Comparison of milk output between mothers of preterm and term infants: the first 6 weeks after birth. *J Hum Lact.* 2005a;21:22–30.

Hill PD, Aldag JC, Chatterton RT, Zinaman M. Primary and secondary mediators' influence on milk output in lactating mothers of preterm and term infants. *J Hum Lact.* 2005b;21:138–150.

Hill PD, Aldag JC, Demirtas H, Zinaman M, Chatterton RT. Mood states and milk output in lactating mothers of preterm and term infants. *J Hum Lact.* 2006;22(3):305–314.

Hills-Bonczyk SG, Avery MD, Savik K, et al. Women's experiences with combining breast-feeding and employment. *J Nurse Midwifery.* 1993;38:257–266.

Human Milk Banking Association of North America, Inc. (HMBANA). Jones F and Tully MR. *Best Practice for Expressing, Storing and Handling Human Milk in Hospitals, Homes and Child Care Settings.* Raleigh, NC: HMBANA; 2006.

International Lactation Consultant Association. Clinical Guidelines for the Establishment of Exclusive Breastfeeding. U.S. Department of Health and Human Services, Maternal/Child Health Bureau; 2005.

Jones E, Dimmock P, Spencer S. A randomised controlled trial to compare methods of milk expression after preterm delivery. *Arch Dis Child Fetal Neonatal Ed.* 2001;85:F91–F95.

Kent JC, Ramsay DT, Doherty D, et al. Response of breasts to different stimulation patterns of an electric breast pump. *J Hum Lact.* 2003;19:179–186;quiz 87–88, 218.

Kyo T. Observation on initiation of breast feeding: the relationship between Okeya's method of breast massage and the quantity of milk secretion. *Josanpu Zasshi.* 1982; 36:548–549. [in Japanese]

Lauwers J, Swisher A. *Counseling the Nursing Mother.* 4th ed. Sudbury, MA: Jones and Bartlett Publishers; 2005.

Lawrence RA, Lawrence T. *Breastfeeding: A Guide for the Medical Profession.* 6th ed. Philadelphia: C.V. Mosby; 2005.

Matthiesen AS, Ransjo-Arvidson AB, Nissen E, Uvnäs-Moberg K. Postpartum maternal oxytocin release by newborns: effects of infant hand massage and sucking. *Birth.* 2001;28:13–19.

Meier PP, Motykowski JE, Zuleger JL. Choosing a correctly-fitted breastshield for milk expression. *Medela Messenger.* 2004;21:1, 8–9.

Mitoulas LR, Lai CT, Gurrin LC, et al. Effect of vacuum profile on breast milk expression using an electric breast pump. *J Hum Lact.* 2002a;18:353–360.

Mitoulas LR, Lai CT, Gurrin LC, et al. Efficacy of breast milk expression using an electric breast pump. *J Hum Lact.* 2002b;18:344–352.

Paul VK, Singh M, Deorari AK, et al. Manual and pump methods of expression of breast milk. *Indian J Pediatr.* 1996;63:87–92.

Prieto CR, Cardenas H, Salvatierra AM, et al. Sucking pressure and its relationship to milk transfer during breastfeeding in humans. *J Repro Fertil.* 1996;108:69–74.

Riordan, J. *Breastfeeding and Human Lactation.* 3rd ed. Sudbury, MA: Jones and Bartlett Publishers; 2005.

Rojansky N, Tsafrir A, Ophir E, Ezra Y. Induction of labor in breech presentation. *Int J Gynaecol Obstet.* 2001;74:151–156. Review.

Slusher T, Slusher I, Biomdo M, et al. Electric breast pump use increases maternal milk volume and decreases time to onset of maternal milk volume in African nurseries [abstract]. *PediatrRes.* 2004;55:445A.

Summers L. Methods of cervical ripening and labor induction. *J Nurse Midwifery.* 1997; 42:71–85. Review.

Uvnäs-Moberg K, Petersson M. Oxytocin, a mediator of anti-stress, well-being, social interaction, growth and healing. *Z Psychosom Med Psychother.* 2005;51:57–80. Review. [in Swedish]

Walker M. Breast pumps and other technologies. In: Riordan J, ed. *Breastfeeding and Human Lactation.* 3rd ed. Sudbury, MA: Jones and Bartlett Publishers; 2005.

Williams-Arnold LD. *Human Milk Storage for Healthy Infants and Children.* Sandwich, MA: Health Education Associates; 2000.

Wilson-Clay B, Hoover K. *The Breastfeeding Atlas.* 3rd ed. Austin, TX: Lactnews Press; 2005.

Zoppou C, Barry SI, Mercer GN. Dynamics of human milk extraction: a comparative study of breast feeding and breast pumping. *Bull Math Biol.* 1997a;59:953–973.

Zoppou C, Barry SI, Mercer GN. Comparing breastfeeding and breast pumps using a computer model. *J Hum Lact.* 1997b;13:195–202.

Suggested Readings

Academy of Breastfeeding Medicine (ABM). Clinical Protocol Number 8. Human milk storage information for home use for healthy full term infants. 2004. Available at: http://www.bfmed.org. Accessed January 20, 2007.

Biancuzzo M. Selecting pumps for breastfeeding mothers. *J Obstet Gynecol Neonatal Nurs.* 1999;28:417–426.

Bowles BC, Stutte PC, Hensley JH. New benefits from an old technique: alternate massage in breastfeeding. *Genesis.* 1987–1988;9:5–9, 17.

Daly SE, Kent JC, Huynh DQ, et al. The determination of short-term breast volume changes and the rate of synthesis of human milk using computerized breast measurement. *Exp Physiol.* 1992;77:79–87.

Daly SEJ, Owens RA, Hartmann PE. The short-term synthesis and infant regulated removal of milk in lactating women. *Exp Physiol.* 1993;78:209–220.

Daly SE, Hartmann PE. Infant demand and milk supply. Part I. Infant demand and milk production in lactating women. *J Hum Lact.* 1995;11:21–25.

Daly SEJ, Hartmann PE. Infant demand and milk supply. Part 2: The short-term control of milk synthesis in lactating women. *J Hum Lact.* 1995;11:27–37.

Groh-Wargo S, Toth A, Mahoney K, et al. The utility of a bilateral breast pumping system for mothers of premature infants. *Neonatal Netw.* 1995;14:31–35.

Hill PD, Aldag JC, Chatterton RT. Breastfeeding experience and milk weight in lactating mothers pumping for preterm infants. *Birth.* 1999b;26:233–238.

Hill PD, Aldag JC. Milk volume on day 4 and income predictive of lactation adequacy at 6 weeks of mothers of nonnursing preterm infants. *J Perinat Neonatal Nurs.* 2005; 19:273–282.

Hill PD, Brown LP, Harker TL. Initiation and frequency of breast expression in breastfeeding mothers of LBW and VLBW infants. *Nurs Res.* 1995;44:352–355.

Hurst NM, Valentine CJ, Renfro L, et al. Skin-to-skin holding in the neonatal intensive care unit influences maternal milk volume. *J Perinatol.* 1997;17:213–217.

Stutte PC, Bowles BC, Morman GY. The effects of breast massage on volume and fat content of human milk. *Genesis.* 1988;10:22–25.

Walker M. *Breastfeeding Management for the Clinician: Using the Evidence.* Sudbury, MA: Jones and Bartlett Publishers; 2006.

Woolridge MW. The anatomy of infant sucking. *Midwifery.* 1986;2:164–171.

Zinaman MJ, Hughes V, Queenan JT, et al. Acute prolactin and oxytocin responses and milk yield to infant suckling and artificial methods of expression in lactating women. *Pediatrics.* 1992;89:437–440.

Breastfeeding Devices and Equipment

Vergie I. Hughes, RN, MS, IBCLC

OBJECTIVES

- Choose the appropriate breastfeeding aids to remedy specific breastfeeding problems.
- List two advantages and two drawbacks of each specific aid.
- Describe the appropriate use of the aid.

Introduction

When mothers experience discomfort while breastfeeding or encounter infants who have difficulty latching on to the breast or gaining weight, interventions might be necessary to correct the problem. The role of the lactation consultant is to identify potential causes of the problem and to offer intervention options in order to remedy the situation. Often, refining the mother's technique (positioning, latch-on, breastfeeding frequency and duration, etc.) is the first strategy toward solving a number of problems. When additional intervention is needed, specific devices and equipment might be helpful. The goal is to establish or return the mother and baby to direct breastfeeding as soon as possible.

I. Nipple Shields

A device placed over the nipple and areola on which the baby sucks; considered a short-term solution until the baby can be transferred to the breast.

A. Types *not* recommended (Wilson-Clay & Hoover, 2005).

1. Thick rubber or latex shields.

a. Can reduce milk transfer by 22% (Lawrence & Lawrence, 2005).

2. Plastic or glass base with a bottle-like nipple attached.

B. Recommended types (Wilson-Clay & Hoover, 2005).

   1. Thin silicone.

   2. One type covers the entire areola.

   3. One type has partial coverage of the areola with the upper portion cut away to allow the infant's nose to touch the mother's skin and smell the areola.

   4. May have ribs on inner surface.

C. Holes in tip.

   1. Shields have from one to five holes; milk flows best through nipple shields that have multiple holes (Nicholson, 1993).

D. Uses. Although nipple shields are not always fully successful, they may be useful in a variety of situations (Barger, 1997; Clum 1996; Frantz, 2000; Marriott, 1997; Walker, 2006; Wilson-Clay & Hoover, 2005), including:

   1. The infant is unable to latch on due to flat or inverted nipples (Drazen, 1998; Elliott, 1996; Powers & Tapia, 2004).

   2. The baby is unable to open his or her mouth wide enough in order to achieve a deep latch.

   3. The baby is unable to draw the nipple/areola into his or her mouth (Meier et al., 2000; Powers & Tapia, 2004).

   4. The mother has an overactive letdown reflex or oversupply where the baby has difficulty handling the flow (Mohrbacher & Stock, 2003; Powers & Tapia, 2004; Wilson-Clay & Hoover, 2005).

   5. The mother's nipples/areola are very sore, damaged, or infected (Brigham, 1996; Drazen, 1998; Powers & Tapia, 2004).

   6. The baby has a weak, disorganized, or dysfunctional suck (Isaacson, 2006; Marmet et al., 2000; Powers & Tapia, 2004; Wilson-Clay, 1996).

   7. There is nipple confusion and/or breast refusal (Powers & Tapia, 2004; Wilson-Clay, 1996; Woodworth & Frank, 1996).

   8. Can be helpful in some circumstances when the baby has certain congenital conditions (cleft palate, Pierre-Robin syndrome, short frenulum) (Powers & Tapia, 2004; Wilson-Clay & Hoover, 2005).

   9. Can be helpful with upper airway problems such as laryngomalacia and tracheomalacia (Walker, 2006).

   10. Mother is considering premature weaning (Walker, 2006).

E. Advantages.

   1. May give immediate results.

   2. Provides shape to a flat or inverted nipple.

3. Helps stretch and improve the elasticity of a flat or inverted nipple when the baby sucks strongly over the shield (Wilson-Clay & Hoover, 2005).

4. Reinforces a wide open mouth position at the breast (Wilson-Clay & Hoover, 2005).

5. Can reduce pain experienced by the mother (Walker, 2006).

6. May help keep the baby at the breast during remediation of the problem (Brigham, 1996).

7. Prolactin levels seem unaffected by the use of the thin silicone shields (Amatayakul et al., 1987; Chertok, Schneider, & Blackburn, 2006).

8. Little or no reduction of milk transfer using thin silicone shield (Chertok et al., 2006; Jackson et al., 1987).

9. Increases milk intake at the breast for some preterm infants (Meier et al., 2000).

10. Can prevent premature weaning (Wilson-Clay, 1997).

F. Disadvantages.

1. Thick rubber shields, bottle-like nipples, and thick latex shields have the capability to reduce milk transfer (Auerbach, 1990; Woolridge, Baum, & Drewett, 1980).

2. Inner ribbed protrusions (if present) can cause discomfort and pain.

3. Complementary feedings may be needed to compensate until milk transfer improves.

4. Use of a breast pump after feedings with the shield may be necessary to initiate and/or maintain an optimal milk supply.

5. Infant may become dependent on the shield (DeNicola, 1986; Hunter, 1999; Johnson, 1997; Newman, 1997).

6. Latex shields carry the risk of inducing a latex allergy in the mother and/or infant.

G. Some institutions require a written consent for the use of nipple shields outlining the concerns with use and the importance of follow-up with a lactation professional (Lactation Education Consultants, 1996).

H. Techniques.

1. Sizing the nipple shield (Wilson-Clay & Hoover, 2005).
   a. Three sizes of nipple shields are available commercially, ranging from 16 mm to 24 mm.
   b. First, size the shield to the infant's mouth.
      i. The teat height should not exceed the length of the infant's mouth from the lips to the junction of the hard and soft palates.
      ii. If the height of the teat is greater than this length, the probability increases that the infant's gum ridges will rest beyond where the tongue

should begin to exert its peristaltic motion. If this situation happens, the nipple and areola might not be drawn into the teat shaft far enough for compression by the infant's tongue, which will reduce the milk transfer.

    iii. In some babies, this excessive length can trigger a gag reflex and an aversion to feeding. In these cases, Wilson-Clay and Hoover (2005) recommend using the shortest available teat with the height under 2 cm.

  c. Second, consider the size of the mother's nipple.

    i. Some small shields are not wide enough at the base to accommodate larger nipples. Wide bases might be too large for some babies who have small mouths. Compromise to find the best fit for both mom and baby.

2. To apply the nipple shield, roll the shield back about one-third of the length of the nipple shank and apply to the breast, unrolling the shield onto the nipple and areola.

3. To ensure the shield remains in place during the feeding.
  a. Moisten the areolar portion of the shield.
  b. Apply small amount of a sticky breast cream.
  c. Warm the shield under hot running water prior to application.

4. Suggestions to place the mother's nipple deeper into the nipple shank (Mohrbacher & Stock, 2003; Wilson-Clay & Hoover, 2005).
  a. May stretch the area near the base of the shank with the fingers and release when placed over the nipple.
  b. The baby can pull the nipple even further into the shield after several minutes of vigorous sucking.

5. If the mother feels pain through the nipple shield, either the nipple is not deeply positioned into the shield or the shield is too small for the nipple.

6. A feeding tube can be used in conjunction with a nipple shield to temporarily increase milk flow (Mohrbacher and Stock, 2003; Walker, 2006; Wilson-Clay, 1996; Wilson-Clay & Hoover, 2005).
  a. Tube placed outside the shield.
    i. Nipple keeps good fit inside the shield.
  b. Tube placed inside the shield.
    i. Easy for mother to position both in infant's mouth.
    ii. May lose suction.
    iii. Baby swallows more air.
    iv. Mom feels less "pulling."

7. The shield can be removed once vigorous sucking is achieved and the infant quickly placed directly on the mother's breast before the nipple/areola loses its shape (Mohrbacher & Stock, 2003; Wilson-Clay & Hoover, 2005).

8. Weaning from the shield.
  a. Start the feeding with the shield, and then remove it. If the baby will not latch, replace the shield and try at the next feeding (Walker, 2006).

   b. Avoid cutting pieces off the tip of the shield in an attempt to wean the baby from it; blunt uncomfortable edges might remain (Mohrbacher & Stock, 2003).

9. Follow-up with a lactation consultant is essential.

10. Have been used long term in some situations (Brigham, 1996).

I. Preterm infants may need to rely on a shield for longer periods of time (2–3 weeks or until term corrected age (Meier et al., 2000).

   1. Typical problems of small preterm infants at the breast include failure to latch-on, sucking for insufficient length of time, immature feeding behaviors, falling asleep as soon as he/she is positioned at the breast, and repeated slipping off the nipple.

   2. Shields have been demonstrated to increase the volume of milk transfer (Meier et al., 2000).

J. Ensure adequate milk intake.

   1. Weigh the baby before and after a feeding with an electronic scale capable of measuring differences of 1–2 grams (Brigham, 1996).

   2. Monitor output.

   3. Monitor weight often.

II. Breast Shells

A two piece plastic device consisting of a dome or cup and a concave backing contoured to fit the shape of the breast; held in place over the nipple/areola by the mother's bra (Frantz, 2000).

A. Types for flat or inverted nipples.

   1. Designed to evert a flat nipple; the part in contact with the breast has a small opening that is just large enough for the nipple to protrude through.

   2. The pressure on the areola was thought to break adhesions that were anchoring the nipple to the base of the areola (Otte, 1975; Riordan, 2005).

   3. The dome has one or more air vents to enable air to circulate around the nipple.

   4. Some brands are constructed with flexible silicone backs.

B. Types for sore nipples.

   1. Most brands have an optional back with a much larger opening to keep the bra off the nipple and enable air to circulate.

   2. Some brands have a cotton liner that surrounds the backing for a comfortable fit.

   3. Some shells have an absorbent cotton pad that is placed in the bottom of the shell under the areola to absorb leaked milk.

C. Uses.

    1. To evert flat or inverted nipples either prenatally or postpartum.

    2. To collect leaking milk.

    3. To relieve engorgement.

    4. For protection of painful, tender nipples.

D. Advantages.

    1. May assist flat or inverted nipples to protrude (Mohrbacher & Stock, 2003).

    2. May protect painful nipples by preventing chafing due to clothing, bra, etc. (Brent et al., 1998).

    3. May encourage milk to leak and help relieve engorgement.
       a. Drip milk should not be fed to the baby (Lawrence, 1999; Mohrbacher & Stock, 2003).

E. Disadvantages.

    1. Theoretical risk of stimulating preterm labor contractions. Discuss with mother's health care provider. May be used in healthy pregnancy with no threat of preterm labor.

    2. Often not effective in everting a flat or retracted nipple (Alexander, Grant, & Campbell, 1992; MAIN Trial Collaborative Group, 1994).

    3. Might cause irritation to the nipple or areola either from contact with the skin or from moisture buildup in the shell and the resulting skin breakdown.

    4. Drip milk can leak out of some shells when the mother leans over.

    5. Some shells are obvious under the bra.

    6. The bra might need to be a cup size larger in order to accommodate the shell.

    7. May cause plugged ducts and mastitis (Mohrbacher & Stock, 2003).

    8. Women who have fibrocystic breasts might experience discomfort from the constant pressure.

    9. Research on effectiveness of breast shells is limited and insufficient to base treatment decisions.

    10. Prenatal use of shells may discourage women from attempting to breastfeed (Alexander et al., 1992).

F. Techniques for use.

    1. Center the opening of the shell over the nipple and apply the bra to hold it in place.

    2. Apply a cotton liner if appropriate.

    3. Wear them for gradually longer periods of time during the day.

    4. Shells should be removed for naps and at bedtime because duct obstruction can occur.

5. In hot weather or if moisture builds up, remove them, allow the breast to dry, and reapply.

III. Nipple Everters

A. Types.

1. A syringe-like device that is placed over the nipple; the plunger is gently pulled to apply suction to the nipple.

2. Commercially available syringe has a soft flexible areolar cone.

3. Noncommercial device can be made from a 10 or 20 ml syringe (Arsenault, 1997; Kesaree et al., 1993).
   a. The end of the barrel is cut off where the needle attaches to form a hollow tube.
   b. The plunger is inserted into the cut end, leaving the smooth side to be placed over the nipple.

4. There is legal concern over adapting medical equipment for a purpose it was not intended.

5. Another commercially available product consists of a thimble-shaped dome placed over the nipple prenatally that generates suction the entire time it is worn (McGeorge, 1994).
   a. Follow manufacturer's instructions for safe use.

B. Uses.

1. Evert a flat or retracted nipple in the prenatal or postpartum period.

2. Form a nipple to make latch-on easier for a baby who is having difficulty grasping and holding the nipple.

C. Advantages.

1. Simple, low-cost technique to aid in latch-on and nipple erection (Kesaree et al., 1993).

2. Mother can control to her level of comfort.

D. Disadvantages.

1. If used too vigorously or incorrectly, has the potential to cause pain or skin damage.

2. The nipple might not remain everted long enough for the baby to achieve latch-on.

3. There is no evidence to demonstrate the effectiveness of these devices.

E. Technique.

1. The mother applies the suction to the nipple and gently pulls back on the plunger to her level of comfort and holds the nipple everted for about 30 seconds (Kesaree et al., 1993).

2. She performs this action prior to each breastfeeding and can repeat between feedings if desired.

IV. Gel Dressings

Three-dimensional networks of cross-linked hydrophilic polymers that are insoluble in water and absorb fluids.

A. Gel dressings promote moist wound healing and are used for nipples that have cracks, fissures, and deep wounds (Cable, Stewart, & Davis, 1997; Cable & Davis, 1998; Dodd & Chalmers, 2003; Wilson, 2001).

B. Absorb excess drainage.

C. Maintain a moist wound surface that enables epidermal cells to migrate across the wound.

D. Provide thermal insulation for improved blood flow.

E. Protect the wound from bacterial invasion or trauma.

F. Types.

    1. Glycerin-based.

    2. Water-based.

    3. Available in gel, gauze, and pre-cut sheet forms.

G. Uses.

    1. Used on nipples for superficial or partial thickness wounds in order to enhance the healing process (Walker, 2006).

H. Advantages.

    1. Provides instant soothing relief of nipple pain.

    2. Speeds wound granulation and healing.

    3. Can be reused for several days.

    4. Non-adherent.

    5. Oxygen permeable.

    6. Maintains a clean, moist environment.

    7. Comfortable and flexible.

    8. May reduce bacterial skin infections (Brent et al., 1998; Dodd & Chalmers, 2003).

I. Disadvantages.

    1. Might macerate peri-wound skin.

    2. Some brands have minimal absorption.

    3. Water-based products can dry out rapidly when exposed to air.

    4. Have the potential in certain situations to contribute to yeast, bacterial overgrowth, or mastitis (Zeimer, Cooper, & Pigeon, 1995).

a. Dressings should not be applied in the presence of a known wound infection.

b. Wound should be inspected frequently for presence of infection and reported to physician.

5. Mixed reviews in the research show that it may not be more effective than lanolin and shells.

6. If the mother forgets that the gel dressing is in place and/or has cut it very small, the baby can suck it into his mouth and choke on it.

7. Can be expensive.

J. Technique for use.

1. Wash hands before handling.

2. The dressing should be cut about one-fourth to one-half inch larger than the wound.

3. Some dressings are manufactured specifically for nipple care and are small and round, not requiring cutting.

4. Remove the backing to the dressing and apply the gel side to the wound.

5. The dressing is removed before nursing and placed on a clean surface, gel side up or in manufacturer's protective covering.

6. The dressing can be chilled and reapplied following each feeding.

7. The breast does not need to be washed prior to nursing.

V. Creams (Cosmetic, Nonmedicated)

Creams have been used to soothe and/or "treat" sore nipples for hundreds of years; most creams have a soothing effect but do not prevent or cure nipple pain (Frantz, 2000; Hewat & Ellis, 1987; Morse, 1989a & b).

A. Types.

1. Purified lanolin or lanolin-predominant creams.

a. Modified lanolin generally has the lowest level of free alcohol and appears to be free of pesticides.

2. Some creams have questionable ingredients and are not recommended.

a. Vitamin E oil, cocoa butter, Bag Balm®, Vitamin A and D ointment, Vaseline®, baby oil.

B. Uses.

1. Reduce nipple pain (especially when used with breast shells).

2. Create a moist wound healing environment (Hinman & Maibach, 1963; Huml, 1995; Huml, 1999;).

C. Advantages.

1. Can speed healing process (Huml, 1995; Pugh et al., 1996; Spangler & Hildebrandt, 1993).

2. Might reduce pain and have a soothing effect.

3. Widely available and inexpensive.

4. Most do not need to be washed off prior to feedings.

5. Might serve to lubricate dry skin and protect it from maceration.

D. Disadvantages.

1. Some products might need to be washed off before each feeding. This wiping off can remove moisture from the skin, create further damage, and slow wound healing.

2. Some combination creams have ingredients that could provoke an allergy in the infant, such as peanut oil.

3. Some have petroleum bases and other ingredients that could irritate nipple skin.

4. Lanolin should have the lowest possible free alcohol content to avoid aggravating a wool allergy in susceptible mothers.

5. Research does not support the use of any types of creams over good positioning and latch-on instruction.

VI. Droppers

A plastic or glass tube with a squeeze bulb at one end.

A. Types.

1. May be made completely of soft plastic; some are glass with a rubber bulb; some are small, child size.

B. Uses.

1. Provide milk incentives at the breast in order to achieve latch-on.
   a. Finger-feed to take the edge off hunger before attempting latch-on.

2. Complementary feeding when breast milk intake is not sufficient.

3. Temporary aid to improve suck organization.

C. Advantages.

1. Avoids the use of artificial nipples.

2. Inexpensive and widely available.

3. Easy to use and teach parents.

4. Quick way for baby to receive small amounts of milk while learning to breastfeed.

5. Baby may be more eager to breastfeed because sucking needs are not met.

D. Disadvantages.

1. Can be difficult to clean.

2. Must be continually refilled.

3. Baby does not learn to suck unless the dropper is used in conjunction with finger feeding.

4. Sucking on the dropper alone will not teach correct sucking patterns.

5. Time consuming.

6. Research on use of droppers for supplementation is very limited.

E. Technique (Marmet & Shell, 1984; Mohrbacher & Stock, 2003; Ross, 1987).

1. If using with a finger, place the filled dropper along the side of the finger as the baby draws the finger into his or her mouth.

2. Allow the baby to suck the milk out of the dropper. If the baby is unable to perform this task, one or two drops can be placed on the baby's tongue to initiate swallowing and sucking.

3. Milk should not be squirted into the baby's mouth.

F. A dropper can be placed into the corner of the baby's mouth while latching on to the breast; one or two drops of milk can then be placed on the tongue to initiate a swallow followed by a suck.

1. The infant must be alert, not sleepy, and have a functioning swallow reflex.

VII. Spoons (Jones, 1998; Mohrbacher & Stock, 2003; Wilson-Clay & Hoover, 2005)

A. Types.

1. Teaspoon, tablespoon, plastic spoon, medicine spoon with a hollow handle, commercially available spoon-shaped device attached to a milk reservoir.

B. Uses.

1. Feed the baby when breastfeeding is interrupted (Darzi, Chowdri, & Bhat, 1996).

2. Complementary feeding when breastfeeding is not sufficient.

3. Feed the baby colostrum that has been hand-expressed or pumped to complement the early feedings and prevent hypoglycemia.

4. Prime the baby for feeding at the breast.

C. Advantages.

1. Avoids the use of artificial nipples.

2. Can be used as a temporary aid to initiate milk intake for the baby who has not yet latched on.

3. Inexpensive and easily available.

4. Easy to use and clean.

5. Baby may be more eager to breastfeed because sucking needs are not met.

6. Can be used to administer small volumes (such as colostrum) efficiently.

D. Disadvantages.

    1. Must be continually refilled.

    2. Does not teach the baby to suck at the breast.

    3. Fluid in the mouth is not associated with sucking.

    4. Does not correct improper sucking patterns.

    5. Research to support spoon feeding is limited.

E. Technique.

    1. Position the baby in a semi-upright position.

    2. Place the spoon just inside the infant's lips over the tongue.

    3. Allow the infant to pace the feeding by sipping or lapping.

    4. *Avoid* pouring the milk into the baby's mouth.

    5. The baby should be alert with a functioning swallow reflex.

VIII. Cups (ABM, 2007; Armstrong 1987; Biancuzzo, 1997; Cloherty et al., 2005; Davis et al., 1948; Fredeen, 1948; Jones, 1998; Kuehl, 1997; Lang, 1994; Mohrbacher & Stock, 2003; Musoke, 1990; Newman, 1990; Wilson-Clay & Hoover, 2005)

A. Types.

    1. 1 oz (28–30 mL) medicine cups, plastic small drinking cups.

    2. Small cups with an extended lip or edge to control the flow of milk.

    3. Flexible silicone cups with a restricted outlet.

    4. Paladai—a small pitcher-shaped device from India.

B. Uses.

    1. Feed the infant when breastfeeding is interrupted.

    2. Complementary feeding when breastfeeding is not sufficient.

    3. Used with both term and preterm infants to avoid bottle nipple preference.

    4. The mother is unavailable to breastfeed.

C. Advantages (Collins et al., 2004; Gupta, Khanna, & Chattree, 1999; Howard et al., 1999; Howard et al., 2003; Kuehl, 1997; Lang, 1994; Mosley, Whittle, & Hicks, 2001; Rocha, Martinez, & Jorge, 2002).

    1. Avoids the use of artificial nipples.

    2. Inexpensive and widely available.

    3. Easy to use and to teach parents to use.

    4. Reduces the incidence of bottle-feeding–associated apnea and bradycardia in preterm infants (Marinelli, Burke, & Dodd, 2001).

5. Noninvasive alternative to gavage feeding; reduces the risk of esophageal perforation and oral aversion (Lang, Lawrence, & Orme, 1994).

6. Baby may be more eager to breastfeed because sucking needs are not met.

7. A quick way to supplement or complement breastfeeding.

8. Physiologic stability.

9. Good weight gain.

10. Promotes breastfeeding in preterm infants. The baby is fed by cup when the mother is not present to breastfeed (Kuehl, 1997).

D. Disadvantages (Dowling et al., 2002; Thorley, 1997).

1. The cup must be frequently refilled.

2. The baby can dribble much milk, reducing intake.
    a. Using a paladai gives greater control and reduces the amount of spilled milk (Malhotra et al., 1999).
    b. If measuring intake is critical, the bib can be weighed before and after feeding to determine the volume lost.

3. The baby does not learn to suck; therefore cups might delay return to the breast.

4. The infant, parents, or health care providers can become dependent on the cup.

5. Risk of aspiration (similar to that of bottle-feeding) if cup feeding is performed improperly.

E. Technique (Biancuzzo, 2002; Healow, 1995; Kuehl, 1997; Lang et al., 1994; Mohrbacher & Stock, 2003; Wilson-Clay & Hoover, 2005).

1. The baby should be in a calm, alert state (not sleepy).

2. Position the baby in a nearly upright position, wrapped so that his/her hands do not bump the cup.

3. Fill the cup about half full.

4. Place the rim of the cup on the baby's lower lip with the cup tilted just to the point of the milk coming into contact with the upper lip.

5. Do not apply pressure to the lower lip.

6. Let the baby pace the feeding by sipping or lapping at the milk (Lang, 1994; Mizuno & Kani, 2005; Rocha et al., 2002).

7. *Do not* pour the milk into the baby's mouth. *Do not* overwhelm the infant with milk.

8. Leave the cup in the same position during the baby's pauses so that he does not need to continually reorganize oral conformation.

9. Refill as needed.

IX. Syringes (Marmet & Shell, 1984; Mohrbacher & Stock, 2003; Riordan, 2005; Ross, 1987)

A. Types.

1. 10 ml to 50 ml capacity; used with a 5 French gavage tube or tubing from butterfly needle (Edgehouse & Radzyminski, 1990; Walker, 2006).

2. Periodontal syringe, 10 ml capacity with a curved tip.

3. Regular syringes (without the needle) are usually not used because the infant might have difficulty forming a complete seal.

B. Uses.

1. To provide an incentive at the breast to encourage latch-on, to initiate suckling, or to aid in sustaining the suckling once started.

2. To provide complementary or supplementary feeding while the infant simultaneously sucks on a caregiver's finger.

C. Advantages (Marmet & Shell, 1984; Riordan, 2005).

1. Avoids the use of artificial nipples and keeps the baby at the breast.

2. Might help improve uncoordinated mouth and tongue movements.

3. Provides a source of milk flow that will work to regulate the suck.

4. Easy to teach parents to do.

D. Disadvantages.

1. Supplies might not be widely available.

2. More intrusive.

3. Infant can become dependent on the method.

4. Infant might demonstrate poor jaw excursion while sucking on an adult finger.

5. Some periodontal syringes have a rough tip that could irritate the baby's mouth.

6. Some have legal concerns about using equipment for a purpose that it was not intended.

7. Research to support syringe feeding is limited.

E. Technique (Mohrbacher & Stock, 2003; Oddy & Glenn, 2003; Ross, 1987; Walker, 1990).

1. At the breast; insert the tip of the syringe (or feeding tube) just inside the infant's lips at the corner of his or her mouth.

2. Give a small bolus of milk (.25–.5 ml) when the infant sucks.
   a. Rate initially: suck:bolus:suck:bolus.
   b. When infant is sucking well, the pattern will be "suck, suck, bolus:suck, suck, bolus" or "suck, suck, suck, bolus: suck, suck, suck, bolus".

3. On the finger: Place the infant in a semi-upright position in the caregiver's arms or in an inclined infant seat.

4. Parents can use a washed finger; the health care provider should wash his or her hands and use a finger cot.

5. Use the finger that is closest in size to the circumference of the mother's nipple.

6. Introduce the finger into the infant's mouth pad up, enabling the baby to pull the finger back to the junction of the hard and soft palate.

7. If the infant resists, withdraw the finger slightly, pause until he or she is comfortable, and then proceed.

8. Place the syringe or tubing next to the finger, making sure that it is positioned so that it will not poke the infant.

9. As the infant sucks, reward correct suckling motions with a small bolus of milk.

10. Use the rate of suck:bolus to entice a reluctant feeder, allowing the infant to gradually suck the milk from the device.

11. Once sustained sucking is achieved, slow rate to suck, suck, suck, bolus.

12. Time frame is about 15 to 20 minutes.

13. If this technique is being used to prime the baby for the breast, place the baby at the breast when he or she demonstrates a sucking rhythm.

14. If the baby stops for more than 10 to 20 seconds, arouse the baby.

15. If the tongue lies behind the lower gum ridge, apply slight pressure to the back of the tongue to stroke it forward over the lower gum ridge.

X. Tube Feeding Devices

Commercially available devices usually consist of a reservoir or container for milk, with one or two thin flexible lengths of tubing attached. The container for milk can be a syringe, a bottle clipped to the shoulder area, a bottle suspended on a cord around the mother's neck, a plastic bag, or a bottle with a regular artificial nipple through which the tubing is threaded. The container might have one or two thin lengths of flexible tubing. Follow the manufacturer's instructions for using larger or smaller tubing sizes.

A. Tubing is usually attached by tape to the mother's nipple/areola or to the finger of the feeder.

B. Uses.

1. To provide complementary feeding to an infant at the breast for low milk supply, inefficient suckling, slow weight gain, adoptive nursing, relactation, preterm infant, or for neurologically affected infants.

2. The tubing can also be attached to a finger for others to feed the baby or to prime the baby for going to the breast.

C. Advantages (Borucki, 2005; Mohrbacher & Stock, 2003; Riordan, 2005; Wilson-Clay & Hoover, 2005).

1. Avoids the use of artificial nipples.

2. Might help improve sucking organization and patterns.

3. Enables delivery of supplements if needed while preserving the breastfeeding.

4. Increasing the flow rate at the breast may encourage a reluctant infant to breastfeed.

D. Disadvantages (Hughes 2005; Sealy, 1996).

1. More intrusive and complex technique to learn and to repeat many times per day; may be rejected by mothers.

2. Supplies might not be widely available.

3. Cost.

4. Infant can become dependent on the method.

5. Infant can learn to prefer faster flow rate at breast.

6. The infant might exhibit shallow jaw excursions while sucking on an adult finger.

7. Time consuming to clean the equipment after each use.

8. Some mothers find it awkward at first to get both the tubing and the nipple into the infant's mouth.

9. If the milk container is positioned too low or the tubing is kinked, the infant might not receive milk.

10. If the milk container is too high, the infant may receive milk without sucking.

11. Some mothers might be allergic to the tape that is used to secure the tubing in place at the breast; consider paper tape or non-allergenic tapes or dressings.

12. Do not allow the infant to suck on the tubing like a straw without the nipple also in her/his mouth.

13. There is little published research on the efficacy of feeding tube devices. Manufacturers are the source of information.

E. Technique (Benakappa, 2002; Hughes, 2005; Jones, 1998; Newman, 1990; Newman, 2006; Walker, 1990; Wilson-Clay & Hoover, 2005).

1. Tube feeding on a finger proceeds in a similar manner as with the syringe feeding (see above).

2. When used at the breast, the milk reservoir can be elevated or lowered to achieve control over the milk flow speed and placed so that the top of the fluid is level with the mother's nipples; the milk should flow only when the baby sucks.

3. The baby should take both the nipple/areola and the tubing into his/her mouth.

4. Tape the tubing so that it enters the infant's mouth in the corner or under the mother's nipple over the infant's tongue.

5. Position the tube so it will not extend beyond the nipple tip when positioned in the infant's mouth.

6. To increase the flow for small or weaker babies, lower the container. If the device has two tubes, open the other tube as a vent or use both tubes on one breast.

7. If the device has a choice of tubing sizes, use the largest size for a preterm baby, a disorganized infant, or one who needs an easier flow; advance the baby to the smaller sizes as sucking improves.

8. Babies need close follow-up for frequent weight checks and to be weaned off the device as soon as possible.

XI. Haberman Feeder

A specialized feeding bottle with a valve and teat mechanism to adjust the milk flow in order to prevent overwhelming or flooding the baby with milk. Three lines on the nipple correspond to three flow rates.

A. Uses.

1. Severe feeding problems, such as Down syndrome, cleft lip/palate, neurological dysfunction, disorganized sucking, preterm infants, cardiac defects, cystic fibrosis (Trenouth & Campbell, 1996).

B. Advantages (Mohrbacher & Stock, 2003; Riordan, 2005; Ross, 1987; Wilson-Clay & Hoover, 2005).

1. May be effective with an infant who is otherwise difficult to feed.

2. If the baby cannot nurse at all or needs assistance, the bottle can be squeezed to release a limited volume of milk.

3. The smaller feeder has a shorter teat for smaller babies.

4. Can be used as a quicker means of complementary or supplementary feedings.

C. Disadvantages.

1. Exposes the infant to an artificial nipple.

2. Might promote a shallow latch-on when the infant goes to the breast.

3. Might be difficult to obtain.

4. Cost.

5. Little research exists regarding the efficacy of Haberman feeders; the manufacturer is the source of information.

D. Technique.

1. Place the nipple onto the infant's lips, allowing him or her to draw it into the mouth if capable.

2. Pull back on the nipple if the baby has a shallow gag reflex or to help her/him to start sucking.

3. Rotate the nipple to adjust the rate of flow to meet the needs and capability of the baby. Follow any particular guidance/instructions for babies with cleft palates.

XII. Pacifiers (Dummies)

A wide variety of shapes of pacifiers are manufactured but generally consist of a nipple shaped tip, a wide guard that rests on the lips and a handle.

A. Uses.

1. Treat delayed swallowing.

2. In non-orally fed infants, pacifiers help maintain oral motor patterns and tactile response that will be necessary to transition to feeding at the breast (Barros et al., 1995; Engebretson & Wardell, 1997).

3. Meets high sucking needs.

4. Frequently used in United States to calm a fussy baby in the absence of the mother.

B. Advantages (Cockburn, Tappin, & Stone, 1996; Measel & Anderson, 1979; Medoff-Cooper & Ray, 1995; Riordan, 2005; Victora et al., 1993; Wilson-Clay & Hoover, 2005).

1. Enables sucking activity for an infant who might otherwise overfeed (Riordan, 2005).

2. Might quiet a crying baby in the absence of the mother.

3. May reduce pain in preterm infants (Pinelli, Symington, & Ciliska, 2002).

4. Non-nutritive sucking in the preterm infant might help in more rapid transition to oral feeding (Drosten, 1997; Gill et al., 1988; Kinneer & Beachy, 1994).

5. Pacifier use when infants are laid down to sleep has been associated with reduced incidence of Sudden Infant Death Syndrome in infants over one month of age (AAP, 2005, Hauck, Omojokun, & Siadaty). However, this finding needs further study and pacifier use continues to be open to debate (Mitchell, Blair, & L'Hoir, 2006).

C. Disadvantages (Aarts, 1999; Drane, 1996; Hill et al., 1997; Howard et al., 1999; Neimela, Uhari, & Mottonen, 1995; Newman & Pitman, 2000; North et al., 1999; Righard, 1998; Righard & Alade, 1997; Schubiger, Schwarz, & Tonz, 1997; Vogel, Hutchison, & Mitchell, 2001; Wilson-Clay & Hoover, 2005).

1. Exposes an infant to an artificial nipple.

2. Displaces sucking from the breast.

3. Might cause drowsiness in the baby and missed feedings.

    4. Increased incidence of otitis media.

    5. Vector for continued fungal infection.

    6. May cause shorter breastfeeding duration (Victora et al., 1993; Victora et al., 1997).

    7. Might see increased rates of malocclusion.

    8. Increases the risk for latex allergy (Venuta et al., 1999).

    9. Pacifiers with balls on the tip enable the baby to maintain the pacifier in the mouth with a weak lick-suck motion, rather than functional sucking activity.

   10. Orthodontic pacifiers might flatten the central grooving of the tongue.

  D. Technique.

    1. Pacifiers should be used with caution.

    2. Non-orally fed infants might benefit from sucking on a number of differently shaped pacifiers to avoid becoming accustomed to only one shape.

    3. Pacifiers should be used for only a few minutes at a time and after the first month of life when breastfeeding is well established (AAP, 2005).

XIII. Artificial Nipples

Bottle nipples come in a wide range of shapes and sizes. No artificial bottle nipple precisely mimics the dynamic qualities of the human breast (Adran, Kemp, & Lind, 1958; Coats, 1990; Davis et al., 1948; Glover & Sandilands, 1990; Henrison, 1990; Jones, 1998; Matthew, 1991; Matthew, 1998; Nowak, Smith, & Erenberg, 1994; Nowak, Smith & Erenberg, 1995; Riordan, 2005; Turgeon-O'Brien et al., 1996; Weber, Woolridge, & Baum, 1986; Woolrich, 1986).

  A. Artificial nipples are made from silicone, rubber, or latex.

  B. Numerous sizes and shapes are available.

  C. Round, cross section nipples tend to be straight and gradually taper to a flared base.

  D. "Orthodontic" nipples have bulb-like ends and narrow necks.

  E. Some have a very wide base to encourage the baby to keep his mouth open wider.

  F. Artificial nipples do not elongate in the mouth as the human breast does.

  G. Types of openings.

    1. Holes.

    2. Crosscuts.

      a. Crosscut nipples do not enable milk to drip from them, but compression on them removes fluid.

    3. Hole size is one of the major determinants of flow rate.

      a. Nipples have high, medium, and low flow rates depending on the number of holes and the size of the holes. Hole diameter may vary from nipple to nipple from the same manufacturer.

b. Some nipples have the hole on the top rather than the tip to avoid milk squirting down the infant's throat.

H. Advantages.

1. Ease and speed of feedings.

2. Some artificial nipples are used in special situations to assist infants in learning sucking patterns (Kassing, 2002; Medoff-Cooper, 2004).

3. Easily obtained.

I. Disadvantages (see Table 31-1).

1. Infant might learn to prefer the bottle nipple (Newman, 1990; Righard 1998; Stein, 1990).

2. Flow might be faster than with breastfeeding, especially likely during the first few days postpartum, so baby becomes accustomed to a quick delivery of milk.

3. Fast flow can contribute to apnea and bradycardia in preterm or stressed infants (Wilson-Clay & Hoover, 2005).

4. Shape is different and consistency is firmer, potentially causing the infant to prefer the stronger stimulus of the artificial nipple (Neifert, Lawrence, & Seacat, 1995; Newman, 1990).

5. Encourages the baby to close his or her mouth, not open wide, and even bite on the narrowed neck of some of the nipples.

6. Orthodontic nipples cause a "squash and fill" type of sucking, remove the central grooving of the tongue, and enable the infant to close his mouth tightly around the nipple (McBride & Danner, 1987; Wilson-Clay & Hoover, 2005).

7. Long nipples might trigger a gag reflex in some babies.

8. Can contribute to latex allergy.

9. Weakens the strength of the suck; reduces the strength of the masseter muscle (Inoue, Sakashita, & Kamegai, 1995; Sakashita, Kamegai, & Inoue, 1996).

10. Muscles involved in breastfeeding are either immobilized, overactive, or mal-positioned during bottle-feeding, which can contribute to abnormal dental and facial development in the child (Palmer, 1998).

11. Bottle-feeding has been positively correlated with finger sucking, which can deform the palate and contribute to malocclusion (Palmer, 1998).

12. Risk of aspiration from a too fast flow (Wilson-Clay & Hoover, 2005).

13. May shorten the duration of breastfeeding (Cronenwett et al., 1992; Kurinij & Shiono, 1991; Righard, 1998; Schubiger et al., 1997; Wright, Rice, & Wells, 1996).

J. Technique (sometimes called *paced bottle feeding*; Coats, 1991, Kassing, 2002; Noble & Bovey, 1997; Wilson-Clay & Hoover, 2005).

1. Select a nipple with a long shank, wide base, and slow flow of milk.

2. Position the infant nearly upright in caregiver's arms (not infant seat).

3. Tickle the infant's lips with the nipple and allow him/her to draw the nipple into the mouth him-/herself.

4. Position the bottle horizontally with just enough angle to keep fluid in the nipple tip.

5. Position the bottle so the infant's jaws are over the wide base.

6. Observe for signs of a milk flow that is too fast or too slow.

7. Pace the feeding to approximately the same suck:swallow ratio as a breastfeeding. If the infant drinks too quickly or does not breathe within three to five sucks, tip the bottle down or remove the bottle to allow a short break (Law-Morstatt et al., 2003).

8. If the bottle is removed, wait for the infant's cues (seeking, open mouth) before replacing it.

Table 31-1   Comparison of Bottle and Breastfeeding

Bottlefeeding	Breastfeeding
Firm nipple	Soft, amorphous shaped nipple
Inelastic nipple	Nipple elongates during sucking
Flow begins instantly	Flow is delayed until the milk ejection reflex occurs
Flow is very fast	Flow is slow, faster during the milk ejection reflex
Feeding is very quick	Feeding a newborn may take 30 to 45 minutes
Sucking on bottle is suction/vacuum	Suckling at breast is peristaltic tongue movement
Tongue is humped in back of mouth	Tongue is forward cupped around the nipple

Source: Adapted from Woolridge, 1986; Weber, Woolridge & Baum, 1986; Medoff-Cooper, 1995, 2004; Ardran, Kemp, & Lind, 1958; Jones, 1998; Wilson-Clay & Hoover, 2005; Riordan, 2005; Walker, 2006.

9. May squeeze the nipple before inverting the bottle; this creates a small amount of suction that slows the flow.

10. Switch sides halfway through the feeding

XIV. Infant Scale

An infant scale that can measure weight changes within 2 g is appropriate for use with a breastfeeding baby to determine intake (Meier et al., 1996). Other researchers question the accuracy of test weights (Savenije & Brand, 2006).

A. Uses.

1. Determine breast milk intake at a feeding session.

2. Determine infant weight gain/loss over time.

3. Milk consumed at the breast can be used to determine if supplementation is necessary (Wilson-Clay & Hoover, 2005).

4. Information may contribute to decision to discharge preterm infant from the hospital.

B. Advantages.

1. Weight gain in grams is equal to volume consumed (Meier et al., 1994).

2. Measures small weight increases (Meier et al., 1994).

3. More accurate than observation of a breastfeeding session by a trained observer (Meier et al., 1996; Meier et al., 1994).

4. Reassuring to mothers of preterm infants of adequate intake (Hurst et al., 2004) but not related to maternal confidence and competence scores (Hall et al., 2002).

C. Disadvantages.

1. Cost of the scale.

2. Must use digital scale, not mechanical or balance scale (Meier et al., 1990).

3. Possibility of error due to tubing or wires attached to infant.

D. Technique (Spatz, 2004).

1. Place scale on a flat surface and ensure the leveling bubble is centered.

2. Periodically check the accuracy of the scale with a reference weight.

3. If the scale is used by many infants, clean it first with disinfectant solution.

4. When weighing an infant, ensure that all parameters are the same for the before-feeding weight and the after-feeding weight; use the same clothing, same diaper, same tubing, and wires if the infant is attached to medical equipment.

5. Do not drape blankets or clothing over the scale that could affect its accuracy.

6. Disconnect any tubing or wires that are safe to temporarily disconnect. Any leads or tubing attached to the baby can be weighed with the baby. Any

tubing that cannot be safely disconnected should be marked with tape so the exact amount of tubing is weighed both times.

a. Do not lift tubing or leads during weighing because this leads to error.

7. Obtain pre-feed weight, two times for accuracy.

8. Remove the infant for feeding.

9. Re-weigh the infant after each breast, or at the end of the feeding, two times for accuracy.

10. Determine the weight gain.

References

Aarts C, Hornell A, Kylberg E, et al. Breastfeeding patterns in relation to thumb sucking and pacifier use. *Pediatrics*. 1999;104:e50. Available at: http://www.pediatrics.org/cgi/ content/full/104/4/e50. Accessed January 22, 2007.

Academy of Breastfeeding Medicine (ABM). Protocol on Supplementation. Available at: http://www.bfmed.org/ace-files/protocol/supplementation.pdf. Accessed January 22, 2007.

Alexander JM, Grant AM, Campbell MJ. Randomized controlled trial of breast shells and Hoffman's exercises for inverted and non-protractile nipples. *BMJ*. 1992;304: 1030–1032.

Amatayakul K, Vutyavanich T, Tanthayaphinat O, et al. Serum prolactin and cortisol levels after sucking for varying periods of time and the effect of a nipple shield. *Acta Obstet Gynecol Scand*. 1987:66:47–51.

American Academy of Pediatrics (AAP). Policy Statement. The changing concept of sudden infant death syndrome: diagnostic coding shifts, controversies regarding the sleeping environment and new variables to consider in reducing risk. *Pediatrics*. 2005;115:1245–1253.

Ardran GM, Kemp FH, Lind J. A cineradiographic study of bottle feeding. *Br J Radiol*. 1958;31:11–22.

Armstrong H. Feeding low birth weight babies: advances in Kenya. *J Hum Lact*. 1987;3:34–37.

Arsenault G. Using a disposable syringe to treat inverted nipples. *Can Fam Phys*. 1997;43:1517–1518.

Auerbach KG. The effect of nipple shields on maternal milk volume. *J Obstet Gynecol Neonatal Nurs*. 1990;19:419–427.

Barger C. Nipple shields: LCs not looking for quick fix. *J Hum Lact*. 1997;13:193–194.

Barros FC, Victoria CG, Semer TC, et al. Use of pacifiers is associated with decreased breastfeeding duration. *Pediatrics*. 1995;95:497–499.

Benakappa A. A new Lact-aid technique. *Indian Pediatr*. 2002;39:1169.

Biancuzzo M. Creating and implementing a protocol for cup feeding. *Mother Baby J*. 1997;2:27–33.

Biancuzzo M. *Breastfeeding the Newborn: Clinical Strategies for Nurses.* 2nd ed. St. Louis: C.V. Mosby; 2002.

Borucki LC. Breastfeeding mothers' experiences using a supplemental feeding tube device: finding an alternative. *J Hum Lact.* 2005;21:4:429–439.

Brent N, Rudy SJ, Redd B, et al. Sore nipples in breast-feeding women: a clinical trial of wound dressings vs conventional care. *Arch Pediatr Adolesc Med.* 1998;152:11: 1077–1082.

Brigham M. Mother's reports of the outcome of nipple shield use. *J Hum Lact.* 1996;12: 91–97.

Cable B, Stewart M, Davis J. Nipple wound care: a new approach to an old problem. *Hum Lact.* 1997;13:313–318.

Cable B, Davis J. Hydrogel dressings not to be used on infected tissue [abstract]. *J Hum Lact.*1998;14:205.

Chertok IR, Schneider J, Blackburn S. A pilot study of maternal and term infant outcomes associated with ultrathin nipple shield use. *J Obstet Gynecol Neonatal Nurs.* 2006;35:265–272.

Cloherty M, Alexander J, Holloway I, et al. The cup-versus-bottle debate: a theme from an ethnographic study of the supplementation of breastfed infants in hospital in the United Kingdom. *J Hum Lact.* 2005;21:151–162.

Clum D, Primomo J. Use of a silicone nipple shield with premature infants. *J Hum Lact.* 1996;12:287–290.

Coats MM. Learning at the conference [abstract]. *J Hum Lact.* 1991;7:4:174.

Coats MM. Bottle-feeding like a breastfeeder: an option to consider. *J Hum Lact.* 1990;6:10–11.

Cockburn F, Tappin D, Stone D. Breastfeeding, dummy use, and adult intelligence. *Lancet.* 1996;347:1765–1766.

Cronenwett L, Stukel T, Kearney M, et al. Single daily bottle use in the early weeks postpartum and breastfeeding outcomes. *Pediatrics.* 1992;90:760–766.

Darzi MA, Chowdri NA, Bhat AN. Breast feeding or spoon feeding after cleft lip repair: a prospective, randomized study. *Br J Plast Surg.* 1996;49:24–26.

Davis HV, Sears RR, Miller HC, Brodbeck AJ. Effects of cup, bottle, and breastfeeding on oral activities of newborn infants. *Pediatrics.* 1948;2:549–558.

DeNicola M. One case of nipple shield addiction. *J Hum Lact.* 1986;2:28–30.

Dodd V, Chalmers C. Comparing the use of hydrogel dressing to lanolin ointment with lactation mothers. *J Obstet Gynecol Neonatal Nurs.* 2003;32:486–494.

Dowling DA, Meier PP, DiFiore J, et al. Cup-feeding for preterm infants: mechanics and safety. *J Hum Lact.* 2002;18:13–20.

Drane D. The effect of use of dummies and teats on orofacial development. *Breastfeeding Rev.* 1996;4:59–64.

Drazen P. Taking nipple shields out of the closet. *Birth Issues.* 1998;7:41–49.

Drosten F. Pacifiers in the NICU: a lactation consultant's view. *Neonatal Netw.* 1997;16:47, 50.

Edgehouse L, Radzyminski SG. A device for supplementing breastfeeding. *Am J Matern Child Nurs.* 1990;15:34–35.

Elliott C. Using a silicone nipple shield to assist a baby unable to latch. *J Hum Lact.* 1996;12:4:309–313.

Engebretson J, Wardell DW. Development of a pacifier for low-birth-weight infants' nonnutritive sucking. *J Obstet Gynecol Neonatal Nurs.* 1997;26:660–664.

Frantz K. *Breastfeeding Product Guide.* Sunland, CA: Geddes Productions; 2000.

Fredeen RC. Cup feeding of newborn infants. *Pediatrics.* 1948:2:544–548.

Gill, N, Behnke ML, Conlon M, et al. Effect of nonnutritive sucking on behavioral state in preterm infants before feeding. *Nurs Res.* 1988;37:347–350.

Glover J, Sandilands M. Supplementation of breastfeeding infants and weight loss in hospital. *J Hum Lact.* 1990;6:163–166.

Gupta A, Khanna K, Chattree S. Cup feeding: an alternative to bottle feeding in a neonatal intensive care unit. *J Trop Pediatr.* 1999;45:108–110.

Hall WA, Shearer K, Mogan J, Berkowitz J. Weighing preterm infants before and after breastfeeding: does it increase maternal confidence and competence? *MCN Am J Matern Child Nurs.* 2002;27:318–326.

Hauck FR, Omojokun OO, Siadaty MS. Do pacifiers reduce the risk of sudden infant death syndrome? A meta-analysis. *Pediatrics.* 2005;116:716–723.

Healow LK. Finger-feeding a preemie. *Midwifery Today Childbirth Educ.* 1995;33:9.

Henrison MA. Policy for supplementary/complementary feedings for breastfed newborn infants. *J Hum Lact.* 1990;6:1–14.

Hewat RJ, Ellis DJ. A comparison of the effectiveness of two methods of nipple care. *Birth.* 1987;14:41–45.

Hill PD, Humenick SS, Brennan ML, et al. Does early supplementation affect long-term breastfeeding? *Clin Pediatr.* 1997;36:345–350.

Hinman CD, Maibach H. Effect of air exposure and occlusion on experimental human skin wounds. *Nature.* 1963;2000:377–388.

Howard CR, de Blieck EA, ten Hoopen CB, et al. Physiologic stability of newborns during cup- and bottle-feeding. *Pediatrics.* 1999;104:1204–1207.

Howard CR, Howard FM, Lanphear B, et al. Randomized clinical trial of pacifier use and bottle-feeding or cupfeeding and their effect on breastfeeding. *Pediatrics.* 2003;111:511–518.

Howard CR, Howard FM, Lanphear B, et al. The effects of early pacifier use on breastfeeding duration. *Pediatrics.* 1999;103:e33. Available at: http://pediatrics.aappublications.org/cgi/content/full/103/3/e33?maxtoshow=&HITS=10&hits=10&RESULTFORMAT=&fulltext=Howard+CR%2C+Howard+FM%2C+Lanphear+B&andorexactfulltext=and&searchid=1&FIRSTINDEX=0&sortspec=relevance&resourcetype=HWCIT.

Hughes V. *Alternative Feeding Methods.* Fairfax, VA: Lactation Education Resources; 2005.

Huml S. Sore nipples: a new look at an old problem through the eyes of a dermatologist. *Pract Midwife.* 1999;2:28–31.

Huml S. Cracked nipples in the breastfeeding mother. Looking at an old problem in a new way. *Adv Nurs Pract.* April 1995.

Hunter HH. Nipple shields. A tool that needs handling with care. *Pract Midwife.* 1999;2:48–52.

Hurst NM, Meier PP, Engstrom JL, Myatt A. Mothers performing in-home measurement of milk intake during breastfeeding of their preterm infants: maternal reactions and feeding outcomes. *J Hum Lact.* 2004;20:178–187.

Inoue N, Sakashita R, Kamegai T. Reduction in masseter muscle activity in bottle-fed babies. *Early Hum Dev.* 1995;42:185–193.

Isaacson LJ. Steps to successfully breastfeed the premature infant. *Neonatal Netw.* 2006;25:77–86.

Jackson D, Woolridge M, Imong SM, et al. The automatic sampling shield: a device for sampling suckled breastmilk. *Early Hum Dev.* 1987;15:295–306.

Johnson SM. Further caution re: nipple shields. *J Hum Lact.* 1997;13:101.

Jones B. Choosing a supplementation method. *J Hum Lact.* 1998;14:245–246.

Kassing D. Bottle-feeding as a tool to reinforce breastfeeding. *J Hum Lact.* 2002;18:1:56–60.

Kesaree N, Banapurmath CR, Banapurmath S, Shamanur K. Treatment of inverted nipples using a disposable syringe. *J Hum Lact.* 1993;9:27–29.

Kinneer M. Beachy P. Nipple feeding premature infants in the neonatal intensive-care unit: factors and decisions. *J Obstet Gynecol Neonatal Nurs.* 1994;23:105–112.

Kuehl J. Cup-feeding the newborn: what you should know. *J Perinatal Neonatal Nurs.* 1997;11:56–60.

Kurinij N, Shiono P. Early formula supplementation of breastfeeding. *Pediatrics.* 1991;88:745–750.

Lactation Education Consultants. *Consent To Use Nipple Shield.* Wheaton, IL: LEC; 1996.

Lang S, Lawrence CJ, Orme RL. Cup feeding: an alternative method of infant feeding. *Arch Dis Child.* 1994;71:365–369.

Lang S. Cup-feeding: an alternative method. *Midwives Chron Nurs Notes.* 1994;107:171–176.

Law-Morstatt L, Judd D, Snyder P, et al. Pacing as a treatment technique for transitional sucking patterns. *J Perinatol.* 2003;23:483–488.

Lawrence RA. Storage of human milk and the influence of procedures on immunological components of human milk. *Acta Paediatr.* 1999;88(Suppl 430):14–18.

Lawrence RA, Lawrence T. *Breastfeeding: A Guide for the Medical Profession.* 6th ed. Philadelphia: C.V. Mosby; 2005.

MAIN Trial Collaborative Group. Preparing for breastfeeding: treatment of inverted and non-protractile nipples in pregnancy. *Midwifery.* 1994;10:200–214.

Malhotra N, Vishwimbaran I, Sundaram KR, Narayanan I. A controlled trial of alternative methods of oral feeding in neonates. *Early Hum Dev.* 1999;54:29–38.

Marinelli KA, Burke GS, Dodd VL. A comparison of the safety of cup feedings and bottle feedings in premature infants whose mothers intend to breastfeed. *J Perinatol.* 2001;21:6:350–355.

Marmet C, Shell E. Training neonates to suck correctly. *Am J Matern Child Nur.* 1984;9:401–407.

Marmet C, Shell E, Aldana S. Assessing infant suck dysfunction: case management. *J Hum Lact.* 2000;16:332–336.

Marriott M. Nipple shields used successfully. *J Hum Lact.* 1997;13:12.

Matthew OP. Science of bottle feeding. *J Pediatr.* 1991;114:511–519.

Matthew OP. Nipple units for newborn infants: a functional comparison. *Pediatrics.* 1998;81:688–691.

McBride MC, Danner SC. Sucking disorders in neurologically impaired infants: assessment and facilitation of breastfeeding. *Clin Perinatol.* 1987;14:190–130.

McGeorge DD. The "Niplette": an instrument for the non-surgical correction of inverted nipples. *Br J Plast Surg.* 1994;47:46–49.

Measel CP, Anderson GC. Nonnutritive sucking during tube feeding: effect on clinical course in premature infants. *J Obstet Gynecol Neonatal Nurs.* 1979;8:265–272.

Medoff-Cooper B. Nutritive sucking research from clinical questions to research answers. *J Perinat Neonat Nurs.* 2004;19:265–272.

Medoff-Cooper B, Ray W. Neonatal sucking behaviors. *Image J Nurs Sch.* 1995;27: 195–199.

Meier PP, Brown LP, Hurst NM, et al. Nipple shields for preterm infants: effect on milk transfer and duration of breastfeeding. *J Hum Lact.* 2000;16:106–114.

Meier PP, Engstrom JL, Crichton CL, et al. A new scale for in-home test-weighing for mothers of preterm and high risk infants. *J Hum Lact.* 1994;10:163–168.

Meier PP, Engstrom JL, Fleming BA, et al. Estimating milk intake of hospitalized preterm infants who breastfeed. *J Hum Lact.* 1996;12:21–26.

Meier PP, Lysakowski TY, Engstrom JL, et al. The accuracy of test weighing for preterm infants. *J Pediatr Gastroenterol Nutr.* 1990;10:62–65.

Mitchell EA, Blair PS, L'Hoir MP. Should pacifiers be recommended to prevent sudden infant death syndrome? *Pediatrics.* 2006;117(5):1755–1758.

Mizuno K, Kani K. Sipping/lapping is a safe alternative feeding method to suckling for preterm infants. *Acta Paediatr.* 2005;94:574–580.

Mohrbacher N, Stock J. *The Breastfeeding Answer Book.* 3rd ed. Schamburg IL: La Leche League; 2003.

Morse J. The hazards of lanolin. *Matern Child Nur.* 1989a;14:204.

Morse J. Lanolin recommended to breastfeeding mothers to prevent nipple discomfort and pain. *Birth.* 1989b;16:35.

Mosley C, Whittle C, Hicks C. A pilot study to assess the viability of a randomized controlled trial of methods of supplementary feeding of breast-fed pre-term babies. *Midwifery.* 2001;17:150–157.

Musoke RN. Breastfeeding promotion: feeding the low birth weight infant. *Suppl Int J Obstet Gynecol.* 1990;(Suppl 31):57–68.

Neifert M, Lawrence R, Seacat J. Nipple confusion: toward a formal definition. *J Pediatr*. 1995;126:S125–S129.

Neimela M, Uhari M, Mottonen M. A pacifier increases the risk of recurrent acute otitis media in children in day care centers. *Pediatrics*. 1995;96:884–888.

Newman J. Caution regarding nipple shields. *J Hum Lact*. 1997;13:12–13.

Newman J. Breastfeeding problems associated with the early introduction of bottles and pacifiers. *J Hum Lact*. 1990;6:59–63.

Newman J. Using a lactation aid. Available at: http://www.obgyn.net/pregnancy-birth/ ?page=/pb/articles/bf_newman5_0599. Accessed January 22, 2007.

Newman J, Pitman T. *Dr. Jack Newman's Guide to Breastfeeding*. Toronto: Harper Collins; 2000.

Nicholson WL. The use of nipple shields by breastfeeding women. *J Aust Coll Midwives*. 1993;6:18–24.

Noble R, Bovey A. Therapeutic teat use for babies who breastfeed poorly. *Breastfeeding Rev*. 1997;5:37–42.

North K, Fleming P, Golding J, et al. Pacifier use and morbidity in the first six months of life. *Pediatrics*. 1999;103:e34 Available at: http://pediatrics.aappublications.org/ cgi/content/full/103/3/e34?maxtoshow=&HITS=10&hits=10&RESULTFORMAT= &fulltext=North+K%2C+Fleming+P%2C+Golding+J&andorexactfulltext= and&searchid=1&FIRSTINDEX=0&sortspec=relevance&resourcetype=HWCIT.

Nowak AJ, Smith WL, Erenberg A. Imaging evaluation of artificial nipples during bottle feeding. *Arch Pediatr Adolesc Med*. 1994;148:40–42.

Nowak AJ, Smith WL, Erenberg A. Imaging evaluation of breastfeeding and bottle feeding systems. *J Pediatr*. 1995;126:S130–S134.

Oddy WH, Glenn K. Implementing the Baby Friendly Hospital Initiative: the role of finger feeding. *Breastfeed Rev*. 2003;11:5–10.

Otte MJ. Correcting inverted nipples—an aid to breastfeeding. *Am J Nurs*. 1975;3: 454–456.

Palmer B. The influence of breastfeeding on the development of the oral cavity: a commentary. *J Hum Lact*. 1998;14:93–98.

Pinelli J, Symington A, Ciliska D. Nonnutritive sucking in high-risk infants: benign intervention or legitimate therapy? *J Obstet Gynecol Neonatal Nurs*. 2002;31: 582–591.

Powers D, Tapia V. Women's experiences using a nipple shield. *J Hum Lact*. 2004;20: 327–333.

Pugh LC, Buchko BL, Bishop BA, et al. A comparison of topical agents to relieve nipple pain and enhance breastfeeding. *Birth*. 1996;23:88–93.

Righard L. Are breastfeeding problems related to incorrect breastfeeding technique and the use of pacifiers and bottles? *Birth*. 1998;25:40–44.

Righard L, Alade MO. Breastfeeding and the use of pacifiers. *Birth*. 1997;24:116–120.

Riordan J. *Breastfeeding and Human Lactation*. 3rd ed. Sudbury, MA: Jones and Bartlett Publishers; 2005.

Rocha N, Martinez F, Jorge S. Cup or bottle for preterm infants: effect on oxygen saturation, weight gain and breastfeeding. *J Hum Lact.* 2002;18:132–137.

Ross M. Back to the breast: retraining infant suckling patterns. In: *The Lactation Consultant Series.* Garden City Park, NY: Avery Publishing Group; 1987.

Sakashita R, Kamegai T, Inoue N. Masseter muscle activity in bottle feeding with the chewing type bottle teat: evidence from electromyographs. *Early Hum Dev.* 1996;45: 83–92.

Savenije OEM, Brand PLP. Accuracy and precision of test weighing to assess milk intake in newborn infants. *Arch Dis Child.* Fetal Neonatal Ed 2006;91(5):F330–332.

Schubiger G, Schwarz U, Tonz O. UNICEF/WHO baby friendly hospital initiative: does the use of bottles and pacifiers in the neonatal nursery prevent successful breastfeeding. *Eur J Pediatr.* 1997;156:874–877.

Sealy CN. Rethinking the use of nipple shields. *J Hum Lact.* 1996;12:29–30.

Spangler A, Hildebrandt H. The effect of modified lanolin on nipple pain/damage during the first 10 days of breastfeeding. *Int J Childbirth Educ.* 1993;8:15–18.

Spatz D. Ten steps for promoting and protecting breastfeeding for vulnerable infants. *J Perinat Neonat Nurs.* 2004;18:385–396.

Stein MJ. Breastfeeding the premature infant: a protocol without bottles. *J Hum Lact.* 1990;6:167–170.

Thorley V. Cup feeding: problems created by incorrect use. *J Hum Lact.* 1997;13:54–55.

Trenouth MJ, Campbell AN. Questionnaire evaluation of feeding methods for cleft lip and palate neonates. *Int J Paediatr Dent.* 1996;6:241–244.

Turgeon-O'Brien H, Lachapelle D, Gragnon PF, et al. Nutritive and non-nutritive sucking habits: a review. *ASDC J Dent Child.* 1996;63:321–327.

Venuta A, Bertolani P, Pepe P, et al. Do pacifiers cause latex allergy? *Allergy.* 1999;54: 1007.

Victora CG, Behague DP, Barros FC, et al. Pacifier use and short breastfeeding duration: cause, consequence, or coincidence? *Pediatrics.* 1997;99:445–453.

Victora C, Tomasi E, Olinto M, Barros F. Use of pacifiers and breastfeeding duration. *Lancet.* 1993;341:404–406.

Vogel AM, Hutchison BL, Mitchell EA. The impact of pacifier use on breastfeeding: a prospective cohort study. *J Paediatr Child Health.* 2001;37:58–63.

Walker M. *Breastfeeding Management for the Clinician: Using the Evidence.* Sudbury, MA: Jones and Bartlett Publishers; 2006.

Walker M. Breastfeeding Premature Babies. In: *Lactation Consultant Series.* Schaumberg, IL: La Leche League; 1990.

Weber R, Woolridge MW, Baum JD. An ultrasonographic study of the organisation of sucking and swallowing by newborn infants. *Dev Med Child Neurol.* 1986;28:19–24.

Wight NE. Cup-feeding. ABM news and views. *Acad Breastfeed Med.* 1998;4:1–5.

Wilson PD. Hydrogel dressing for treatment of sore nipples during early lactation: should we be promoting these products? *J Hum Lact.* 2001;17:4:295–297.

Wilson-Clay B. Clinical use of silicone nipple shields. *J Hum Lact.* 1996;12:655–658.

Wilson-Clay B. Nipple shields: just another tool. *J Hum Lact.* 1997;13:194. Comment 1997;12:279–285.

Wilson-Clay B, Hoover K. *The Breastfeeding Atlas.* 3rd ed. Austin, TX: LactNews Press; 2005.

Woodworth M, Frank E. Transitioning to the breast at six weeks: use of a nipple shield. *J Hum Lact.* 1996;12:305–307.

Woolridge MW. The "anatomy" of infant sucking. *Midwifery.* 1986;2;164–171.

Woolridge MW, Baum JD, Drewett RF. Effect of a traditional and of a new nipple shield on sucking patterns and milk flow. *Early Hum Dev.* 1980;4:57–64.

Wright A, Rice S, Wells S. Changing hospital practices to increase the duration of breastfeeding. *Pediatrics.* 1996;97:669–675.

Zeimer M, Cooper DM, Pigeon JG. Evaluation of a dressing to reduce nipple pain and improve nipple skin condition in breastfeeding women. *Nurs Res.* 1995;44:347–351.

Suggested Readings

Billet J. Aids to breastfeeding: a look at some of the products. *Prof Care Mother Child.* 1994;4:19–20.

Bodley V, et al. Long-term nipple shield use—a positive perspective. *J Hum Lact.* 1996; 12:301–304.

Brown SJ. Nipple shields—never a good thing? *Pract Midwife.* 2003;6:42.

Brown SH, Alexander J, Thomas P. Feeding outcome in breast-fed term babies supplemented by cup or bottle. *Midwifery.* 1999;15:2:92–96.

Bull P, Barger J. *Fingerfeeding with the SNS.* Medela Inc: Rental Roundup 1987; Summer.

Collins C, Phillip R, Crowther A, et al. Effect of bottles, cups and dummies on breast feeding in preterm infants: a randomized controlled trial. *BMJ.* 2004;329:193–198.

Jackson JM, Mourino AP. Pacifier use and otitis media in infants twelve months of age or younger. *Pediatr Dent.* 1999;21:256–261.

Lang S. *Breastfeeding Special Care Babies.* 2nd ed. London: Baillière Tindall; 2002.

Lennon I, Lewis B. Effect of early complementary feeds on lactation failure. *Breastfeeding Rev.* 1987;11:25–26.

Wolf LS, Glass RP. *Feeding and Swallowing Disorders in Infancy.* Tucson, AZ: Therapy Skill Builders; 1992.

INDUCED LACTATION AND RELACTATION

Virginia Thorley, OAM, DipEd, MA, IBCLC
with contributions from Ruth Worgan, RN, CM, IBCLC

OBJECTIVES

- Define induced lactation and relactation.
- Discuss the historical basis and cultural issues of induced lactation and relactation.
- List indications for inducing lactation and for relactation.
- Describe factors related to the infant that influence the outcome of induced lactation.
- Describe the necessary hormonal and physiological changes required for lactation to occur nonpuerperally.
- Describe physical and non-pharmaceutical actions that can assist in inducing lactation and relactation.
- List the action of medications prescribed to induce lactation and/or relactate.
- Describe management of induced lactation and relactation.

Introduction

Breast development and maturation during pregnancy are the usual precursors to lactation. However, both the historical and contemporary literature demonstrate that a woman can produce milk without the preparatory effect of pregnancy and birth, that is, *nonpuerperally.* After breast and nipple stimulation is commenced, many women experience breast fullness and tenderness. Induced lactation and relactation have occurred and continue to occur with unknown prevalence in indigenous societies (Basedow, 1925; Kramer, 1995; Nemba, 1994; Slome, 1956; Wieschhoff, 1940), in developing countries (Abejide et al., 1997; Banapurmath, Banapurmath, & Kesaree, 1993a; Brown, 1977; De et al., 2002; Kesaree, 1993) and also in the developed world (ABA, 2004; Auerbach and Avery, 1980; Boyle, 1993; Hormann, 1977; Phillips, 1993; Raphael, 1973; Scantlebury, 1923). Nonpuerperal lactation has also been described in animals, both female and male, in response to suckling (Anon., 1845; Archer, 1990; Creel et al., 1991).

Where the society or the family has a strong breastfeeding culture, relactation is part of lactation, with some women resuming lactation after a gap for a number of reasons (Datta et al., 1993; Marquis et al., 1998; Phillips, 1993). Indeed, Mobbs and Babbage (1971) considered nonpuerperal lactation to be a normal physiological response of the breasts to suckling. Interest in induced lactation and relactation appears to have paralleled the increased interest in breastfeeding in developed countries. Where breastfeeding is accepted as the norm, the normal course of lactation in individual women may differ from the stereotype of exclusive breastfeeding, followed sequentially by mixed feeding and weaning. Breastfeeding may follow a number of other patterns (Table 32-1), with the first weaning followed by one of more episodes of partial or exclusive breastfeeding (Datta et al., 1993; Marquis et al., 1998; Phillips, 1993).

Table 32-1   Patterns in Human Lactation

Pattern	Type
EBF → MF → W	(1)
MF → W	(2)
MF → EBF → MF → W	(3)
EBF → MF → W^n → MF → W	(4)
EBF → MF → W → MF → W	(5)
EBF → MF → EBF → MF → W	(5)
MF → W → MF → EBF → MF → W	(5)
MF → W → MF → W	(5)
NBF → MF → EBF → MF → W	(6)
NBF → MF → W	(6)

Abbreviations: EBF, exclusive breastfeeding; MF, mixed feeding/part breastfeeding; W, weaned; NBF, never breastfed.
(1) Classic physiological breastfeeding pattern after delivery of an infant.
(2) Initial difficulties followed by weaning.
(3) Progression to classic pattern after initial difficulties.
(4) Data from pattern observed by Marquis et al., 1998, with one or more temporary weanings (W^n), followed by relactation.
(5) Other patterns involving relactation (space prevents every variation of these patterns being tabulated here).
(6) Two patterns associated with both adoptive breastfeeding and establishing breastfeeding for the mother's biological child who was not initially breastfed.

I. Definitions

A. *Induced lactation.* The purposeful stimulation of lactation where it was previously absent, usually in the absence of a pregnancy in the months immediately prior to the induction of lactation (*nonpuerperally*). The term also includes adoptive breastfeeding where a woman who is not breastfeeding induces lactation, whether or not she has ever breastfed in the past (Thorley, 2006; Waletzky, 1976).

B. *Relactation.* Properly, relactation means induced lactation in a mother who has previously breastfed the index baby (that is, reversing weaning), but the term also is used where a mother induces lactation for a biological child she has never breastfed following the suppression of lactation postpartum. The term is loosely used as a generic term for any type of induced lactation (Thorley, 2006). Some authors include reversing a significant decrease in breast milk production in their definition of relactation (Lakhkar, Shenoy, & Bhaskaranand, 1999; Seema, Patwari, & Satyonarayana, 1997).

C. *Nursing.* Used here to mean *breastfeeding.*

D. *Mother.* Used here as any woman inducing lactation, whether she is the biological, adoptive, or foster mother.

II. Physiological Mechanisms

A. The hormonal influences on the development of secretory tissue in the breast during a pregnancy and the events triggered by the delivery of the placenta are described in Chapter 14.

B. The physiology of induced lactation is not as well understood; however, it is known that:

1. In the absence of a pregnancy, mammary stimulation, especially nipple stimulation, facilitates proliferation of secretory tissue, enabling milk secretion to occur.

C. Suckling or expression, or other nipple stimulation, stimulates prolactin secretion and the release of oxytocin (Hill, Aldag, & Chattereton, 1996; Hormann & Savage, 1998; Zinaman et al., 1992); it is milk removal that continues milk secretion.

D. Confidence-building is important to the release of oxytocin by the posterior pituitary, a process that can be inhibited by stress.

E. Oxytocin release can become a conditioned response (Hill, Chatterton, & Aldag, 1999).

F. Clinical indications.

1. Induced lactation and relactation have been practiced in most cultures and for a variety of reasons.

   a. When a mother adopts or fosters a baby (or child of any age) and desires to breastfeed (sometimes referred to as *adoptive breastfeeding*).

    b. When a relation/friend stimulates lactation to nourish an infant if the biological mother is unable (for example, in the case of maternal human immunodeficiency virus, maternal death, the maternal inability to breastfeed because of a physical abnormality, or maternal absence (Hormann & Savage, 1998; Slome, 1956).

    c. When emergency situations exist following a natural disaster, warfare, or civil strife (Brown, 1978; Gribble, 2005b; Hormann & Savage, 1998).

    d. When an adoptive child seeks the comfort of the breast, or the mother or grandmother finds nursing at the breast calms an emotionally labile child (Gribble, 2005a; Gribble, 2005c; Gribble, 2006; Slome, 1956).

2. Relactation has been practiced:

    a. When the mother wishes to recommence breastfeeding after weaning, to enhance maternal-infant bonding.

    b. To ameliorate an infant health problem that followed weaning, such as:

      i. Proven or suspected intolerance or allergy to artificial baby milks (ABM, 2004; Avery, 1973).

      ii. Constipation.

3. The situation that led to weaning, or to failure to initiate breastfeeding, has been overcome or ameliorated.

    a. Maternal breast or nipple conditions (Kesaree et al., 1993; Seema et al., 1997), illness, or maternal-infant separation (Brown, 1978).

    b. Unsupportive hospital practices that have prevented the initiation of breastfeeding in the postnatal period (De, 2003).

    c. Infant conditions such as prematurity (Thompson, 1996), oral-facial anomalies (Menon & Mathews, 2002), severe dehydration (Sofer, Ben-Ezer, & Dagan, 1993), or hospitalization (Auerbach & Avery, 1979a; Auerbach & Avery, 1979b).

4. The child initiates breastfeeding following weaning (Phillips, 1993; Thorley, 1997).

5. Emergency or disaster situations exist following a natural disaster, warfare, or civil strife (Brown, 1977; Gribble, 2005b; Hormann & Savage, 1998).

III. Induced Lactation: Clinical Practice

A. Assessment.

  1. History.

    a. Previous pregnancies and endocrine history.

      i. How many?

      ii. Duration of pregnancies?

      iii. How long ago?

    b. Does she have a history suggestive of hormonal imbalance or anomalies?

      i. Reason for adoption (for instance, related to obstetrical or hormonal difficulties).

      ii. History of infertility (for example, hormonal, polycystic ovary syndrome).

      iii. Other hormonal abnormalities (such as thyroid or pituitary disorders).

2. Previous breastfeeding experience.

   a. Has the mother breastfed previous children, and if so, for how long?

   b. Did she have any breastfeeding difficulties? If so, what, and were they resolved?

   c. What were her reason(s) for weaning and the age of the child?

   d. How long is the lactation gap (length of time from last breastfeeding to commencing induction of lactation)?

      i. A longer lactation gap has been associated with a longer time to achieve a milk flow (De et al., 2002; Lakhkar et al., 1999).

      ii. A long lactation gap, even years, has not been an obstacle in some case series (Banapurmath et al., 1993a; Lakhkar, 2000; Nemba, 1994; Slome, 1956).

      iii. Women who had never previously lactated experienced more difficulty in inducing a milk flow in some studies (Auerbach & Avery, 1979c); in others, there was no disadvantage (Marieskind, 1973; Nemba, 1994).

   e. Was the previous breastfeeding experience with an adopted baby? The experience with a different adopted baby may be different (Mobbs & Babbage, 1971).

   f. Assess the mother's education on breastfeeding in general (Auerbach & Avery, 1979c), such as reading, classes, and videos, irrespective of presence or absence of previous breastfeeding experience.

B. Cultural influences.

1. Assess the mother's support system.

2. Determine her expectations about her ability to make breast milk.

3. Determine her expectations about her ability to introduce her baby to the breast.

4. Assess her concerns regarding modesty.

5. Does she hold religious beliefs regarding breast milk and breastfeeding that affect family relationships, including relationships of this baby with other children?

6. In an indigenous culture, is this a traditional adoption where the baby will go from the birth mother to the adoptive mother at or soon after birth? If so, the baby may be able to be breastfed by the biological mother while the adoptive mother is establishing lactation (Nemba, 1994).

C. Reasons for wanting to breastfeed an adopted baby.

1. To normalize the arrival of a child and to simulate the experience of biological motherhood.

2. To enhance the mother-infant relationship and increase the opportunity for close attachment.

3. To optimize the baby's health.

4. To ensure that the baby will not miss out on the experience.

5. To give a debilitated infant a chance at survival (e.g., during a natural disaster).

IV. Prior to Receiving the Infant

A. Requirements, essential (Brown, 1977).

1. A healthy woman, with intact pituitary, motivated to establish lactation.

2. A baby willing to suckle, or a mother willing to do milk expression (manual or mechanical) for breast stimulation.

3. A support network that may be:
   a. Family and friends.
   b. Mother-support group (breastfeeding specific).
   c. Internet Web sites supportive of adoptive breastfeeding (Gribble, 2001; Table 32-2).
   d. Professional support.

4. Confidence, or confidence-building (Banapurmath, Banapurmath, & Kesaree, 2003; Nemba, 1994).

5. Rehydration therapy, if induced lactation is undertaken for a dehydrated or ill infant (Brown, 1977).

B. Requirements, desirable.

1. Preparation by reading or other education on induction of lactation (Auerbach & Avery, 1979c; Nemba, 1994; Thearle & Weissenberger, 1984).

2. Reading (Auerbach & Avery, 1979c) or education on the normal management of breastfeeding if the mother has limited experience of observing others breastfeeding.

C. Questions to be addressed.

1. How long will it be until the mother receives the child to be breastfed?
   a. The mother should be warned of difficulty in predicting the date when she will receive her adopted baby, especially with overseas adoptions.
   b. She may receive her baby on short notice, reducing the expected preparation time, or
   c. She may have a longer wait than anticipated.
   d. Few mothers today will receive their adoptive babies at or soon after birth. Exceptions may be:

      i. Following the birth of the baby to a surrogate mother.

      ii. Traditional adoptions; for instance, in some indigenous cultures or within a family.

  2. Approximately how old does she expect the child to be (for example, newborn, over six months, over 12 months?).

  3. What type of milk is the child being fed at present?

  4. How is the child currently being fed (for example, wet nursed, fed by bottle, fed by cup)?

D. Infant's age.

  1. Newborns and babies younger than 8 weeks are most likely to suckle willingly (Auerbach & Avery, 1979c); this may be because suck is initially reflexive and changes to a voluntary action by about three months (Walker, 2006).

  2. Adopted infants over two months may be as likely to reject as to respond when put to the breast (Auerbach & Avery, 1980) and may require similar techniques to resolve breast refusal as for an infant born to the mother.

  3. Early rejection of the breast need not mean the baby will always refuse (Auerbach & Avery, 1979c; Seema et al., 1997; Thearle & Weissenberger, 1984).

  4. Babies who are older than six months are likely to require patience in the gradual process of introducing the breast.

  5. The older the child is when introduced to the breast, the less willing he or she may be to suckle (Auerbach & Avery, 1979c), unless he or she has previously been breastfed or is being breastfed by the biological mother or a foster mother at the time of the adoption.

  6. For a baby older than nine months, factors influencing willingness to accept breastfeeding attempts include quality foster care prior to adoption (vs. negative care with little physical contact) and the child's personality (ABA, 2004).

E. Breasts and nipples

  1. Assess physical characteristics of the breasts that may make inducing a milk supply a greater challenge.
    a. Anomalies, scars, history of any surgical procedures.
    b. Breast size and shape (for example, tubular, asymmetrical, or pendulous (Huggins, Petok, & Mireles, 2000).

  2. Assess the size and shape of the nipples and areola.
    a. Normal, inverted, flat, and retracted.
    b. Nipple anomalies and supernumerary nipples.
    c. Areola anomalies.
    d. The direction the nipple points; this will influence the position of the baby's mouth.

Table 32-2 Selected Internet Resources on Adoptive Breastfeeding for Professionals and Clients*

Source and Description	Web Site
Protocols	
Academy of Breastfeeding Medicine	http://www.bfmed.org/ace-files/protocol/prot9galactogoguesEnglish.pdf
Protocol #9: Use of galactogogues in initiating or augmenting maternal milk supply.	
Goldfarb L, Newman J	http://www.asklenore.info/breastfeeding/induced_lactation/intro.html
The Newman-Goldfarb protocols for induced lactation.	
Breastfeeding Aids	
Lact-Aid	http://www.lact-aid.com/uses.htm
A tube-type feeding system that permits the baby to learn to breastfeed safely by supplementing at the breast.	
Supplemental Nursing System	http://www.medela.ch/ISBD/en/breastfeeding/products/nursing.php?navid=54
Long-term supplemental tube feeding system enabling the baby to stay on the breast.	
Support	
La Leche League International	http://www.lalecheleague.org/NB/NBadoptive.html
Frequently asked questions; Online articles from LLLI publications, New Beginnings and Leaven.	

Adoption Media LLC	http://breast-feeding.adoption.com
Resources, articles, forums, Chat line, community outreach. Adoption procedures for US, Canada, UK.	
Yahoo Groups	http://groups.yahoo.com/group/adoptivebreastfeeding
Adoptive Breastfeeding; an online chat group and links to other supports.	
The Adoptive Breastfeeding Resource Website	http://www.fourfriends.com/abrw
Naomi B. Duane Resources, milk calculator, articles, news, message boards, support.	

Compiled by Virginia Thorley with input from Noreen Siebanaler, MSN, RN, IBCLC.
*Note: Web sites change over time. These URLs were valid as of January 28, 2007.

V. Planning

A. Expected outcome.

1. Counseling.
   a. Explain to the mother that two partners are involved, mother and baby.
   b. Ascertain her expectations and how she defines *breastfeeding success*.
   c. Emphasize the breastfeeding relationship and realistic levels of achievement (Riordan, 2005).
      i. *Success* is best defined as how the individual mother feels about the experience (Auerbach & Avery, 1979c).
      ii. Center upon the baby's willingness to nurse at the breast.
      iii. Confidence, a factor in lactation success following a pregnancy (Blyth et al., 2002; Dennis, 1999), is also an important factor in inducing lactation nonpuerperally.
   d. Low confidence and lack of support and infrequent suckling have been associated with poorer outcomes (Lakhkar, 2000).
   e. While full lactation/exclusive breastfeeding might never be achieved by some mothers, many mothers and their adopted babies have continued supplemented breastfeeding for extended periods.
   f. The breast can be a place of comfort, where the baby feels safe.
   g. Build trust, especially with an older baby, before attempting to offer the breast (ABA, 2004).
   h. Breast milk may be offered as a drink or mixed in other food, even if the child never accepts nursing at the breast.
2. The first milk drops in the absence of a baby can be expected after a few days to a few weeks of preparation.
3. If the baby is suckling, then breast milk may be evident as early as a few days to two weeks, but there is wide individual variation. Consequently, it is advisable not to give the mother a number value for how long this will take.

B. Support for the mother.

1. Support from family and friends (Avery, 1973; Hormann, 1977; Lakhkar, 1999), including psychological support and household assistance.
2. Support, encouragement, and appropriate information from the lactation consultant or other professional caregiver, with an emphasis on confidence-building (Banapurmath et al., 2003; De et al., 2002).
3. Access to an online support group for adoptive breastfeeding mothers, to normalize the experience (Gribble, 2001; see Table 32-2).
4. Mothers may receive little support or outright discouragement from adoption agencies, family, and friends. Mothers need to be prepared for addressing this issue.

VI. Establishing Lactation

A. Expressing.

1. Assess the mother's comfort with manual or mechanical expressing.

2. Teach and assess her ability to hand-express the breasts.

3. Discuss the types of manual and electric breast pumps available and the mother's ability to access them (see Chapter 30).

   a. Simultaneous bilateral (double) pumping with a portable, hospital-grade electric pump is more efficient than other pumping options (Siebenaler, 2002).

4. Assess the mother's ability to use these technologies correctly.

5. Assess the mother's ability to achieve expression frequency.

   a. Ideally, as frequently as a newborn would breastfeed (8–12 times per 24 hours; Hormann & Savage, 1998), *OR*

   b. Two-hourly (Lakhkar, 2000), with one or more expressions at night, *OR*

   c. At least six times per 24 hours, at 15 minutes per expression.

6. Discuss expression strategies while traveling, if the mother is required to travel to another country in the case of an overseas adoption.

   a. Manual expression.

   b. Does the electric pump have a manual mode and does the mother know how to use it?

   c. Power adaptors for countries with incompatible power.

   d. Can the pump run on batteries, and does the mother have sufficient batteries with her?

B. Stimulation to induce breast milk production.

1. Nipple stimulation (through nipple exercises or stroking, suckling, or expressing) for development and maturation of breast tissue prior to breastfeeding (Auerbach & Avery, 1979c).

2. Many women have induced lactation solely by expressing or by nursing the baby, or combining this with nipple stimulation (Auerbach & Avery, 1979c; Banapurmath et al., 1993a; Cohen, 1971; Kleinman et al., 1980; Lakhkar, 2000).

   a. Limit milk expression sessions to 15 to 25 minutes.

   b. Simultaneous expression of both breasts is believed to enhance prolactin secretion (Hill et al., 1999; Zinaman et al., 1992).

3. Breast and nipple stimulation has been reported to include the following:

   a. Nipple exercises for about four weeks prior to receiving the baby, every three to four hours (Auerbach & Avery, 1979c).

   b. Breast massage or application of warmth (Auerbach & Avery, 1979c; Phillips, 1969).

   c. The baby nursing at the breast, as the sole or main stimulus (ABA, 2004; Lakhkar, 2000).

    d. Use of a tube feeding device that delivers milk while the baby is simultaneously suckling at the breast (ABA, 2004; Auerbach & Avery, 1979c; Hormann & Savage, 1998; Kulski et al., 1981).

4. Some mothers may not have breast secretions prior to putting the baby to the breast.
   a. Mothers who have previously breastfed are more likely to have milk after manual or mechanical stimulation prior to putting the adopted baby to the breast, although the difference is not always significant.
   b. Tandem breastfeeding does not guarantee a full milk supply for the newly adopted baby (Auerbach & Avery, 1979c).

5. Galactagogues (medications or other substances believed to increase milk yield).
   a. Priming medications.
      i. Estrogen and progesterone (Auerbach & Avery, 1979c; Kramer, 1995; Nemba, 1994; see Table 32-2 for induced lactation protocols available online).
      ii. Caution is advised, because of the risk of deep vein thrombosis associated with high doses.
   b. Prolactin secretion, necessary for lactogenesis, is set in motion by stimulation of sensory nerves in the breast, via neural pathways. Additional stimulation of prolactin, in addition to breastfeeding or expressing (Gabay, 2002; McNeilly et al., 1974), is provided by the use of drugs that are dopamine antagonists.
      i. Metoclopramide (ABM, 2004; Auerbach & Avery, 1980; Banapurmath, Banapurmath, & Kesaree, 1993b; Bose et al., 1981; Brown, 1973; Budd et al., 1993; Hale, 2006; Kauppila, Kivinen, & Ylikorkala, 1983).
      ii. Domperidone (Brown, 1978; Hale, 2006; Hofmeyr & van Iddekinge, 1983; Hoffmeyr, Iddekinge, & Blott, 1985); available outside the USA, but may sometimes be obtained from compounding pharmacies in the USA (ABM, 2004).
      iii. Sulpiride, in low doses, because it is not dose-dependent (Aono et al., 1982; Cheales-Siebenaler, 1999; Hale, 2006; Ylikorkala et al., 1984); unavailable in some countries.
   c. Less-used pharmaceutical galactagogues include:
      i. Thyrotropin-releasing hormone; (Emery, 1996; Hill et al., 1999; Peters, Schulaze-Tollert, & Schuth, 1991); not advised for general use (Hormann & Savage, 1998).
      ii. Chlorpromazine (Ehrenkranz & Ackerman, 1986); has side effects (Hale, 2006; Sousa et al., 1975).
      iii. Human growth hormone (Hofmeyr et al., 1985; Milsom et al., 1992).

6. The hormone oxytocin stimulates the milk-ejection reflex.
   a. Synthetic forms of this hormone should be used only after there is milk present to be ejected and the mother's milk-ejection reflex is ineffective.

    b. Oxytocin is usually available as an intranasal spray (Syntocinon); not available in some countries, in the United States it can be mixed at a compounding pharmacy (Walker, 2006).

    c. Hale (2006) suggests the intranasal spray be limited to the first week postpartum. In induced lactation, it would be reasonable to extrapolate this to the first week after milk is present beyond a few drops, although this has not been studied.

    d. Bucal oxytocin may not have any affect on actual milk yield (Ylikorkala et al., 1984).

    e. The oxytocin nasal spray, also, may not have any effect on actual milk yield (Fewtrell et al., 2006).

    f. Because oxytocin release can become a conditioned response (Hill et al., 1999), the mother may find that developing a ritual or routine just prior to breastfeeding or expressing will trigger this response.

7. Herbal galactagogues, dietary supplements, and alternative medicine have been used in most cultures as galactagogues.

    a. Most information is anecdotal.

    b. It is common for mothers who are inducing lactation to improve their own diets and increase fluid intake (similarly to women who are lactating following childbirth) (Auerbach & Avery, 1979c; De et al., 2002).

    c. Many mothers believe that dietary supplements or increasing fluid intake will stimulate milk production, but evidence that special foods or herbal products will enhance milk synthesis is lacking. Those that have been used include:

        i. Brewer's yeast (may cause fussiness in some infants).

        ii. Beer; alcohol may, however, both inhibit the milk ejection reflex and reduce the baby's suckling behavior and sleep (Mennella, 2001; Mennella & Beauchamp, 1993; Mennella, Pepino, & Teff, 2005).

        iii. Fenugreek, fennel, and anise (not star anise) have been used as herbal galactagogues; they may be allergenic in susceptible individuals (Humphrey, 2003).

        iv. Fenugreek; generally regarded as safe, but may have a hypoglycemic effect on the mother (Bryant, 2006; Hale, 2006).

        v. Fennel; considered safe, but no documentation of galactogoguic effects (Hale, 2006).

        vi. Acupuncture, through enhancing prolactin secretion (Clavey, 1996; Jenner & Filshie, 2002; Sheng & Xie, 1989).

        vii. Hypnosis (Auerbach & Avery, 1979c).

    d. So-called "natural" treatments should be used with caution because some herbal products have been found to be detrimental to infant health (Rosti et al, 1994).

C. The most common problems adoptive mothers might encounter (Auerbach & Avery, 1979c).

1. Lack of preparation time.
2. Maintaining the newly stimulated breast milk supply while traveling to collect the baby.
3. Getting the baby to nurse, or experiencing breast refusal through infant frustration.
   a. Rewarding the baby with supplemental milk through the *drop and drip* technique (dripping donor breast milk or artificial baby milk (ABM) onto the areola) or through a supplemental feeding tube device can reduce frustration (Lakhkar et al., 1999).
4. Worry about the baby getting enough milk (Auerbach & Avery, 1979c) or self-doubt leading to stress (Bose et al., 1981).
5. Fatigue.
6. Uncertainty about decreasing supplements.
   a. Regular contact with relevant members of the health care team (lactation consultant, physician, child health nurse) for guidance.
   b. Emotional support/reassurance.
7. Expressing/feeding equipment difficulties.
8. Finding the time to initiate lactation due to competing demands of other children or employment.

D. Physiological responses to induced lactation and related discomforts (Auerbach & Avery, 1979c).
   1. Nipple pain (Seema et al., 1997), which should be addressed by:
      a. Reassurance and attention to the baby's attachment and positioning (Banapurmath et al., 2003).
      b. Selection of appropriate diameter of the breast pump flange and correct use of it.
   2. Breast pain.
   3. Nipple and breast changes, including fullness (ABA, 2004; Riordan, 2005).
   4. Signs of milk ejection.
   5. Menstrual cessation or irregularities (Hormann, 1977; Riordan, 2005).
   6. Increased appetite (Auerbach & Avery, 1979c).
   7. Weight changes; Auerbach & Avery (1979c) reported either gain or loss.

E. Infant suckling.
   1. Skin-to-skin contact.
      a. Begin skin contact when the baby is not hungry and is contented.
      b. Older babies not used to being held close may at first find skin-to-skin threatening, so patience and respect for the baby's feelings are needed.

2. Establish breastfeeding.
    a. Facilitate good attachment and positioning.
    b. Encourage the mother to begin to nurse the infant on the side on which he or she is used to being fed (for example, if bottle-fed on the left side, begin breastfeeding on the left breast).
    c. Facilitate short, frequent breastfeeds (8–12 each 24 hours).
    d. The infant should not be forced to the breast or to breastfeed.
        i. Early refusal is not predictive; infants who reject the breast initially may later learn to accept it (Auerbach & Avery, 1980).
    e. To encourage a reluctant baby, teach the mother to:
        i. Assuage hunger with partial feeding before breastfeeds, using a cup, syringe, or bottle, or finger feeding with a feeding tube.
        ii. Use the drop and drip method to encourage suckling; that is, dribble milk onto the areola while the baby is attached (Kesaree, 1993; Lakhkar, 2000). The milk can be dropped from a spoon, dropper, syringe, or bottle.
        iii. Breastfeed when the baby is drowsy.
        iv. Breastfeed in a darkened, quiet room.
        v. Use a supplemental feeding tube device to deliver milk while the baby is suckling at the breast (Auerbach & Avery, 1980; Bryant, 2006); placing the device's milk container higher will initially allow for a faster flow.
        vi. Some babies will take the breast without the supplementer at night.
        vii. Some babies will latch and stay attached if the mother walks around; wearing the baby in a sling may facilitate breastfeeding.
    f. Teach the mother to recognize milk transfer.
    g. Do not allow the infant to cry at the breast; the breastfeeding experience should be pleasurable.
        i. Remove a crying baby from the breast and soothe or divert her/him in other ways.
        ii. Talk or sing to the baby while at the breast.
    h. Begin with short, frequent breastfeeding attempts, extending the time as the child indicates willingness.
    i. Once the child accepts the breast, expressing can be discontinued and replaced with frequent suckling.

3. Supplementation.
    a. Supplementation is essential for the baby's well-being while the mother's milk supply is being established.
    b. If banked human milk is unavailable, the ABM that the baby was already drinking should be continued, unless there is good reason to change it.
    c. Eliminate/decrease the use of bottles and artificial nipples, including pacifiers, by putting the child to the breast frequently and providing

whatever additional nourishment is needed via feeding tube device at the breast, or by cup or syringe after breastfeeding.

d. If a supplemental feeding tube device is not being used and milk has been observed:
   i. Offer the supplement only after the baby has nursed at the breast.
   ii. Offer the ABM after every second feed, provided breastfeeds are approximately two-hourly.
   iii. Feed the baby on the breast alone at night, if the mother and baby are sleeping in close proximity and able to breastfeed ad lib.
e. If a cup is used for supplements, teach the mother to cup-feed the baby in an upright position (see Chapter 33).
f. If supplements are given by bottle, bottle-feed on both the left and right side to avoid a one-sided preference.
g. If the baby is accustomed to being fed by bottle with a fast flow, introduce bottle nipples with a slower flow to accustom the baby to receiving milk more slowly.
h. Gradually decrease ABMs and other foods as appropriate, using infant output and growth as guides. However,
   i. Do not keep the baby hungry in an attempt to encourage suckling at the breast; this is counterproductive because the baby becomes weak and less effective at nursing (Avery, 1973).
   ii. Do not dilute the supplementary milk, for similar reasons.
   iii. Do not restrict the amounts of supplements.
   iv. If the baby's output lessens or growth falters, temporarily increase the supplement.
i. Replace milk expression/pumping with additional breastfeeds; however, expression after some feeds may be necessary for additional stimulation if the baby is weak and suckles poorly.
j. Gradually reduce any galactagogue being used.
k. Some babies will require supplementation for as long as the mother nurses.

F. Evaluation.
1. Mother-infant relationship.
   a. Skin-to-skin contact is facilitating bonding.
   b. A harmonious mother-infant relationship is developing, with mother-infant dyad happy and contented.

2. Infant breastfeeding.
   a. Infant suckling at the mother's breast.
   b. The infant is contented to suckle at the breast for increasing periods.

3. Mother is producing breast milk.
   a. Mother is producing breast milk in increasing quantities.
   b. Milk secretion observed on expression.

4. Infant indicators of breast milk intake.
   a. Evidence of milk transfer/swallowing.
   b. Changes in stools, which may vary through the day.
   c. Milk/food intake from other sources diminishing, while the urinary output (diaper count) remains normal.
   d. Pre- and post-feed weights to assess amounts of milk obtained directly from the breasts, if necessary.
   e. Weight checks every three to five days and then weekly, to assess that adequate growth continues.

G. Infant taking all nutrition from breast.

   1. Infant receiving only breast milk.
      a. Cessation of supplementary ABM/foods.
      b. Cessation of use of feeding tubes, bottles, cups, or other devices.
      c. Other stimulation (expressing, galactagogues) no longer needed.
      d. Milk production maintained by infant's breastfeeding.

   2. Infant receiving only breast milk and age-appropriate complementary (solid) foods.
      a. As above, except for the inclusion of solid foods.

VII. Relactation

A. Definition.

   1. Relactation is similar in many aspects to induced lactation and to lactation generally.

   2. Information in this section applies in situations where relactation is initiated by the mother.

   3. In the less usual situation where relactation is initiated by an older baby or child who is an experienced breastfeeder (Phillips, 1993), and who is eating semi-solid complementary foods daily, little assistance may be required other than reassurance.

B. Assessment.

   1. History.
      a. Refer to section III.
      b. Questions that apply when a mother is relactating for her biological child.
         i. Did the mother breastfeed this child at all?
         ii. If so, then for how long?
         iii. What was the reason for weaning/not breastfeeding (Phillips, 1992)?
         iv. Were there any breastfeeding difficulties? Is so, were they:
            (1) Infant-related (for instance, prematurity, tongue tie, other oral anomalies, hypertonic bite, developmental lag) *OR*

(2) Mother-related (such as inverted nipples, illness).

v. How and what is the infant currently being fed?

C. Infant's current health status.

1. Birth details (for example, normal vaginal, forceps, vacuum extraction, cesarean, birth asphyxia).

2. Infant's health history, and current growth and developmental status.

3. Is the infant strong enough to suckle?

4. Have factors related to previous feeding difficulties been addressed (Phillips, 1992)?

5. Age of infant.

a. Babies who are fewer than two or three months old may be more willing to accept the breast, as at this stage suckling is reflexive.

b. Babies older than this may respond to measures appropriate to breast refusal.

c. Children who are older than 12 months and who have a long history of breastfeeding may remember how to breastfeed effectively (Phillips, 1993).

D. Cultural influences.

1. Refer to Section III.

E. Breast and nipple assessment.

1. Refer to Section III.

2. Breast milk production.

a. Is the mother producing any breast milk at present?

b. How long has it been since the last breastfeed or expression of milk?

c. A very short lactation gap may mean a short time to achieving a flow of milk (De et al., 2002).

F. Planning.

1. Expected outcome.

a. Encourage a focus on the breastfeeding relationship.

2. Counseling.

a. Emphasize the breastfeeding relationship, facilitated by skin-to-skin contact.

b. Center upon having the baby nurse at the mother's breast.

3. Breastfeeding confidence is important for relactation, just as it is for lactation immediately following a delivery (Blyth et al., 2002).

4. Confidence-building support from a knowledgeable health worker has been recommended by various authors (Banapurmath et al., 2003; De et al., 2002; Gribble, 2001; Seema et al., 1997).

5. Two parties are involved in relactation: the mother and her baby.

6. Realistic levels of achievement. While some mothers fully relactate, some mothers may never achieve full lactation but are able to breastfeed, with supplementation, for an extended period (Riordan, 2005).

7. Is the mother employed and working at the moment?
   a. If so, is she able to reduce her hours temporarily?
   b. What are her goals? For some mothers, mixed feeding may be an achievable goal while employed; that is, giving the baby breast milk, with some ABM or age-appropriate complementary foods.

8. Regular telephone contact may be an appropriate form of professional support.

9. If the baby is suckling at very frequent intervals, a flow of breastmilk can appear in a few days to a few weeks. It is unwise to suggest a specific time frame.

G. Support from family and friends.

   1. Psychological support and household assistance.

   2. Appropriate information, support, and encouragement from a knowledgeable health worker (Seema et al., 1997).

   3. Ongoing support from a mother's support group or breastfeeding counselor.

H. Re-establishing lactation/weaning reversal.

   1. Stimulation to induce breast milk production.
      a. Many women have achieved relactation simply by nursing the baby intensively, with or without manual stimulation of the breast and nipples (Banapurmath et al., 2003; Kesaree et al., 1993; Marquis et al., 1998; Scantlebury, 1923; Seema et al., 1997; Taylor, 1995).
      b. Banapurmath et al. (1993b) and Lakhker et al. (1999) found no difference in relactation outcomes between mothers who used breast/nipple hyperstimulation (very frequent suckling) and those who used metoclopramide.

I. Infant suckling at the breast (see Section VI).

J. Expressing.

   1. Expression of the breasts by hand or with an electric or manual pump, if mother and baby are separated or the baby is reluctant to nurse.
      a. Provides stimulus to the breasts.
      b. Allows milk production to be initiated, which, in turn, increases the infant's willingness to nurse.

   2. Teach and assess the skill of hand expression.

   3. Assess the effectiveness of the breast pump of her choice and her ability to use it.

   4. Assess the mother's ability to achieve expression frequency in the case of a non-nursing baby (minimum six times in 24 hours/15 minutes each expression; two-hourly if possible).

K. Galactagogues.

   1. Increases in prolactin secretion through stimulation of the sensory nerves of the breast during breastfeeding or expression (Auerbach & Avery, 1981) may be enhanced by certain drugs.

a. Metoclopramide (Auerbach & Avery, 1980; Bose et al., 1981; Brown, 1973; Ehrenkranz & Ackerman, 1986; Hale, 2006; Kauppila, Kivinen, & Ylikorkala, 1981).

b. Domperidone (Brown, 1978; Budd et al., 1993; Hale, 2006; Hofmeyr et al., 1985).

c. Sulpiride (Ylikorkala et al., 1982; Ylikorkala et al., 1984); not available in the United Sates (Emery, 1996).

2. Stimulation of oxytocin for the milk ejection reflex.

a. Skin-to-skin contact.

b. Syntocinon nasal spray (Hormann & Savage, 1998); available from compounding pharmacies in the United States.

c. The nasal spray may have no effect on actual milk yield (Fewtrell et al., 2006).

3. Nonpharmaceutical treatments and "natural" galactogogues (see Section VI, B).

L. Evaluation.

1. Refer to Section VI, F.

M. Problems.

1. Relactation is not always easy, nor is it necessarily easier than induced lactation.

2. While for some mother-baby dyads a flow of milk is soon established, for others it may take weeks to increase the milk yield.

3. Baby not accepting the breast, or refusing out of frustration before there is a milk flow.

4. Unreliable milk ejection reflex.

5. Baby not getting enough to eat.

6. Fatigue.

VIII. Milk Composition Following Induced Lactation and Relactation

A. Milk composition following induced lactation has been shown in other species (for example, bovine and rat) to be similar to breast milk produced after a pregnancy and delivery (Lawrence & Lawrence, 2005).

B. Case series and case studies have repeatedly noted normal growth on human milk produced after induced lactation/relactation (Abejide et al., 1997; Banapurmath et al., 1993a; De et al., 2002; Mobbs & Babbage, 1971; Nemba, 1994; Scantlebury, 1923; Seema et al., 1997).

C. Relactation has been used to correct poor growth in weaned infants (Marquis et al., 1998).

D. Few papers have been published specifically on the nutritional and immunological composition of milk produced in induced lactation or relactation.

1. Investigations of the milk composition of adoptive mothers involve only a handful of cases.

2. Breast milk composition following relactation or unweaning of a biological child has yet to be investigated, literature searches being unsuccessful in finding published sources.

3. Research on breast milk after induced lactation is still very limited and contradictory, because methodology differs.

   a. Kulski et al. (1981) included two adoptive mothers who had induced lactation in their case series of nonpuerperal lactation, with other cases involving galactorrhea due to pathologies.

      i. Total protein concentrations in the first milk of the adoptive mothers approximated those of transitional milk following a pregnancy, with no colostral phase.

      ii. The proportions of proteins differed from that of the biological mothers, with lower IgA and higher α-lactalbumin than colostrum, though the values were between those of transitional and mature milk.

      iii. Concentrations of lactose, potassium, and chloride in the first milk of nonbiological mothers approximated those of the transitional or mature milk of the biological mothers.

   b. Kleinman et al. (1980) compared the breast secretions of five adoptive mothers who had induced lactation with those of five biological mothers.

      i. A colostral phase was absent in the milk of the nonbiological mothers.

      ii. The total protein values of the first milk resembled that of the transitional and mature milk of biological mothers.

References

Abejide OR, Tadese MA, Babajide DE, et al. Non-puerperal induced lactation in a Nigerian community: case reports. *Ann Trop Paediatr*. 1997;17:109–114.

Academy of Breastfeeding Medicine (ABM). Protocol #9: Use of galactogogues in initiating or augmenting maternal milk supply. July 30, 2004.

Anon. *Lancet*. 1845;1:38.

Aono T, Aki T, Koike K, Kurachi K. Effect of sulpiride on poor puerperal lactation. *Am J Obstet Gynecol*. 1982;143:927–932.

Archer M. Coming to grips with male nipples. *Australian Natural History*. 1990;23: 494–495.

Auerbach KG, Avery JL. Relactation after an untimely weaning: report from a survey. Denver, CO: Resources in Human Nurturing International, Monograph Number 2; 1979a.

Auerbach KG, Avery JL. Relactation after a hospital-induced separation: report from a survey. Denver, CO: Resources in Human Nurturing International, Monograph Number 4; 1979b.

Auerbach KG, Avery JL. Nursing the adopted infant: report from a survey. Denver, CO: Resources in Human Nurturing International, Monograph Number 5; 1979c.

Auerbach K, Avery J. Relactation: a study of 366 cases. *Pediatrics.* 1980;65:236–242.

Auerbach K, Avery J. Induced lactation: a study of adoptive nursing and counseling in 240 women. *Am J Dis Child.* 1981;135:340–334.

Australian Breastfeeding Association (ABA). *Relactation and Adoptive Breastfeeding.* 2nd ed. East Malvern, Australia: ABA; 2004.

Avery JL. *Induced Lactation: A Guide for Counseling and Management.* Denver, CO: J.J. Avery; 1973.

Banapurmath CR, Banapurmath S, Kesaree N. Successful induced non-puerperal lactation in surrogate mothers. *Indian J Pediatr.* 1993a;60:639–643.

Banapurmath CR, Banapurmath SC, Kesaree N. Initiation of relactation. *Indian Pediatr.* 1993b;30:1329–1332.

Banapurmath S, Banapurmath CR, Kesaree N. Initiation of lactation and establishing relactation in outpatients. *Indian Pediatr.* 2003;40:343–347.

Basedow H. *The Australian Aboriginal.* Adelaide, South Australia: F.W. Preece & Sons; 1925:125.

Blyth R, Creedy DK, Dennis CL, et al. Effect of maternal confidence on breastfeeding duration: an application of breastfeeding self-efficacy theory. *Birth.* 2002;29:278–284.

Bose CL, D'Ercole J, Lester AG, et al. Relactation by mothers of sick and premature infants. *Pediatrics.* 1981;67:565–569.

Boyle D. Adoptive nursing. *Leaven.* 1993; Jan-Feb:3–5, 10.

Brown R. Breastfeeding in modern times. *Am J Clin Nutr.* 1973;26:556–562.

Brown R. Relactation: an overview. *Pediatrics.* 1977;60:116–120.

Brown RE. Relactation with reference to application in developing countries. *Clin Pediatr.* 1978;17:333–337.

Bryant CA. Nursing the adopted infant. *J Am Board Fam Med.* 2006;19:374–379.

Budd S, Erdman S, Long D, et al. Improved lactation with metoclopramide. *Clin Pediatr.* 1993;32:53–57.

Cheales-Siebenaler NJ. Induced lactation in an adoptive mother. *J Hum Lact.* 1999;15:41–43.

Clavey S. The use of acupuncture for the treatment of insufficient lactation (Que Ru). *Am J Acupunct.* 1996;24:35–46.

Cohen R. Breast feeding without pregnancy. *Pediatrics.* 1971;48:996–997.

Creel SR, Monfort SL, Wildt DE, et al. Spontaneous lactation is an adaptive result of pseudopregnancy. *Nature.* 1991;351:660–662.

Datta P, Embree JE, Kreiss JK, et al. Resumption of breast-feeding in later childhood: a risk factor for mother to mother immunodeficiency virus type 1 transmission. *Pediatr Infect Dis J.* 1993;11:974–976.

De NC, Pandit B, Mishra SK, et al. Initiating the process of relactation: an institute based study. *Indian Pediatr.* 2002;39:173–178.

De NC. Baby friendly hospitals: how friendly are they? *Indian Pediatr.* 2003;40:378–379.

Dennis CL. Theoretical underpinnings of breastfeeding confidence: a self-efficacy framework. *J Hum Lact.* 1999;15:195–2001.

Ehrenkranz RA, Ackerman BA. Metoclopramide effect on faltering milk production by mothers of premature infants. *Pediatrics.* 1986;78:614–620.

Emery MM. Galactagogues: drugs to induce lactation. *J Hum Lact.* 1996;12:55–57.

Fewtrell MS, Loh KL, Blake A, et al. Randomised double blind trial of oxytocin nasal spray in mothers expressing breast milk for preterm infants. *Arch Dis Child.* 2006; 91:F169–F174.

Gabay MP. Galactogogues: medications that induce lactation. *J Hum Lact.* 2002;18: 274–279.

Gribble KD. Mother-to-mother support for women breastfeeding in unusual circumstances: a new method for an old model. *Breastfeed Rev.* 2001;9:13–19.

Gribble K. Breastfeeding a medically fragile foster child. *J Hum Lact.* 2005a;21:42–46.

Gribble KD. Infant feeding in the post Indian ocean tsunami context: reports, theory and action. *Birth Issues.* 2005b;14:121–127.

Gribble KD. Post-institutionalized adopted children who seek breastfeeding from their new mothers. *Journal of Prenatal & Perinatal Psychology and Health.* 2005c;19:217–235.

Gribble KD. Mental health, attachment and breastfeeding: implications for adopted children and their mothers. *Int Breastfeed J.* 2006;1:5.

Hale T. *Medications and Mothers' Milk: A Manual of Lactational Pharmacology.* 12th ed. Amarillo, TX: Hale Publishing; 2006.

Hill PD, Aldag JC, Chatterton RT. The effect of sequential and simultaneous breast pumping on milk volume and prolactin levels: a pilot study. *J Hum Lact.* 1996;12:193–199.

Hill PD, Chatterton RT, Aldag JC. Serum prolactin in breastfeeding: state of the science. *Biol Res Nurs.* 1999;1:65–75.

Hofmeyr G, van Iddekinge B. Domperidone and lactation. *Lancet.* 1983;1:647.

Hofmeyr G, van Iddekinge B, Blott JA. Domperidone: secretion in breast milk and effect on puerperal prolactin levels. *Br J Obstet Gynaecol.* 1985;92:141–144.

Hormann E. Breastfeeding the adopted baby. *Birth Fam J.* 1977;4:165–172.

Hormann E, Savage F. Relactation: Review of Experience and Recommendations for Practice. Geneva: World Health Organization; 1998.

Huggins KE, Petok ES, Mireles O. Markers of lactation insufficiency: a study of 34 mothers. In: *Current Issues in Clinical Lactation 2000.* Sudbury, MA: Jones and Bartlett Publishers; 2000:25–35.

Humphrey S. *The Nursing Mother's Herbal.* Minneapolis: Fairview Press; 2003.

Jenner C, Filshie J. Galactorrhoea following acupuncture. *Acupunct Med.* 2002; 20:107–108.

Kauppila A, Kivinen S, Ylikorkala O. Metoclopramide and breastfeeding: transfer into milk and the newborn. *Eur J Clin Pharmacol.* 1983;25:819–823.

Kauppila A, Kivinen S, Ylikorkala O. A dose response relation between improved lactation and metoclopramide. *Lancet.* 1981;1:1175–1177.

Kesaree N. Drop and drip method. *Indian Pediatr.* 1993;30:277–278.

Kesaree N, Banapurmath CR, Banapurmath S, Shamanur K. Treatment of inverted nipples using a disposable syringe. *J Hum Lact.* 1993;9:27–29.

Kleinman R, Jacobson L, Hormann E, Walker W. Protein values of milk samples from mothers without biologic pregnancies. *J Pediatr.* 1980;97:612–615.

Kramer P. Breastfeeding of adopted infants (letter). *BMJ.* 1995;311:188–189.

Kulski J, Hartmann P, Saint W, et al. Changes in milk composition of nonpuerperal women. *Am J Obstet Gynecol.* 1981;139:597–604.

Lakhkar BB. Breastfeeding in adopted babies. *Indian Pediatr.* 2000;37:1114–1116.

Lakhkar BB, Shenoy VD, Bhaskaranand N. Relactation–Manipal experience. *Indian Pediatr.* 1999;36:700–703.

Lawrence RA, Lawrence RM. *Breastfeeding: A Guide for the Medical Profession.* 6th ed. St Louis: C.V. Mosby; 2005.

Marieskind H. Abnormal lactation. *J Trop Pediatr Environ Child Health.* 1973;19:123–128.

Marquis GS, Diaz J, Bartolini R, et al. Recognizing the reversible nature of child-feeding decisions: breastfeeding, weaning and relactation patterns in a shanty town community of Lima, Peru. *Soc Sci Med.* 1998;47:645–656.

McNeilly A, Thorner M, Volans G, Besser GM. Metoclopramide and prolactin. *BMJ.* 1974;2:729.

Mennella JA. Sleep disturbances after acute exposure to alcohol in mother's milk. *Alcohol.* 2001;25:153–158.

Mennella J, Beauchamp G. Beer, breastfeeding and folklore. *Dev Psychobiol.* 1993;26:459–466.

Mennella JA, Pepino MY, Teff KL. Acute alcohol consumption disrupts the hormonal milieu of lactating women. *J Endocrinol Metab.* 2005;90:1970–1985.

Menon J, Mathews L. Relactation in mothers of high-risk infants. *Indian Pediatr.* 2002;39:983–984.

Milsom S, Breier B, Gallaher B, et al. Growth hormone stimulates galactopoesis in healthy lactating women. *Acta Endocrinol.* 1992;127:337–343.

Mobbs GA, Babbage NF. Breast feeding adopted children. *Med J Aust.* 1971;2:436–437.

Nemba K. Induced lactation: a study of 37 non-puerperal mothers. *J Trop Pediatr.* 1994;40:240–242.

Peters F, Schulaze-Tollert J, Schuth W. Thyrotrophin-releasing hormone: a lactation promoting agent? *Br J Obstet Gynecol.* 1991;98:880–985.

Phillips V. Non-puerperal lactation among Australian Aboriginal women. Part I. Nursing Mothers' Association of Australia News; 1969;5(4). Repr as NMAA Res Bull No. 1.

Phillips V. Relactation and high needs infants. *J Hum Lact.* 1992;8:64.

Phillips V. Relactation in mothers of children over 12 months. *J Trop Pediatr.* 1993;39:45–47.

Raphael D. Breastfeeding the adopted baby. Chapter 9, in *The Tender Gift: Breastfeeding.* Englewood Cliffs, NJ: Prentice-Hall; 1973;89–96, 105–115.

Riordan J. *Breastfeeding and Human Lactation.* 3rd ed. Sudbury, MA: Jones and Bartlett Publishers; 2005:467–470.

Rosti L, Nardini A, Bettinelli ME, Rosti D. Toxic effects of a herbal tea mixture in two newborns. *Acta Paediatr.* 1994;83:683.

Scantlebury V. The establishment and maintenance of breastfeeding. In: *Transactions of 1923 Australasian Medical Congress;* 1923:190–191.

Seema, Patwari AK, Satyanarayana L. Relactation: an effective intervention to promote exclusive breastfeeding. *J Trop Pediatr.* 1997;43:213–216.

Sheng PL, Xie QW. Relationship between effect of acupuncture on prolactin secretion and central catecholamine and R-aminobutyric acid. *Zeng Ci Yan Jiu.* 1989;14: 446–451. (Abstract in English.)

Siebenaler N. Adoptive mothers and breastfeeding. In: Walker M, ed. *Core Curriculum for Lactation Consultant Practice.* Sudbury, MA: Jones and Bartlett Publishers; 2002:416–421.

Slome C. Non-puerperal lactation in grandmothers. *J Pediatr.* 1956;49:550–552.

Sofer S, Ben-Ezer D, Dagan R. Early severe dehydration in young breast-fed newborn infants. *Isr J Med Sci.* 1993;29:85–89.

Sousa PLR, Barros FC, Pinheiro GNM, Gazalle RV. Re-establishment of lactation with metoclopramide. *J Trop Pediatr.* 1975;321:214–215.

Taylor R. Relactation on the Peloponnese. *Midwives.* 1995;108:152.

Thearle MJ, Weissenberger R. Induced lactation in adoptive mothers. *Aust NZ J Obstet Gynaecol.* 1984;24:283–286.

Thompson NM. Relactation in a newborn intensive care setting. *J Hum Lact.* 1996;12: 233–235.

Thorley V. Relactation: what the exceptions can tell us. *Birth Issues.* 1997;6:24–29.

Thorley V. *Relactation and Induced Lactation: Bibliography and Resources,* rvsd. Brisbane, Australia: Thorley; 2006.

Waletzky L, Herman E. Relactation. *Am Fam Pract.* 1976;14:69–74.

Walker M. *Breastfeeding Management for the Clinician: Using the Evidence.* Sudbury, MA: Jones and Bartlett Publishers; 2006.

Wieschhoff HA. Artificial stimulation of lactation in primitive cultures. *Bull Hist Med.* 1940;8:1403–1415.

Ylikorkala O, Kauppila A, Kivinen S, et al. Sulpiride improves inadequate lactation. *BMJ.* 1982;285:249–251.

Ylikorkala O, Kauppila A, Kivinen S, et al. Treatment of inadequate lactation with oral sulpiride and bucal oxytocin. *Obstet Gynecol.* 1984;63:57–60.

Zinaman MJ, Hughes V, Queenan JT, et al. Acute prolactin and oxytocin responses and milk yield to infant suckling and artificial methods of expressing in lactating women. *Pediatrics.* 1992;89:437–440.

Donor Human Milk Banking

Mary Rose Tully, MPH, IBCLC

OBJECTIVES

- List appropriate uses of donor human milk.
- Describe similarities and differences between donor milk banking operations in different countries.
- List benefits and costs of using donor milk for at-risk infants.
- Discuss the risks of informal milk sharing.
- Discuss the history of donor milk banking.

Introduction

Donor human milk banking is the process of providing human milk to a recipient other than the donor's own child. It involves recruiting and screening donors, storing, treating, and screening donated milk, and distributing the milk on physician order (HMBANA, 2007; Springer, 1997; UKAMB, 2003). Donor milk banking should not be confused with storage and handling of mother's own milk for her own child in any setting (HMBANA, 2007).

In hospitals where donor milk is used, it is often prescribed as a supplement to a mother's own supply until she has sufficient milk for her baby(ies)'s needs, to feed the baby whose mother cannot lactate, to feed the baby whose mother's milk cannot be used temporarily, or for feeding an adopted baby (HMBANA, 2007; Table 33–1). It is also used for feeding an infant who is not being breastfed and is not thriving on human milk substitutes, as a short-term therapy after gastrointestinal surgery (Rangecroft, de San Lazaro, & Scott, 1978), to provide a source of Immunoglobulin A (IgA) for an infant who is not being breastfed, or an older child or adult suffering from IgA deficiency (Merhav et al., 1995; Tully, 1990).

Donor milk is never intended to replace mother's own, but to provide human milk where there is a medical need. In the United States and Canada, donor milk is occasionally used for infants whose mothers cannot provide it when the parents desire to use human milk and can afford the processing fee. Health insurance will not cover

Table 33-1   Diagnoses for Which Donor Milk Has Been Prescribed

Infants

    Prematurity

    Feeding/formula intolerance

    Failure to thrive

    Allergies

    Immunologic deficiencies

    Postoperative nutrition

    Treatment of infectious diseases such as rotovirus

    Treatment of some inborn errors of metabolism

Older children and adults

    Cancer therapy (experimental)

    IgA deficiency (including liver transplant patients)

    Treatment of infectious diseases such as rotovirus

    Gastrointestinal disorders such as severe reflux and Crohn's disease

Source: Data are from the Human Milk Banking Association of North America (HMBANA, 2006).

the fee if the baby does not have a medical need. An order from the infant's physician is still required. Donor milk is mentioned by both the World Health Organization (WHO, 2003) and the American Academy of Pediatrics (Gartner et al., 2005) as an alternative when mother's own milk is not available.

A compelling argument can be made to support the investment necessary to make donor milk available to every preterm or sick infant due to the body of evidence citing sufficient risks to not feeding human milk (Gartner et al., 2005). The Convention on the Rights of the Child, Article 24 (United Nations, 1990), recognizes the right of every child to "the enjoyment of the highest attainable standard of health and to facilities for the treatment of illness and rehabilitation to health." Ethically, the question becomes one of offering the highest standard of care to all infants, regardless of the individual mother's ability to provide her own milk.

I. Research Findings

    A. Research and clinical practice have shown that preterm infants fed human milk, including banked donor milk, have improved outcomes related to the nutritional qualities, ease of digestibility, and immunological components of human milk (Wight, 2001). Wight (2001) estimates that because of the reduction in length of stay, necrotizing enterocolitis (NEC), and sepsis there is a relative savings of approximately $11 to the hospital or health care plan for each $1 spent for donor milk obtained from a nonprofit bank.

    1. A multi-center study in the United Kingdom (UK) found that infants fed at least some human milk in the first month of life (donor or mother's own, all by gavage) had higher IQs at 7.5 to 8 years of age, even when controlling for psychosocial influences (Lucas et al., 1992).

    2. Further studies of this cohort as they reached adolescence showed that the children who were fed donor human milk have lower cholesterol and better high-density lipoprotein to low-density lipoprotein ratios than those children fed preterm formula (Singhal, Cole, & Lucas, 2001).

B. A meta-analysis of randomized controlled trials comparing incidence of NEC, a devastating bowel disease that is frequently fatal for preterm infants, showed that use of donor human milk compared to human milk substitutes (formula) was protective.

    1. Although none of the individual studies showed a significant risk to using formula, in aggregate the studies showed that infants who were fed donor milk when mother's own was not available were four times less likely to develop confirmed NEC (McGuire & Anthony, 2003).

    2. A recent paper by Schanler et al. (2005) reported that donor milk "offered little observed short-term advantage over [preterm formula] for feeding extremely premature infants."

    3. However, as Wight pointed out (2005), this study did show a significantly lower incidence of chronic lung disease among the babies fed mother's own and donor milk compared to those fed preterm formula as well as a trend toward fewer days on a ventilator.

C. A U.S. study at a large neonatal unit showed that using fortified mother's own milk was related to decreased infections and more rapid achievement of full feeds with no untoward effects related to slower weight gain, because the feedings were better tolerated (Schanler, Shulman, & Lau, 1999). Many clinicians who regularly use donor milk find the same to be true with donor milk.

D. There are several case reports in the literature describing the use of donor milk for treatment of a variety of conditions or to provide immunologic support and appropriate nutrition to full-term infants and older children (Tully, Lockhart-Borman, & Updegrove, 2004) as well as some adults.

    1. Infants with chronic renal failure (Anderson & Arnold, 1993), metabolic disorders (Arnold, 1995), IgA deficiency, and allergy (Tully, 1990) have been fed donor milk as adjunct to other treatments.

2. Milk banks report many cases of feeding intolerance and allergy that have been treated with donor milk but not reported in the literature, including infants who have failed to thrive on anything but human milk. Donor milk is typically a treatment of last resort in these cases, primarily because of the expense.

3. Some adult conditions respond to human milk, including hemorrhagic conjunctivitis (MMWR, 1982), IgA deficiency in liver transplant recipients (Merhav et al., 1995), and gastrointestinal problems, such as severe reflux (Wiggins & Arnold, 1998).

II. Therapeutic Components of Human Milk for Adults

A. Certain proteins unique to human milk are being investigated for their therapeutic value for adults.

1. Human milk contains a unique protein, multimeric alpha-lactalbumin, which induces apoptosis (programmed cell death) in certain cancer cells (Gustafsson et al., 2005; Hakansson et al., 1995).

2. Human alpha-lactalbumin made lethal to tumor cells made by treating human milk is currently being investigated in a rat model as a very specific treatment for human glioblastomas (brain tumors) (Gustafsson et al., 2005).

3. Alpha-lactalbumin-oleic acid isolated from human milk has been found to be successful as a topical treatment for skin papillomas resistant to traditional treatment (Gustafsson et al., 2004).

III. Acceptance of Donor Milk

A. Generally donor milk is acceptable to the families of the recipient babies, but in most cultural settings, parents do need to understand how the donors are screened and the milk is processed and tested (Ighogboja et al., 1995).

1. A few families request donor milk for an adopted baby or a baby whose mother cannot lactate simply because of the advantages of human milk feeding for all infants. Again, cost becomes a factor if there are no medical reasons for needing the donor milk and, in some countries, donor milk is dispensed only to infants in the hospital.

2. Milk donors are anonymous except in special circumstances.
   a. Few milk banks are set up to do directed donations.
   b. However, among Muslims, it is important that the recipient mother and donor mother meet, because the Koran decrees that all babies who receive milk from the same mother are siblings and it would be an act of incest for the two women's children to marry when they are older (al-Naqeeb et al., 2000).

IV. Donor Milk Banking Worldwide

A. Donor human milk banks are found in most parts of the world and are typically associated with a neonatal intensive care unit (NICU).

B. The use of donor milk is more common in some countries than in others.

   1. Central and South America.

      a. With 186 active donor milk banks, Brazil has the most extensive national network of donor milk banks in the Americas and possibly in the world (www.redeblh.fiocruz.br, accessed 2/4/2007).

         i. These milk banks all operate under quality control from the national standard bank at Fiocruz University in Rio de Janeiro, and all milk bank personnel go through a 40-hour training course established by the national standard bank.

         ii. Donor milk is the feeding of choice for all infants who do not have mother's own milk to meet their needs in Brazilian hospitals (Gutiérrez & de Almeida, 1998).

         iii. The national network of donor milk banks is also the organization charged with promoting breastfeeding and offering clinical care and services to breastfeeding mothers and babies.

         iv. Many other countries in South and Central America have established donor milk bank networks, or at least individual banks, based on the Brazilian model and have relied on the Brazilian central bank to provide training for personnel.

   2. North America.

      a. In 2006, the United States had 10 nonprofit donor milk banks with more hospitals considering opening banks. These 10 milk banks serve both inpatients and outpatients across the country and accept donations from mothers across the country. Milk can be shipped frozen by overnight express.

      b. Canada has one active donor milk bank with two more in the development stages.

   3. Europe.

      a. The UK has 17 donor milk banks, located in hospitals in England, Scotland, and Ireland (www.ukamb.org, accessed 2/27/2007).

      b. All of the Scandinavian countries have donor milk banks and while the use of donor milk is common, it is not universal (personal communication, Tully, 1991).

      c. In the former East Germany, donor milk banking is more common than in the former West Germany (Springer, 1997; Springer, 2000; Springer, 2003).

      d. In France, there are donor milk banks across the entire country and milk is shipped as needed (Voyer, Nobre, & Magny, 2000). Some of the milk banks lyophilize (freeze dry) milk after pasteurization (Voyer et al., 2000).

e. Italy has 18 donor milk banks associated with NICUs primarily in the northern part of the country (di Nisi, 2000).

f. Poland has donor milk banks in NICUs (Penc, 1996).

4. Asia and Africa.

a. India has developed milk banking guidelines and is establishing donor milk banks in NICUs (R. Deolankar, MD, National Institute of Virology, Pune, India, personal communication 1999; Fernandez, Mondkar, & Vaz, 1990; Fernandez, Mondkar, & Nanavati, 1993; N. Munshi, MD, K.G. Patel Children's Hospital, Karelibaug, Baroda, India, personal communication, 2000).

b. China has donor milk banks in many hospitals (Arnold, 1996).

c. Kuwait has one donor milk bank (al-Naqeeb et al., 2000).

d. Donor milk banking has recently started in South Africa.

i. In a presentation at the International Congress of the Human Milk Banking Association of North America (HMBANA), Anna Coutsoudis, an acquired immune deficiency syndrome (AIDS) researcher, described the development of the first donor milk bank to feed orphan infants who were wasting from AIDS, emphasizing the dramatic effect the donor milk has had on their lives (Coutsoudis, 2005).

e. The opening of the first donor milk bank in Australia was announced in 2006.

V. Donor Compensation

Typically, donors are not paid for their milk; however, in some countries, donors are compensated at the end of their donation sufficiently to cover the cost of electric pump rental (Tully, 1991). Most donors have altruistic motives of helping others and sharing with babies who are not as healthy as their own. Donating milk also can be an important and therapeutic part of the grieving process for mothers whose babies have died (*HMBANA Matters*, January 2006; Tully, 1999).

A. The HMBANA guidelines, which are used in the United States and Canada, prohibit compensation to donors, as do the Brazilian government guidelines (Gutiérrez & de Almeida, 1998; HMBANA, 2007).

B. A few European banks do compensate donors nominally.

1. Usually the compensation is sufficient to cover pump rental (A. Grovslien, personal communication 2005; Tully, 1991).

2. Some milk banks loan breast pumps to donors during the period of donation (Voyer et al., 2000).

C. Buying and selling donor milk as a commodity is discouraged for several reasons.

1. The mother may feel economic pressure to sell her milk rather than feeding her own baby.

2. It is difficult to ensure quality of screening of the potential donor.

3. It is difficult to ensure the quality of the milk purchased (that is, has it been diluted or contaminated?).

4. There is no long-term follow-up of recipients or donors or valid recordkeeping.

VI. Milk Bank Operation

A. In developed countries, donors typically use electric breast pumps at home; however, in developing countries, milk is often hand expressed, or the donor goes to the milk bank daily to pump.

B. Donor milk banks usually operate in a hospital within the NICU, the food service department, or the blood or tissue banking department (Tully, 1991; Weaver, 1999).

1. Some milk banks are free-standing (Flatau & Brady, 2006).

2. In some countries, they are regulated by the government as are blood banks (Gutiérrez & de Almeida, 1998; Voyer et al., 2000; N. Munshi, MD, K.G. Patel Children's Hospital, Karelibaug, Baroda, India, personal communication, 2000).

C. Milk banks are staffed by a Milk Bank Director/Coordinator who oversees day-to-day operations and supervises donor recruiting and screening as well as milk processing and dispensing, and a Medical Director who may or may not do a physical exam on each donor and her infant, but supervises medical decisions.

1. The Milk Bank Director/Coordinator may be an International Board Certified Lactation Consultant, nurse, physician, or a trained milk bank coordinator.

2. Frequently a trained technician does the milk processing.

3. The Medical Director is often (but not always) a neonatologist and is responsible for clinical decisions and oversight of the milk banking operations.

4. In Brazil, there is a 40-hour training course required for milk bank personnel, and many countries in Central and South America use this same course for training milk bank personnel (Giugliani & de Almeida, 2005).

5. Most donor milk banks are also sources of breastfeeding support and counseling. In many developing countries they are a part of implementation of the Baby Friendly Hospital Initiative (Giugliani & de Almeida, 2005).

D. Some countries, including Brazil (Giugliani & de Almeida, 2005), France (Voyer et al., 2000), India (N. Munshi, personal communication, 2000), Norway (A. Grovslien, personal communication, 2005), and Poland (Penc, 1996), have national milk banking regulations through the ministry of health. However, others, including the United States, Canada, and the UK, are regulated through professional organizations, or general tissue banking guidelines (HMBANA, 2007; UKAMB, 2003).

1. Cost to recipient varies by country and by service setting. With nonprofit banks, if there is a charge, it is to cover the expense of screening the donors and processing the milk, not for the milk itself. For example, in France the cost

is set by the ministry of health at about $2.45 per ounce (30 mL), in North America the cost ranges from $2.90 to $4 per ounce depending on the milk bank, and in Central and South America the milk is used only with hospitalized patients and is a part of the care, so there is no charge to the patient.

VII. Screening and Storage

A. Milk donors and the donor milk are carefully screened, just as with other donor human tissues.

1. In developed countries donors are serum screened for such communicable diseases as human immunodeficiency virus (HIV), human T-lymphoma virus (HTLV), hepatitis B and C, and syphilis (HMBANA, 2006; al-Naqeeb et al., 2000; Springer, 1997; UKAMB, 2003; Voyer et al., 2000).

   a. Since blood banks screen for all of these diseases, so do donor milk banks even though HIV and HTLV are the only diseases known to be potentially transmitted via human milk.

B. The cost of serum screening is born by the milk bank or the national health system, not the donor.

C. Most milk banks require a form completed by the donor's physician and her infant's physician.

D. Some milk banks have physicians on staff who do a physical on each mother and her infant.

E. Because cost is prohibitive in developing countries and the donor milk is so vital, some banks do a verbal/written screening to eliminate high-risk donors, and rely on heat treatment to kill viruses and other pathogens (Coutsoudis, 2005; Giugliani & de Almeida, 2005).

F. All donor milk is screened for bacteria before it is dispensed.

1. In Norway and Germany, after donor screening, milk is screened for bacteria and dispensed raw (Springer, 1997; A. Grovslien, personal communication, 2005).

2. It may be stored refrigerated or frozen until it is dispensed, depending on the length of time it is stored.

3. HMBANA Guidelines (2007) allow for dispensing of milk raw in rare circumstances in North America; however, since 1988 no bank has reported a request for raw milk in the United States or Canada.

G. In most other countries, the donor milk is stored frozen at −20° C until it is heat processed and used, and it is refrozen after processing until it is distributed.

1. Although freezing preserves most of the nutritional, immunologic, hormonal, and other unique properties of the milk, it does not destroy many pathogens.

2. Careful heat treatment with Holder pasteurization (62.5° C timed for 30 minutes after the center container reaches temperature) preserves as many of the properties of the milk as possible (see Table 33–2; Tully, Jones, & Tully, 2001).

Table 33-2   Selected Components of Human Milk After Freezing and Pasteurization

	Function	Percentage Activity	References
IgA and sIgA*	Binds microbes in the baby's digestive tract to prevent their passage into other tissues	67–100	19,27,30
IgM*	Antibodies specifically targeted against pathogens to which the mother has been exposed	0	30,33
IgG*	Antibodies specifically targeted against pathogens to which the mother has been exposed	66–70	30,34
Lactoferrin (iron-binding capacity)*	Binds iron required by many bacteria and thus retards bacterial growth	27–43	19,33,34
Lysozyme*	Attacks bacterial cell walls and thus destroys many bacteria	75	33,34
Lipoprotein lipase*	Partly responsible for lipolysis of milk triglycerides to release monoglycerides and free fatty acids	0	23,38
Bile salt activated lipase*	Partly responsible for lipolysis of milk triglycerides to release monoglycerides and free fatty acids	0	23,38
Monoglycerides produced by lipolysis of milk triglycerides*	Disrupts the membrane coating of many viruses and protozoans, destroying them	100	37,38,39
Free fatty acids produced by lipolysis of milk triglycerides**	Disrupts the membrane coating of many viruses and protozoans, destroying them	100	37,38,39
Linoleic acid (18:2n6)**	Essential fatty acid; metabolic precursor for prostaglandins and leukotrienes	100	37,38,39
α-linolenic acid (18:3n3)**	Essential fatty acid; metabolic precursor for docosahexaenoic acid; important for eye and brain development	100	37,38,39

*These biologically active components do not occur in commercial formula.
**Some manufacturers are now adding docosahexaenoic acid and other supplemental fats to selected infant formula preparations.
Source: Used with permission from Tully, DB, Jones, F, and Tully, MR. Donor Human Milk: What's In It and What's Not. *Journal of Human Lactation,* 2001;17:152.

H. Either a commercial human milk pasteurizer (HMBANA, 2007; UKAMB, 2003) or a standard laboratory shaking water bath is used (HMBANA, 2007).

1. The shaking water bath is considerably less expensive but more time intensive because the milk containers must be physically moved to a vat containing an ice slurry for quick chilling after heat treatment (Tully, 2000).

2. In Brazil, the central standards bank has developed a chart for processing time based on container volume, which minimizes even further the damage to the milk components (J.A. Guerra de Almeida, PhD, Coordinator of the National Reference Center for Human Milk Banks, Fiocurz University, Rio de Janeiro, Brazil, personal communication, 2000).

I. Milk banks use a wide variety of containers for processing and storing milk. Some decisions have been based on scientific investigation and others are based on convenience (HMBANA, 2006; J.A. Guerra de Almeida, PhD, Coordinator of the National Reference Center for Human Milk Banks, Fiocurz University, Rio de Janeiro, Brazil, personal communication, 2000).

J. Most milk banks will accept initial donations in whatever container the donor has been using but will then provide containers for the future donations.

VIII. Records

A. Donor milk bank records allow tracking of milk from donor to recipient. They also include each donor's screening profile and data on each batch of milk screened, processed, and dispensed.

1. Just as with other donor human tissue, it is important to be able to track milk from the time it arrives at the bank through the batch in which it is processed, screened, and dispensed.

B. Records on each individual batch of milk are maintained, including the processing and bacterial screening results.

C. Once a batch of milk is dispensed to a hospital, it is the hospital's responsibility to maintain accurate records of which patients received donor milk, from which bank, and from which batch(es).

D. In most countries such records must be maintained until all recipients would have reached age of majority plus three years.

References

Anderson A, Arnold LD. Use of donor breast milk in the nutrition management of chronic renal failure: three case histories. *J Hum Lact.* 1993;9:263–264.

Arnold LD. Use of donor milk in the treatment of metabolic disorders: glycolytic pathway defects. *J Hum Lact.* 1995;11:51–53.

Arnold LD. Donor milk banking in China: the ultimate step in becoming baby friendly. *J Hum Lact.* 1996;12:319–321.

Coutsoudis A. Use of donor milk for AIDS orphans: South Africa's experiences (oral presentation) in Human Milk Banking: A Global Perspective on Best Practice. Sponsored by HMBANA; October 17–18, 2005, Alexandria, VA.

Fernandez A, Mondkar J, Vaz C. Experiences with milk banking in Bombay. *Indian J Pediatr.* 1990;57:375–379.

Fernandez A, Mondkar J, Nanavati R. The establishment of a human milk bank in India. *J Hum Lact.* 1993;9:189–190.

Flatau G, Brady S. *Starting a Donor Human Milk Bank: A Practical Guide.* 2006; Raleigh, NC: HMBANA.

Gartner LM, Morton J, Lawrence RA, et al. Breastfeeding and the use of human milk. *Pediatrics.* 2005;115:496–506.

Giugliani E, de Almeida J. The role of donor milk banking in breastfeeding promotion: Brazil's experience (oral presentation) in Human Milk Banking: A Global Perspective on Best Practice. Sponsored by HMBANA; October 17–18, 2005; Alexandria, VA.

Gustafsson L, Hallgren O, Mossberg AK, et al. HAMLET kills tumor cells by apoptosis: structure, cellular mechanisms, and therapy. *J Nutr.* 2005;135:1299–1303.

Gustafsson L, Leijonhufvud I, Aronsson A, et al. Treatment of skin papillomas with topical alpha-lactalbumin-oleic acid. *N Engl J Med.* 2004;350:2663–2672.

Gutiérrez D, de Almeida JA. Human milk banks in Brazil. *J Hum Lact.* 1998;14:333–335.

Hakansson A, Zhivotovsky B, Orrenius S, et al. Apoptosis induced by a human milk protein. *Proc Natl Acad Sci U S A.* 1995;92:8064–8068.

HMBANA Matters. A donor mom's story from the Mothers' Milk Bank of Ohio. *HMBANA Matters.* January 2006:4.

Human Milk Banking Association of North America (HMBANA). Guidelines for the Establishment and Operation of a Donor Human Milk Bank. Raleigh, NC: HMBANA; 2007.

Ighogboja IS, Olarewaju RS, Odumodu CU, Okuonghae HO. Mothers' attitudes towards donated breastmilk in Jos, Nigeria. *J Hum Lact.* 1995;11:93–96.

Lucas A, Morley R, Cole TJ, Lister G, Leeson PC. Breast milk and subsequent intelligence quotient in children born preterm [see comments]. *Lancet.* 1992;339:261–264.

McGuire W, Anthony MY. Donor human milk versus formula for preventing necrotising enterocolitis in preterm infants: systematic review. *Arch Dis Child Fetal Neonatal Ed.* 2003;88:F11–F14.

Merhav HJ, Wright HI, Mieles LA, Van Thiel DH. Treatment of IgA deficiency in liver transplant recipients with human breast milk. *Transplant Int.* 1995;8:327–329.

Morbidity and Mortality Weekly Report (MMWR). Acute hemorrhagic conjunctivitis–American Samoa. *MMWR.* 1982:1.

al-Naqeeb NA, Azab A, Eliwa MS, Mohammed BY. The introduction of breast milk donation in a Muslim country. *J Hum Lact.* 2000;16:346–350.

di Nisi G. Indagine fra le banche del latte umano in Italia. In: di Nisi G, ed. La Banca del Latte Materno. Trento, Italy: new MAGAZINE; September 2000. (in Italian)

Penc B. Organization and activity of a human milk bank in Poland. *J Hum Lact.* 1996; 12:243–246.

Rangecroft L, de San Lazaro C, Scott JE. A comparison of the feeding of the postoperative newborn with banked breast-milk or cow's-milk feeds. *J Pediatr Surg.* 1978;13:11–12.

Schanler RJ, Lau C, Hurst NM, Smith EO. Randomized trial of donor human milk versus preterm formula as substitutes for mothers' own milk in the feeding of extremely premature infants. *Pediatrics.* 2005;116:400–406.

Schanler RJ, Shulman RJ, Lau C. Feeding strategies for premature infants: beneficial outcomes of feeding fortified human milk versus preterm formula [comment]. *Pediatrics.* 1999;103:1150–1157.

Singhal A, Cole TJ, Lucas A. Early nutrition in preterm infants and later blood pressure: two cohorts after randomised trials. *Lancet.* 2001;357:413–419.

Springer S. Human milk banking in Germany. *J Hum Lact.* 1997;13:65–68.

Springer S. News about human milk banking in Germany. *Adv Exp Med Biol.* 2000; 478:441–442.

Springer S. [Breastfeeding and human milk for preterm infants]. *Zentralbl Gynakol.* 2003;125:44–47. (in German)

Tully MR. Banked human milk in treatment of IgA deficiency and allergy symptoms. *J Hum Lact.* 1990;6:75–76.

Tully MR. Human milk banking in Sweden and Denmark. *J Hum Lact.* 1991;7:145–146.

Tully MR. Donating human milk as part of the grieving process. *J Hum Lact.* 1999;15: 149–151.

Tully MR. Cost of establishing and operating a donor human milk bank. *J Hum Lact.* 2000;16:57–59.

Tully DB, Jones F, Tully MR. Donor milk: what's in it and what's not. *J Hum Lact.* 2001; 17:152–155.

Tully MR, Lockhart-Borman L, Updegrove K. Stories of success: the use of donor milk is increasing in North America. *J Hum Lact.* 2004;20:75–77.

United Kingdom Association for Milk Banking (UKAMB). Guidelines for the Establishment and Operation of Human Milk Banks in the UK. 3rd ed. London: UKAMB; 2003.

United Nations. Convention on the Rights of the Child. 1990. Available at: http://www.unicef.org/crc/index_framework.html. Accessed February 26, 2007.

Voyer M, Nobre R, Magny JF. Human milk banks organization in France: legal proceedings and their consequences on milk bank activities. In: De Nisi G, ed. La Banca Del Latte Materno. Trento, Italy: new MAGAZINE; 2000:21–28.

Weaver G. Every drop counts: news from the United Kingdom Association for Milk Banking. *J Hum Lact.* 1999;15:251–253.

Wiggins PK, Arnold LD. Clinical case history: donor milk use for severe gastroesophageal reflux in an adult. *J Hum Lact.* 1998;14:157–159.

Wight NE. Donor human milk for preterm infants. *J Perinatol.* 2001;21(4):249–254.

Wight NE. Donor milk: down but not out. *Pediatrics.* 2005;116:1610; author reply, 116:1610–1611.

World Health Organization (WHO). Global Strategy for Infant and Young Child Feeding. Geneva: WHO; 2003.

Breastfeeding Problem Solving: Maternal and Infant Issues

PREGNANCY, LABOR, AND BIRTH COMPLICATIONS

Marsha Walker, RN, IBCLC
Revised by Sue Cox, AM, RN, RM, IBCLC

OBJECTIVES

- Describe several maternal problems that can occur in the perinatal period.

- Plan for how breastfeeding can continue under adverse situations.

- Ascertain whether any of these conditions are present when working with a breastfeeding problem.

- Discuss how these situations can impact the baby and breastfeeding.

Introduction

While pregnancy, labor, and birth are normal and natural processes, occasional problems arise that might have an impact on breastfeeding. These complications can change a mother's birth plan and might affect access to her infant after delivery. The lactation consultant will benefit from knowledge of the more common alterations in maternal health and strategies in order to circumvent any impediment to breastfeeding that might be present.

I. Hypertensive Disorders of Pregnancy

These include preeclampsia, severe preeclampsia, eclampsia (toxemia), and HELLP syndrome.

  A. Preeclampsia.

    1. Determined by increased blood pressure after 20 weeks of gestation (pregnancy-induced hypertension) accompanied by proteinuria, edema, or both.

    2. Occurs in 3% to 5% of otherwise normal pregnancies (Dietl, 2000; Higgins & de Swiet, 2001) and more frequently in women who have chronic renal or

vascular diseases such as diabetes, collagen vascular disease, or chronic hypertension.

3. Preterm delivery usually occurs in order to improve the mother's condition and decrease infant morbidity associated with growth retardation and fetal asphyxia.

B. Severe preeclampsia.

1. A progression to higher blood pressure, increased proteinuria (protein in the urine), oliguria (decreased urine output), cerebral or visual changes, severe headaches, epigastric pain, pulmonary edema, or cyanosis.

C. Eclampsia.

1. If the baby is not delivered as severe preeclampsia continues, then it can progress to eclampsia (toxemia).

2. *Eclampsia* denotes the occurrence of convulsions not caused by neurologic disease and usually occurs after 32 weeks gestation.

3. Seizures can occur even after the baby is delivered.

4. Women who have severe preeclampsia are usually hospitalized and placed on seizure precautions.

5. The mother might be sedated and given antihypertensive medications and anticonvulsive medications, such as magnesium sulfate.
    a. Magnesium sulfate is compatible with breastfeeding (Hale, 2006).
    b. Magnesium sulfate given to the mother prior to delivery may lead to neonatal neuromuscular blockage with hypotonia and urine retention (Blackburn, 2003:394).

6. Breastfeeding will depend on the condition of the mother and the baby.

7. Because it is important to reduce stress and other noxious stimuli that could provoke a seizure, breastfeeding with mother and baby in skin-to-skin contact might actually be therapeutic due to the calming and sedating effects of prolactin and oxytocin (Light et al., 2000; Uvnäs Moberg & Petersson, 2005).

8. If the baby cannot go to the breast, arrangements need to be made for expressing breast milk within hours of the birth.

9. Medications might continue after the baby is born.

D. HELLP syndrome.

1. H (intravascular hemolysis), EL (elevated liver enzymes: aspartate aminotransferase and alanine aminotransferase, LP (low platelets).

2. A very small percentage (0.1%) of women who have preeclampsia develop HELLP syndrome (Abraham et al., 2001).

3. It occurs most often early in the third trimester and is thought to result from a circulating immunologic component.

4. Management is still controversial. To improve maternal and fetal prognosis, two approaches are usually considered.

    a. Immediate delivery after stabilization of the clinical condition (Haram et al., 2000) but with the risk of fetal complications related to prematurity.

    OR

    b. Conservative treatment using corticosteroids (Haram et al., 2000), which are associated with higher stillbirth rate (Curtin & Weinstein, 1999) and with the maternal risk of complications related to hematologic disorders (Visser & Wallenburg, 1995).

5. Women who develop HELLP might also experience disseminated intravascular coagulation (DIC) and require intensive medical care.

    a. DIC is caused by a process that consumes the plasma's clotting factors and platelets so that hemorrhage occurs.

    b. Severe hemorrhage associated with DIC may result in pituitary necrosis (Sheehan syndrome), a well recognized cause of lactation failure (see Section IV) (Kelestimur, 2003).

II. Cesarean Delivery

A. The most frequently performed surgery in industrialized societies around the world.

1. Usually performed under epidural or spinal anesthesia.

2. Breastfeeding should not be delayed unless the conditions of the mother and/or baby preclude it.

B. Occasionally, a mother will receive general anesthesia.

1. Mother can breastfeed as soon as she is awake and able to respond.

2. General anesthetic agents such as thiopental sodium and halothane are considered to be usually compatible with breastfeeding (Hale, 2006).

C. Compatible with skin-to-skin contact and breastfeeding.

1. Mother can nurse her infant as soon as she feels ready, including in the recovery room (Cox, 2006).

2. Most incisions are a lower uterine segment transverse, enabling the mother to more comfortably position her baby for breastfeeding across her lap.

3. Vertical incisions are usually done when other surgery is indicated at the same time or in emergency deliveries.

D. Full-term healthy babies and mothers can and should recover together after cesarean delivery in skin-to-skin contact in the recovery room (Spear, 2006).

E. Medications.

1. Mothers who are receiving pain relief intrathecally (around the spine) are usually quite comfortable and ready to breastfeed soon after surgery.

2. Regular pain relief needs to be given to ensure no breakthrough pain occurs and that the mother is comfortable to breastfeed whenever her baby requires, and to allow her to become ambulatory.

3. Pain medication is usually required for 72 hours.

    a. Most common postoperative pain medications require no interruption or delay in breastfeeding, with morphine (Duramorph, Infumorph) being preferred due to absence of pediatric side effects.

    b. In comparison, meperidine (Demerol/Pethidine) has been shown to cause pediatric sedation and poor sucking (Hale, 2006).

F. An unexpected cesarean delivery can be a significant disappointment to the mother, and time needs to be made for debriefing.

1. Some mothers experience anger, resentment, remorse, grief, or relief at this point.

2. Skin-to-skin contact and the concomitant release of extra oxytocin may alleviate both her pain and disappointment (Uvnäs-Moberg & Petersson, 2005) and need to be instituted as soon as possible after the surgery.

G. An urgent cesarean may result in delayed lactogenesis II (Dewey, 2001) and skin-to-skin contact following surgery (Uvnäs-Moberg & Petersson, 2005) and/or frequent hand expressing may assist in overcoming this early delay.

H. Some babies might be lethargic at first, especially if the mother has labored, the labor was protracted, and it involved long exposure to analgesia or anesthesia (Kuhnert, Kennard, & Linn, 1998; Rosenblatt et al., 1991; Sepkoski et al., 1994; Scherer & Holzgreve, 1995; Volikas et al., 2005).

I. Suctioning of the mouth and throat might cause breastfeeding problems because it may temporarily cause infant oral defensiveness (Widstrom et al., 1987).

J. Finding a comfortable position in which to breastfeed can be worrisome to mothers.

1. Placing the baby between the mother's breasts as she lies on her back, with a pillow behind her head, will allow the baby time to follow pre-feeding cues and self latch (Matthiessen et al., 2001) as the mother watches.

2. If the mother lies on her side, it is often easier for the baby to be placed so that the baby's nose is opposite the top breast. The mother can draw the baby forward with her free top arm, so the baby's chin touches the breast and he or she can self-latch.

3. When the mother is sitting up, a pillow may be used to cover her cesarean incision area and to rest the baby on once he or she has latched.

4. Fathers and other helpers should be encouraged to lift and change the baby and help position the baby at the breast.

K. The mother should breastfeed her baby 8 to 12 times each 24 hours including at night, when the infant demonstrates readiness to feed, and refrain from sending her baby to the nursery for long periods of time. Separation of mother and baby decreases opportunities for frequent breastfeeding and increases the likelihood of supplemental feedings, both of which will adversely affect maternal milk production and the baby's interest in feeding at the breast.

L. In the early days, mothers who have had a cesarean need their rest; visitors are best limited to allow for napping and breastfeeding during the day.

M. Low-grade maternal fever (> 99°F [37°C] but < 100°F [37.8°C]) can occur. In the absence of other symptoms such as tachycardia, tachypnea, and wound redness/ oozing, low-grade fever should not interrupt breastfeeding.

   1. Even with antibiotic therapy, breastfeeding should continue, since antibiotics are "usually compatible with breastfeeding" (Hale, 2006).

N. If the baby is born preterm or will be unable to breastfeed for some time, the mother should hand express and/or use a hospital-grade breast pump with a double collection kit to stimulate milk production (see Chapter 30).

O. If the baby is temporarily unable to latch on to the breast, the mother can hand express colostrum into a spoon or cup and feed it to the baby (Collins et al., 2004; Dowling et al., 2002).

P. Mothers might be given antibiotics, placing them at a higher risk for *Candida* overgrowth.

III. Postpartum Hemorrhage

A. The most common obstetric emergency (5% of deliveries) and is life-threatening (Reynders et al., 2006).

B. Considerable blood volume may be lost and intravenous fluids, including blood transfusion, may be necessary.

C. Oxytocic agents such as ergonovine maleate (Ergotrate, Ergometrine) or pitocin (Syntocinon or Syntometrine) are given intravenously and if use is prolonged may affect milk production (Hale, 2006).

D. The mother will need assistance with positioning her baby for easy latch while she has an intravenous infusion and her blood pressure is low.

E. The mother will be exhausted and needs to be told that she will have low energy levels for between 6 weeks and 12 weeks while she is replacing her red blood cells.

   1. During this period, breastfeeding will be an excellent time for her to rest.

   2. She will need assistance with her baby's care.

IV. Sheehan Syndrome

A. Caused by a severe postpartum hemorrhage and hypotension often associated with disseminated intravascular coagulation (Kelestimur, 2003).

   1. The decreased blood flow to the pituitary gland leads to an infarction and necrosis or other complications.

B. At the end of pregnancy, the pituitary is very sensitive to decreased blood flow because of its vascularity and increased size.

C. With no prolactin secretion, the alveoli can involute and lactation might be suppressed.

D. Prolactin-stimulating drugs such as metoclopramide (Reglan, Maxolon) or supleride (Lawrence & Lawrence, 1999) have been used to treat this condition (Hale, 2006).

E. Mild cases of pituitary disruption can occur with a delay in lactogenesis II and during this period there may be a need to offer supplementary fluid to the infant, preferably donor milk if available.

V. Episiotomy

A. A surgical incision of the perineum made to facilitate birth as the fetal head distends the perineum.

1. A midline episiotomy, which is a straight line incision toward the rectum. *OR*

2. A mediolateral episiotomy, which is angled down and off to one side, usually the right.

B. This procedure is often done routinely in industrialized countries.

C. Current research does not support routine episiotomies (Hartmann et al., 2005).

D. Usually done therapeutically for shoulder dystocia to allow more room for manual maneuvers to free the impacted shoulders of the infant.

E. Also used with forceps to provide more room for their application.

F. Naturally occurring lacerations involve less tissue and muscle impairment than do episiotomies, are less painful, and heal well without suturing (Lundquist et al., 2000).

G. Complications include: excessive blood loss, infection of the incision, necrotizing fasciitis, extension of the midline episiotomy into a third degree tear (into the rectal sphincter), and further extension into a fourth-degree perineal laceration (into the anterior rectal wall).

H. Can be extremely painful, and if pain is not controlled it could interfere with the milk ejection reflex, impeding milk flow to the baby.

1. To lessen the need for medications, ice therapy is frequently used.

2. Cold packs are usually applied immediately following delivery, and iced sitz baths are also used for pain and to hasten healing; are more effective for pain relief than warm sitz baths (Ramler & Roberts, 1986).

3. Extreme pain may require analgesic rectal suppositories such as diclofenac (Voltaren) that transfers in extremely low levels into breast milk (Hale, 2006).

4. Topical preparations have not been shown to hasten healing or decrease pain (Minassian et al., 2002).

I. Positioning to alleviate pain.

    1. Mothers who have episiotomies may have pain lasting up to two weeks or longer and often find it very hard to assume a comfortable position, especially when sitting upright.

    2. Therefore, mothers may need assistance to position themselves and their babies in a side-lying position or, if sitting up, with a soft cushion under their buttocks.

J. Mothers can be counseled during the prenatal period to request that an episiotomy not be done unless absolutely necessary.

VI. Assisted Birth or Operative Vaginal Delivery

A. Forceps use has declined in many countries.

    1. They can cause trauma to the baby, such as bruising to the face where the blades are applied, facial nerve paralysis, or cephalhematoma (hemorrhage into the subperiosteum which does not cross a suture line) that can be associated with intracranial bleeding or skull fracture.

B. Vacuum extraction does not need more room in the vagina than forceps do for application and therefore episiotomies are rarely done.

    1. Some babies who undergo this procedure have marked bleeding of the scalp and face, with associated increased bilirubin levels, and poor feeding (Hall et al., 2002).

VII. Retained Placenta

A. Sub-involution of the uterus due to retained placental fragments is typically diagnosed after the mother has been discharged from the hospital.

B. It might present itself as bleeding that is uncharacteristic for the length of time post-delivery: normal change from rubra (red) loss on day 3, to serosa (serous) loss until day 9, and then alba (pale creamy-brownish loss).

C. Placental retention can inhibit lactogenesis II by keeping inhibitory hormones at levels that are representative of pregnancy (Neifert, McDonough, & Neville, 1981).

    1. Mothers might experience little to no breast fullness by days 3 to 5 and might still be producing colostrum when transitional milk should be seen.

    2. Failure to see breast fullness might occur prior to excessive bleeding or hemorrhage (Anderson, 2001).

    Curettage might be required, after which spontaneous milk flow should commence (Neifert et al., 1981).

D. Retained placenta can be suspected (Anderson, 2001) if the mother complains of:

    1. Little to no breast fullness by day five.

2. A colostrum stage of milk that persists beyond day four.

3. Continued bright-red vaginal bleeding that continues to be heavy after 3 days.

4. A uterus that might be painful to palpation and larger than expected.

5. With an infant who:
   a. Is not satisfied at the breast.
   b. Has less than the normal amount of wet and soiled diapers per day.
   c. Is possibly showing visible signs of jaundice.

VIII. Venous Thrombosis

A. Defined as the formation of a blood clot inside a blood vessel.

B. A reduction in this complication has been seen because of:

1. Early ambulation following delivery.

2. Fewer operative deliveries using general anesthesia.

3. Better health of women during pregnancy.

4. Routine use of subcutaneous enoxoprin (Clexane, Lovenox) anticoagulant therapy daily for three days after caesarean section; enoxoprin is compatible with breastfeeding (Hale, 2006).

C. Deep vein thrombosis is serious because pulmonary embolism can result if thrombi formed in the legs migrate to the lungs.

D. A pulmonary embolism can be fatal.

E. Procedures to establish a diagnosis and systemic medications involved in treatment are considerations during lactation.

1. Scans using radio contrast media might be necessary to confirm a diagnosis.
   a. Interruption or delay in breastfeeding is not necessary if radio-opaque or radiocontrast agents are used (Hale, 2006).

2. Radioactive materials vary in their half-lives, with some requiring little disruption to breastfeeding and others requiring pumping and discarding milk for up to two weeks; the lactation consultant should ascertain the contrast medium being used, its half-life if radioactive, and when breastfeeding can recommence.

3. Anticoagulant treatment may involve heparin, warfarin, or a newer, lower-molecular-weight fraction of heparin, enoxoprin (Clexane, Lovenox), all of which are considered compatible with breastfeeding (Hale, 2006).

4. If long-term anticoagulant therapy is initiated, prothrombin (clotting) time in the infant is usually monitored monthly and the infant might be given extra vitamin K if necessary.

F. Some mothers can experience a lengthy hospital stay or readmission and possible separation from their baby.

1. Plans must be made for continued breastfeeding and/or for the expressing of breast milk.

G. Some hospital units enable babies to room with their mothers if an adult caretaker is available to be responsible for the infant.

1. Because the mother might be on bed rest and pain medication, a helper is usually needed for baby care and to provide infant access to the mother.

IX. Postpartum Infection

A. Infection processes might remain localized in the reproductive or genital area, urinary tract, or breasts, or it might progress, resulting in metritis, endometritis, peritonitis, or parametritis.

B. Prenatal risk factors associated with postpartum infections include preexisting infections, chronic diseases, anemia, diabetes, obesity, and poor nutritional status.

C. Intrapartum risk factors include prolonged rupture of the membranes, frequent vaginal examinations, intrauterine fetal monitoring, intrauterine manipulation, lacerations in the reproductive tract, operative delivery, retained placental fragments, manual removal of the placenta, hematomas, postpartum hemorrhage, and improper aseptic technique.

D. Portals for bacterial entry include the placental site, the episiotomy, cesarean incision, the vagina, the urinary tract, the breasts, and the lymphatic system along the uterine veins.

E. Perineal, vaginal, and cesarean incision infections are usually easily treated with antibiotics that are compatible with breastfeeding; these infections, however, are a source of significant discomfort for the mother (making positioning for breastfeeding cumbersome; see Section II).

F. *Endometritis*, an infection of the lining of the uterus, is the most frequent cause of postpartum infection.

1. Early endometritis occurs within 48 hours of the delivery.

2. Mothers usually experience elevated temperatures, considerable pain, and malaise.
   a. Note: Early temperature rises are also seen with epidural anesthesia/analgesia (Philip et al., 1999).

3. The most important risk factor is premature rupture of the membranes or nonelective cesarean section after the onset of labor with rupture of the membranes.

4. Treatment is usually with broad spectrum antibiotics that are compatible with breastfeeding.

5. The mother's condition will determine how breastfeeding proceeds.

G. Parametritis (also known as pelvic cellulitis) is an extension of the infectious process beyond the endometrium into the broad ligaments.

1. Typically occurs during the second week postpartum.

2. Mothers usually experience a persistent high fever, malaise, chills, lethargy, and marked pain over the affected area.

3. The lactation consultant will need to remember to ask whether pain is present in areas other than the breasts, because some of these infections present with symptoms similar to mastitis.

4. Intravenous antibiotics are used; needle aspiration or surgery might be required to drain an abscess.

   a. The baby needs to feed or the mother pump just before surgery so that breastfeeding/pumping can resume as soon as the mother is conscious after the surgery.

   b. Antibiotics and anesthetic agents are compatible with breastfeeding (Hale, 2006).

5. Separation and interrupted breastfeeding might occur.

   a. Arrangements for access to the baby and/or a breast pump will need to be made.

H. Urinary tract infections (UTIs) caused by urine retention after childbirth are common.

1. Causes include: trauma to the base of the bladder, use of regional anesthesia, increased capacity and decreased sensitivity of the puerperal bladder, and the use of oxytocin infusion after birth, which induces potent antidiuretic effects. Once the oxytocin is discontinued, rapid diuresis follows.

2. Catheterization is a frequent cause of UTIs because the insertion of the catheter introduces residual urine and bacteria into the bladder.

3. Mothers can experience fever and considerable pain.

4. Treatment includes antibiotic therapy that is compatible with breastfeeding, urinary alkalinizers, increased fluid intakes, and proper nutrition.

I. Cesarean incision infections occur in 10% of mothers following cesarean section (Johnson, Young, & Reilly, 2006) even with the use of prophylactic antibiotics (Bagratee et al., 2002).

1. The most common symptom is fever occurring on about the fourth day.

2. Treatment is with antibiotics usually compatible with breastfeeding (Hale, 2006) and less frequently with surgical drainage.

X. Side Effects of Labor Medications That Can Affect Breastfeeding

A. In optimal birth settings mothers are encouraged to have uninterrupted skin-to-skin contact and rooming-in options, which minimize effects of labor medications on lactation success (Halpern et al., 1999; Righard & Alade, 1990).

B. Both mothers and babies are affected by labor medications in the early postpartum period.

   1. Some mothers feel drugged or "hung over" or may be immobilized by the epidural.

   2. Babies may show poor feeding abilities during the early postpartum period.

   3. Mothers may need assistance to position and latch their babies.

   4. Mothers who are affected by analgesia/anesthesia and whose babies are in skin-to-skin contact should be under constant supervision until the medications are no longer effective.

C. Epidural medications are measurable in the fetal circulation within 10 minutes of administration (Hale, 2006). Following birth:

   1. Babies who are separated from their mothers after medicated labors show a delayed and depressed sucking and rooting behavior (Righard & Alade, 1990).

   2. Babies' feeding abilities may be affected by the metabolite of meperidine (normeperidine) for 63 hours after administration (Quinn, cited in Hale, 2006).

   3. Babies have poor neonatal alertness and orientation when their mothers have postnatal intravenous patient-controlled analgesia with meperidine (Wittels, cited in Hale, 2006).

D. Metabolites of some medications, particularly meperidine/demerol (pethidine) (regardless of route of administration) and intrathecal fentanyl, may affect the baby until they are excreted (Scherer & Holzgreve, 1995).

   1. Fentanyl: Has a short half-life and is found in very low concentrations in colostrum (Hale, 2006). High-dose fentanyl epidurals have been shown to impede the establishment of breastfeeding (Jordan et al., 2005) or lead to early cessation in breastfeeding in women who have breastfed previous babies (Beilin et al., 2005).

   2. Bupivicaine (Marcaine): Due to its lack of effect on neonates and low levels of detection in breast milk (Naulty, cited in Hale, 2006), it has become the most commonly used epidural and local anesthetic in labor (Hale, 2006).

E. Prenatal education needs to include advice to women that epidurals increase the length of labor and lead to higher levels of instrumental delivery (Rosenblatt et al., 1991).

References

Abraham KA, Connolly G, Farrell J, Walshe JJ. The HELLP syndrome, a prospective study. *Ren Fail.* 2001;23:705–713.

Anderson AM. Disruption of lactogenesis by retained placental fragments. *J Hum Lact.* 2001;17:142–144.

Bagratee JS, Moodley J, Kleinschmidt I, Zawilski W. A randomized controlled trial of antibiotic prophylaxis in elective caesarean delivery. *BJOG.* 2002;109:1423–1424.

Beilin Y, Bodian CA, Weiser J, et al. Effect of labor epidural analgesia with and without fentanyl on infant breast-feeding: a prospective, randomized, double-blind study. *Anesthesiology.* 2005;103:1111–1112.

Blackburn ST. *Maternal, Fetal and Neonatal Physiology: A Clinical Perspective.* 2nd ed. Basel: Elsevier Science; 2003.

Collins CT, Ryan P, Crowther CA, et al. Effect of bottles, cups, and dummies on breast feeding in preterm infants: a randomised controlled trial. *BMJ.* 2004;329:193–198.

Cox SG. *Breastfeeding with Confidence.* New York: Meadowbook Press, Simon & Schuster; 2006.

Curtin WM, Weinstein L. A review of HELLP syndrome. *J Perinatol.* 1999;19:138–143.

Dewey KG. Maternal and fetal stress are associated with impaired lactogenesis in humans. *J Nutr.* 2001:131:3012S–3015S.

Dietl J. Pathogenesis of pre-eclampsia—new aspects. *J Perinat Med.* 2000;28:464.

Dowling DA, Meier PP, DiFiore JM, et al. Cup-feeding for preterm infants: mechanics and safety. *J Hum Lact.* 2002;8:13–20.

Hale TW. *Medications and Mothers' Milk.* 12th ed. Amarillo, TX: Hale Publishing; 2006.

Hall RT, Mercer AM, Teasley SL, et al. A breastfeeding assessment score to evaluate the risk for cessation of breastfeeding by 7 to 10 days of age. *J Pediatr.* 2002;141:659–664.

Halpern SH, Levine T, Wilson DB, et al. Effect of labor analgesia on breastfeeding success. *Birth.* 1999;26:8388; comment in 26:275–276.

Haram K, Bjorge L, Guttu K. Tidsskr Nor Laegeforen. (HELLP syndrome). 2000; 120:1433–14336 (in Norwegian; abstract in English).

Hartmann K, Visawanthan M, Palmieri R, et al. Outcomes of routine episiotomies: a systematic review. *JAMA.* 2005;293:2141–2148.

Higgins JR, de Swiet M. Blood pressure measurement and classification in pregnancy. *Lancet.* 2001;357:131–135.

Johnson A, Young D, Reilly J. Caesarean section surgical site infection surveillance. *J Hosp Infect.* 2006;64(1):30–35.

Jordan S, Emery S, Bradshaw C, et al. The impact of intrapartum analgesia on infant feeding. *BJOG.* 2005;112:927–934.

Kelestimur F. Sheehan's syndrome. *Pituitary.* 2003;6:181–188.

Kuhnert BR, Kennard MJ, Linn PL. Neonatal behaviour after epidural anesthesia for caesarean section: a comparison of bupivacaine and chloroprocaine. *Anaesth Analg.* 1998;67:64–68.

Lawrence RA, Lawrence RM. *Breastfeeding: A Guide to the Medical Profession.* 5th ed. St. Louis: C.V. Mosby; 1999.

Light KT, Smith TE, Johns JM, et al. Oxytocin responsivity in mothers and infants: a preliminary study of relationships with blood pressure during laboratory stress and normal ambulatory activity. *Health Psychol.* 2000;90:560–567.

Lundquist M, Olsson A, Nissen E, Norman M. Is it necessary to suture all lacerations after a vaginal delivery. *Birth*. 2000;27:79–85.

Matthiessen A-S, Ransjo-Arvidsson A-B, Nissen E, Uvnäs-Moberg K. Postpartum maternal oxytocin release by newborns: effects of infant hand massage and sucking. *Birth*. 2001;28:13–19.

Minnassian VA, Jazayeri A, Prien SD, et al. Randomized trial of lidocaine ointment versus placebo for the treatment of postpartum perineal pain. *Obstet Gynecol*. 2002;100:1239–1243.

Neifert M, McDonough SL, Neville MC. Failure of lactogenesis associated with placental retention. *Am J Obstet Gynecol*. 1981;140:477–478.

Philip, J, Alexander, JM, Sharma, SK, et al. Epidural analgesia during labor and maternal fever. *Aneasthesiology*. 1999;(90)3:1250–1252.

Ramler D, Roberts J. A comparison of cold and warm sitz baths for relief of postpartum perineal pain. *J Obstet Gynecol Neonatal Nurs*. 1986;15:471–474.

Reynders FC, Senten L, Tjalma W, Jacquemyn Y. Postpartum hemorrhage: practical approach to a life threatening complication. *Clin Exp Obstet Gynecol*. 2006;33:81–84.

Righard L, Alade MO. Effect of delivery room routines on success of first breast-feed. *Lancet*. 1990;336:1105–1107.

Rosenblatt D, Belsey E, Lieberman BA, et al. The influence of maternal analgesia on neonatal behaviour. II. Epidural bupivicaine. *Br J Obstet Gynaecol*. 1991;88:407–413.

Scherer R, Holzgreve W. Influence of epidural analgesia on fetal and neonatal well-being. *Eur J Obstet Gynecol Reprod Biol*. 1995;59(Suppl):S17–S19.

Sepkoski CM, Lester BM, Ostheimer GW, Brazelton TB. The effects of maternal epidural anaesthesia on neonatal behaviour during the first month. *Dev Med Child Neurol*. 1994;36:91–92.

Spear HJ. Policies and practices for maternal support options during childbirth and breastfeeding initiation after caesarean in south-eastern hospitals. *J Obstet Gynecol Neonatal Nurs*. 2006;35(5):634-643.

Uvnäs-Moberg K, Petersson M. Oxytocin, a mediator of anti-stress, well-being, social interaction, growth and healing. *Z Psychomon Med Psychother*. 2005;51:51–80 (in German; abstract in English).

Visser W, Wallenburg HC. Maternal and perinatal outcome of temporizing management in 254 consecutive patients with severe preeclampsia remote from term. *Eur J Obstet Gynecol Reprod Biol*. 1995;63:147–154.

Volikas I, Butwick A, Wilkinson C, et al. Maternal and neonatal side-effects of remifentanil patient controlled analgesia in labour. *Br J Anaesth*. 2005;95:504–509.

Widstrom AM, Ransjo-Arvidson AB, Christensson K, et al. Gastric suction in healthy newborn infants. Effects on circulation and developing feeding behaviour. *Acta Paediatr Scand*. 1987;76:566–572.

Congenital Anomalies, Neurologic Involvement, and Birth Trauma

Marsha Walker, RN, IBCLC
Revised by Catherine Watson Genna, BS, IBCLC

OBJECTIVES

- Discuss how congenital anomalies, neurologic impairments, and birth trauma can affect early breastfeeding.
- List strategies for assisting these babies with initiating breastfeeding.

Introduction

A number of conditions presenting at birth or shortly thereafter can have a significant impact on the initiation and duration of breastfeeding. Some of these conditions are temporary while others will remain for a lifetime. Compromised babies especially benefit from the provision of breast milk and/or breastfeeding. A few babies will be unable to feed at the breast, but provision of breast milk for them can and should continue as long as possible. Some of these conditions will first be brought to the attention of a health care provider because of poor feeding, with the inability to breastfeed being a marker or symptom of the problem. Mothers of these babies can experience an enormous range of emotions. They might be frightened, frustrated, anxious, fatigued, angry, or depressed. Their emotional well-being should not be neglected in the flurry of activity surrounding the baby.

I. Postmature Infants, Those Born at the Onset of Week 42 of Gestation

A. Fully mature infants who have remained in utero beyond the time of optimal placental function.

B. Aging of the placenta and reduced placental function impairs nutrient and oxygen transport to the fetus, placing the fetus at risk for a lower tolerance to the stresses of labor and delivery, including hypoxia.

1. In response to hypoxia, meconium might be passed, increasing the risk for meconium aspiration.

2. Amniotic fluid might be decreased, increasing the risk for meconium aspiration and umbilical cord compression.

C. If the placenta continues to function well, the baby might become large for gestational age (LGA) and thereby increase the risk for shoulder dystocia and possible fractured clavicle.

D. Post-mature infants are characterized by the following:

1. Loss of weight in utero.

2. Dry, peeling skin that appears to hang due to the loss of subcutaneous fat and muscle mass.

3. A wrinkled, wide-eyed appearance.

4. Lack of vernix caseosa (the waxy or cheese-like substance coating the newborn's skin; composed of sebum and skin sloughed in utero).

5. Reduced glycogen stores in the liver.

E. These babies might be at higher risk for hypoglycemia due to low glycogen reserves.

1. Early, frequent breastfeeding, or feeding of colostrum if not latching, can help maintain blood sugar levels.

F. These babies might feed poorly, appear lethargic, and require considerable incentives to sustain suckling, including alternate massage/breast compression, expressed colostrum incentives, skin-to-skin contact (because their body temperature is quite labile), and avoidance of crying episodes, which can further drop their blood glucose levels.

II. Birth Trauma

A. Forceps use might result in small areas of ecchymosis (bruising) on the sides of the face where the blades were placed.

B. Trauma to the facial nerves can occur; any muscles innervated by these nerves might be temporarily hypotonic, making latching and sucking difficult; observe for an asymmetric movement of the mouth, a drooping mouth, or a drooping eyelid.

C. Vacuum-assisted deliveries can pose an increased risk of cranial hemorrhage (FDA, 1998; Ng, 1995).

1. Extracranial hemorrhage (bleeding between the skin and cranial bone).
   a. Caput succedaneum, hemorrhagic edema of the soft tissues of the scalp, usually resolves within the first week of life.

    b. Cephalhematoma, bleeding that is contained within the subperiosteal space, preventing it from crossing suture lines.

    c. Subgaleal hemorrhage can represent a significant blood loss to the infant.

        i. It presents as a fluctuant area of the scalp, sometimes increasing in size to the point of blood dissecting into the subcutaneous tissue of the back of the neck (Cavlovich, 1994).

        ii. These babies will need special help in positioning to keep pressure off the hemorrhagic area.

        iii. Some infants feed poorly or not at all until some of the hemorrhage has resolved, a condition that presents an increased risk for high bilirubin levels as the body breaks down the red blood cells and recycles the hemoglobin.

  2. Intracranial hemorrhage (not visible externally).

    a. The baby might present with common signs such as sleepiness, feeding intolerance, and decreased muscle tone.

    b. Subdural hemorrhage is the most common intracranial hemorrhage resulting from a traumatic delivery (Steinbach, 1999).

    c. Some of the signs and symptoms become evident following discharge; babies who have a history of vacuum extraction that demonstrate lethargy, feeding problems, hypotonia, increased irritability, diffuse swelling of the head, and pallor need an immediate follow-up (Davis, 2001).

    d. Ability to suck, swallow, and root are sensitive to neurologic insults (Katz-Salamon, 1997).

D. Fractured clavicle.

  1. Can occur with an LGA infant or with malpresentations of the baby.

  2. The baby might display a decreased movement of the arm or distress with arm movements; the arm and shoulder will be immobilized and special positioning might be needed in order to breastfeed the baby.

  3. Some babies are not diagnosed until after discharge when certain positions are noted to cause crying in the baby; the clutch hold or placing the baby on the unaffected side at each breast might be helpful.

III. Inborn Errors of Metabolism

A. Galactosemia.

  1. Caused by a deficiency of the enzyme galactose-1-phosphate uridyltransferase, causing an inability in the infant to metabolize galactose.

  2. Infant can have severe and persistent jaundice, vomiting, diarrhea, electrolyte imbalance, cerebral involvement, and weight loss.

  3. These babies are weaned from the breast to a lactose- and galactose-free formula.

B. Phenylketonuria (PKU).

1. The most common of the amino acid metabolic disorders.

2. An autosomal, recessive, inherited disorder where the amino acid, phenylalanine, accumulates due to the absence of the enzyme phenylalanine hydroxylase, which converts phenylalanine to tyrosine for further breakdown.

3. Newborn screening for PKU is done in all 50 states in the United States and in more than 30 other countries.

4. Babies need some phenylalanine.

5. Infants who have PKU can continue to breastfeed when a balance is maintained between the use of a phenylalanine-free formula and breast milk (van Rijn et al., 2003).

6. Human milk has lower levels of phenylalanine than standard commercial formulas (Duncan, 1997).

7. The amount of phenylalanine-free formula and breast milk can be calculated by weight, age, blood levels, and the need for growth.

8. Another approach is to feed the baby 10 to 30 mL of the special formula followed by breastfeeding.
   a. As long as phenylalanine levels are properly maintained, the exact calculations of breast milk and formula might not need to be made.
   b. Breast milk might be more than half of the diet, improving the baby's exposure to the trophic (tissue building), immune, and immunomodulating functions of human milk.

9. Breastfeeding before diagnosis and dietary intervention has been shown to produce a 14 point higher IQ than babies who are artificially-fed pre-diagnosis (Riva et al., 1996).

IV. Other Genetic Disorders

A. Cystic fibrosis (CF).

1. A congenital disease involving a generalized dysfunction of exocrine glands due to a mutation in the transmembrane conductance regulatory protein.

2. The glands produce abnormally thick and sticky secretions that block the flow of pancreatic digestive enzymes, clog hepatic ducts, and affect the movement of the cilia in the lungs.

3. Increased sodium chloride in the child's sweat is frequently the first indicator of the condition; the baby tastes salty when nuzzled.

4. Another early indicator of CF is intestinal obstruction or ileus.
   a. The meconium blocks the small intestine, resulting in abdominal distension, vomiting, and failure to pass stools (resulting in the failure to gain weight).

5. Babies who have CF produce normal amounts of gastric lipase, which combined with the milk lipase in breast milk enhances fat absorption.

6. Breastfed infants with CF are less likely to need intravenous antibiotics (Parker et al., 2004).

7. Breastfed infants with CF may present with protein malnutrition (edema) and reduced weight gain, but may escape the characteristic infections, confounding diagnosis.

   a. Pancreatic enzymes can be given to the baby to improve protein metabolism (Cannella et al., 1993).

8. There is no need to interrupt breastfeeding (Luder et al., 1990).

B. Neurologic disorders.

1. Infants who have neurologic impairments often have extremely complex needs.

2. The infant's nervous system can be damaged, abnormally developed, immature, or temporarily incapacitated from insults such as asphyxia, sepsis, trauma, or drugs.

3. Infants can have an absent or depressed rooting response, gag reflex, sucking reflex, and/or may have difficulty swallowing (dysphagia).

4. Giving a bottle to a baby who is to be breastfed provides inconsistent sensory input that additionally disorganizes the nervous system.

5. A depressed or absent suck reflex, where infants might exhibit a limited response to stimulation to the palate and tongue; these babies might have decreased muscle tone.

6. A weak or poorly sustained sucking reflex.

   a. Denotes an oral musculature weakened to the point of an inability to sustain a rhythmic suck.

   b. The rhythm is interrupted by irregular pauses and sometimes a lack of the 1:1 suck/swallow cycle.

   c. Adequate negative intraoral pressure is not generated, causing the nipple to fall out of the mouth.

   d. Lips do not form a complete seal.

   e. The hypotonic tongue might remain flat, not cupping around the breast.

7. Uncoordinated sucking includes a mistiming of the component muscle movements of the suck/swallow cycle.

   a. The lactation consultant might see extraneous movements of the mouth, head, or neck.

   b. Hypersensitivity or hyposensitivity might be seen in other areas of the body.

   c. Infant might have dysfunctional tongue movements and uncoordinated swallowing, increasing risk of aspiration.

C. Down syndrome.

1. Results from an extra chromosome 21 (Trisomy 21).

a. Common characteristics that relate to feeding include the following:
  i. A flaccid tongue that appears too large for the mouth due to reduced growth of the mandible (lower jaw).
  ii. Generalized hypotonia, including the oral musculature.
  iii. Heart defects that decrease aerobic capacity for feeding and might require surgery.
  iv. Incomplete development of the gastrointestinal (GI) tract.
  v. Hyperbilirubinemia is common.
  vi. Infant is especially prone to infection.
  vii. Might have a depressed sucking reflex or a weak suck, or both.
b. Some babies have no problem sucking while others might exhibit initial sucking difficulties.
c. The Dancer hand position (Danner, 1992) can benefit many of these babies because it stabilizes the jaw and supports the masseter muscles, which decreases the intra-oral space and enhances the generation of negative pressure.
  i. The breast is supported by the third, fourth, and fifth fingers so that the webbing between the thumb and index finger forms a U-shaped cup on which the baby's chin rests.
  ii. The thumb and index finger support the cheeks with gentle traction toward the corner of the lips.
  iii. The baby should be in a quiet, alert state in order to feed.
  iv. The infant might need hindmilk supplementation in order to gain weight and may benefit from the use of a supplementer to deliver it.
D. Fetal distress and hypoxia (decreased levels of oxygen).
  1. Infants can be compromised in utero or during delivery from low levels of oxygen due to the following:
  a. Insufficient placental reserve.
  b. Umbilical cord compression.
  c. Umbilical cord prolapse.
  2. Newborns are vulnerable to brain cell death from hypoxia.
  a. Neonatal encephalopathy is the current term for altered level of consciousness, seizures, apnea, and reduced brain stem function, including feeding ability.
  b. Recovery begins after three to four days; some infants remain compromised and may develop cerebral palsy or other neurologic deficits.
  c. Low Apgar scores combined with inability to suck requiring tube feeding is the most sensitive indicator of later disability, followed by seizures and need for mechanical ventilation (Moster, Lie, & Markestad, 2002).
  d. Colostrum is very important to this baby because his or her GI tract might have suffered hypoxic damage; colostrum should be expressed and used as

soon as the baby can tolerate feedings by mouth; mothers should frequently hand express or pump during this time.

e. Hypoxia decreases the motility of the gut and reduces the gut-stimulating hormones.

f. These infants might have a depressed suck that is not well coordinated with the swallow, and they may have difficulty bottle-feeding.

g. A supplementer device, cup, or other feeding device might be needed initially until the infant's feeding skills recover. Mothers need to express milk about eight times daily when their infant is unable to remove milk to drive the supply effectively (Academy of Breastfeeding Medicine, 2005).

h. The hypotonic (low muscle tone) baby might breastfeed better in a clutch hold with the trunk stabilized against mother's side or while swaddled in flexion (McBride & Danner, 1987).

i. The hypertonic (high muscle tone) baby should be held in a flexed, well supported position to reduce the overall extensor patterning.

j. Breastfeeding interventions are similar to those for the baby who has Down syndrome, including cheek and jaw support (Dancer hand position).

k. These infants have increased effort of feeding, fatigue easily, and may require very short frequent feedings.

l. Recovery usually proceeds for many months, and infants who are not able to breastfeed at birth may develop the skills later, especially if oral motor therapy is provided.

E. GI tract disorders.

1. Esophageal atresia (EA).

a. A congenital defect of the esophagus. In most cases the upper esophagus does not connect with the lower esophagus and stomach. May be associated with other birth defects.

b. Tracheoesophageal fistula (TEF) occurs when the esophagus is connected to the trachea and is a common variation of EA. Occurs in 1 of every 3,000–5,000 live births.

c. Usually detected in the first few hours of life and is considered a surgical emergency.

d. Symptoms can include excess amniotic fluid during pregnancy and difficulties with feeding such as coughing, spilling fluid from the lips, gagging, choking, and cyanosis.

e. There is no research to justify test feeds of sterile or glucose water to diagnose TEF or EA. Water or low-chloride fluids in the neonatal airway have the potential to cause prolonged apnea (Thach, 1997).

2. Gastroesophageal reflux (GER).

a. A persistent, nonprojectile regurgitation (spitting-up) seen after feeds.

b. Can be mild and self-limiting, requiring no modification or interventions.

    c. Can be more severe, with worsening regurgitation and weight gain or loss problems.

    d. Can present as follows:

      i. Fussiness at the breast as stomach contents contact the lower section of the esophagus.

      ii. Might be more apparent in certain side-lying positions at the breast.

      iii. Mothers might report increased fussing at the breast, a baby who arches off or pulls away from the breast, or a baby who cries until placed upright.

      iv. Baby mouths refluxed milk between feedings ("cud chewing").

      v. Upper respiratory infections and congestion may occur from chronic aspiration of refluxing fluid (ascending aspiration).

      vi. Feeding refusal.

      vii. Micro- and macroaspiration, may manifest as nasal congestion that increases throughout the feeding, coughing, or wheezing during or between feeds (Catto-Smith, 1998).

    e. Mothers are encouraged to keep providing breast milk, nurse the baby in an upright position (in clutch hold or straddled across her lap), nurse on one breast at each feeding to keep from overdistending the stomach, feed frequently, and keep the baby upright for 10-20 minutes after feedings (Boekel, 2000).

    f. Reflux needs to be differentiated from hyperlactation with overfeeding or lactose overload.

      i. Generally, if the infant is gaining rapidly, has signs of gut irritation and rapid intestinal transit time (green, mucousy stools), and is fussy, maternal hyperlactation might be responsible.

      ii. Reducing milk production by gradually increasing the amount of time before changing breasts is generally successful.

    g. If the reflux is severe, the baby might undergo diagnostic tests and be placed on medication.

3. Pyloric stenosis.

    a. A stricture or narrowing of the pylorus (muscular tissue controlling the outlet of the stomach) caused by muscular hypertrophy, more common in non-breastfed infants (Pisacane et al., 1996).

    b. It usually occurs between the second and sixth week of life, although it can occur any time after birth.

    c. Vomiting is characteristic, intermittent at first, progressing to after every feeding, and projectile in nature. Baby usually begins to refuse feeds.

    d. Dehydration, electrolyte imbalance, and weight loss can occur in extreme situations.

    e. If the baby does not outgrow the condition or if it is severe, surgery can be performed after rehydration and correction of electrolyte balance.

       i. A breastfed baby can resume breastfeeding earlier than a bottle-fed baby who is consuming formula due to the faster stomach emptying time and zero curd tension of human milk.

      ii. Mothers should feed with one breast initially after surgery to prevent overfilling of the baby's stomach; these limited feedings gradually expand the stomach and can be advanced as the baby tolerates it.

     iii. Mothers can position the baby upright in a straddle position to avoid stress on the incision.

F. Congenital heart defects.

  1. Seen along a continuum of mild with no symptoms to severe with cyanosis, rapid breathing, shortness of breath, and lowered oxygen levels (desaturation) that requires surgical correction.

  2. Cardiac disease is not a medical indication to interrupt or cease breastfeeding (Barbas & Kelleher, 2004).

  3. Feeding at the breast presents less work for the baby, keeps oxygen levels higher than with bottle-feeding, and keeps heart and respiratory rates stable when the baby is at the breast (Marino, O'Brien, & LoRe, 1995).

  4. A baby who has more serious heart involvement might be either unable to sustain sucking at the breast or might need to pause frequently in order to rest; if intake is inadequate, the baby will not gain weight or will exhibit weight loss.

  5. Infants with cardiac disease often have increased caloric requirements.

  6. Mothers might describe these babies in any number of ways, including the following:

    a. Able to sustain sucking for only short periods of time.

    b. Pulling off the breast frequently.

    c. Turning blue around the lips (circumoral cyanosis).

    d. Rapid breathing or panting; rapid heart rate.

    e. Sweating while at the breast.

    f. Requires very frequent feedings.

  7. If surgery is planned, it is typically scheduled after the baby reaches a predetermined weight and/or age.

    a. Small, frequent feeds might be necessary.

    b. If additional calories are needed, consider hindmilk supplementation at the breast with a supplementer device.

G. Sudden infant death syndrome (SIDS) or sudden unexplained infant death.

  1. Also known as *crib death* or *cot death,* is the leading cause of death in infants in developed countries who are older than one month; rates vary worldwide.

  2. The etiology is unknown; it seems multicausal; parental smoking is the greatest risk factor.

3. The sleeping position dramatically affects the rates; babies placed on their backs (supine) are less prone to SIDS.

4. The majority of deaths occur between 2 and 6 months of age with a peak at about 10 weeks of age.

5. Artificially fed infants might have higher risk of SIDS than breastfed infants.
   a. Breastfeeding offers dose-response protection across race and socioeconomic levels; it is associated with a 50% reduction in risk on meta-analysis, but the quality of existing studies is deficient (McVea, Turner, & Peppler, 2000).
   b. The exact protective mechanism is not well understood.
      i. Breastfeeding reduces minor infections such as acute upper-respiratory infections and diarrheal infections that are frequently associated with SIDS.
      ii. Breastfeeding and breast milk enhance the development of the central nervous system and the brain stem, which might also provide protection.
   c. The American Academy of Pediatrics (AAP) SIDS Task Force did not find compelling evidence to indicate that breastfeeding is protective against SIDS (AAP, 2005).

6. The AAP's 2005 statement on SIDS recommended against bedsharing and for pacifier use during sleep for infants over one month of age.
   a. Lactation consultants can help ensure that pacifier use is delayed and does not unduly impact breastfeeding, while continuing to call for higher quality studies that recognize mother-baby togetherness and breastfeeding as the human norm.

H. Respiratory disorders.

1. Common features.
   a. Increased effort of breathing leaves less energy for feeding.
   b. Increased baseline respiratory rate reduces the amount of swallowing that can be done, because swallowing inhibits breathing (Glass & Wolf, 1994).
   c. Short sucking bursts are typical signs of respiratory disorders.
   d. Very careful pacing of the feed (making sure the infant can control the speed of milk flow), head extension to reduce airway resistance to air flow (Ardran & Kemp, 1968; Wolf & Glass, 1992), and more frequent feedings are generally helpful.
   e. Growth should be monitored closely, and expressed milk provided by slow flow methods if the infant is unable to meet needs at breast.

2. Laryngomalacia.
   a. Epiglottis lacks normal stiffness and collapses into airway on inspiration, causing inspiratory stridor, suprasternal retractions, and increased work of breathing, particularly during crying, feeding, and supine positioning.
   b. Strongly associated with GER due to increased pressure on the lower esophageal sphincter.

    c. Head extension and prone positioning during feeding reduces airway resistance; short frequent feeds may be necessary to prevent failure to thrive (Wolf & Glass, 1994).

    d. Generally outgrown by 6 to 18 months as the neck elongates and structures become anatomically separated.

3. Tracheomalacia.

    a. Cartilage rings in trachea may be malformed and are insufficiently stiff, rapid air flow during expiration (and inspiration as well in newborns) causes partial collapse of trachea (Wiatrak, 2000).

    b. Can be seen as sternal retraction and heard as stridor.

    c. Increases work of respiration.

    d. Same strategies are helpful as for laryngomalacia; also is outgrown in the first year of life.

4. Laryngeal webs.

    a. Persistence of tissue in the lumen of the airway that can cause significant respiratory distress.

    b. Infant may have great difficulty feeding; very careful pacing of feeding is necessary to prevent hypoxia.

5. Vocal fold paralysis.

    a. Usually unilateral from injury to fold or nerve.

    b. Hoarse cry.

    c. Reduces airway protection on the affected side.

    d. Infant will usually coordinate swallowing and breathing better if the paralyzed cord is oriented upward.

6. Velopharyngeal insufficiency/incompetence.

    a. Hypoplasia or dysfunction of the soft palate and pharyngeal constrictor muscles that prevent milk from entering the nasopharynx, sometimes due to submucous cleft palate.

    b. Nasal regurgitation, harsh respiration in feeding pauses, apnea from milk in the nasopharynx, feeding resistance.

    c. Careful pacing, upright positioning (straddle) may help.

References

Academy of Breastfeeding Medicine. Breastfeeding Is Associated with a Lower Risk of SIDS. Los Angeles: Breastfeeding Task Force of Greater Los Angeles; 2005. Available at: http://www.breastfeedingtaskforla.org/SIDS/AAP-SIDS-ABM-response.htm. Accessed January 28, 2007.

Academy of Breastfeeding Medicine supplementation protocol #3. Available at: http://www.bfmed.org/ace-files/protocol/supplementation.pdf). Accessed February 16, 2007.

American Academy of Pediatrics. Task Force on Sudden Infant Death Syndrome. The Changing Concept of Sudden Infant Death Syndrome: Diagnostic Coding Shifts, Controversies Regarding Sleeping Environment, and New Variables to Consider in Reducing Risk. *Pediatrics.* 2005;116:1245–1255.

Ardran G, Kemp F. The mechanism of changes in form of the cervical airway in infancy. *Med Radiogr Photogr.* 1968;44:26–38, 54.

Barbas KH, Kelleher DK. Breastfeeding success among infants with congenital heart disease. *Pediatr Nurs.* 2004;30:285–289.

Boekel S. *Gastroesophageal Reflux Disease (GERD) and the Breastfeeding Baby.* Independent Study Module. Raleigh, NC: International Lactation Consultant Association; 2000.

Cannella PC, Bowser EK, Guyer LK, et al. Feeding practices and nutrition recommendations for infants with cystic fibrosis. *J Am Diet Assoc.* 1993;93:297–300.

Catto-Smith AG. Gastroesophageal reflux in children. *Aust Fam Physician.* 1998;27:465–473.

Cavlovich FE. Subgaleal hemorrhage in the neonate. *J Obstet Gynecol Neonatal Nurs.* 1994;24:397–404.

Danner SC. Breastfeeding the neurologically impaired infant. NAACOG's clinical issues in perinatal and women's health nursing. *Breastfeeding.* 1992;3:640–646.

Davis DJ. Neonatal subgaleal hemorrhage: diagnosis and management. *CMAJ.* 2001; May 15;164(10):1452–1453.

Duncan LL, Elder SB. Breastfeeding the infant with PKU. *J Hum Lact.* 1997;13:231–235.

Food and Drug Administration (FDA) Public Health Advisory: Need for caution when using vacuum assisted delivery devices. Washington, DC: USFDA. May 21, 1998.

Glass RP, Wolf LS. Incoordination of sucking, swallowing and breathing as an etiology for breastfeeding difficulty. *J Hum Lact.* 1994;10:185–189.

Katz-Salamon M. Perinatal risk factors and neuromotor behaviour during the neonatal period. *Acta Paediatr Suppl.* 1997;419:27–36.

Luder E, Kattan M, Tanzer-Torres G, et al. Current recommendations for breastfeeding in cystic fibrosis centers. *Am J Dis Child.* 1990;144:1153–1156.

Marino BL, O'Brien P, LoRe H. Oxygen saturations during breast and bottle feedings in infants with congenital heart disease. *J Pediatr Nurs.* 1995;10:360–364.

McBride MC, Danner SC. Sucking disorders in neurologically impaired infants. *Clin Perinatol.* 1987;14:109–130.

McVea KLSP, Turner PD, Peppler DK. The role of breastfeeding in sudden infant death syndrome. *J Hum Lact.* 2000;16:13–20.

Moster D, Lie RT, Markestad T. Joint association of Apgar scores and early neonatal symptoms with minor disabilities at school age. *Arch Dis Child Fetal Neonatal Ed.* 2002;86:F16–F21.

Ng PC. Subaponeurotic haemorrhage in the 1990s: a 3-year surveillance. *Acta Paediatr.* 1995;84:1065–1069.

Parker EM, O'Sullivan BP, Shea JC, Regan MM, Freedman SD. Survey of breast-feeding practices and outcomes in the cystic fibrosis population. *Pediatr Pulmonol.* 2004;37:362–367.

Pisacane A, et al. Breast feeding and hypertrophic pyloric stenosis: population based case-control study *BMJ.* 1996;312:745–746.

Riva E, Agostoni C, Biasucci G, et al. Early breastfeeding is linked to higher intelligence quotient scores in dietary treated phenylketonuric children. *Acta Paediatr.* 1996;85: 56–58.

Steinbach MT. Traumatic birth injury–intracranial hemorrhage. *Mother Baby J.* 1999; 4:5–14.

Thach, BT. Reflux associated apnea in infants: Evidence for a laryngeal chemoreflex. *Am J Med.* 1997;103(5A):120–124.

van Rijn M, Bekhof J, Dijkstra T, et al. A different approach to breast-feeding of the infant with phenylketonuria. *Eur J Pediatr.* 2003;162:323–326.

Wiatrak B. Congenital anomalies of the larynx and trachea. *Otolaryngol Clin North Am.* 2000;33:91–110.

Wolf LS, Glass RP. *Feeding and Swallowing Disorders in Infancy: Assessment and Management.* Tucson, AZ: Therapy Skill Builders; 1992.

Wolf LS, Glass RP. Feeding and Oral Motor Skills. In: Case Smith J, ed. *Pediatric Occupational Therapy and Early Intervention.* Los Angeles: Butterworth-Heinemann; 1993.

BREAST PATHOLOGY

Angela Smith, RN, RM, BA, IBCLC
Joy Heads, OAM, RM, MHPEd, IBCLC

OBJECTIVES

- Describe common breastfeeding problems related to the lactating breast.
- Describe preventative and prophylactic measures for these problems.
- Differentiate between common presenting signs and symptoms.
- Identify appropriate interventions by the lactation consultant.
- Identify relevant educational issues for the mother with a breastfeeding problem.

Introduction

There are a number of common problems related to the lactating breast. While most can either be prevented or improved, early recognition, prompt treatment and/or referral, and close follow-up are required in order to preserve the breastfeeding experience. Some of these problems can be painful and extend over a period of time, which can be disappointing and frustrating to the new mother. Many lactation consultants use a number of therapeutic interventions that are based on long years of clinical experience rather than on randomized, controlled trials. Most have a particular set of treatment options they have come to prefer, but these strategies likely vary from region to region and country to country. Some are commonly seen in daily practice and others are used more rarely. All solutions to problems depend on careful assessment and management plans developed in conjunction with the mother.

I. Differentiation Between Normal and Engorged Breasts

A. Normal fullness.

   1. Engorgement is generally a preventable postpartum complication.

   2. Many women experience normal fullness when the milk increases during lactogenesis II.

3. The increase in blood flow to the breast, triggered by the prolactin surge, is accompanied by an increase in milk volume and interstitial tissue edema; this results in normal fullness in most women.

4. Normal fullness can be differentiated from problematic engorgement.
   a. The normally full breast will be larger, warmer, and uncomfortable; milk flow will be normal.
   b. The engorged breast will look tight and shiny and feel painful; milk flow may be compromised.

5. Restrictive feeding practices, suboptimal attachment, and/or ineffective sucking will compromise milk removal and result in pathologic engorgement (Woolridge, 1986a; Woolridge, 1986b).

B. Engorgement.

1. When milk production increases rapidly, the volume of milk in the breast can exceed the capacity of the alveoli to store it.

2. If the milk is not removed, overdistention of the alveoli can cause the milk-secreting cells to become flattened and drawn out; tight junction permeability is increased (Humenick, Hill & Anderson, 1994; Nguyen & Neville, 1998).

3. The distention can partly or completely occlude the capillary blood circulation surrounding the alveolar cells, further decreasing cellular activity. This distention can partly or completely occlude the oxytocin-rich capillary blood reaching the myoepithelial complex.

4. Congested blood vessels leak fluid into the surrounding tissue space, contributing to interstitial edema, which further compresses and impedes the milk flow. A cycle of congestion/edema/poor flow/congestion can occur easily.

5. Pressure and congestion obstruct the lymphatic drainage of the breasts, stagnating the system that rids the breasts of toxins, bacteria, and cast-off cell parts, thereby predisposing the breast to mastitis (both inflammatory and infectious).

6. It is also thought that a protein called the *feedback inhibitor of lactation (FIL)* accumulates in the mammary gland during milk stasis, further reducing milk production (Daly & Hartmann, 1995; Peaker & Wilde, 1996).

7. Accumulation of milk and the resulting engorgement are a major trigger of apoptosis, or programmed cell death, that causes involution of the milk secreting gland, milk reabsorption, collapse of the alveolar structures, and the cessation of milk production (Marti et al., 1997).

8. Engorgement has also been classified as involving only the areola, only the body of the breast, or both.

9. Areolar engorgement in its simple form may occur with large pendulous breasts or women with generalized edema from intravenous fluids or hypertension.

C. Prevention of engorgement requires efficient, thorough, and frequent milk removal (Glover, 1998).

   1. Good approaches to prevention.
      a. Optimal attachment/latch.
      b. Early and frequent feedings.
      c. Feeding according to need (i.e., on cue of baby).
      d. Not restricting frequency or length of feeds.
      e. Finishing the first breast before offering the second.

   2. The degree/duration of engorgement that poses an unrecoverable situation is unknown. The breast compensates to a point as milk production in the unaffected areas continues normally.

   3. Predicting an individual mother's risk for engorgement might not be possible, but some general principles can be of help in anticipating situations that predispose women to a higher risk (Hill & Humenick, 1994; Moon & Humenick, 1989; Newton & Newton, 1951).
      a. Failure to prevent or resolve milk stasis resulting from infrequent or inadequate drainage of the breasts.
      b. Women who have small breasts (other than hypoplastic and tubular) due to lack of space.
      c. Mothers with high rates of milk synthesis (hyperlactation), because milk stasis magnifies whenever milk volume significantly exceeds milk removal.

II. Treatment Modalities

A. Common treatment modalities.

   1. Warmth. Where a milk ejection reflex is thought to be compromised or slow, warmth has been shown to improve oxytocin uptake (Uvnäs-Moberg, 1998).

   2. Softening the areola prior to attachment helps achieve optimal attachment.

   3. If areolar edema is apparent, gentle massage of the interstitial fluid away from the nipple will help shape the areola, reveal the nipple, and improve milk flow.
      a. Originally referred to as *feathering* by British midwives, this technique has been redefined and described by Miller and Riordan (2004) as *areolar compression* and by Cotterman (2004) as *reverse pressure softening*.

   4. Cold therapy (cryotherapy).
      a. Cold applications in the form of ice packs, gel packs, frozen bags of vegetables, frozen wet towels, and so on have been studied under various application conditions.
      b. Cold application triggers a cycle of vasoconstriction during the first 9 to 16 minutes (Hocutt et al., 1982).

    c. Where blood flow is reduced, local edema decreases, and lymphatic drainage is enhanced.

    d. This condition is followed by a deep tissue vasodilation phase lasting 4 to 6 minutes that prevents thermal injury (Barnes, 1979).

  5. Chilled cabbage leaves.

    a. Rosier (1988) anecdotally describes the use of chilled cabbage leaves in a small sample of women as having a rapid effect on reducing edema and increasing milk flow.

    b. Nikodem et al. (1993) showed a nonsignificant trend in reduced engorgement in mothers who were using cabbage leaves.

    c. Roberts (1995) compared chilled cabbage leaves and gel packs, showing similar significant reduction in pain with both methods with two-thirds of the mothers preferring the cabbage due to a stronger, more immediate effect.

    d. Roberts, Reiter, and Schuster (1998) studied the use of cabbage extract cream applied to the breasts, which had no more effect than the placebo cream.

  6. Expressing milk.

    a. Refraining from expressing milk because the mother will "just make more milk" cannot be justified.

    b. Hand expressing or pumping *to comfort* reduces the buildup of FIL, decreases the mechanical stress on the alveoli (preventing the cell death process), prevents blood circulation changes, alleviates the impedance to lymph and fluid drainage, decreases the risk of mastitis and compromised milk production, and feels good to the mother (Peaker & Wilde, 1996; Prentice, Addey, & Wilde, 1989).

B. Plugged ducts.

  1. Compromised milk drainage from the breast is thought to occur from external pressure to the breast. For example: a tight fitting bra, baby carrier straps, mother's fingers, or baby's fist.

  2. Ineffective drainage of the breast by factors such as: ineffective or inefficient sucking, suboptimal attachment, disorganized or dysfunctional sucking, skipped or irregular feeds, or hyperlactation.

  3. The section of the breast behind this blockage might experience a focal area of engorgement; an older name for this was *caked breast.*

  4. The mother might complain of tenderness, heat, or possibly redness over a palpable lump; the lump has well-defined margins and no fever is present.

  5. Management is by hot compresses and gentle massage before the feed. During the breastfeed, gentle pressure behind the blockage may improve milk flow. Alternating the baby's position at the breast may assist in milk removal; however, optimal attachment is still the most crucial component.

6. A blocked nipple pore is another potential cause of *milk stasis.*
   a. Frequently described as a solitary bleb/white dot or pressure cyst on the tip of the nipple (Lawrence & Lawrence, 2005).
   b. It is shiny, smooth and less than 1 mm in diameter and causes pinpoint pain.
   c. The bleb blocks the terminal opening for drainage of one of the lobes of the breast and as such could contribute to milk stasis in a larger area of the breast.
   d. Warm soaks and optimal attachment sometimes resolve the problem.
   e. After removal, the initial flow of milk is often gritty followed by normal milk.
   f. The bleb may require a health professional to open it with a sterile needle; it often reforms and requires repeated opening; the mother may need to be shown how to remove it herself.
7. Corpora amylacia (*ALCA News,* 1992).
   a. Described as white crystals caused by the aggregation and fusion of casein micelles in the alveoli to which further materials are added, which hardens them.
8. Other descriptions of milk expressed from blocked areas of the breast include strings that look like spaghetti or lengths of fatty-looking material.
   a. This type of blockage might account for the ropy texture of an obstructed area and the thought that thickened milk could be responsible for the blockage.
   b. Lawrence and Lawrence (2005) describe improvement in this condition when the mother's diet contains only polyunsaturated fats and a lecithin supplement is added to meals.

C. Mastitis.
   1. A preventable but common lactation complication (Fetherston, 1998; Foxman et al., 2002).
   2. Approximately 10% of women with mastitis wean due to the debilitating nature of the condition (Fetherston, 1997a; Wambach et al., 2005).
   3. Onset is usually in the first three weeks postpartum or with abrupt weaning or sudden changes in breast usage (Foxman et al., 2002).
   4. An inflammatory process that may or may not progress to a breast infection.
      a. The initial cause of mastitis is an unresolved increase in the intraductal pressure, first causing a flattening of the secretory cells and an increase in permeability of the tight junctions.
      b. A paracellular pathway then may occur between the cells, which allows the passage of some of the components in breast milk to leak into the interstitial tissue, resulting in an inflammatory response.
      c. This inflammatory response and resultant tissue damage can be a precursor to infective mastitis.

d. Studies have suggested that an elevated sodium/potassium ratio, an increase in sodium chloride, increased immunoglobulins, and a decrease in lactose with consequent decrease in milk volume are early signs of mastitis, which is often demonstrated by infant breast refusal (Fetherston, 2001). This is commonly referred to as subclinical mastitis (Michie, Lockie, & Lynn, 2003; Willumsen et al., 2000)

5. Usually is associated with lactation, can be acute or chronic, and often occurs as a result of poor breastfeeding techniques.

6. Can progress to an infection and provoke serious sequelae, such as an abscess and early unnecessary weaning if it is treated inappropriately (WHO, 2000).

7. Incidence varies among studies; it is estimated to occur in 24% to 33% of lactating women (Fetherston, 2001).

8. Mastitis has a variety of definitions that usually describe different aspects of the problem and are often based on the symptoms or ultimate treatment approach (Freed, Landers, & Schanler, 1991; Niebyl, Spence, & Parmley, 1978).

9. Lawrence and Lawrence (2005) differentiate two types of mastitis.
   a. Acute puerperal mammary cellulitis, a nonepidemic mastitis involving interlobular connective tissue, is the most common form of mastitis.
   b. Acute puerperal mammary adenitis, which was epidemic with an outbreak of skin infections in infants (a rare occurrence).

10. Most clinicians simply use a cluster of signs and symptoms to diagnose mastitis (the infection).
    a. Fever > 38°C (100.4°F).
    b. Chills.
    c. Increased pulse.
    d. Flu-like body aches.
    e. Pain/swelling at the site.
    f. Red, tender, hot area.
    g. Increased sodium levels in the milk (the baby might reject the breast due to the salty taste of the milk).
    h. Red streaks extending toward the axilla.

11. Thomsen et al. (1983) microscopically examined the milk itself to differentiate between milk stasis, inflammation, and infection; all of the mothers in their study complained of tender, red, hot, and swollen breasts.
    a. Diagnosis of a breast infection was made by counting (not culturing) leukocytes and bacteria in milk samples taken from the affected breast and studied under a microscope (Thomsen et al., 1983).
    b. Three clinical states were identified.
       i. Milk stasis < 106 leukocytes and < 103 bacteria/mL of milk.

      ii. Noninfectious inflammation > 106 leukocytes and < 103 bacteria/mL of milk.

     iii. Infectious mastitis > 106 leukocytes and > 103 bacteria/mL of milk.

12. The highest occurrence is generally at two to three weeks postpartum (WHO, 2000).

13. The upper, outer quadrant of the breast is the most frequent site for infection to occur (Riordan & Nichols, 1990).

14. There seems to be a fairly equal distribution of cases between the right and left breasts. Bilateral mastitis occurs much less frequently (usual organism, *Streptococcus*).

15. Breast milk is not sterile.

    a. The vast majority of confirmed cases of mastitis show *S. aureus* as the causative organism.

    b. Although lactating women potentially have pathogenic bacteria on their skin or in their milk, most do not go on to develop infectious mastitis (the infection) (Matheson et al., 1988).

    c. Conversely, in many women who actually develop an infection, pathogenic bacteria cannot be cultured in their milk.

16. Buescher and Hair (2001) found that mastitis milk has the same anti-inflammatory components and characteristics of normal milk, with elevations in selected components that may help protect the infant from developing clinical illness due to feeding from the affected mastitis breast.

17. Contributing factors.

    a. Milk stasis.

      i. If the pressure rises high enough, as with severe, unrelieved, and prolonged engorgement, small amounts of milk components will be forced out from the tight junctions between the epithelial cells that line the ductal system into the surrounding breast tissue.

      ii. This triggers a localized inflammatory response, which involves pain, local swelling, redness, and heat over the affected area and/or a general response of a rise in body temperature and pulse rate.

     iii. Once the integrity of these tight junctions has been disrupted, it may be easier for it to happen again when similar circumstances increase the pressure in the breast; this situation might help explain why women who have had mastitis in a previous lactation have a greater chance of a recurrence of mastitis in the same or next lactation compared to women who have never had mastitis.

     iv. The disruption of the tight junction integrity can also provide a partial explanation for why women develop recurrent mastitis within a particular lactation.

      v. If milk components also leak into the vascular channels, capillaries, and bloodstream, it can account for the systemic/autoimmune response of fever, aches, fatigue, and general malaise that accompany mastitis (the infection).

      vi. The body's response to both the inflammatory agents in the milk (interleukin-1) and the antigenic response to the milk proteins (which are recognized as foreign) are thought to contribute to the flu-like symptoms above.

      vii. If milk stasis is allowed to persist, it might be the condition that provides the medium that is needed for bacterial overgrowth and that may provoke an infection.

    b. Inefficient milk removal.

18. Conditions and situations contributing to inefficient emptying of the breast and hence milk stasis (Fetherston, 1997b; Foxman, Schwartz, & Looman, 1994).

    a. Scheduled, interrupted, or erratic feeding patterns.

    b. Baby with a neurologic impairment.

    c. A sudden change in the number of feeds.

    d. Mother's or baby's illness.

    e. Baby sleeping longer at night.

    f. Overabundant milk supply (hyperlactation).

    g. Sucking at breast displaced by pacifiers or bottles.

    h. Separation of mother and baby.

    i. Breastfeeding technique (switching too soon from the first breast to the second before the baby has adequately drained the first side).

    j. Abrupt weaning.

    k. Baby's oral anatomy that leads to inefficient emptying of the breast (for example, short frenulum, cleft palate, Pierre Robin syndrome).

    l. Cracked or damaged nipples that prevent effective milk removal (Evans & Heads, 1995; Foxman et al., 2002).

    m. Breast pump use (Foxman et al., 2002).

19. Hyperlactation.

    a. Livingstone et al. (1996) describe several factors of maternal hyperlactation consisting of a high rate of milk synthesis and an abundant milk supply.

20. Cracked or damaged nipples.

    a. Cracked or damaged nipples that prevent effective milk removal are often thought to contribute to mastitis (Evans & Heads, 1995).

    b. Research suggests the possibility of an ascending infection (Livingstone et al., 1996).

    c. However, studies by Kawada et al. (2003) found that methicillin-resistant *S. aureus* (MRSA) or methicillin-sensitive *S. auerus* may be transmitted between healthy lactating mothers without mastitis and their infants by breastfeeding.

21. Maternal stress and/or fatigue.
   a. Riordan and Nichols (1990) state that the most common factor that women associated with mastitis was fatigue; this retrospective recall helps identify a facilitating condition rather than a cause.
   b. Wambach (2003) also identified the burden mastitis places on women.
22. Use of nipple creams.
   a. It has been hypothesized that the use of creams and lotions alters the pH of the nipple and areolar epithelium, blocks the glands of Montgomery, or alters their secretions, thus reducing the natural protective factors of the areola.
   b. Use also may indicate the presence of sore or damaged nipples and could appear as one of a cluster of situations or conditions simply associated with mastitis.
   c. Jonsson and Pulkkinen (1994) found that the use of a nipple cream several times a day was associated with an increased incidence of mastitis.
   d. Brent et al. (1998) discontinued the study on moist wound healing because of significantly more infections in the study group using hydrogel dressings.

D. Recurrent mastitis.
   1. Usually caused by delayed or inadequate treatment of the initial mastitis.
   2. Condition most frequently recurs when:
      a. Bacteria are resistant or not sensitive to the prescribed antibiotic.
      b. Antibiotics are not continued long enough.
      c. Mother stopped nursing on the affected side.
      d. The initial cause of the mastitis was not addressed (such as milk stasis).
   3. Clinicians can recommend that the mother continues to feed (or pump) on the affected side, that she take a full 10- to 14-day course of antibiotics, and that the cause or precipitating factors be identified and remedied (Hale & Berens, 2002).
   4. At the first recurrence, Lawrence and Lawrence (2005) recommend milk cultures as well as cultures of the infant's nasopharynx and oropharynx.
      a. Other family members can be cultured as necessary to identify the source of the bacteria to keep it from re-infecting the mother.
      b. Culture and sensitivity testing is important to determine that the proper antibiotic is given.
      c. Nasal carriers of S. aureus should be identified and can be treated with mupirocin 2% (Bactroban nasal ointment) (Amir, 2002).
      d. Lawrence and Lawrence (2005) also state that if the infection is chronic, low-dose antibiotics can be instituted for the duration of the lactation (erythromycin 500 mg/day).
      e. Mothers with a history of mastitis in previous lactations need to be especially vigilant in preventing milk stasis and in ensuring optimal positioning and latch-on of the baby.

f. Ultrasound examination of the breast is used when either a cyst or an abscess is suspected. If the breast shows a fluid-filled cavity, an abscess is likely to be present.

E. Prevention of mastitis.

1. Begins with accurate breastfeeding education and information.
   a. The lactation consultant needs to enable the mother to be able to confidently feed her infant and to recognize and implement management of problems such as mastitis.

2. Such education should include:
   a. Importance of early, frequent, unrestricted access to the breast.
   b. Optimal positioning of the baby at the breast.
   c. Individual mother's unique breast storage capacity and feeding pattern.
   d. Early signs and symptoms of mastitis.
   e. Common predisposing factors.

3. Twenty-four-hour rooming in at the hospital, which promotes the prompt recognition of infant feeding cues, reduces skipped feedings (especially at night), and leads to more frequent breast drainage during the early days.

4. Avoiding the use of pacifiers, which displaces sucking from the breast; this situation causes the breasts to remain full of milk as the time between breastfeeds increases.

5. Recognition and prompt attention of early warning signs that lead to milk stasis.

6. Plugged milk ducts can be massaged during the feed/expression to encourage the removal of the plug and enhance milk flow.

7. If a baby remains an inefficient feeder for whatever reason, the mother may need to hand express or pump following feeds to ensure adequate breast drainage and to provide additional milk for the baby. The mother can also use alternate massage/breast compression to improve milk drainage if the infant is unable to drain the breast adequately.

8. Adequate rest, help around the house and with other children, good nutrition, and proper hand washing before manual expression are common guidelines that can contribute to better overall health of the mother.

9. Limited milk expression might be needed if the baby abruptly starts sleeping for longer periods at night or if there is a substantial decrease in the number of breastfeedings for any reason.

10. Mothers who have a history of mastitis in previous lactations or women who have undergone breast surgery will need to be especially vigilant in preventing milk stasis and in ensuring proper positioning and latch-on of the baby.

F. Management of mastitis.

1. While antibiotics treat the infection, they do not treat the underlying cause of mastitis.
   a. If a mother develops infectious mastitis, then symptomatic treatments and antibiotic therapy must be joined by the third part of the intervention plan: identification and treatment of the underlying cause.
   b. Failure to do so can lead to recurrent mastitis.

2. Clinical assessment.
   a. Because milk stasis is the primary contributor to both inflammation and infection in the lactating breast, a lactation history is crucial in determining the underlying cause.
   b. Feed assessment should ensure optimal attachment and milk transfer.

3. Management plan.
   a. Supportive counseling.
   b. Bed rest as much as can be managed.
   c. Increase fluid intake.
   d. Analgesic/antipyretic (Acetaminophen, Paracetamol).
   e. A more rapid reduction of inflammation may be seen by treatment with a nonsteroidal anti-inflammatory drug such as ibuprofen.
   f. Warm compresses prior to feeds if milk release appears to be delayed.
   g. Continue feeding on both breasts, including MRSA mastitis (Lawrence, 2005).
      i. Begin the feed on the affected side unless the breast is so painful that latch is impossible.
      ii. The rationale for this is that most babies will suck more vigorously and effectively on the first side.
   h. Use warm moist packs or cold/cabbage compresses between feeds, whichever gives greatest comfort (WHO, 2000).
   i. If there is no improvement within 12 to 24 hours, if her symptoms worsen, or the woman has multiple risk factors such as bilateral nipple damage, previous mastitis history, or unwell baby, then the mother needs immediate referral to her physician for antibiotic therapy. Ensure that an appropriate length of antibiotic treatment is prescribed to prevent recurrence or possible abscess formation.
   j. Other comfort measures.
      i. Immersing the affected breast in warm water before feeding.
      ii. Utilizing gravity by lying in a bath of hot water with the affected breast hanging.
      iii. Feeding in a hands-and-knees body position.
      iv. Ultrasound's efficacy is more likely to be from the radiant heat or massage than from the ultra-wave emitting crystal (McLachlan et al., 1991).

G. Microbiology.

1. Breast milk is seldom obtained for routine culture and sensitivity testing for appropriate antibiotic prescribing.

2. Culture and sensitivity testing should be undertaken if the following situations occur:

   a. There is no response to antibiotics within two days.

   b. If the mastitis recurs more than twice.

   c. If it occurs while the mother is still in hospital. Globally, MRSA is becoming more common both in the hospital setting and in the community.

3. Severe or unusual cases.

   a. Because *S. aureus* is most commonly associated with breast infections, choices of antibiotics are generally penicillinase-resistant penicillins or cephalosporins, which are effective against *S. aureus*.

   b. Common drugs of choice are dicloxacillin and flucloxacillin; other antibiotics that may be used include erythromycin, nafcillin, and clindamycin.

   c. In streptococcal infections (often bilateral mastitis), penicillin might be preferable.

   d. In the case of a penicillin allergy, erythromycin would be the drug of choice.

4. Mothers who are treated with antibiotics for mastitis might subsequently develop Candidiasis (Amir & Hoover, 2002; Amir et al., 1996).

H. Breast abscess.

1. Can be a complication of mastitis.

2. Almost always follows inappropriate/ineffective management of mastitis (Brodribb, 2004; WHO, 2000).

3. An abscess is a localized collection of pus that the body walls off; once encapsulated, it must be surgically drained/aspirated (Benson, 1989; O'Hara & Dexter, & Fox, 1996).

4. Risk factors.

   a. Prior mastitis.

   b. A delay in therapy.

   c. Noncompliance of antibiotic therapy.

   d. Inappropriate choice of antibiotics or insufficient length of treatment.

   e. Antibiotic resistance.

   f. Failure to drain the affected breast.

   g. Avoiding breastfeeding on the affected side.

   h. Abrupt weaning.

5. Benson and Goodman (1970) classified abscesses as follows:

   a. Subareolar (superficial and near the nipple) 23%.

   b. Intramammary unilocular (a single area of pus deep in the breast and away from the nipple) 12%.

   c. Submammary multilocular (having multiple sites of pus within the abscess) 65%.

6. The most common offending organism is *S. aureus*, although other organisms are occasionally cultured from an abscess.

7. Prevention of an abscess resides on a continuum.
   a. Efficient milk transfer from breast to baby.
   b. Avoidance and/or intervention for milk stasis.
   c. Quick relief of breast inflammation.
   d. The prompt treatment of breast infection, which includes continued and frequent nursing or pumping on the affected side.
   e. Maternal education regarding gradual rather than abrupt weaning.
   f. Health professional and maternal education regarding type, duration, and compliance with antibiotic prescribing.

8. It is not always possible to confirm or exclude the presence of an abscess by clinical examination alone.

9. Mammography might not reveal an abscess due to extreme tenderness of the breast and very dense tissue.

10. Ultrasound (diagnostic).
   a. Can exclude the presence of an abscess and thereby avoid unnecessary surgery (Christensen et al., 2005).
   b. Can confirm the existence of the abscess and indicate a suitable site for the incision/aspiration (Hayes, Michell, & Nunnerley, 1991).
   c. Ultrasound-guided aspiration is less invasive than traditional surgery and has a high rate of success (Christensen et al., 2005; Dixon, 1988; Karstrup et al., 1993).
   d. Mothers can breastfeed throughout the course of ultrasound-guided needle aspiration drainage and possibly avoid surgery, admission to the hospital, and separation from their baby and families.

11. Surgical drainage of a breast abscess in some cases may be the necessary method of management.

12. Weaning or inhibiting lactation might hinder the rapid resolution of the abscess by producing increasingly viscid fluid that tends to promote rather than reduce breast engorgement.

13. The baby is not affected with continued breastfeeding unless the surgical site prevents optimal attachment/latch; pumping may be initially necessary.
   a. Some babies, however, might refuse to feed from the affected side due to a change in the taste of the milk.

b. Following the onset of mastitis, changes in protein, carbohydrate, and electrolyte concentrations of milk from the affected breast have been observed.

c. In particular, there is a decreased level of lactose and a marked rise in the concentrations of sodium and chloride; this situation has the temporary effect of causing the milk to taste salty.

d. The decreased level of lactose will also cause a decrease in volume of breast milk produced (Connor, 1979; Prosser & Hartmann, 1983).

I. Galactocele.

1. A benign cyst in the ducts of the breast that contains a milky fluid; often called a *milk retention cyst.*

2. Presence of a galactocele should not interrupt breastfeeding (Merewood & Philipp, 2001).

3. Contents of the cyst at first are pure milk but change to a thickened cheesy or oily consistency.

4. Cyst is smooth and rounded and might cause milk to ooze from the nipple when it is pressed.

5. Thought to be caused by the blockage of a milk duct.

6. Cyst can be aspirated but usually refills with milk.

7. If deemed necessary, it can be surgically removed under local anesthesia without interfering or interrupting breastfeeding; some spontaneously resolve.

8. Diagnosis can be made with ultrasound (Stevens et al., 1997).

J. Duct ectasia.

1. Also known as comedo mastitis, varicocele tumor, or granulomatous mastitis (Dixon et al.,1996).

2. Most common cause of a bilateral, multiduct, multicolored, intermittent sticky nipple discharge (Brodribb, 2006).

3. Starts as dilatation of the terminal ducts (within 2–3 cm of the nipple); can occur in pregnancy, but is most commonly seen between 35 and 40 years of age.

4. An irritating lipid forms in the ducts, producing an inflammatory reaction and nipple discharge.

5. Women complain of burning, itching, pain, and swelling of the nipple and areola, which must be differentiated from symptoms of *Candida.*

6. A palpable, wormlike mass might develop as the condition progresses that mimics cancer, with chronic inflammation leading to fibrosis.

7. Surgery is not indicated unless the condition becomes severe and bleeding commences from the nipple.

8. Lactation can aggravate this condition but is not contraindicated.

K. Fibrocystic disease.

1. Also known as benign breast disease, cystic mastitis, mammary dysplasia, fibrocystic mastopathy, and chronic cystic mastopathy (Coomes & McIntyre, 1994; Norwood, 1990; Olsen & Gordon, 1990).

2. This condition is benign.

3. Palpable irregularities in breast tissue can be felt in varying degrees in response to the normal menstrual cycle.
   a. These occur as proliferations of the alveolar system under hormonal influence.

4. Women might experience pain, tenderness, palpable thickenings, and nodules of varying sizes.

5. This condition might regress during pregnancy and does not contraindicate breastfeeding.

6. Some women describe varying degrees of relief from the condition when they eliminate caffeine from their diet and take vitamin E supplements.

L. Other lumps, cysts, and discharges.

1. Intraductal papilloma is a benign tumor or wart-like growth on the lining of a duct that bleeds as it erodes.

2. The discharge is usually spontaneous from a single duct, and a nontender lump might be felt under the areola.

3. After serious disease has been ruled out, breastfeeding can continue.
   a. Mothers are usually advised to pump the affected breast until the milk is clear of blood and continue breastfeeding on the other side.
   b. If the baby tolerates the milk, many can simply continue breastfeeding.
   c. The baby's stools might contain black flecks or become discolored and tarry temporarily.

4. If the discharge does not stop, the affected duct can be surgically removed.

5. Sometimes the first sign of this condition is when the baby spits up blood or when a mother who is pumping sees blood or pink-tinged milk.

6. This condition is extremely upsetting to the mother; infant disease can be ruled out by checking the regurgitated blood for fetal or adult hemoglobin (Apt test) to determine from whom the blood came.

M. Breast cancer.

1. Inflammatory breast cancer must be differentiated from mastitis and plugged ducts.

2. Lumps that do not disappear in a couple of days, that are fixed with no clearly defined margins, and a pink slightly swollen breast that does not resolve with frequent breastfeeding or anti-inflammatory/antibiotic medications should be evaluated by a physician.

3. The majority of nipple discharges in women of childbearing age are not clinically concerning and require no specific treatment.

4. Serous or blood-stained discharges, especially if the discharge is coming from one duct only, need prompt referral and evaluation.

5. Approximately 1% to 3% of masses diagnosed during pregnancy and lactation are malignant.

6. Ductal carcinoma in situ may present as bloodstained nipple discharge with abnormal cells identified on cytology.

7. Paget disease of the nipple is a superficial manifestation of an underlying breast malignancy and is about 1% to 3% of all breast cancers.
   a. It appears as a unilateral, well demarcated, red, scaly plaque involving the nipple or areola.
   b. The mother might also complain of a serous or blood-tinged discharge, pain, crusting, itching, burning, skin thickening, redness, ulceration, or nipple retraction.
   c. There is an underlying breast mass about 60% of the time.
   d. Lesion tends to appear on the nipple first and then spread to the areola.

8. Prominent masses need prompt evaluation; mammography might be difficult to interpret; fine needle biopsy can be performed with minimal problems during lactation; ultrasound or magnetic resonance imagery can be used to confirm a solid mass.

9. Treatment might include surgery, chemotherapy, and radiation therapy.

10. Infants are usually weaned from the breast if chemotherapy is necessary.

11. Young women who are treated with breast-conserving therapy and radiation for early stage cancer might experience subsequent full-term pregnancies and successful breastfeeding on the untreated breast, and some women may successfully breastfeed on the treated breast.

12. The milk volume of the treated breast might be diminished.

13. Sometimes a baby will refuse to nurse from a cancerous breast, which is the first clue that a problem exists.

14. There is compelling evidence that breastfeeding is protective against developing premenopausal and probably postmenopausal breast cancer (Zheng et.al., 2000).
   a. There is convincing evidence of a dose-response effect, with longer duration and more exclusive breastfeeding being more protective.
   b. A review of 47 studies carried out in 30 countries indicated that the relative risk of breast cancer decreased by 4.3% for every 12 months of breastfeeding (Beral, 2002).

N. Augmentation mammoplasty.

1. Implants for breast augmentation are done for a variety of reasons, such as asymmetric breasts, hypoplastic breasts, breast reconstruction from surgery, or more commonly to simply have bigger breasts.

2. Breasts undergoing augmentation might lack functional breast tissue, so the reason for the augmentation will impact breastfeeding management.

3. Some augmentation procedures are done on adolescents.

4. Lactation success will depend on the surgical technique used and if the breasts have sufficient functional breast tissue.
   a. Infrasubmammary procedure, where the incision is made under the breast.
   b. Periareolar, where the incision goes around the areola.
   c. An axillary incision near the armpit.
   d. Women who have a periareolar incision are at the highest risk for milk insufficiency.

5. All women who have had augmentation surgery face the possibility of this problem, not only from the site of the incision but also from nerve disruption and pressure from the implant on breast structures.

6. Mothers need close follow-up and strong encouragement to breastfeed early and often, paying close attention to engorgement and infant weight gain, especially in mothers who have insufficient glandular tissue.

7. Women who received silicone implants are usually concerned about the leakage of silicone into breast milk.
   a. For the most part, silicone implants seem to pose little hazard to the breastfed baby (Hale, 2006).
   b. Silicon measurements of infant formula show vastly higher amounts in artificial baby milks than in breast milk from women who have implants.
   c. Most implants used currently are saline-filled, but silicone implants will reappear, since the U.S. Food and Drug Administration has cleared them for use.

O. Breast reduction mammoplasty.

1. Women may have breast reduction for aesthetic reasons or because of large breasts that cause shoulder and back pain that interfere with normal activities and relationships.

2. Full breastfeeding might not always be possible after reduction surgery, depending on the amount of tissue removed and the surgical technique used (Harris, Stevens, & Frieberg, 1992; Marshall, Callam, & Nicholson, 1994; Neifert et al., 1990).

3. Mothers have the best chance of lactation with the least amount of tissue removed, if the fourth intercostal nerve that branches to the breast and areola is left intact, and if the pedicle technique is used during surgery.

4. Two techniques are commonly used for breast-reduction surgery.
   a. The pedicle technique leaves the nipple and areola attached to the breast gland on a stalk of tissue. A wedge is removed from the undersides of the breast because, for the most part, the breast tissue, blood supply, and some nerves remain intact, and breastfeeding might have varying degrees of success.
   b. The free nipple technique (autotransplantation of the nipple) involves removing the nipple/areola entirely so that larger amounts of breast tissue can be removed; the blood supply to the nipple/areola is severed and nerve damage occurs; this situation might result in diminished sensations in the nipple/areola.

5. Full breastfeeding is a possibility with the pedicle technique but not with the free nipple technique.

6. Mothers who have breast reduction surgery should be encouraged to breastfeed early and frequently to stimulate the breasts to provide as much breast milk as possible.
   a. Babies might need to be supplemented.
   b. Supplementation can often be done at the breast with a tube feeding device so that the mother and baby can enjoy each other and the breastfeeding experience.

P. Dermatitis.

1. Dermatitis may affect any area of skin on the body including the breasts (Whitaker-Worth et al., 2000).

2. Dermatitis may be caused by contact with an allergen, viral dermatitis may be caused by herpes simplex infection, and bacterial dermatitis may occur with impetigo (Thorley, 2000) or staphylococcus infection.

3. There is also a case report of a mother developing dermatitis on the nipple and areola after having developed an allergy to her infant's saliva (Kirkman, 1997).

4. Nipple eczema.
   a. Tends to present with redness, crusting, oozing, scales, fissures, blisters, excoriations (slits), or lichenification.
   b. Mothers might complain of burning and itching, and the eczema can extend onto and beyond the areola.
   c. This condition is usually treated with topical steroids and can occur on both nipples.
   d. When eczema appears on just one nipple, referral should be considered to rule out Paget's disease, a superficial manifestation of underlying breast malignancy.

5. Allergic contact dermatitis.
   a. Can present in a similar manner.

b. Arises from the use of lanolin, emollients, or ointments containing beeswax or chamomile.

c. The lactation consultant should ask what is being put on the nipples that might be causing this problem.

6. Psoriasis can affect any area of the breast and can present as a pink plaque that appears moist with minimal or no scale.

7. Seborrheic dermatitis can occur on the breast, most commonly in the mammary folds.

   a. It exhibits a greasy white or yellow scale on a reddened base and can be treated topically with ketoconazole, zinc, or selenium sulfide preparations.

8. Herpes simplex with active oozing lesions on the nipple or areola requires a culture of the lesions and immediate treatment.

   a. Breastfeeding on that side should be interrupted until the lesions heal.

Q. Mammary candidiasis (*thrush*).

1. The offending organism *Candida albicans* is a commensal organism, that is, we live in harmony with this organism until a change disrupts the balance between the fungus and its host, the human body.

   a. The best example of this disruption is the use of antibiotics and the often-resultant vaginal overgrowth of *Candida* (Amir & Hoover, 2002).

   b. It can affect the breastfeeding dyad in many ways (Heinig, Francis, & Pappagianis, 1999).

   c. The organism *C. albicans*, found frequently in the vagina and gastrointestinal tract, is the most frequent cause of thrush in the oral cavity of a baby and for the superficial and ductal infection of the breast.

2. Diagnosis is frequently based on a cluster of symptoms rather than on laboratory evidence or a standard technique.

3. Intact dry skin is protective against *C. albicans*, while the warm moist nipple possibly damaged or eroded from poor position or improper sucking is a perfect host for colonization and infection.

4. *C. albicans* can exist in a number of forms, from the spherical cells on the surface of the nipple to the invasive form that is capable of penetrating cell walls.

5. Infant symptoms of oral thrush range from no visible symptoms to a white plaque coating of the tongue to cottage cheese-like fungal colonies on the tongue, buccal mucosa, soft palate, gums, or tonsils.

6. These plaques, if wiped, might reveal a reddened or bleeding base.

7. A fiery red diaper/nappy rash with glistening red patches, clear margins, and pustules that enlarge, appear outside the rash, and rupture, resulting in scaly and peeling skin, might be present on the baby.

8. An infected nipple might appear red, shiny, and have sloughing skin or be merely pink; the areola might have irregular shiny confluences.

9. Mothers complain of burning, itching, and stinging pain in the nipples that persists between feedings for many days and that is unresponsive to position changes or sucking corrections.

10. Some mothers also complain of burning and shooting pain in the breasts, which needs to be differentiated from a bacterial infection or nipple vasospasm that can cause the same symptoms (Amir et al., 1996; Anderson, Held, & Wright, 2004).

11. Skin swabs of the nipple/areola can be examined under a microscope in a potassium hydroxide wet mount for the presence of superficial candidiasis.

12. This examination enables the proper use of antifungals, because their excessive use has produced resistant strains.
    a. Culturing can confirm the *Candida* species.
    b. Milk cultures are difficult because milk components can inhibit fungal growth.
    c. A new laboratory technique that uses the addition of iron to counteract the action of lactoferrin has been shown to reduce the likelihood of false-negative results and improve the accuracy of detecting *Candida* in human milk (Morrill et al., 2003).

13. Both mother and baby should be treated simultaneously, even if the baby shows no signs in his or her mouth.

14. More than 40% of *Candida* strains are resistant to topical Nystatin (usually the first medication prescribed); other topical treatments can follow, including clotrimazole and miconazole (Amir & Hoover, 2002).
    a. Gentian Violet (*Methylrosanilinium Chloride*). Gentian Violet is classified as a disinfectant/germicide. The previously used common practice of painting the baby's mouth and the mother's nipple with Methylrosanilinium Chloride (Gentian Violet) has been discontinued in some countries (e.g., Australia, United Kingdom [UK]). In the UK it is recommended that methylrosanilinium chloride not be applied to mucous membranes or open wounds. "Topical application of methylrosanilinium chloride can produce irritation and ulceration of mucous membranes" (Micromedex Healthcare Series, 2007). In the United States and Canada some authors continue to recommend 0.5–1.0% solutions applied once daily for 3–5 days as a simple, effective treatment for both the baby and the mother (Hale, 2006; Newman, 2003).

15. Pacifiers are a continuous source of reinfection, so all items coming into contact with the baby's mouth need to be boiled, bleached, or washed daily (Amir & Hoover, 2002).

16. Iatrogenic factors increase the risk of *Candida*, including the use of antibiotics, oral contraceptives, and steroids.

17. If all topical medications fail to bring relief, systemic oral fluconazole can be prescribed for 14 to 28 days.

R. Abnormal nipple tenderness (sore) and damage.

 1. In late pregnancy and early breastfeeding, there is normal tenderness as nipple sensitivity is heightened. This peaks on days 3 to 6 postpartum and is relieved as the volume of milk increases.

 2. Women feel nipple discomfort as the collagen fibers are stretched with early sucking. This decreases as nipple flexibility increases.

 3. Increased vascularity of the nipple and normal epithelial denudement can occur with optimal latch but will increase initial tenderness.

 4. Transient latch-on pain may occur from lack of established keratin layer on the nipple epithelium.

 5. Prior to milk ejection, unrelieved negative pressure will increase nipple tenderness. This is relieved with milk ejection (Heads & Higgins, 1995).

 6. Protracted tenderness that lasts longer than a week and is felt throughout a feed is not normal and requires intervention.

 7. Skin color, hair color, prenatal preparation, or limiting sucking time at the breast are not related to the discomfort experienced (Renfrew, Woolridge, & Ross McGill, 2000). Pain during a feed is most commonly a result of incorrect latch.

 8. Nipple pain/protractility and baby's oral anatomy and functional suck will require assessment, review, and/or correct positioning.

 9. Eliminate diagnosis of impetigo, eczema, C. albicans overgrowth.

 10. Observance of nipple shape as the baby detaches is diagnostic and may present as:
     a. Horizontal or vertical red or white stripes.
     b. Asymmetrical stretching.
     c. Blisters.
     d. Fissures, cracks, or bleeding.
     e. Sharp pain experienced in one or both nipples post-feed.
     f. Blanching (vasospasm).

 11. Nipple pain will be aggravated by engorgement and the level of existing nipple damage.

 12. The individual response of the mother will mediate nipple pain.

 13. Some mothers will present with a long history of acutely sensitive nipples prior to pregnancy.

 14. Sexual abuse and domestic violence may be a complicating factor (Kendall-Tackett, 1998).

 15. Nipple shields should not be considered as a part of routine management for nipple damage but may be a useful tool if maternal and infant anatomy prevent optimal latch or if the history of acute sensitivity and/or sexual abuse is a complicating factor in degree of nipple pain experienced.

16. Vasospasm of the nipple (a Raynaud-like condition of the nipple).
   a. Described as causing extreme pain, stinging and burning of the nipple.
   b. The shape of the nipple post-feed can indicate proper latch but pain is evident.
   c. Nipple appears blanched post-feed, then the classic triphasic color change of white to blue to red is apparent.
   d. Babies who bite at the breast, clench their jaw, or chew on the nipple can cause nipple spasms (spasms of the blood vessels within the nipple).
   e. Symptomatic management of vasospasm that has shown to be of benefit (Anderson et al., 2004; Lawlor-Smith & Lawlor-Smith, 1997) includes:
      i. Initiate the milk ejection reflex or express drops of colostrum before putting the baby to the breast.
      ii. Feed on the less tender side first.
      iii. Review and/or correct positioning.
      iv. Warm compresses.
      v. Avoid cold air.
      vi. Reduction of nicotine and caffeine intake.
      vii. Pain relief.
      viii. Vitamin B_6.
      ix. Calcium supplementation.
      x. Magnesium supplementation.
      xi. Nifedipine.

References

ALCA News. White spots (Corpora amylacia). 1992;3:8–9.

Amir L, Hoover K. Candidiasis and breastfeeding. In: *Lactation Consultant Series Two, Unit 6*. Schaumburg, IL: La Leche League International; 2002.

Amir L. Breastfeeding and *Staphylococcus aureus*: three case reports. *Breastfeeding Rev.* 2002;10:15–18.

Amir LH, Garland SM, Dennerstein L, Fariah SJ. *Candida albicans*: is it associated with nipple pain in lactating women? *Gynecol Obstet Invest.* 1996;41:30–34.

Anderson JE, Held N, Wright K. Raynaud's phenomenon of the nipple: a treatable cause of painful breastfeeding. *Pediatrics.* 2004;113:360–364.

Barnes L. Cryotherapy: putting injury on ice. *Physician Sports Med.* 1979;7:130–136.

Benson EA. Management of breast abscesses. *World J Surg.* 1989;13:753–756.

Benson EA, Goodman MA. Incision with primary suture in the treatment of acute puerperal breast abscess. *Br J Surg.* 1970;57:55–58.

Beral V. Breast cancer and breastfeeding: collaborative reanalysis of individual data of 47 epidemiological studies in 30 countries, including 50,302 women with breast cancer and 96,973 women without the disease. *Lancet.* 2002;360:187–195. Comments in *Lancet.* 2002; 360:203–210; 2003:361:176–177.

Brent N, Rudy SJ, Redd B, Rudy TE, Roth LA. Sore nipples in breast-feeding women: a clinical trial of wound dressings vs conventional care. *Arch Pediatr Adolesc Med.* 1998;152:1077–1082.

Brodribb W, ed. *Breastfeeding Management in Australia.* 3rd ed. Malvern, Victoria, Australia: Australian Breastfeeding Association; 2004.

Brodribb W. Nipple Discharge. Hot Topic. Malvern, Victoria, Australia: Australian Breastfeeding Association, Lactation Resource Centre. Available at: http://www.lrc.asn.au/publications.html. Accessed July 22, 2006.

Buescher ES, Hair PS. Human milk anti-inflammatory component contents during acute mastitis. *Cell Immunol.* June 15, 2001;210(2):87–95.

Christensen AF, Al-Suliman N, Nielsen KR, et al. Ultrasound-guided drainage of breast abscesses: results in 51 patients. *Br J Radiol.* 2005;78:186–188.

Connor AE. Elevated levels of sodium and chloride in milk from mastitic breasts. *Pediatrics.* 1979;63:910–911.

Coomes F, McIntyre E. Fibrocystic breast disease. In: *Topics in Breastfeeding Set VI.* Melbourne, Australia: Lactation Resource Centre; 1994.

Cotterman JK. Reverse pressure softening: a simple tool to prepare areola for easier latching during engorgement. *J Hum Lact.* 2004;20:227–237.

Daly SEJ, Hartmann PE. Infant demand and milk supply. Part 2: The short-term control of milk synthesis in lactating women. *J Hum Lact.*1995;11:27–37.

Dixon JM. Repeated aspiration of breast abscesses in lactating women. *Br Med J.* 1988;297:1517–1518.

Dixon JM, Ravisekar O, Chetty U, Anderson TJ. Periductal mastitis and duct ectasia: Different conditions with different aetiologies. *Br J Surg.* 1996;83:820–822.

Evans M, Heads J. Mastitis: Incidence, prevalence and cost. *Breastfeeding Rev.* 1995;3:65–72.

Fetherston C. Characteristics of lactation mastitis in a Western Australian cohort. *Breastfeeding Rev.* 1997a;5:5–11.

Fetherston C. Management of lactation mastitis in a Western Australian cohort. *Breastfeeding Rev.* 1997b;5:13–19.

Fetherston C. Risk factors for lactation mastitis. *J Hum Lact.* 1998;14:101–109.

Fetherston C. Mastitis in lactating women: physiology or pathology? *Breastfeeding Rev.* 2001;9:5–12.

Foxman B, Schwartz K, Looman SJ. Breastfeeding practices and lactation mastitis. *Soc Sci Med.* 1994;38:755–761.

Foxman B, D'Arcy H, Gillespie B, et al. Lactation mastitis: occurrence and medical management among 946 breastfeeding women in the United States. *Am J Epidemiol.* 2002;155:103–114.

Freed GL, Landers S, Schanler RJ. A practical guide to successful breastfeeding management. *Am J Dis Child.* 1991;145:917–921.

Glover R. The engorgement enigma. *Breastfeeding Rev.* 1998;6:31–34.

Hale TW. *Medications and Mothers' Milk*. 12th ed. Amarillo, TX: Hale Publishing; 2006:753–754.

Hale TW, Berens P. *Clinical Therapies in Breastfeeding Patients*. Amarillo, TX: Pharmasoft Publishing; 2002.

Harris LMD, Stevens FM, Frieberg A. Is breastfeeding possible after reduction mammoplasty? *J Plast Reconstr Surg*. 1992;89:836–839.

Hayes R, Michell M, Nunnerley HB. Acute inflammation of the breast—the role of breast ultrasound in diagnosis and management. *Clin Radiol*. 1991;44:253–256.

Heads J, Higgins L. Perceptions and correlates of nipple pain. *Breastfeeding Rev*. 1995;3:59–64.

Heinig MJ, Francis J, Pappagianis D. Mammary candidosis in lactating women. *J Hum Lact*. 1999;15:281–288.

Hill PD, Humenick SS. The occurrence of breast engorgement. *J Hum Lact*. 1994;10:79–86.

Hocutt JE, Jaffe R, Rylander CR, Beebe JK. Cryotherapy in ankle sprains. *Am J Sports Med*. 1982;10:317–319.

Humenick SS, Hill PD, Anderson MA. Breast engorgement: patterns and selected outcomes. *J Hum Lact*. 1994;10:87–93.

Jonsson S, Pulkkinen MO. Mastitis today: Incidence, prevention and treatment. *Ann Chir Gynaecol Suppl*. 1994;208:84–87.

Karstrup S, Solvig J, Nolsoe CP, et al. Acute puerperal breast abscess: US-guided drainage. *Radiology*. 1993;188:807–809.

Kawada M, Okuzumi K, Hitomi S, Sugishita C. Transmission of *Staphylococcus aureus* between healthy, lactating mothers and their infants by breastfeeding. *J Hum Lact*. 2003;19:411–417.

Kendall-Tackett K. Breastfeeding and the sexual abuse survivor. *J Hum Lact*. 1998; 14:125–130.

Kirkman W. Breast dermatitis. *Le Leche League News, Great Britain*. 1997;97:6–7.

Lawlor-Smith LS, Lawlor-Smith CL. Vasospasm of the nipple: a manifestation of Raynaud's phenomenon; case reports. *BMJ*. 1997;314:644–645.

Lawrence RA, Lawrence RM. *Breastfeeding: A Guide for the Medical Profession*. 6th ed. St. Louis: Elsevier/C.V. Mosby; 2005.

Livingstone VH, Willis CE, Berkowitz J. Staphylococcus aureus and sore nipples. *Can Fam Physician*. 1996;42:654–659.

Marshall DR, Callam PP, Nicholson W. Breastfeeding after reduction mammoplasty. *Br J Plast Surg*. 1994;47:167–169.

Marti A, Feng Z, Altermatt HJ, Jaggi R. Milk accumulation triggers apoptosis of mammary epithelial cells. *Eur J Cell Biol*. 1997;73:158–165.

Matheson I, Aursnes I, Horgen M, et al. Bacteriological findings and clinical symptoms in relation to clinical outcome in puerperal mastitis. *Acta Obstet Gynecol Scand*. 1988;67:723–726.

McLachlan Z, Milne J, Lumley J, Walker B. Ultrasound treatment for breast engorgement: a randomised double blind trial. *Austr J Physiother*. 1991;37:23–29.

Merewood A, Philipp BL. *Breastfeeding Conditions and Disease: A Reference Guide.* Amarillo, TX: Pharmasoft Publishing; 2001.

Michie C, Lockie F, Lynn W. The challenge of mastitis. *Arch Disease in Childhood.* 2003; 88:818–821.

MICROMEDEX Healthcare Series, 2007. Drug Information Service. Available at: http:// www.micromedex.com.

Miller V, Riordan J. Treating postpartum breast edema with areolar compression. *J Hum Lact.* 2004;20:223–226.

Moon JL, Humenick SS. Breast engorgement: contributing variables and variables amenable to nursing intervention. *J Obstet Gynecol Neonatal Nurs.* 1989;18:309–315.

Morrill JM, Pappagianis D, Heinig MJ, et al. Detecting *Candida albicans* in human milk. *J Clin Microbiol.* 2003;41:475–478.

Neifert M, DeMarzo S, Seacat J, et al. The influence of breast surgery, breast appearance, and pregnancy-induced breast changes on lactation sufficiency as measured by infant weight gain. *Birth.* 1990;17:31–38.

Newman Jack. Handout #6: Using Gentian Violet. 2003. Available at: http://www. breastfeedingonline.com/6pdf.pdf. Accessed March 13, 2007.

Newton M, Newton N. Postpartum engorgement of the breast. *Am J Obstet Gynecol.* 1951;61:664–667.

Nguyen DD, Neville MC. Tight junction regulation in the mammary gland. *J Mammary Gland Biol Neoplasia.* 1998;3:233–246.

Niebyl JR, Spence MR, Parmley TH. Sporadic (non-epidemic) puerperal mastitis. *J Repro Med.* 1978;20:97–100.

Nikodem VC, Danziger D, Gebka N, et al. Do cabbage leaves prevent breast engorgement? A randomized, controlled study. *Birth.* 1993;20:61–64.

Norwood S. Fibrocystic breast disease: an update and review. *J Obstet Gynecol Neonatal Nurs.* 1990;129:116–121.

O'Hara RJ, Dexter SPL, Fox JN. Conservative management of infective mastitis and breast abscess after ultrasonographic assessment. *Br J Surg.* 1996;83:1413–1414.

Olsen G, Gordon R. Breast disorders in nursing mothers. *Am Fam Physician.* 1990;45:1509–1516.

Peaker M, Wilde CJ. Feedback control of milk secretion from milk. *J Mammary Gland Biol Neoplasia.* 1996;1:307–314.

Prentice A, Addey CVP, Wilde CJ. Evidence for local feedback control of human milk secretion. *Biochem Soc Trans.* 1989;15:122.

Prosser CG, Hartmann PE. Comparison of mammary gland function during the ovulatory menstrual cycle and acute breast inflammation in women. *Aust J Exp Biol Med Sci.* 1983;61:277–286.

Renfrew MJ, Woolridge MW, Ross McGill H. *Enabling Women to Breastfeed; a Review of Practices Which Promote or Inhibit Breastfeeding—with Evidence-based Guidance for Practice.* Leeds, UK: The Stationary Office, University of Leeds; 2000.

Riordan JM, Nichols FH. A descriptive study of lactation mastitis in long-term breastfeeding women. *J Hum Lact.* 1990;6:53–58.

Roberts KL. A comparison of chilled cabbage leaves and chilled gelpaks in reducing breast engorgement. *J Hum Lact.* 1995;11:17–20.

Roberts KL, Reiter M, Schuster D. Effects of cabbage leaf extract on breast engorgement. *J Hum Lact.* 1998;14:231–236.

Rosier W. Cool cabbage compresses. *Breastfeeding Rev.* 1988;12:28–31.

Stevens K, Burrell HC, Evans AJ, Sibbering DM. The ultrasound appearance of galactocoeles. *Br J Radiol.* 1997;70:239–241.

Thomsen AC, Housen KB, Moller BR. Leukocyte counts and microbiologic cultivation in the diagnosis of puerperal mastitis. *Am J Obstet Gynecol.* 1983;146:938–941.

Thorley V. Impetigo on the areola and nipple. *Breastfeeding Rev.* 2000;8:25–26.

Uvnäs-Moberg K. Oxytocin may mediate the benefits of positive social interaction and emotions. *Psychoneuroendocrinology.* 1998;23:(8):819–835.

Wambach KA. Lactation mastitis: a descriptive study of the experience. *J Hum Lact.* 2003;19:24–34.

Wambach K, Campbell SH, Gill SL, et al. Clinical lactation practice: 20 years of evidence. *J Hum Lact.* 2005;21:245–258.

Whitaker-Worth DL, Carlone V, Susser WS, et al. Dermatologic diseases of the breast and nipple. *J Am Acad Dermatol.* 2000;43:733–754.

Willumsen JF, Filteau SM, Coutsoudis A, Uebel KE, Newell ML, Tomkins AM. Subclinical mastitis as a risk factor for mother-infant HIV transmission. *Adv Exp Med Biol.* 2000;478:211–223.

Woolridge MW. Aetiology of sore nipples. *Midwifery.* 1986a;2:172–176.

Woolridge MW. The 'anatomy' of infant sucking. *Midwifery.* 1986b;2:164–171.

World Health Organisation (WHO). Mastitis: causes and management. Geneva: WHO; 2000.

Zheng T, Duan L, Liu Y, et al. Lactation reduces breast cancer risk in Shandong Province, China. *Am J Epidemiol.* 2000;152:1129–1135.

Suggested Readings

Brodribb W, ed. *Breastfeeding Management in Australia.* 3rd ed. Malvern, Victoria, Australia: Australian Breastfeeding Association; 2004.

Dixon JM, Mansel RE. ABC of breast disease. Symptoms, assessment and guidelines for referral. *Br Med J.* 1994;309:722–726.

Walia HS, Abraham TK, Shaikh H. Fungal mastitis: case report. *Acta Chir Scand.* 1987;153:133–135.

Walker M. Mastitis in Lactating Women. In: *Lactation Consultant Series 2*, revised. Schaumburg, IL: La Leche League International; 2004.

Hyperbilirubinemia and Hypoglycemia

Sallie Page-Goertz, MN, CPNP, IBCLC

OBJECTIVES

- Define and differentiate the characteristics of physiologic jaundice, breastfeeding-associated jaundice, pathologic jaundice, and breast milk jaundice.
- Describe the breastfeeding management of the infant who is experiencing jaundice.
- List strategies for the prevention of breastfeeding-associated jaundice.
- List the criteria for referral for medical evaluation.
- List the risk factors for the development of hypoglycemia.
- Describe breastfeeding management of an infant who has hypoglycemia.
- List measures for preventing hypoglycemia in a newborn infant.

Introduction

During the newborn period, two problems impact and are impacted by breastfeeding management: hyperbilirubinemia and hypoglycemia. Appropriate breastfeeding routines, awareness of the risk factors, and the continuous assessment of a newborn are critical elements in preventing or reducing morbidity from these two concerns.

Background Information

Hyperbilirubinemia is the presence of elevated bilirubin. *Jaundice* is the term used when there is yellow staining of the skin and sclera caused by abnormally high blood levels of the bile pigment bilirubin, irrespective of the cause.

Sections I through VI discuss issues related to indirect (unconjugated) hyperbilirubinemia, where increased bilirubin levels are caused by either increased bilirubin production, or decreased bilirubin metabolism/excretion. The terms *bilirubin* and *hyperbilirubinemia* refer to indirect bilirubin, unless indicated otherwise. Direct (conjugated) hyperbilirubinemia is caused by hepatocellular disorders such as hepatitis and biliary tree abnormalities such as biliary atresia. These disorders are considered if an infant/child has persistent hyperbilirubinemia, with an elevation of the direct bilirubin component, and are outside the scope of this discussion.

A spectrum of bilirubin-induced neurologic dysfunction results from bilirubin levels, which can cause damage primarily to the basal ganglia, central and peripheral neurologic pathways, hippocampus, brain stem nuclei for oculomotor function and the cerebellum). Damage can be minimal to severe. Extremely high levels of bilirubin can lead to *kernicterus*, which is chronic, irreversible brain damage. Clinical sequelae include movement disorders (dystonia and athetosis), abnormalities of gaze and other visual difficulties, auditory disorders (hearing loss, processing disorders) and dysplasia of the enamel of deciduous teeth (Bhutani, Johnson, & Keren, 2005). Fortunately, for many children who experience marked hyperbilirubinemia, sequelae may resolve over time (Harris et al., 2001). However, others may suffer irreversible neurologic damage as described above (Ip et al., 2004). Kernicterus should be a "never event" because it is completely preventable when evidence-based newborn care is provided.

Reports in the United States literature of infants experiencing complications from hyperbilirubinemia as well as concurrent dehydration and excessive weight loss are increasing (Hall, Simon, & Smith, 2000; Haberal & Gurakan, 2005; Seidman et al., 1995). The vast majority of the babies in these reports were breastfeeding (apparently ineffectively). In the majority of cases, recommended preventive care, monitoring, and/or follow-up care was not provided. Such cases are preventable when the mother-infant dyad receives evidence-based newborn care. Cases were also reported, although with less frequency, from other industrialized countries such as Canada, Denmark, Holland, and New Zealand (Kaplan & Hammerman, 2004). Neonatal hyperbilirubinemia causes significant morbidity/mortality in Africa as well (Udoma et al., 2001).

The American Academy of Pediatrics' (2004) updated guideline for prevention and treatment of hyperbilirubinemia recommends that all newborns have either a formal risk assessment performed, or a bilirubin level obtained prior to hospital dismissal. The guideline includes a risk stratification nomogram to assist the health care provider in evaluating the individual infant's potential of developing bilirubin levels that might require intervention (Figure 37-1). This risk nomogram requires a total serum bilirubin (or transcutaneous bilirubin [TcB] equivalent) along with the exact hour of age of the infant at the time of obtaining the sample. Petersen et al. (2005) reported that after the institution of a policy of obtaining a TcB prior to discharge, the mean number of readmissions for hyperbilirubinemia decreased significantly from 4.5 to 1.8 per 1000 births per month. It is not known at this time if these guidelines are appropriate for populations or systems of care dissimilar to that in the United States (Kaplan & Hammerman, 2005; Manning, 2005). Furthermore, performing a TcB on every newborn leads to a cost of $9,191,352 for prevention of one case of kernicterus in the United States (Suresh & Clark, 2004). If clinical guidelines for appropriate policies and practices of newborn care were in fact implemented, this type of expense could be avoided.

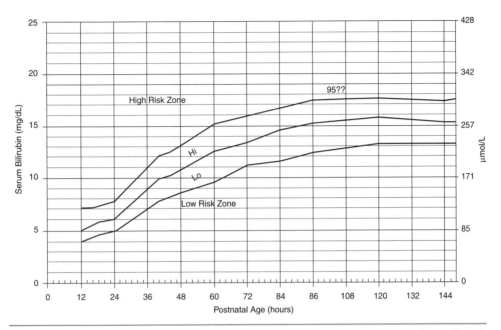

Figure 37-1   Risk Nomogram for Infants > 35 Weeks' Gestation. *Source*: Reproduced with permission from the American Academy of Pediatrics Subcommittee on Neonatal Hyperbilirubinemia. Management of hyperbilirubinemia in the newborn infant 35 or more completed weeks of gestation. *Pediatrics*. 2004:114:301.

Often, the lactation consultant is asked to evaluate and manage the breastfeeding of an infant who has hyperbilirubinemia during the first few days of life. Table 37-1 describes the most common causes of hyperbilirubinemia in the newborn. Jaundiced infants might present to the consultant's practice with family members who are unaware of the significance of jaundice. In certain situations, a jaundiced infant might also have excessive weight loss and other underlying health problems contributing to his or her problems with feeding. There might even be life-threatening situations due to associated dehydration and hypernatremia. The lactation consultant must work in collaboration with the infant's medical care provider in the management of the infant with hyperbilirubinemia.

Section VII examines hypoglycemia in newborn infants. It is of concern because of the detrimental effect that sustained hypoglycemia may have on the infant's neurologic/ developmental outcome. The definition of hypoglycemia is controversial because there are no firmly established guidelines establishing a specific blood glucose value for hypoglycemia. Cornblath and colleagues (2000) offer operational thresholds below which intervention should be considered; these are followed by many health care providers. Operational thresholds as recommended by Cornblath et al. may not

Table 37-1   Comparison of Common Causes of Indirect Hyperbilirubinemia in the Term Newborn Infant

	Physiologic Jaundice	Breastfeeding-Associated Jaundice	Breast-Milk Jaundice
Onset of clinical jaundice	48–72 hours	48–72 hours	5–10 days of age
Peak	Day 3–5	Day 3–5+	Day 15
Rate of rise	2 mg/dL/day	5 mg/dL/day	1–2 mg/dL/day
Cause	RBC breakdown	Starvation/delayed defecation	Unknown
Condition of infant	Thriving; normal weight loss; normal output; clinically jaundiced	Lethargic/fussy; excessive weight loss; ineffective feeding; scant urine/stool output; signs of dehydration	Thriving; clinically jaundiced
Breastfeeding management	Monitor in order to ensure effective breastfeeding and initiation of normal weight gain	Increase caloric intake; intervene to establish effective breastfeeding; assist with supplementation; stimulate milk supply	No intervention needed
Medical Management	Monitor; return visit at 72 hours of age; phototherapy per guidelines (seldom needed)	Phototherapy per guidelines; supplementation if indicated	Monitor bilirubin until stable; consider brief interruption of mother's milk feedings (preferable to avoid this strategy)

Source: Adapted from Page-Goertz, S and McCamman, S. *Hyperbilirubinemia in the Breastfed Infant, Lectures To Go.* Overland Park, Kansas: Best Beginnings Productions, 1996. Used with permission from Best Beginnings Productions.

be applicable to breastfed infants because of differences in metabolism. Despite their lower caloric intake, they have higher concentrations of ketone bodies than formula-fed babies that serve as alternative fuel (Cornblath et al., 2000).

Effective breastfeeding provides the normal newborn infant with sufficient calories to prevent hypoglycemia (Diwakar & Sasidhar, 2002). Healthy, large-for-gestational-age infants do not appear to be harmed by transient mild hypoglycemia (Brand et al., 2005). Certain infants have a higher risk for experiencing hypoglycemia. If risk factors are present, the infant's effective breastfeeding and intake of normal amounts of colostrum might not be sufficient to support the newborn's unusual metabolic demands; in these cases, a supplement might be required. The baby's primary health care provider will determine whether calories are best supplied as an oral supplement or by using intravenous glucose infusion.

Hypoglycemia is most likely to occur after the first two to three hours of birth, before fat metabolism has begun, and particularly if any other risk factors are present (Hoseth et al., 2000). Infants who are born prior to 38 completed weeks have limited glycogen reserves. Infants who are intrauterine growth-retarded or who are small for gestational-age have limited fat reserves. Infants of diabetic mothers quickly deplete their glycogen stores after birth due to hyperinsulinism, which is caused by producing large amounts of insulin in response to maternal hyperglycemia while in utero. Newborns who have persistent hypoglycemia in the first days of life require evaluation to determine the cause.

Incidence of hypoglycemia in healthy term infants is difficult to determine because a standard definition of hypoglycemia has not been used across studies. Reported rates using 1.8 mmol/L (32 mg/dL) range from 0.4% to 34%. Rates using 2.2 mmol/L (40 mg.dL) range from 4% to 40% (Hoseth et al., 2000).

Reports of admissions to a regional hospital in Kenya noted that of 280 neonatal admissions, 23% were hypoglycemic. Eighty-one percent of the hypoglycemic infants were under seven days of age (English et al., 2003). Hypoglycemia was correlated with weight of < 2500 grams and inability to breastfeed effectively. Infants with hypoglycemia (blood glucose less than 2.2 mmol (40 mg/dL) had much higher mortality as well.

A Nepalese study looked at incidence of hypoglycemia in nearly 600 infants born at the largest maternity hospital. In this hospital, maintaining a neutralthermic environment was problematic. Forty-one percent of newborn infants had mild hypoglycemia (< 2.6 mmol/L) and 11% had moderate hypoglycemia (< 2 mmol/L). Risk factors included delayed initiation of breastfeeding, and cold ambient temperatures. Feeding delay increased the risk of hypoglycemia at age 12 to 24 hours of age (Pal et al., 2000).

I. Bilirubin Physiology in the Normal Newborn

A. Red blood cells (RBCs) break down after birth with the transition to a higher-oxygen environment.

B. Bilirubin is one of the break-down products of these RBCs; it is released into the bloodstream.

C. Bilirubin is then bound to albumin in the bloodstream and carried to the liver, where it is conjugated with glucuronide.

D. Conjugated bilirubin is then excreted via the bile duct into the intestine.

E. Bilirubin is excreted through the stool.

II. Physiologic and Pathologic Hyperbilirubinemia

A. Physiologic jaundice is the normal increase in bilirubin associated with RBC breakdown after birth and immaturity of bilirubin metabolism systems. It is unusual for bilirubin levels in purely physiologic jaundice to reach the high risk zones (Herschel & Gartner, 2005).

1. Age and bilirubin.
   a. Bilirubin levels in normal newborns of at least 35 weeks gestation increase the most rapidly in the first 6 to 18 hours of life, and then less rapidly from 18 to 42 hours of life, followed by a slower increase until the peak is reached at 3 to 5 days of age.
   b. Decreased gestational age and exclusive breastfeeding were associated with higher bilirubin levels at 24, 48, 72, and 96 hours of age (Maisels & Kring, 2006).
   c. Near term infants (35–37 completed weeks) may have bilirubin levels that peak later, on day 5 to 7, and are more likely to develop significant hyperbilirubinemia compared to those of 38 to 42 weeks (Sarici et al., 2004).

2. Ethnicity and bilirubin.
   a. Babies of Caucasian and Asian descent have higher physiologic bilirubin levels than babies of African descent (Maisels,1995).
   b. Johnson and colleagues (1986) reported that Navajo infants had exaggerated levels of bilirubin as well.
   c. Newer research demonstrates a genetic difference in Asians that may account for the increased propensity of about 20% of Asian infants for severe neonatal indirect hyperbilirubinemia (Akakba et al., 1998).

B. Neonatal pathologic hyperbilirubinemia.

1. A result of either overproduction of bilirubin or lack of effective excretion of bilirubin, or both, resulting in bilirubin levels requiring active intervention to prevent complications.

2. Infants with pathologic jaundice must be under the care of a primary health care provider in addition to receiving assistance from a lactation consultant.

3. Suspect pathologic jaundice if:
   a. Infant has onset of jaundice within the first 24 hours of life.
   b. Bilirubin levels are rising rapidly; or the infant is jaundiced beyond three weeks of life *AND* not thriving (AAP, 2004).

4. Causes of increased production/presence of circulating bilirubin beyond the liver's capability to metabolize it.

    a. Hemolysis due to pathologic causes such as ABO or Rh incompatibility, congenital RBC disorders such as spherocytosis and glucose 6-phosphate dehydrogenase (G6PD) deficiency.

    b. Polycythemia (placenta-to-infant or twin-to twin transfusion).

    c. Birth trauma with resultant bruising (AAP, 2004), such as cephalohematoma or bruising elsewhere, seen especially with vacuum- or forceps-assisted vaginal deliveries.

5. Interference with the liver's capability to metabolize bilirubin.

    a. Genetic variants/disorders of conjugation such as Gilbert syndrome, Crigler-Najjar syndrome.

    b. Hypothyroidism.

    c. Genetic mutations (Akakba et al., 1998).

6. Interference with the body's ability to excrete bilirubin via stooling.

    a. Inadequate intake due to ineffective feeding (for example, breastfeeding-associated jaundice) and resultant delayed stooling.

    b. Intestinal obstruction such as meconium ileus, other congenital intestinal anomalies.

    c. Possibly breast milk jaundice due to an increase in intestinal absorption of biblirubin (Alonso, 1991).

III. Risk Factors for Hyperbilirubinemia

A. Maternal factors.

1. Factors that may result in insufficient milk or ineffective feeding.

    a. Diabetes and other endocrinopathies (Neubauer et al., 1993).

    b. Anatomic breast abnormality (Huggins, Petok, & Mreles, 2000; Neifert et al., 1990).

    c. Breast surgery, especially breast reduction/periareolar incision (Neifert et al., 1990).

    d. Retained placenta (Anderson, 2001).

    e. Hypertension/eclampsia.

    f. Mother-infant separation (Yamauchi & Yamanouchi, 1990a).

    g. Delayed first feeding (Yamauchi & Yamanouchi, 1990a).

2. Factors that may increase the infant's risk for congenital disorders of bilirubin metabolism.

    a. Family history of RBC disorders (such as spherocytosis, G6PD deficiency, or Gilbert syndrome).

B. Labor and delivery factors may result in increased RBC breakdown (*hemolysis*).

1. Epidural analgesia due to the associated increased risk of interventional delivery using forceps or vacuum extraction (Thorp & Breedlove, 1996) and associated bruising of the infant.

2. Birth trauma and associated bruising.

C. Infant risk factors.

1. Factors associated with ineffective feeding/inadequate intake.
   a. Sleepy infant/infrequent feedings (Yamauchi & Yamanouchi, 1990b).
   b. Congenital oral-facial anomalies, such as cleft palate, ankyloglossia, or Pierre Robin syndrome (Marques et al., 2001).
   c. Congenital heart disease/neurologic impairment, such as an infant with Trisomy 21 or large ventricular septal defect.
   d. Oral motor difficulties, such as difficulties with attachment or effective suckling.
   e. Small for gestational age/preterm.

IV. Approach to the Jaundiced Infant

A. Quick appraisal to determine the immediate need for a medical evaluation.

1. Lethargic, unable to be aroused.

2. Refusal to feed.

3. Excessive weight loss ($\geq$ 10%; AAP, 2004).

4. Vomiting.

5. Inadequate urine or stool output for the infant's age.

6. Visible jaundice in the first 24 hours, or jaundice extending below the shoulders/upper chest at any time (AAP, 2004).

B. History.

1. Infant history.
   a. Assess for presence of the risk factors previously listed.
   b. Know what the child's risk level is based on the use of the AAP risk nomogram (Figure 37–1) if bilirubin levels are available. Confer with the medical provider if the child is in an elevated risk category.
   c. Assess color of urine; it should be yellow and not orange.
   d. Presence of uric acid crystals in the urine (brick dust appearance in the diaper); this may indicate dehydration but is also common in the first few days of life.
   e. Assess infant's behavior over the past 24 to 48 hours.
      i. Waking to feed?
      ii. Content after feedings?
      iii. Fussy or unsatisfied with feedings?

2. Maternal history.
   a. Health history; underlying risk factors (see Section III).
   b. Breast health history; underlying risk factors (see Section III).
   c. Evidence of breast changes; occurrence of breast fullness by days 3 to 4.

    d. Breast/nipple pain or discomfort.

    e. Evidence of milk ejection reflex.

  3. Feeding history.

    a. Frequency of feeds.

    b. Length of active feeding.

    c. Swallows present.

    d. Number of voids and stools per 24 hours.

      i. First 24 hours: 1 wet diaper and ≥ 1 meconium stool(s).

      ii. Day 2: 2 to 3 wet diapers and ≥ 1 meconium stool(s).

      iii. Day 3: 4 to 6 wet diapers and transitional stools.

      iv. Day 4: 4 to 6 wet diapers and transitional stools.

      v. Day 5: ≥ 6 wet diapers and 3 to 4 yellow stools.

    e. Mother's perception of breast fullness (lactogenesis II).

C. Physical assessment.

  1. Infant.

    a. General appearance of the infant.

    b. Level of vigor: alert/active versus difficult to arouse/lethargic.

    c. Evidence of dehydration.

      i. Check capillary refill by pressing the infant's finger or toe to blanch it, and observing how quickly it becomes pink again (this should take only 1–2 seconds).

      ii. Capillary refill longer than 2 seconds is the most sensitive indicator of dehydration (other than weight loss).

      iii. Check skin turgor by pulling up on the skin and observing the elasticity. It should immediately recoil, with no tenting.

      iv. Check mucous membranes for moistness.

    d. Presence of any congenital oral-facial anomalies or other syndromes that might interfere with effective breastfeeding.

    e. Current weight and the percent of weight loss.

    f. Assess the extent of jaundice.

      i. When jaundice extends beyond the upper chest, visual inspection is *NOT* accurate for judging degree of jaundice at the upper extremes (Szabo et al., 2004).

      ii. The infant should be referred for evaluation by the medical provider.

  2. Feeding assessment.

    a. Latch-on technique.

    b. Presence/frequency and length of bursts of swallows.

    c. Impact of change of feeding positions on the quality of feeding.

    d. Consider obtaining pre- and post-feeding test weights if weight loss greater than 8% has occurred.

      i. Although a test weight documents intake for a single feeding, one cannot be sure if it represents the best or worst feeding effort the infant is capable of.

ii. Therefore, whether or not test weighing is done, a follow-up weight check within 24 hours must be obtained to ensure the infant's safety.

3. Maternal breast assessment.

a. Evidence of scars, marked asymmetry, inverted/flat nipples, tubular breasts, or widely spaced breasts.

b. Evidence of nipple trauma.

D. Table 37-1 summarizes and compares the findings related to different causes of jaundice in newborn infants.

E. Breastfeeding management.

1. Infant with hyperbilirubinemia who demonstrates appropriate weight for age.

a. No interruption of breastfeeding (with the exception of galactosemia).

b. Continued exclusive breastfeeding.

c. No supplementation.

2. Infant who has excessive weight loss or inadequate weight gain (see Chapter 40).

a. Establish effective breastfeeding techniques and routines.

b. Provide supplemental fluid/calories at the breast or by other methods as indicated with expressed mother's milk or a human milk substitute.

c. Initiate additional stimulation of the milk supply.

d. Monitor bilirubin per primary care provider's instruction.

e. Weight check within 24 hours, with repeat checks until appropriate weight gain established.

f. If supplement is used, reduce or increase the amount based on weight gain, hydration status, and the infant's breastfeeding capabilities.

g. The child's primary health care provider will make a decision regarding the need for phototherapy or other medical intervention.

h. Although medical therapy might be effective in reducing the bilirubin levels, the infant still needs a careful feeding evaluation and assessment in order to ensure adequate hydration, weight gain, and restoration of effective breastfeeding as well as sufficient maternal milk supply.

F. Medical management of hyperbilirubinemia (see Table 37-1).

1. Establishment of a definitive cause.

2. Treatment based on the definitive cause.

3. Interventions to decrease bilirubin levels if they are at potentially dangerous or high levels.

a. Phototherapy.

i. Under the influence of phototherapy lights, photo-isomers of bilirubin are formed that are more easily excreted by the liver (see Figure 37-2).

ii. Phototherapy lights or fiberoptic blankets are used.

iii. Phototherapy lights are preferred for efficient management of significant hyperbilirubinemia.

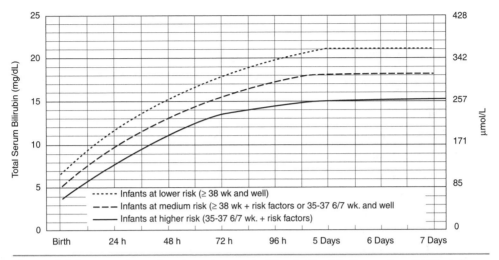

Figure 37-2 Guidelines for Phototherapy in Hospitalized Infants of > 35 Weeks' Gestation. *Source:* Used with permission from the American Academy of Pediatrics Subcommittee on Neonatal Hyperbilirubinemia. Management of hyperbilirubinemia in the newborn infant 35 or more completed weeks of gestation. *Pediatrics.* 2004;114:304.

    b. Exchange transfusion.
       i. Rarely needed.
      ii. Used only in the case of extremely high bilirubin levels.
     iii. When not responding to intensive phototherapy; more likely to occur in a preterm infant.
  4. New treatments being researched.
    a. Tin-mesoporphyrin.
       i. A metal that inhibits bilirubin formation (Kappas, 2004; Martinez et al., 1999).
      ii. One or two injections are administered to the infant, usually resulting in a rapid fall in bilirubin levels without the need for phototherapy.
     iii. This medication is not approved by the Food and Drug Administration in the United States at this time but may be available under compassionate use protocol for Jehovah's Witnesses whose child would otherwise require exchange transfusion.
    b. L-aspartic acid.
       i. Being studied for its ability to prevent the occurrence of high bilirubin levels without disrupting breastfeeding.
      ii. Infants receiving six oral doses of this beta glucuronidase inhibitor had significantly lower peak bilirubin levels (Gourley et al., 2005).

G. Danger signs that indicate an immediate need for referral to the primary care medical provider.

   1. Excessive weight loss of $\geq$ 10% of birth weight.

   2. History of brick dust urine or inadequate urine output for the age of the infant.

   3. Vomiting.

   4. Refusing to feed.

   5. Excessive sleeping or continued fretfulness.

   6. Jaundiced color below the upper chest.

H. Education and counseling.

   1. Remember that families view hyperbilirubinemia and its treatment as a threat to their infant (Hannon, Willis, & Scrimshaw, 2001; Willis, Hannon, & Scrimshaw, 2002).

   2. Expect that parents may have ongoing feelings of concern that they caused the baby's illness and will need continued support to continue exclusive breastfeeding.

   3. Explain to the family the reason for the jaundiced color and the implications related to breastfeeding (see Section IV. F.).

   4. Teach the family how to determine if the infant is feeding effectively.

   5. Provide the family with written information regarding the clinical indicators of sufficient intake and infant danger signals.

   6. Assist the mother with techniques for the stimulation of milk supply when appropriate.
      a. Frequent, effective feeding; hand or mechanical milk expression as an adjunct if a supplement has been recommended.

   7. If phototherapy is required, advocate the avoidance of mother-infant separation.

   8. If a supplement is required, teach the family how to obtain additional mother's milk.

   9. Work with the primary care provider to develop a feeding plan that is individualized to the infant-mother dyad's particular need.

   10. Provide families with a feeding diary to record feedings, supplement amounts, and the infant's output.

   11. Ensure that the family understands the need for frequent, close follow-up.

I. Evaluation.

   1. The infant's weight will be normal, with 20 to 28 g weight gain/day after day of life 4 (Lawrence & Lawrence, 2005).

2. For the baby with breastfeeding-associated jaundice (see Section V), bilirubin levels will decrease with the onset of effective feeding and resultant stooling. There may be a rapid fall in the bilirubin level if effective feeding is established within 12 to 24 hours, which might eliminate the need for medical therapy.

3. Maternal milk supply will develop normally, or increase if it had been insufficient as evidenced by infant weight/hydration/stool patterns and the ability to decrease or eliminate the supplement.

4. The breastfeeding relationship will be maintained and strengthened based on the previous parameters.

5. Failure of the infant to improve within 12 to 24 hours indicates other underlying problems and a need for reappraisal of the infant by the primary care health provider. Further exploration of reasons for insufficient milk supply is also indicated.

V. Breastfeeding-Associated Jaundice (Also Called Starvation Jaundice, Lack of Breastfeeding Jaundice, Non-Breastfeeding Jaundice)

A. One of the significant causes of hyperbilirubinemia.

1. Lack of intake leads to delayed stooling and recirculation of bilirubin.

2. Is one of the most common situations the lactation consultant will encounter.

3. Breastfeeding does not cause the jaundice; rather, a *lack* of effective breastfeeding causes the problem.

4. Infants who have hyperbilirubinemia due to lack of appropriate intake might be significantly dehydrated as well, occasionally presenting to the practitioner in a life-threatening condition.

5. Quick appraisal and timely referral to the primary health care provider is a critical component of the lactation consultant's responsibilities.

B. Pathophysiology.

1. An infant who is not feeding effectively may experience jaundice in part related to the delay in the passage of meconium, and in part due to dehydration.

2. Meconium contains conjugated bilirubin.

3. If the meconium is not passed in a timely manner, then the bilirubin is reabsorbed from the intestine back into the bloodstream where it must be conjugated by the liver again to attempt to excrete it (this is *recirculation* of bilirubin).

C. Health implications for the infant.

1. Ineffective feeding is associated with inadequate fluid intake and resultant dehydration.

2. Severe hypernatremic dehydration can result from the lack of fluid intake as well as from the increased sodium content noted in breast milk of women whose babies are feeding ineffectively (so-called *weaning milk*); this is potentially life-threatening.

3. Insufficient caloric and fluid intake results in excessive weight loss > 8% of birth weight.

4. Kernicterus may occur if bilirubin levels remain greater than 25 to 30 mg/dL in the term infant.

D. Typical infant with breastfeeding-associated jaundice.

1. History.
   a. Onset of jaundiced appearance at 48 to 72 hours of age.
   b. Delayed or scant meconium output.
   c. Scant urine output.
   d. Either infrequent, ineffective feeds or frequent, ineffective feedings.
   e. Either lethargic with few requests for feedings or very fussy and not content after feedings.

2. Physical assessment.
   a. Thin, jaundiced infant.
   b. Lethargic, difficult to arouse or fussy, and difficult to console.
   c. Excessive weight loss or lack of appropriate interval weight gain for age.

3. Feeding assessment.
   a. Problems with latch-on.
   b. Scant swallows noted during the feeding.
   c. Maternal engorgement might be noted.

E. Feeding management (see section IV. E).

F. Prevention.

1. *Clinical Guidelines for the Establishment of Exclusive Breastfeeding* (ILCA, 2005) enumerates practices that prevent breastfeeding-associated jaundice, among other breastfeeding complications.

2. Early initiation of breastfeeding.

3. Frequent breastfeeding (de Carvalho, Klans, & Merkatz, 1982; Yamauchi & Yamanouchi, 1990b).

4. Avoidance of water supplement/complement (de Carvalho, Hall, & Havey, 1981).

5. Effective breastfeeding.

6. Early follow-up with the primary care provider (within 48–72 hours of birth or sooner if high risk) for an assessment of the weight, hydration, breastfeeding effectiveness, and cardiovascular assessment (AAP, 2004).

G. Education and counseling (see Section, IV. H).

H. Evaluation (see Section IV. I).

VI. Breast Milk Jaundice

A. Overview.

    1. Infants who have breast milk jaundice are healthy breastfed infants who have no pathologic cause of indirect hyperbilirubinemia. They are breastfeeding effectively, have good weight gain, and have no other signs or symptoms of illness. Some consider this another component of physiologic jaundice (Gartner & Herschel, 2001).

    2. Diagnosis is made by excluding other causes of delayed-onset hyperbilirubinemia either by history or laboratory testing before assuming that breast milk jaundice is the cause of the persistent hyperbilirubinemia. The infant may have clinically perceptible jaundice for up to three months. If jaundice persists beyond this time, other causes need to be considered.

B. Introduction.

    1. Physiology.
        a. Not well understood.
        b. Some assume that there is an element in breast milk that leads to this condition, yet no element has yet been identified (Gartner & Herschel, 2001).
        c. There is speculation as to whether there is a difference in the infant's capacity for metabolizing or excreting bilirubin, but such a difference has not yet been identified (Gartner & Herschel, 2001).

    2. Tends to recur in subsequent infants in the family.

    3. No other health implications/risks for the infant.

C. History.

    1. Breast milk jaundice may appear between 5 to 10 days of age after physiologic jaundice has peaked and declined.

    2. Positive family history of late-onset jaundice.

    3. Infant is vigorous, feeding well, and gaining weight appropriately.

D. Physical assessment.

    1. Assess level of jaundice.

    2. Assess alertness.

    3. Assess the weight status.

E. Breastfeeding assessment.

    1. Expect effective breastfeeding.

F. Management.

    1. Ensure continued, effective breastfeeding.

    2. The health provider will decide on the frequency of bilirubin monitoring.
        a. Typically, bilirubin levels may be monitored until the level plateaus.

b. An infant who has additional risk factors, such as prematurity or ethnicity, might experience levels high enough to require phototherapy.

c. Some health care providers will advise interruption of breastfeeding for 12 to 24 hours, although this is not the preferred approach.

   i. Bilirubin levels will drop precipitously.

   ii. This strategy serves as a diagnostic method; if the bilirubin level indeed drops, then one does not have to look further for the cause of the jaundice.

   iii. It is not thought to be necessary by most experts (Gartner & Lee, 1999).

   iv. Interruption of breastfeeding might jeopardize the breastfeeding relationship between the mother and her infant.

   v. Risks and benefits of breastfeeding interruption need to be carefully assessed.

d. If phototherapy is required, advocate for the avoidance of mother-infant separation.

G. Education and counseling.

1. Reassure the family that the infant is not seriously ill.

2. Work with the primary care provider to develop a breastfeeding plan.

3. If breastfeeding is interrupted, teach the mother how to maintain her milk supply.

H. Evaluation.

1. Maintenance of the breastfeeding relationship.

2. Continued, normal weight gain.

3. A gradual decrease in jaundiced appearance in the infant over 3 to 12 weeks of age.

VII. Hypoglycemia

A. The fetus receives energy continuously via the placenta.

B. Glycogen reserves that are available for conversion to glucose during the immediate neonatal period are laid down during the later part of the third trimester.

C. Newborns have a greater demand for glucose than children and adults due to their large brain-to-body weight.

D. Preterm infants have an even greater demand for glucose and have limited to absent glycogen reserves.

E. Glucose is the primary nutrient for brain metabolism, and the placentally derived supply terminates at birth.

F. Neonatal physiology.

1. At birth, there is a transition period as glucose homeostasis is established by the infant.

2. Change in glucoregulatory hormones as follows:
   a. Increased epinephrine.
   b. Increased norepinephrine.
   c. Increased glucagon.
   d. The net effect is mobilization of glycogen and fatty acids.

G. The collective activities that maintain glucose homeostasis are called *counterregulation*, which consist of the following:

   1. *Glycogenolysis*: mobilization and release of glycogen from body stores to form glucose.

   2. *Gluconeogenesis*: production of glucose by the liver and kidneys from non-carbohydrate substrates such as fatty acids and amino acids.

H. The rate of glucose production is 4 to 6 mg/kg/minute (Eidelman, 2001).

   1. 3.7 mg/kg/minute is needed to meet the requirements of the brain.

   2. About 70% is provided by glucose oxidation with the rest being provided from alternative fuels.

   3. Alternative brain fuels are also produced, such as ketone bodies.

I. Dietary intake and gluconeogenesis.

   1. After 12 hours, the baby is dependent on glucose made from dietary intake of milk components (20%–50%) and gluconeogenesis to maintain blood glucose (galactose, amino acids, glucerol, lactate) as well as free fatty acids from fat stores and milk.

   2. Breast milk is more ketogenic than formula, enabling the breastfed baby to create high levels of alternative fuels until the milk supply increases sufficiently to draw upon milk components for glucose synthesis (de Rooy & Hawdon, 2002).

   3. High levels of ketone bodies enable breastfed babies to demonstrate lower measured blood glucose levels, but still maintain the optimal production of brain fuels (de Rooy & Hawdon, 2002).

   4. Glycogen stores are converted to glucose (*glycogenolysis*), rapidly depleting glycogen stores over the first hours of life; liver glycogen stores are 90% depleted by three hours and gone by 12 hours.

   5. Fat metabolism provides a glucose substrate beginning at two to three days of age.

J. Definition.

   1. No consensus on the definition of hypoglycemia in a full-term infant; hypoglycemia is a continuum of falling blood glucose levels, not an arbitrary number (Cornblath et al., 1990; 2000).

   2. Serum glucose below 36 to 45 mg/dL (2.0–2.5 mmol/L in the newborn is considered the threshold for intervention (Cornblath et al., 2000).

K. Testing for hypoglycemia.

1. Recommendations for glucose screening (AAP, 2005; ABM, 2006; Williams, 1997).
   a. Universal screening is not recommended.
   b. Screen infants who are at risk.

2. Which infants should be screened?
   a. Any infant who is symptomatic.
      i. Weak cry, apnea, cyanosis, hypothermia, irritability, lethargy, feeding problems, and tremors or seizures.
      ii. Infants meeting high-risk criteria: large or small for gestational age, infant of a diabetic mother, babies who have been asphyxiated, those with sepsis, intrauterine growth retardation, cold stress, Rh disease, or with congestive heart failure.
      iii. Jitteriness is a very common, nonspecific finding. Linder (1989) suggests that if jitteriness ceases with suckling, there is no need to be concerned about hypoglycemia or hypocalcemia (another cause of newborn tremor).

3. Which screening method?
   a. Bedside screening devices are in general not designed to be accurate in the lower ranges, but rather in the normal and higher ranges.
      i. For newborns, the greatest need is for accuracy in the hypoglycemia ranges.
      ii. A comparison of 5 different "point of care" devices found that none was satisfactory as the only measuring device (Ho, Yeung, & Young, 2004).
   b. Reagent strips are of limited accuracy in newborns. Visual interpretation of test strip results is highly inaccurate and is not recommended.
   c. Accuracy depends on following the directions precisely.
   d. Significant variability of the results have been noted.
   e. Results from most point of care devices are affected by the infant's hemoglobin status.

4. Confirm abnormal screening results with a serum glucose level sent to a laboratory.

5. If an infant has galactosemia, some screening tests will give falsely high glucose results.
   a. If screening glucoses are high, also confirm these with serum glucose level, because the infant may in fact be profoundly hypoglycemic (Newman, Ramsden, & Balazs, 2002).

6. Do not delay treatment while waiting for the serum glucose results (AAP, 2004).

L. Health implications for a breastfed infant.

1. Hypoglycemia is linked to later developmental difficulties.

2. Delay in first feeding and ineffective breastfeeding can contribute to the development of hypoglycemia, even in low-risk infants (Moore & Perlman, 1999).

M. Risk factors for hypoglycemia in a full-term newborn.

    1. Gestational diabetes; women are not always aware of their glycemic status (Simmons, Thompson, & Conroy, 2000).

    2. Diabetes, type I or II (insulin- or noninsulin-dependent).

    3. Anatomic or physiologic disorders affecting lactogenesis.

    4. Hypertension (pregnancy-induced or essential).

N. Labor and delivery management factors (Williams, 1997).

    1. Maternal intravenous fluids using dextrose and water solutions.

    2. Cool room temperature.

    3. Infant separation from mother.

    4. Delayed feeding.

    5. Crying that is not quickly attended to.

O. Infant.

    1. Large for gestational age (more than 4,000 g).

    2. Small for gestational age (under 2,500 g).

    3. Intrauterine growth retardation.

    4. Preterm ($<$ 37 completed weeks of gestation).

P. Prevention of hypoglycemia in newborns.

    1. *Clinical Guidelines for the Establishment of Exclusive Breastfeeding* (ILCA, 2005) is a guide for prevention of hypoglycemia as well as other newborn complications.

    2. Labor and delivery management.

        a. If intravenous fluids are used for the laboring woman, choose balanced electrolyte solutions rather than dextrose and water to reduce the risk of hyperinsulinism in the infant.

        b. Provide a neutral thermal environment.

        c. Avoid cold stress in the infant.

           i. Towel dry.

           ii. Place baby in skin-to-skin contact with the mother and cover the dyad.

           iii. Babies separated from their mother have lower body temperatures, cry more, and have lower blood glucose levels (Christensson et al., 1992; Williams, 1997).

        d. Prevent infant crying because crying rapidly depletes glycogen stores.

    3. Feeding routine.

        a. Early first feeding.

           i. Hypoglycemia is *NOT* associated with lack of feeding in the first 6 hours of life in healthy infants who are appropriate for gestational age (Diwakar & Sasidhar, 2002).

        ii. However, this finding does not negate the importance of early first feeding for the establishment of exclusive breastfeeding.

    b. Frequent feeding (Hawdon, Ward Platt, & Annsley-Green, 1992).

        i. After the first few hours, the major determinant of blood glucose concentration is the interval between feeds.

    c. Ensure effective feedings.

    d. Avoid dextrose water complement or supplemental feedings because this leads to rebound hypoglycemia (AAP, 2004).

  4. Post-discharge follow-up.

    a. Perform an early follow-up at 48 hours of age to ensure the well-being and establishment of effective breastfeeding.

    b. Teach families the early symptoms of hypoglycemia.

Q. Implementation and planning.

  1. Monitor the infant closely to assess for signs of hypoglycemia.

  2. Notify the primary health care provider if the infant is symptomatic.

  3. Ensure effective breastfeeding.

  4. If breastfeeding has been effective and infant's glucose level is still low, provide an appropriate supplement per order of the health care provider.

  5. If breastfeeding is ineffective and the infant's glucose levels are low, initiate supplementation according to the health care provider's recommendation (expressed mother's milk or human milk substitute is preferred to glucose water for the prevention of rebound hypoglycemia).

  6. If supplementation is required it is preferred to supplement at the breast if the infant is able to breastfeed effectively.

  7. If the infant is unable to sustain suckling at the breast, feed away from the breast by using a method that is best suited to the infant's capabilities and the parents' and provider's preference.

    a. The mother can hand express colostrum into a spoon and spoon-feed it frequently to her baby.

    b. The protein and fat in colostrum provide substrates for gluconeogenesis, enhance ketogenesis, and increase gut motility and gastric emptying time, which causes a rapid absorption of nutrients.

  8. The health care provider might use intravenous glucose if the initial feedings are not sufficient to increase the infant's serum glucose level.

  9. All infants require close monitoring after discharge by either home or office visits with a health care provider at 48 to 72 hours of age in order to assess well-being.

    a. Case reports describe breastfed infants who had no other risk factors yet became symptomatic of hypoglycemia on the third day of life, presenting with seizures at home (Moore & Perlman, 1999). Each of these infants was experiencing feeding difficulties.

    b. Hume, McGreechan and Burchell (1999) reported on preterm infants (gestation of < 37 weeks) who were at risk for hypoglycemia at the time of discharge. Their findings stressed the importance of timely feedings to avoid hypoglycemia at home.

R. Education and counseling.

    1. Explain to the family the short-term feeding implications for an infant who has low blood sugar.

       a. Need for short-term supplementation; importance of frequent feedings.

       b. Need for blood tests to monitor glucose levels until normoglycemia is established.

    2. If supplementation is needed, assist the mother with initiating milk expression.

    3. Assist the mother in administering oral supplementation if ordered.

    4. Ensure that the family understands the importance of a timely return visit to the health care provider.

    5. Teach the family the indicators of effective breastfeeding.

    6. Teach the family the symptoms of hypoglycemia.

S. Evaluation.

    1. The infant will be able to maintain blood glucose without the need for supplementation.

    2. Breastfeeding will be established prior to discharge from the birthing site.

References

Academy of Breastfeeding Medicine (ABM). Clinical Protocol #1: Guidelines for Glucose Monitoring and Treatment of Hypoglycemia in Breastfed Neonates. 2006. Available at: http://www.bfmed.org. Accessed March 10, 2007.

Akakba K, Kimura T, Sasaki A, et al. Neonatal hyperbilirubinemia and mutation of the bilirubin uridine diphosphate-glucuronosyltransferase gene: a common missense mutation among Japanese, Koreans, and Chinese. *Biochem Mol Biol Int.* 1998;46:21–26.

Alonso EM, Whitington PF, Witington SH, et al. Enterohepatic circulation of nonconjugated bilirubin in rats fed with human milk. *J Pediatr.* 1991;118:425–430.

American Academy of Pediatrics (AAP) Subcommittee on Neonatal Hyperbilirubinemia. Management of hyperbilirubinemia in the newborn infant 35 or more completed weeks of gestation. *Pediatrics.* 2004;114:297–316.

American Academy of Pediatrics (AAP) Policy Statement on Breastfeeding and the Use of Human Milk. *Pediatrics.* 2005;115:496–506. Available at: http://www.aap.org/advocacy/releases/feb05breastfeeding.htm. Accessed March 10, 2007.

Anderson AM. Disruption of lactogenesis by retained placental fragments. *J Hum Lact.* 2001;17:142–144.

Bhutani VK, Johnson LH, Keren R. Treating acute bilirubin encephalopathy before it is too late. *Contemp Pediatr.* 2005;22:57–74.

Brand PLP, Molenaar NLD, Kaaijk C, Wierenga WS. Neurodevelopmental outcome of hypoglycaemia in healthy, large for gestational age, term newborns. *Arch Dis Child.* 2005;90:78–81.

Christensson K, Siles C, Moreno L, et al. Temperature, metabolic adaptation and crying in healthy full-term newborns cared for skin-to-skin or in a cot. *Acta Paediatr.* 1992;81:488–493.

Cornblath M, Schwartz R, Aynsley-Green A, Lloyd JK. Hypoglycemia in infancy: the need for a rational definition. *Pediatrics.* 1990;85:834–837.

Cornblath M, Hawdon JM, Williams AF, et al. Controversies regarding definition of neonatal hypoglycemia: suggested operational thresholds. *Pediatrics.* 2000;105:1141–1145.

de Carvalho M, Hall M, Havey D. Effects of water supplementation on physiological jaundice in breastfed babies. *Arch Dis Child.* 1981;56:568–569.

de Carvalho M, Klaus MH, Merkatz RB. Frequency of breastfeeding and serum bilirubin concentration. *Am J Dis Child.* 1982;136:737–738.

de Rooy L, Hawdon J. Nutritional factors that affect the postnatal metabolic adaptation of full-term small- and large-for-gestational-age infants. *Pediatrics.* 2002;109:E42.

Diwakar KK, Sasidhar MV. Plasma glucose levels in term infants who are appropriate size for gestation and exclusively breast fed. *Arch Dis Child Fetal Neonatal Ed.* 2002;87:F46–F48.

Eidelman AI. Hypoglycemia and the breastfed neonate. *Pediatr Clin N Am.* 2001;48:377–387.

English M, Ngama M, Musumba C, et al. Causes and outcome of young infant admissions to a Kenyan district hospital. *Arch Dis Child.* 2003;88:438–443.

Gartner, LM, Lee K. Jaundice in the breastfed infant. *Clin Perinatol.* 1999;26:431–445.

Gartner LM, Herschel M. Jaundice and breastfeeding. *Pediatr Clin North Am.* 2001;48:389–399.

Gourley GR, Zhanhai K, Kreamer BL, Kosorok MR. A controlled, randomized, double blind trial of prophylaxis against jaundice among breastfed newborns. *Pediatrics.* 2005;116:385–391.

Haberal A, Gurakan B. Weight loss and hypernatremia in breast-fed babies: frequency in neonates with non-hemolytic jaundice. *J Paediatr Child Health.* 2005;41:484–487.

Hall RT, Simon S, Smith MT. Readmission of breastfed infants in the first 2 weeks of life. *J Perinatol.* 2000;20:432–437.

Hannon PR, Willis SK, Scrimshaw SC. Persistence of maternal concerns surrounding neonatal jaundice: an exploratory study. *Arch Pediatr Adolesc Med.* 2001;155:1357–1363.

Harris MC, Bernbaum JC, Polin JR, et al. Developmental follow-up of breastfed term and near-term infants with marked hyperbilirubinemia. *Pediatrics*. 2001;107:1075–1080.

Hawdon MJ, Ward Platt MP, Annsley-Green A. Patterns of metabolic adaptation for term and preterm infants in the first neonatal week. *Arch Dis Child*. 1992;67:357–365.

Herschel M, Gartner L. Jaundice and the breastfed baby. In: Riordan J, ed. *Breastfeeding and Human Lactation*. Sudbury, MA: Jones and Bartlett Publishers; 2005:311–321.

Ho HT, Yeung WKY, Young BWY. Evaluation of "point of care" devices in the measurement of low blood glucose in neonatal practice. *Arch Dis Child Fetal Neonatal Ed*. 2004;89:F356–F359.

Hoseth E, Joergensen A, Ebbesen J, Moeller M. Blood glucose levels in a population of healthy, breast fed, term infants of appropriate size for gestational age. *Arch Dis Child Fetal Neonatal Ed*. 2000;83:F117–F119.

Huggins KE, Petok ES, Mreles O. Markers of lactation insufficiency: a study of 34 mothers. *Curr Issues Clin Lact*. 2000:25–35.

Hume R, McGeechan A, Burchell A. Failure to detect preterm infants at risk of hypoglycemia before discharge. *J Pediatr*. 1999;134:499–502.

International Lactation Consultant Association (ILCA). *Clinical Guidelines for the Establishment of Exclusive Breastfeeding*. Raleigh, NC: ILCA; 2005.

Ip S, Chung M, Kulig J, et al. An evidence-based review of important issues concerning neonatal hyperbilirubinemia. *Pediatrics*. 2004;114:130–153.

Johnson JD, Angelus P, Aldrich M, Skipper BJ. Exaggerated jaundice in Navajo neonates. *Am J Dis Child*. 1986;140:889–890.

Kaplan M, Hammerman C. Understanding and preventing severe hyperbilirubinemia: is bilirubin neurotoxicity really a problem in the developed world? *Clin Perinatol*. 2004;31:555–575.

Kaplan M, Hammerman C. American Academy of Pediatrics guidelines for detecting neonatal hyperbilirubinemia and preventing kernicterus: are there worldwide implications? *Arch Dis Child Fetal Neonatal Ed*. 2005;90:F448–F449.

Kappas A. A method for interdicting the development of severe jaundice in newborns by inhibiting the production of bilirubin. *Pediatrics*. 2004;113:119–123.

Lawrence RA, Lawrence RM. *Breastfeeding. A Guide for the Medical Profession*. 6th ed. St. Louis: Mosby, Inc.; 2005.

Linder N, Moser AM, Asli I, et al. Suckling stimulation test for neonatal tremor. *Arch Dis Child*. 1989;64:44–46.

Maisels MJ, Kring E. Transcutaneous bilirubin levels in the first 96 hours in a normal newborn population of ≥ 35 weeks' gestation. *Pediatrics*. 2006;117:1169–1173.

Maisels MJ. Clinical rounds in the well-baby nursery: treating jaundiced newborns. *Pediatr Ann*. 1995;10:547–552.

Manning D. American Academy of Pediatrics guidelines for detecting neonatal hyperbilirubinemia and preventing kernicterus: Are they applicable in Britain? *Arch Dis Child Fetal Neonatal Ed*. 2005;90:F450–F451.

Marques IL, de Sousa TV, Carneiro AF, et al. Clinical experience with infants with Robin Sequence: a prospective study. *Cleft Palate-Craniofac J.* 2001;38:171–178.

Martinez JC, Garcia HO, Otheguy LE, et al. Control of severe hyperbilirubinemia in full-term newborns with the inhibitor of bilirubin production Sn-mesoporphyrin. *Pediatrics.* 1999;103:1–5.

Moore AM, Perlman M. Symptomatic hypoglycemia in otherwise healthy, breastfed term newborns. *Pediatrics.* 1999;103:837–839.

Neifert M, De Marzo S, Seacat J, et al. The influence of breast surgery, breast appearance, and pregnancy-induced breast changes on lactation sufficiency as measured by infant weight gain. *Birth.* 1990;17:31–38.

Neubauer SH, Ferris AM, Chase CG, et al. Delayed lactogenesis in women with insulin-dependent diabetes mellitus. *Am J Clin Nutr.* 1993;58:54–60.

Newman JD, Ramsden CA, Balazs NDH. Monitoring neonatal hypoglycemia with the Accu-chek Advantage II glucose meter: the cautionary tale of galactosemia. *Clin Chem.* 2002;48:2071.

Pal DK, Manandhar DS, Rajbhandari S, et al. Neonatal hypoglycaemia in Nepal 1. Prevalence and risk factors. *Arch Dis Child Fetal Neonatal Ed.* 2000;82:F46–F51.

Petersen JR, Okorodudu AO, Mohammad AA, et al. Association of transcutaneous bilirubin testing in hospital with decreased readmission rate for hyperbilirubinemia. *Clin Chem.* 2005;51:540–544.

Sarici SU, Sedar MA, Korkmaz A, et al. Incidence, course, and prediction of hyperbilirubinemia in near-term and term newborns. *Pediatrics.* 2004;113:775–780.

Seidman DS, Stevenson DK, Ergaz Z, Gale R. Hospital readmission due to neonatal hyperbilirubinemia. *Pediatrics.* 1995;96:727–729.

Simmons D, Thompson CF, Conroy C. Incidence and risk factors for neonatal hypoglycaemia among women with gestational diabetes mellitus in South Auckland. *Diab Med.* 2000;17:830–834.

Suresh GK, Clark RE. Cost-effectiveness of strategies that are intended to prevent kernicterus in newborn infants. *Pediatrics.* 2004;114:917–924.

Szabo P, Wolf M, Bucher HU, et al. Detection of hyperbilirubinemia in jaundiced full-term neonates by eye or by bilirubinometer? *Eur J Pediatr.* 2004;163:722–727.

Thorp JA, Breedlove G. Epidural analgesia in labor: an evaluation of risks and benefits. *Birth.* 1996;23:63–83.

Udoma EJ, Udo JJ, Etuk SJ, Duke ES. Morbidity and mortality among infants with normal birth weight in a new born baby unit. *Niger J Paediatr.* 2001;28:13.

Williams A. *Hypoglycaemia of the Newborn.* Geneva: World Health Organization (WHO); 1997.

Willis SK, Hannon PR, Scrimshaw SC. The impact of the maternal experience with a jaundiced newborn on the breastfeeding relationship [abstract]. *J Fam Pract.* 2002;51:465.

Yamauchi Y, Yamanouchi I. The relationship between rooming-in/not rooming-in and breast-feeding. *Acta Paediatr Scand.* 1990a;79:1017–1022.

Yamauchi Y, Yamanouchi I. Breastfeeding frequency during the first 24 hours after birth in full-term neonates. *Pediatrics.* 1990b;86:171–175.

Suggested Readings

Cole MD, Peevy K. Hypoglycemia in normal neonates appropriate for gestational age. *J Perinatol.* 1994;14:118–120.

Committee on the Fetus and Newborn. Routine evaluation of blood pressure, hematocrit, and glucose in newborns. *Pediatrics.* 1993;92:474–476.

Duvanel C, Fawer CL, Cotting J, et al. Long-term effects of neonatal hypoglycemia on brain growth and psychomotor development in small-for-gestational-age preterm infants. *J Pediatr.* 1999;134:492–498.

Holtrop BC. The frequency of hypoglycemia in full-term large and small for gestational age newborns. *Am J Perinatol.* 1993;10:150–154.

Nylander G, Lindemann R, Helsing E, Bendvold R. Unsupplemented breastfeeding in the maternity ward. *Acta Obstet Gynecol Scand.* 1991;70:205–209.

Samson LF. Infants of diabetic mothers: current perspectives. *J Perinat Neonat Nurs.* 1992;6:61–70.

Schwartz R. Neonatal hypoglycemia: back to basics in diagnosis and treatment. *Diabetes.* 1991;40(suppl 2):71–73.

Stevenson DK, Dennery PA, Hintz SR. Understanding newborn jaundice. *J Perinatol.* 2001;21(suppl 1):S21–S24.

Wight N, Marinelli KA, Academy of Breastfeeding Medicine. ABM Clinical Protocol #1: Guidelines for glucose monitoring and treatment of hypoglycemia in breastfed neonates. *Breastfeeding Medicine.* 2006;1(3):178–184.

MATERNAL ACUTE AND CHRONIC ILLNESS

Marsha Walker, RN, IBCLC

OBJECTIVES

- Describe the influence of acute and chronic maternal illness on breastfeeding and lactation.
- Identify breastfeeding management strategies to preserve breastfeeding under adverse situations.
- Discuss contraindications to breastfeeding.

Introduction

Not only has there been an increase in the number of women choosing to breast-feed, but more women now than ever have been able to conceive and carry a pregnancy to term or near term under a variety of acute and chronic health conditions. Almost all of these mothers can breastfeed partially or totally, even if they are taking medications or are experiencing viral or bacterial infections. The lactation consultant should gain familiarity with a number of the more common health challenges in order to better provide lactation care and services when confronted with maternal health problems.

I. Pituitary Disorders

A. Sheehan's syndrome (panhypopituitarism).

1. Caused by severe postpartum hemorrhage and hypotension; this can lead to the failure of the pituitary gland to produce gonadotropins.

2. Symptoms of severe Sheehan's syndrome include weight gain and then loss postpartum, loss of pubic and axillary hair, intolerance to cold, low blood pressure, and vaginal and breast tissue atrophy.

3. Milder cases might see a delay in milk synthesis; frequent breastfeeding or pumping would be required in order to stimulate the number and sensitivity of breast prolactin receptors and to take advantage of what little prolactin might be available.

4. The role of the pituitary gland might be permissive rather than completely responsible for the success of lactation; women who have varying levels of prolactin have been shown to produce adequate amounts of milk for their infants (Cox, Owens, & Hartmann, 1996).

5. The breast and body have compensatory mechanisms that make lactation a robust activity; autocrine control of milk production can fill in for a less-than-optimal hormonal environment (Cregan, DeMello, & Hartmann, 2000).

B. Prolactinomas; prolactin-secreting adenomas.

1. Prolactin-secreting tumors that can produce amenorrhea and galactorrhea do not show a correlation with milk production (DeCoopman, 1993).

2. Women can breastfeed with this condition (Verma, Shah, & Faridi, 2006).

3. Chronic, high levels of prolactin also can be caused by certain medications, excessive breast manipulation, hypothyroid states, hyperthyroid disease, chronic renal failure, and several less-frequently seen syndromes (Verhelst & Abs, 2003).

II. Diabetes

A. Diabetes is a chronic disease of impaired carbohydrate metabolism.

1. Type 1 diabetes, also termed insulin-dependent diabetes mellitus (insufficient insulin).

2. Type 2 diabetes, also termed late-onset or noninsulin dependent diabetes that is usually not insulin dependent (inefficient use of insulin).
   a. Reduced by breastfeeding (see Chapter 10).

3. Gestational diabetes is a glucose intolerance that is seen in about 7% of pregnancies.
   a. Women who have gestational diabetes during a pregnancy are more likely to develop Type 2 diabetes if they do not breastfeed the baby (Kjos et al., 1993).

B. The breast has insulin-sensitive tissue and requires insulin to initiate milk production.

1. There can be a 15- to 28-hour delay in lactogenesis II as the mother's body competes with the breasts for the available insulin (Arthur, Kent, & Hartmann, 1994; Hartmann & Cregan, 2001).

C. Lactation has an insulin-sparing effect on the mother.

1. This can cause lower insulin requirements during lactation.

   2. The constant conversion of glucose to galactose and lactose during milk synthesis lowers the insulin requirement.

   3. The diabetic mother also needs extra calories while lactating.

D. Diabetic mothers should be encouraged to breastfeed.

   1. Their infants might be large and are prone to hypoglycemia, so very frequent feedings of colostrum are necessary; if mother and baby are separated, pumping should be initiated as soon as possible (ABM, 2007; California Diabetes and Pregnancy Program, 2002).

   2. Some babies of diabetic mothers are observed in a nursery for a number of hours following birth.
      a. Separation increases the chances for supplemental feeding and delayed initiation of breastfeeding.
      b. Hand-expressed colostrum can stabilize blood sugar levels; colostrum (or breast-milk substitutes in the absence of colostrum) can be offered to the baby by cup, spoon, dropper, or tube feeding device.
      c. Mothers can hand express colostrum into a spoon and spoon feed it to the baby.
      d. Mothers with diabetes can express colostrum during the prenatal period, freeze it, and bring it to the hospital for use if necessary instead of infant formula (Cox, 2006).

   3. Insulin is a large molecule that does not pass into the milk of a mother on insulin replacement therapy.

E. Mothers who have diabetes might be more prone to infection, mastitis, and overgrowth of *Candida albicans*.

   1. Hypoglycemia in the mother might increase the release of epinephrine, reducing milk production and interfering with the milk ejection reflex (Asselin & Lawrence, 1987).

   2. The presence of acetone signals the need for more calories and carbohydrates; acetone can be transferred to the milk and stress the newborn's liver (Lawrence & Lawrence, 2005).

III. Thyroid Disease

A. The thyroid gland controls the body's metabolism and is involved with the hormones of pregnancy and lactation.

B. Because untreated hypothyroidism has a low probability for the maintenance of a pregnancy, most mothers who have this condition are already receiving thyroid replacement therapy (which is compatible with breastfeeding).

C. Low thyroid levels have been associated with low milk production and insufficient weight gain in some babies and should be examined in these situations.

D. Hypothyroidism has also been identified in postpartum mothers who have prolonged "baby blues," a new onset of depression, or extended fatigue.

E. Hyperthyroidism is an excess amount of thyroid hormone that can result in rapid weight loss, increased appetite, nervousness, heart palpitations, and a rapid pulse at rest.

   1. The ability to lactate is not compromised by this condition.

   2. Hyperthyroidism with bulging eyes is called Graves' disease.

   3. Laboratory examination of a blood sample can usually diagnose this condition; sometimes radioiodine studies are recommended. The lactation consultant should identify the compound being used and decide whether breastfeeding needs to be interrupted.

   4. Treatment is usually an antithyroid drug that is safe for the infant.

   5. Sometimes the baby's thyroid function is measured periodically.

IV. Cystic Fibrosis (CF)

A. CF is characterized by the dysfunction of the exocrine glands and includes chronic pulmonary disease, obstruction of the pancreatic ducts, and pancreatic enzyme deficiency.

B. Formerly, life expectancy was short with few women reaching adulthood.

C. In early stages, more sophisticated treatments are now enabling women to live into adulthood, reproduce, and breastfeed.

D. Concerns center on the mother maintaining her own weight and her health status, rather than quality or quantity of her breast milk.

   1. Mothers who have CF usually need plenty of extra calories and supplements to their own diet in order to maintain their weight.

E. Individuals who have CF are chronic carriers of pathologic bacteria such as *Staphylococcus aureus* and *Pseudomonas*.

   1. Breast milk lymphocytes are sensitized to these pathogens carried by the mother and are passed to the baby in breast milk, protecting him or her from infections by these agents (Larson, 2004).

V. Phenylketonuria (PKU)

A. PKU is an inborn error of metabolism whereby the body lacks the enzyme to break down the amino acid phenylalanine, which can result in lowered intelligence.

B. Because of widespread newborn screening for this situation and early treatment, many women with PKU are reaching their childbearing years with normal intelligence.

   C. Dietary restrictions should not be discontinued at any age, especially in women (Lee et al., 2005).

     1. Blood phenylalanine levels should be ≤ 4 mg in women (Matalon, Michals, & Gleason, 1986).

     2. Breastfeeding is compatible with the condition (Matalon et al., 1986).

     3. The milk of mothers who have PKU is of normal composition (Fox-Bacon et al., 1997).

VI. Systemic Lupus Erythematosus (SLE)

   A. SLE is an autoimmune disease of the connective tissue primarily affecting women of childbearing age.

   B. Symptoms are diverse, exacerbated by pregnancy, and include the following: fatigue, fibromyalgia, joint redness and swelling, and a butterfly rash on the cheeks and nose.

   C. Women who have SLE experience higher rates of miscarriage and delivery of preterm infants.

   D. Raynaud's phenomenon is present in about 30% of cases.

   E. Insufficient milk supply is the most frequent complaint during lactation.

     1. Infant weight gain must be carefully watched, and babies might need supplementation.

     2. Fatigue and some medications may contribute to faltering milk production.

   F. Nonsteroidal anti-inflammatory medications and corticosteroids are frequent medications that are given to handle symptoms.

   G. Breastfeeding is especially beneficial to mothers who have SLE because it enables them to rest while feeding the baby and helps space out pregnancies.

VII. Osteoporosis

   A. Osteoporosis is a condition of bone thinning that is generally associated with older, postmenopausal women.

   B. Normal lactation-associated bone mineral mobilization takes place and does not require drug therapy or nutritional supplements.

   C. Bone loss can be measurable during lactation but returns to normal baseline following weaning (Eisman, 1998).

   D. Because a lactating woman's body is more efficient in energy use and nutrient uptake, lumbar bone density actually increases the longer a woman breastfeeds and the more infants she nurses (Kalkwarf & Specker, 1995; Kalkwarf et al., 1996).

   E. Age, diet, body frame size, and weight-bearing exercise all contribute to good (or poor) bone health.

VIII. Seizure Disorders (Epilepsy)

A. Mothers who have epilepsy can successfully breastfeed and should be encouraged to do so.

B. The major concern is the sedating effect on the baby of maternal medications.

C. Antiepileptic drugs tend to make a baby sleepy and depress his or her sucking in the early days following birth until he or she is better able to handle drug clearance (Hale, 2006).

   1. It is important that mothers pump milk following feedings or if the baby feeds poorly in order to provide breast stimulation in the absence of adequate sucking by the baby during the early days.

D. Some mothers have been advised not to breastfeed because they might drop the baby if they have a seizure while breastfeeding; this situation is no more likely to occur during breastfeeding than during bottle-feeding.

IX. Migraine Headaches

A. These severe episodic headaches tend to be worse during the first trimester of pregnancy and are sensitive to hormones and other triggers.

B. Many remedies, both pharmacologic and of a biofeedback nature, are used to help this condition.

C. It does not preclude breastfeeding.

D. When a mother experiences this type of headache and if it is severe enough, she might not feel well enough to breastfeed (although pumping may not be much of a relief).

E. Mothers might want some extra milk in the freezer in case others need to feed the baby.

X. Raynaud's Phenomenon of the Nipple

A. Raynaud's phenomenon is an intermittent ischemia (narrowing of the blood vessels) usually affecting the fingers and toes, especially when exposed to cold and more commonly seen in women.

B. In some women, this condition shows indications of blanching of the nipple before, during, or after breastfeedings.

C. These nipple spasms also have been seen clinically as a result of babies biting at the breast, jaw clenching, and in the presence of severe nipple damage; such sucking variations need to be corrected to help eliminate the trigger to the spasms (Lawlor-Smith & Lawlor-Smith, 1997).

D. The mother feels extreme pain during this nipple spasm, which might continue to spasm and relax for up to 30 minutes after a feeding.

E. Exposure to cold can exacerbate this problem.

F. Some maternal medications, such as fluconazole and oral contraceptives, might be associated with vasospasm.

G. Mothers usually feel relief from warm compresses to the breasts or a heating pad.

H. Other anecdotal remedies for this condition that have not been thoroughly studied include the following:

    1. Ibuprofen.

    2. Nifedipine (5 mg 3×/day for one week; Anderson, Held, & Wright, 2004).

    3. Supplemental calcium (2000 mg/day).

    4. Supplemental magnesium (1000 mg/day).

XI. Surgery

A. Breastfeeding can continue through almost all situations that require surgery.

B. Mothers can usually breastfeed upon arousal from anesthesia.

C. Concern is over anesthetic and pain medications, the mother's ability to hold and feed the baby, access to the baby, access to a breast pump, and the ability to pump on a regular basis.

D. Babies might be able to room with the mother during her hospital stay as long as an assistant is present to care for the baby.

    1. Otherwise, the baby can be brought to the hospital for feedings.

    2. If this situation is not possible, the mother should have access to a hospital-grade electric breast pump with a double collection kit.

    3. If she is physically unable to pump, then the nurse or caretaker can pump the breasts for her.

E. With elective surgery, the mother has time to arrange for access to the baby, a private room, and perhaps pump extra milk and freeze it for use any time she is unavailable to feed.

XII. Viral Infections (Pickering, 2006)

A. Breastfeeding is rarely contraindicated in maternal infection.

B. Exceptions relate to specific infectious agents with strong evidence of transmission and to the association of increased morbidity and mortality in the infant.

C. Cytomegalovirus (CMV; one of the human herpes viruses).

    1. Congenital infections are usually asymptomatic but can result in later hearing loss or learning disability.

2. Infections in full term infants acquired at birth from maternal cervical secretions or breast milk are usually not associated with symptoms (Lawrence & Lawrence, 2005).

3. Infants who have congenital or acquired CMV do better if they are breastfed because of the antibody protection delivered through breast milk.

4. Nonbreastfed infants can be infected through other secretions, including saliva, and receive no protective antibodies or other host resistance factors that are present in breast milk.

    a. They can have significant health effects from the disease, including microcephaly and mental retardation.

    b. High rates of transmission occur in child care centers.

5. Term infants can be fed breast milk when the mother is shedding virus in her milk because of the passively transferred maternal antibodies (Lawrence, 2006).

6. Preterm infants can develop the disease, even from breast milk; recommendations include freezing the breast milk for three to seven days at −20°C, which decreases infectivity but does not totally eliminate the virus (Lawrence, 2006).

D. Herpes simplex virus.

1. Infection in the early neonatal period is serious and can be fatal.

2. The infection is most frequently transmitted to the baby through the birth canal.

3. Only lesions on the breast would require a temporary interruption of breastfeeding on that breast until the lesions have completely cleared (Lawrence, 1997).

4. Active lesions elsewhere on the body should be covered, and the mother should be instructed to wash her hands before handling the infant; breastfeeding is not affected.

5. A mother who has cold sores on her lips should refrain from kissing and nuzzling the baby until the lesions have crusted and dried.

E. Herpes varicella zoster (chickenpox).

1. If maternal chickenpox occurs within six days of delivery and no lesions are present in the mother or the baby, mother and baby should be isolated from each other.

2. When the mother becomes noninfectious (6–10 days), she can be with her baby.

3. The mother will need to pump breast milk only while she remains clinically infectious. The breastmilk can and should be given to the baby as long as there are no active lesions on the breast (Lawrence & Lawrence, 2005).

F. Respiratory syncytial virus (RSV).

    1. RSV is a common cause of respiratory illness in children.

    2. Mortality can be high in neonates, especially preterm babies or ill full-term babies.

    3. There is no reason to stop breastfeeding during maternal RSV infection; in fact, breast milk might be protective against severe RSV (Lawrence & Lawrence, 2005).

    4. Infants who have RSV should breastfeed.

G. Human immunodeficiency virus 1 (HIV-1).

    1. HIV-1 can be transmitted through breast milk, but the relative risk is not well quantified.

    2. HIV-1 antibodies also occur in the breast milk of infected women.

    3. A major dilemma in estimating the risk from breastfeeding is in the difficulty in determining when the HIV infection actually occurs in the infant.

    4. Current standards of the Occupational Safety and Health Administration do not require gloves for the routine handling of expressed human milk.

       a. Health workers should wear gloves in situations where exposure to expressed breast milk would be frequent or prolonged, such as in milk banking (Nommsen-Rivers, 1997).

    5. Expressed breast milk from HIV-positive mothers can be made safe for infant consumption and should be carefully considered for use, especially in areas of the world where breast-milk substitute use would pose a grave threat to the life of the infant.

    6. Refer to Chapter 19.

H. Hepatitis.

    1. The varying types of hepatitis carry different risks of contagion, pathways of exposure, treatments, and preventive measures.

    2. Hepatitis A is an acute illness and is usually transmitted through food-borne and water-borne routes as well as commonly in child care settings through fecal contamination.

       a. A newborn can be infected by vertical transmission from an infected mother during delivery.

       b. The baby should be isolated from other babies in the nursery (such as rooming-in).

       c. Gamma globulin is given to the baby if the mother developed the disease within two weeks of the delivery.

       d. The mother will also receive gamma globulin.

       e. Breastfeeding should proceed as usual.

3. Hepatitis B can cause a wide variety of infections, from asymptomatic conversion to fulminant fatal hepatitis.
   a. Mandatory prenatal testing reveals the mother's status prior to delivery.
   b. Infants who are born to mothers who have the active disease or who are active carriers receive hepatitis B specific immunoglobulin (HBIG) at birth or soon after, followed by an immunization program.
   c. As soon as HBIG is given, breastfeeding should begin (Lawrence & Lawrence, 2005).

4. Hepatitis C infection has an insidious onset, with many people not aware that they are affected.
   a. The risk of infection via breast milk has not been documented (Lawrence, 1997).
   b. Concern arises if a mother has a co-infection, such as HIV.
   c. The virus might be inactivated in the infant's gastrointestinal tract or neutralized in colostrum; mothers who have hepatitis C can and should breastfeed.

5. Hepatitis D, E, and G.
   a. Not much is known about transmission of these forms of hepatitis through breastfeeding.
   b. Hepatitis D is usually a co-infection or superimposed on a hepatitis B infection.
   c. Once immunoglobin has been given and the vaccine has begun, breastfeeding should proceed as usual.
   d. Hepatitis E is self-limited and is not a chronic disease (usually associated with water contamination).
   e. Breastfeeding has not been shown to transmit this disease and should proceed as usual.
   f. Hepatitis G seems associated with blood transfusions but has not been shown to be transmitted through breast milk.
   g. Reports of infected mothers breastfeeding infants are few, but no clinical infections have been reported.

XIII. Tuberculosis

A. Breastfeeding is not contraindicated in women who have previously positive skin tests and no evidence of disease.

1. A mother who has had a recent conversion to a positive skin test should be evaluated for the disease, and if there is no sign of disease, breastfeeding should begin or continue.

2. If a mother has suspicious symptoms, she might need to pump milk and have it fed to the baby until a diagnosis is made.

3. In developed countries where there is easy access to an electric breast pump, mothers might need to pump milk during the time they are being evaluated.

4. If there is confirmation of the disease, the mother needs to be treated and breastfeeding can begin or resume after two weeks of maternal therapy.

5. In developing countries where nonbreastfed infants have a high mortality rate, breastfeeding is not interrupted.

6. If it is safe for the mother to be in contact with her baby, then it is safe to breastfeed.

References

Academy of Breastfeeding Medicine. Hypoglycemia. Available at: http://www.bfmed.org/ace-files/protocol/hypoglycemia.pdf. Accessed February 2, 2007.

Anderson JE, Held N, Wright K. Raynaud's phenomenon of the nipple: a treatable cause of painful breastfeeding. *Pediatrics.* 2004;113:e360–e364.

Arthur PG, Kent JC, Hartmann PE. Metabolites of lactose synthesis in milk from diabetic and non-diabetic women during lactogenesis II. *J Pediatr Gastroenterol Nutr.* 1994; 19:100–108.

Asselin BL, Lawrence RA. Maternal disease as a consideration in lactation management. *Clin Perinatol.* 1987;14:71–87.

California Diabetes and Pregnancy Program. *Guidelines for Care: Sweet Success Express.* Sacramento, CA: Maternal and Health Branch, Department of Health Services; 2002.

Cox DB, Owens RA, Hartmann PE. Blood and milk prolactin and the rate of milk synthesis in women. *Exp Physiol.* 1996;81:1007–1020.

Cox SG. Expressing and storing colostrum antenatally for use in the newborn period. *Breastfeeding Rev.* 2006;14:11–16.

Cregan MD, DeMello TR, Hartmann PE. Pre-term delivery and breast expression: consequences for initiating lactation. *Adv Exp Med Biol.* 2000;478:427–428.

DeCoopman J. Breastfeeding after pituitary resection: support for a theory of autocrine control of milk supply? *J Hum Lact.* 1993;9:35–40.

Eisman J. Relevance of pregnancy and lactation to osteoporosis? *Lancet.* 1998;352: 504–505.

Fox-Bacon C, McCamman S, Therou L, et al. Maternal PKU and breastfeeding: case report of identical twin mothers. *Clin Pediatr.* 1997;36:539–542.

Hale TW. *Medications and Mothers' Milk.* Amarillo, TX: Hale Publishing; 2006.

Hartmann PE, Cregan M. Lactogenesis and the effects of insulin-dependent diabetes mellitus and prematurity. *J Nutr.* 2001;3016S–3020S. Available at: http://jn. nutrition.org/cgi/content/full/131/11/3016S. Accessed February 2, 2007.

Kalkwarf HJ, Specker BL. Bone mineral loss during lactation and recovery after weaning. *Obstet Gynecol.* 1995;86:26–32.

Kalkwarf HJ, Specker BL, Heubi JE, et al. Intestinal calcium absorption of women during lactation and after weaning. *Am J Clin Nutr.* 1996;63:526–531.

Kjos SL, Henry O, Lee RM, et al. The effect of lactation on glucose and lipid metabolism in women with recent gestational diabetes. *Obstet Gynecol.* 1993;82:451–455.

Larson LA. *Immunobiology of Human Milk: How Breastfeeding Protects Babies.* Amarillo, TX: Pharmasoft Publishing; 2004.

Lawlor-Smith L, Lawlor-Smith C. Vasospasm of the nipple—a manifestation of Raynaud's phenomenon: case reports. *Br Med J.* 1997;314:844–845.

Lawrence RA. A review of the medical benefits and contraindications to breastfeeding in the United States (Maternal and Child Health Technical Information Bulletin). Arlington, VA: National Center for Education in Maternal and Child Health; 1997.

Lawrence RA, Lawrence RM. *Breastfeeding: A Guide for the Medical Profession.* 6th ed. St. Louis: Mosby, Inc.; 2005.

Lawrence RM. Cytomegalovirus in human breast milk: risk to the premature infant. *Breastfeeding Med.* 2006;1:99–107.

Lee PJ, Ridout D, Walter JH, Cockburn F. Maternal phenylketonuria: report from the United Kingdom Registry 1978–97. *Arch Dis Child.* 2005;90:143–146.

Matalon R, Michals K, Gleason L. PKU: strategies for dietary treatment and monitoring compliance. *Ann NY Acad Sci.* 1986;477:223–230.

Nommsen-Rivers L. Universal precautions are not needed for health care workers handling breast milk. *J Hum Lact.* 1997;13:267–268.

Pickering LK, ed. *2006 Red Book: Report of the Commission on Infectious Diseases.* 27th ed. Elk Grove Village, IL: American Academy of Pediatrics; 2006.

Verhelst J, Abs R. Hyperprolactinemia: pathophysiology and management. *Treat Endocrinol.* 2003;2:23–32.

Verma S, Shah D, Faridi MM. Breastfeeding a baby with mother on Bromocriptine. *Indian J Pediatr.* 2006;73:435–436.

INSUFFICIENT MILK SUPPLY

Kay Hoover, MEd, IBCLC, and Lisa Marasco, MA, IBCLC

OBJECTIVES

- Explain normal milk production.
- Delineate between a real and a perceived insufficient milk supply.
- Discuss the etiology of insufficient milk.
- Describe potential indicators of insufficient milk.
- List options for improvement of an insufficient milk supply.

Introduction

An insufficient supply of breast milk continues to be the major reason given by mothers worldwide for the discontinuation of breastfeeding during the first six to eight weeks postpartum. This reason is also commonly given around four months of age. Whether the problem is real or perceived is addressed by a careful history and breastfeeding assessment. True low milk supply can be caused by a number of factors and is often a combination of these factors (termed *overlapping etiologies*). Perceived low milk supply is a mother's misinterpretation of infant behaviors such as frequent feedings or apparent unsettledness after a feed. Many mothers reporting infant fussiness after breastfeeding will give the baby a bottle of formula to "satisfy" the infant. Supplementing the baby usually begins a downward spiral to real insufficient milk unless interrupted. The percentage of mothers reporting insufficient milk in the literature varies, with many reports not differentiating between real and perceived insufficiency.

I. Normal Milk Production

A. Normal milk production begins with successful mammogenesis.

1. Three important periods of mammary gland development: embryo/fetal, puberty, and pregnancy (Knight & Sorenson, 2001).

2. While growth hormone is essential for puberty, estrogen has primary influence on the breast gland, causing ductal growth into the mammary fat pad. Progesterone, the second major hormone of mammary gland development, stimulates development of alveoli along the ducts and ductules (Lawrence & Lawrence, 2005).

3. With each successive menstrual cycle, estrogen rises during the first half while progesterone dominates the second half of the cycle, continuing on a minute level to stimulate glandular growth until approximately age 30 (Hartmann et al., 1996; Lawrence & Lawrence, 2005).

4. Generally speaking, lactation capability is reached approximately halfway through pregnancy. At this time, colostrum begins to be made and the substrates for milk production are laid down (*lactogenesis I*).

5. With premature deliveries between 22 and 34 weeks, mammogenesis may or may not be sufficiently complete for full lactation (Cregan, 2007).

6. The major stimulating hormones during pregnancy include: estrogen, progestererone, human placental lactogen (HPL), prolactin, and chorionic gonadotropin (Lawrence & Lawrence, 2005).

7. Change in breast volume is most closely associated with concentration of HPL (Cox et al., 1999). The additional placenta present in multiple pregnancies stimulates greater mammogenesis (Knight & Sorenson, 2001), while placental insufficiencies can negatively impact mammary development during pregnancy.

8. During weaning, unneeded alveoli are destroyed and the breast involutes until it returns to its pre-pregnancy state.

9. Potential interferences with normal mammary gland development.
   a. Genetic aberrations such as Poland syndrome.
   b. Inappropriate hormonal exposure, such as, too much testosterone during critical windows, can affect development.
   c. Environmental disruptor theory implicating environmental contaminants such as TCDD, BPA, PCBs, and PCAHs (Fenton et al. 2002; Guillette et al., 2006; Hond et al., 2002; Lewis et al. 2001; Markey et al., 2003; Vorderstrasse et al., 2004).

B. Initiation of milk production is hormonally (endocrine) controlled.

1. Onset is triggered by separation of placenta from uterus, removing progesterone interference with prolactin receptors and allowing lactogenesis II to begin.

2. Key hormones necessary for initiation of lactation are prolactin, insulin, and cortisol (Lawrence & Lawrence, 2005).

3. Under normal circumstances, change to more copious milk production usually begins in 30 to 40 hours (Chapman & Perez-Escamilla, 1999) and is usually noticed by mothers between days 2 and 4.

4. Milk production at five days is highly variable, with mothers producing between 200 and 900 g/24 hours (Woolridge, 1996).

5. Early milk removal (within first 48 hrs) is associated with higher milk output. (Hill, Aldag, & Chatterton, 2001; Neville & Morton, 2001) Milk production will begin to shut down if milk removal does not begin at the onset of copious milk production (typically 3–4 days).

C. Transition to autocrine control begins over the following three to five weeks as milk output is progressively calibrated to the baby's needs, increasing in most cases but sometimes decreasing (Woolridge, 1996). *Lactogenesis III* is the maintenance of long-term milk production.

1. Milk removal is the key factor to calibration of milk production. If milk production is to be sustained, milk must be consistently and effectively removed.
   a. The emptier the breast, the faster the rate of milk synthesis. The fuller the breast, the slower the rate of synthesis.
   b. Unremoved milk exerts an inhibitory effect on milk production, down-regulating the amount produced through:
      i. Chemical means: feedback inhibitor of lactation (Wilde et al., 1995).
      ii. Physical means: pressure atrophy of milk secreting cells.
   c. Inhibition of oxytocin/milk ejection can affect ability to remove milk.

2. Overall, the rate of increase in milk production is about 175 g/week; after about six weeks, the rate of milk increase slows to about 4 g/week.

3. 750 g/24 hours meets the needs of the average infant, even beyond six weeks; the range of milk production for a singleton baby in the first six months is approximately 788 ± 169 g (Kent et al., 1999; Kent et al., 2006).
   a. Total milk required is a function of a combination of baby's sex, baby's metabolic needs, and caloric content of the milk.
   b. Boys take in more than girls on average; thus, mothers of boys make more milk than mothers of girls on average (Kent et al., 2006).
   c. After one month and again around six months, a baby's energy requirements per kilogram of body weight decreases (Butte, 2005).

4. Milk output is not constrained at 750 g/24 hours because mothers of twins are quite capable of outputs of 1500 g/24 hours (Saint, Maggiore, & Hartmann, 1986).

5. It is normal for one breast to make more milk, even significantly more, than the other; this effect has been found to be independent of the infant (Engstrom, Meier, & Jegier; Kent et al., 2006).

6. Prolactin receptor theory: Successful transition to autocrine control may rely in part on continued development of prolactin receptors, which appears to be influenced by frequency of feeding (Woolridge, 1996).

D. Interference with the calibration of the breasts during the early days can cause the breasts to calibrate at an inappropriate level. Such interference may include the following:

1. Iatrogenic.
   a. Supplemental feeds of water or formula.
   b. Unnecessarily interrupted or delayed breastfeeding for a variety of reasons without concomitant removal of milk (pumping of the breasts).
      i. Hyperbilirubinemia.
      ii. Hypoglycemia.
      iii. Maternal medications.
      iv. Maternal illness.
      v. Infant illness.
   c. Necessary interruption or delay of breastfeeding without concomitant removal of milk.
   d. A baby who does not efficiently remove milk from the breast (see Chapters 5 and 40).
   e. Unrelieved engorgement; a mother might have been engorged and mistakenly told not to pump milk because she would just make more milk (low milk production is the result of such advice).
   f. A mother might have been encouraged to send her baby to the nursery at night, leading to undermining situations such as mother-baby separation, infant introduction to artificial nipples or infant dissatisfaction with colostrum after larger boluses of formula, that can start a downward spiral of supplementation and down-regulation of milk production.
   g. Hormonal birth control before six weeks (oral, injectable, implants, transdermal patch, vaginal ring, or emergency contraceptives; Smith & Valentine, 2006).

2. Maternal misunderstanding of the process.
   a. A mother of a preterm infant who does not express her milk to her peak yield, but just to the transient limited needs of the small baby at the time, causing a low calibration of milk yield.
   b. A limited number of feedings.
   c. Feedings that are not long enough.
   d. An infant sucking on pacifiers, fingers, thumbs, or nipple shield (Auerbach, 1990; Woolridge, Baum, & Drewett, 1980)

3. Something goes wrong internally when the system switches from endocrine to autocrine control.
   a. Might have seen evidence of higher milk output at an earlier stage, but output has inexplicably dropped despite good management.
   b. Hormonal problem may or may not be easily pinpointed.

4. Baby is not capable of sufficient milk removal to maintain adequate supply.

5. Potential risk factors.
   a. Mothers who are less informed about breastfeeding.
   b. Making the decision to breastfeed later in pregnancy.
   c. Intending to breastfeed for a short or limited period of time.
   d. Planning to "do both" (mixed feeding).
   e. Initiation of milk removal > 48 hours and/or low frequency of milk removal when baby is unable to feed (Hill et al., 2001).
   f. Being less confident about their ability to breastfeed; mothers who are tentative and say that they are going to "try" to breastfeed.
   g. Being sensitive to a lack of privacy.
   h. Receiving less encouragement from male partner, mother, and/or mother-in-law.
   i. Having a poorer health status and more problems with illness while breastfeeding.
6. After six weeks, this condition might be more difficult to reverse.

II. Unsubstantiated Low Milk Supply (Perceived Insufficiency)

A. The vast majority of "insufficient milk supply" is perceived rather than real.

1. Some newborns may desire to nurse very frequently until the milk increases with lactogenesis II. Mothers may interpret this as "not enough milk" and "starving the baby" and initiate supplemental feeds prior to full lactogenesis II.

2. Mothers often describe an unsettled baby who fusses after feedings; a baby who feeds for long periods at the breast; or a baby who feeds constantly at the breast and fusses when put down. While this may be due to low supply, it also may be due to infant discomfort or high sucking needs. This behavior can also be seen when the baby is sucking at the breast but not swallowing milk (i.e., impaired milk ejection reflex).

3. Normal newborn pattern of wakefulness and feeding more often at night may be misinterpreted as the result of low supply.

4. Perceptions by the mother that her supply is low due to softer breasts, normal decrease in size of the breasts, breasts feeling less full, cessation of leakage, or a change in the sensation of the milk ejection.

5. Mothers simply doubt their ability to make sufficient milk.

6. Sometimes the symptoms of oversupply (baby pulling away from the breast and crying, fussy baby who still wants to nurse) may be mistaken for insufficient milk production.

B. Teach mothers about normal physiologic breastfeeding.

1. Successful nursing dyads generally breastfeed 8–12 or more times in 24 hours (de Carvalho et al., 1982; Kent et al., 2006).

2. Clustered or bunched feedings in the late afternoon and early evening are normal. Cluster feedings may occur at any time, one or more times a day. Each feed in the "cluster" contributes to the 8 to 12 feeds expected in the 24-hour period.

3. Frequency days can occur anytime, and the baby should be fed whenever he or she wants.

4. The baby should drain the first breast before being offered the second.

5. There should be no arbitrary time limitations at the breast, such as five minutes on the first side so that the baby will take both sides. Mother should feed the baby until the baby comes off the first side in a relaxed manner, and then feed on the second breast if the baby so desires.

6. The baby should feed at night; breastfeeding should not be skipped at night.

7. Avoid the use of sleep-through-the-night baby training programs that do not enable night feeds.

8. Avoid parenting programs that attempt to control how frequently a baby can be breastfed.

9. Ensure that the cause of nipple pain is addressed (positioning or ineffective sucking patterns).

10. Advise mothers not to decrease the number of breastfeedings to "let the breasts fill."

C. Early help for problems that may lead to insufficient feeds and low milk supply increases the rate of successful breastfeeding.

1. Nipple pain.

2. Breast pain (engorgement, mastitis).

3. Discomfort in positioning from cesarean surgery or episiotomy.

4. Any other maternal problems.

D. Support and encouragement.

1. Is beneficial to educate family members, especially the father of the baby and grandmothers of the baby, regarding breastfeeding norms in order to eliminate the pressure to give bottles or to not breastfeed as much as is necessary.

2. Frequent weight checks will help to reassure the family.

3. Family can be involved in household chores and care of other children.

E. Sociological problems.

1. Too busy mother who is not breastfeeding enough.
   a. Unusual stress or fatigue.
   b. More than one child younger than 5 years.
   c. Many caregiving responsibilities such as elderly parents or relatives, pets, or farm animals.

d. Logistics of returning to work or school and maintaining adequate milk removal and stimulation.

2. Mother concerned she is not eating well enough.
   a. Deposits of fat during pregnancy subsidize lactation.
   b. Breastfeeding women need at least 1500 calories per day.
   c. Lesser intakes have been related to reductions in milk production (Institute of Medicine, 1991).
      i. Minimum caloric requirements vary according to individual metabolism and level of activity (Picciano, 2003).
      ii. Generally speaking, an extra 500 kcal/day over normal are needed the first 6 months; this drops to 400 kcal/day from 7 to 9 months (Picciano, 2003).
   d. History of an eating disorder is rarely a problem unless the disorder is active.
      i. One case study showed no problem (Bowles & Williamson, 1990).
      ii. Active binge/purge of bulimia can cause lower prolactin levels; implications are unknown (Monteleone et al., 1998; Weltzin et al., 1991).
   e. Severe restriction of food intake during pregnancy or lactation may cause milk supply problems (Motil, Sheng, & Montandon, 1994; Paul, Muller, & Whitehead, 1979).
   f. Gastric bypass surgery (GBS) (Grange & Finlay, 1994; Martens, Martin, & Berlin, 1990; Wardinsky et al., 1995).
      i. Must also consider underlying cause of obesity leading to GBS.
      ii. If mother still in high caloric restriction phase, risk for problems are higher (Stefanski, 2006).
      iii. High risk of poor absorption of nutrients essential to milk composition, most especially vitamin B_{12} (Fussy, 2005).
      iv. Recommend at least 65 grams of protein daily (Stefanski, 2006).

F. Psychological concerns.

1. Social support.
   a. How do the people around her feel about breastfeeding?
   b. Is she being pressured to breastfeed?

2. Postpartum depression (O'Brien et al., 2004).

3. Emotional problems.
   a. How does she feel about being a mother?
   b. How does she feel about breastfeeding?
   c. Is she embarrassed when she breastfeeds?

4. Was this a planned pregnancy?

5. Severe psychological issues may affect oxytocin release and impair milk ejection, which can lead to low supply if chronic (rare).
   a. Post-traumatic stress syndrome; nursing may awaken unwanted memories or fears.
   b. History of sexual abuse.

G. Medications and foods.

    1. Reports of sage, parsley, and mint reducing milk supply (anecdotal; no formal research).

    2. Cigarette smoking.

        a. Interpretations of research are conflicting (Amir, 2001; Amir & Donath, 2003; deMello, Pinto, & Botelho, 2001).

        b. Reduces the length of breastfeeding (Amir, 2001).

        c. Believed to reduce prolactin secretion (Andersen et al., 1982).

        d. Lower milk yield (Hopkinson et al., 1992; Vio, Salazar, & Infante, 1991).

        e. Lower total lipid levels and docosahexaenoic acid content of milk (Agostoni et al., 2003; Hopkinson et al., 1992).

    3. Some over-the-counter and prescription medicines reduce milk supply.

        a. Pseudoephedrine (a nasal decongestant; Aljazaf et al., 2003; Hale et al., 2004).

        b. Bromocriptine, cabergoline, ergotamine.

        c. Hormonal birth control.

        d. Bupropion (antidepressant; smoking deterrent; case reports, Hale, 2006).

        e. Medicines to treat Parkinson's disease.

        f. Blood pressure medicine; methyldopa suppresses prolactin (Lawrence & Lawrence, 2005:590).

        g. Marijuana may reduce milk supply (Djulus, Moretti, & Koren, 2005).

           i. Women who use marijuana should not breastfeed because it may be harmful to the baby (Astley & Little, 1990; Djulus et al., 2005).

    4. Overdoses of vitamin B_6 may reduce milk for some women (conflicting research).

    5. Alcohol consumption.

        a. Prolactin response to suckling after ingestion of alcohol is greater, but the higher the prolactin level, the longer the time to milk ejection (Mennella, Pepino, & Teff, 2005).

        b. Oxytocin response to suckling is lower after ingestion of alcohol, with slowed milk ejection (Cobo, 1973; Mennella, 2001; Minella et al., 2005).

        c. Babies transfer less milk during the immediate hours after maternal ingestion of alcohol, though they are able to make up for it later when the affects of the alcohol have worn off (Mennella, 2001).

        d. Frequent ingestion of alcohol can cause lowered milk production (Mennella, 2001; de Araújo Burgos, Bion, & Campos, 2004).

III. Pathophysiologic Lactation Failure

A. Presentation.

    1. Mothers can present with an infant who shows slow or static weight gain or weight loss.

    2. May have had previous babies with problems gaining weight.

B. Delayed lactogenesis II, full milk production > 72 hours (Dewey et al., 2003).

  1. Temporary problem, usually self-resolving.

  2. Risk factors.

    a. Stress during labor.

    b. Second stage of labor over one hour (Dewey et al., 2003).

    c. Significant edema, especially when onsets or worsens during/after delivery (anecdotal).

    d. Cesarean birth, especially when urgent (Chapman & Perez-Escamilla, 1999; Leung, Lam, & Ho, 2002).

    e. Forceps or vacuum delivery (Leung et al., 2002).

    f. Epidural analgesia affects duration of breastfeeding (Henderson et al., 2003).

    g. Augmentation of labor with pitocin (Dewey et al., 2003).

    h. Flat or inverted nipples (Dewey et al., 2003).

    i. Hypertension (Hall et al., 2002).

    j. Type 1 diabetes (average 24 hr delay) (Hartmann & Cregan, 2001; Miyake et al.,1989; Neubauer et al., 1993; Ostrom & Ferris, 1993).

    k. Obesity (Chapman & Perez-Escamilla, 1999); Maternal body mass index greater than 27 kg/m2 (Dewey et al., 2003).

  3. Other causes of delayed lactation:

    a. Gestational ovarian theca lutein cysts—a rare condition that causes high testosterone levels during pregnancy. In a few cases it may also cause virilization (balding, deepening of the voice, facial or abdominal hair growth, pimples on the face or back, or enlargement of the clitoris). High testosterone gradually resolves days to weeks after birth on its own. With continued breast stimulation some women eventually have produced a full milk supply, though it has taken as long as 30 days before milk dramatically increased in volume (Betztold, Hoover, & Snyder, 2004; Hoover, Barbalindo, & Platia).

    b. Retained placental tissue.

  i. May continue to issue progesterone and interfere with full milk production until passed or removed (Anderson, 2001; Neifert, McDonough, & Neville, 1981).

    ii. Placenta accreta/increta/percreta; the more severe forms are more difficult to resolve.

    iii. Medications used to treat these conditions may suppress lactation (Arabin, Ruttgers, & Kubli, 1986).

C. Maternal nipple anomalies.

  1. Large (Caglar, Ozer, & Altugan, 2006).

  2. Long.

  3. Meaty/non-pliable.

  4. Flat or inverted (Caglar, Ozer, & Altugan, 2006; Cooper et al., 1995; Dewey et al.,

2003; Lawrence & Lawrence, 2005; Livingstone et al., 2000; Neifert et al., 1990; Wilson-Clay and Maloney, 2002; Yaseen, Salem, & Darwich, 2004).

    5. Few or no patent ducts through nipple.

D. Maternal breast anatomy and physiology.

    1. Surgery.
       a. Breast milk insufficiency has been particularly noted when periareolar incisions are used (Hurst, 1996; Neifert et al., 1990; Souto et al., 2003).
       b. Augmentation.
       c. Reduction (Harris, Morris, & Freiberg, 1992).
       d. Cyst removal.
       e. Biopsy.
       f. Cancer.
          i. Lumpectomy.
          ii. Mastectomy.
       g. Chest tube as preterm baby (Rainer et al., 2003).
       h. Nipple surgery.
       i. Abscess.
       j. Galactocele.

    2. Pathologic engorgement.

    3. Trauma, burns, radiation.

    4. Spinal cord injuries.
       i. Breast innervated T4–T6; if damage occurs T6 or above, lactation may be affected (Halbert, 1998).
       ii. Lactation often falters after 3 months, but case report suggests that aiding milk ejection via visualization or synthetic oxytocin spray may help sustain lactation (Cowley, 2005).

E. Maternal breast anatomy: insufficient glandular tissue (IGT).

    1. Defined as insufficient lactation tissue to produce enough milk to support adequate infant growth and development (Neifert & Seacat, 1987; Neifert, Seacat, & Jobe, 1985).

    2. "Classic" or more obvious insufficient mammary tissue.
       a. Frequently asymmetric in size and/or shape.
       b. One or both breasts may be conical/tubular in shape.
       c. Breasts may be completely underdeveloped.
          i. Hypoplasia.
          ii. Amastia (congenital absence of the breast and nipple; Lawrence & Lawrence, 2005).
          iii. An endocrine disorder resulting in faulty development, or lack of development of secondary sex characteristics.
       d. Breasts may be large, even pendulous, but palpate as soft fatty tissue.

3. Risk factors for IGT/poor lactation (Huggins, 2000).
   a. Little or no breast enlargement either during pregnancy or early postpartum.
   b. Greater than 1.5 inches (3.8 cm) between breasts.
   c. Lack of significant visible veining on breasts.
   d. Stretch marks (striae) on breast in the absence of breast growth.
   e. Higher risk for poor lactation, but may produce more milk over time with sustained effort, and may produce more milk with subsequent pregnancies.

4. IGT not always evident visually, but most evident on palpation. Some breasts present with normal dimensions except their appearance suggests a failure to respond normally to pregnancy hormones.

5. Assessing breast tissue.
   a. Degree of changes during pregnancy (growth, sensitivity, areolar enlargement, darkening).
   b. Enlargement postpartum.
   c. Palpate for granular versus smooth tissue.

F. Maternal issues.

1. Illness of mother.
   a. Infection (including mastitis).
   b. Anemia (Henly et al., 1995).

2. Chronic condition.
   a. Lupus erythematosus (Ferris & Reese, 1994).
   b. Diabetes. (Ferris & Reese, 1994).
   c. Allergies (pseudoephedrine reduces milk supply).
   d. Parkinson's disease (medicines inhibit milk production).
   e. Autoimmune disease.
   f. Connective tissue disease.
   g. Renal failure.
   h. Hypopituitarism.

3. Birth experience.
   a. Hemorrhage after birth, especially causing large sudden drop in blood pressure and/or requiring blood transfusion (< 500 mL loss is normal). (Willis & Livingstone, 1995)
      i. May cause damage to pituitary, ranging from mild insult to major infarction.
      ii. Severe hemorrhage and drop in blood pressure may result in necrosis of the anterior pituitary (Sheehan's syndrome, Sheehan & Murdoch, 1938). This is the "only commonly recognized endocrine disorder associated with lactation failure" (Lawrence & Lawrence, 2005).

4. Diabetes especially when poorly controlled (Lau, Sullivan, & Hazelwood, 1993; Miyake et al., 1989.

a. Decreases prolactin and placental lactogen in the rat (Botta et al., 1984).

b. Thyroid dysfunction may occur concomitantly (Gallas et al., 2002).

5. Hypertension, pregnancy-induced hypertension, hemolysis elevated liver, low platelets (HELLP) syndrome.

6. Obesity (Baker et al., 2004, Elliott et al., 1997, Hilson, Rasmussen, & Kjolhede, 1997; Hilson, Rasmussen, & Kjolhede, 2004; Lovelady, 2005; Kugyelka, Rasmussen, & Frongillo, 2004; Rasmussen, Hilson, & Kjolhede, 2001; Rasmussen et al., 2006).

a. Can blunt prolactin response in some women (Rasmussen & Kjolhede, 2004).

b. May also be related to underlying metabolic cause of obesity.

7. Age older than 35 years (Escobar et al., 2002).

8. Radiation to the brain.

9. Hormone-related issues and risk factors.

a. Risk factors for milk production problems.

   i. History of irregular menses or very late menarche.

   ii. Infertility with underlying hormonal imbalance or deficiency.

   iii. Required fertility medications to achieve pregnancy.

   iv. In vitro fertilization pregnancy.

b. History of polycystic ovary syndrome (PCOS) (Marasco, Marmet, & Shell, 2000).

   i. Can present with a number of hormonal aberrations, such as low progesterone levels, insulin resistance, elevated estrogen levels, and high levels of testosterone and androstenedione (with their possible effect of down-regulating estrogen and prolactin receptors).

c. Pregnancy during lactation.

d. Hormone patch for postpartum depression.

e. Hormonal birth control (Kennedy, Short, & Tully, 1997)

   i. Emergency contraception, DepoProvera, implant, patch, ring.

   ii. Estrogen reduces the milk supply (Ball & Morrison, 1999). Progesterone may reduce milk supply in early weeks/months (Kennedy et al., 1997; Smith & Valentine, 2006).

f. Endocrine issues.

   i. Low progesterone could affect breast development.

   ii. Prolactin deficiency—rare cases of familial deficiencies reported (Zargar et al., 1997).

   iii. Prolactin resistance (theorized; Zargar et al., 2000).

g. High testosterone can suppress lactation, probably via prolactin receptors.

h. Thyroid dysfunction—may affect both oxytocin and prolactin (Marasco 2006).

   i. Hypothyroidism (case study, Stein, 2002; rat research, Hapon et al., 2003, 2005).

    ii. Thyroid surgery.

    iii. Hyperthyroid; rat studies show problems with impaired oxytocin and milk ejection as well as lipid metabolism (Rosato, Gimenez, & Jahn, 1992).

    iv. Postpartum thyroiditis (Stagnaro-Green, 2002).

    v. Thyroid dysfunction risk higher with PCOS, type 1 diabetes and smoking (de Mello et al., 2001; Janssen et al., 2004).

    vi. Subclinical and/or borderline thyroid dysfunction may present through lactation problems; lab values may not always be clear (Marasco, 2006).

    vii. Hormone receptor problems; not well researched for lactation, but if there are not enough receptors (down-regulated) or they are resistant to binding, then even if there is a normal amount of hormone, the hormone cannot have an effect.

IV. Infant Problems

A. Take a thorough infant history.

    a. Gestational age (Wight, 2003).

    b. Near-term infants may not suckle well enough for adequate milk removal.

B. Consider normal variants of growth.

    1. Small parents so baby is growing to his or her genetic potential.

    2. Premature babies do not grow at the same rate as age-matched peers.

    3. Large-at-birth baby may have postnatal "catch down" growth.

C. Assess the baby.

    1. Check the baby's oral and facial anatomy (Abadie et al., 2001).

       a. General.

         i. Cheeks: thick sucking pads.

         ii. Comfortable mouth (no scratches or punctures from suctioning).

         iii. Lips: intact, no blisters, no tight frenum, flanged at breast, good tone.

         iv. Philtrum: well defined.

         v. If chin is receding, latch with chin very close to breast or use a prone position.

         vi. Mandibular asymmetry/torticollis (Wall & Glass, 2006).

       b. Palate.

         i. High, bubble, channel (Burke-Snyder, 1997).

         ii. Partial or complete cleft of soft or hard palate (Glenny et al., 2005; Wilton, 1998).

         iii. Submucosal cleft can interfere with ability to create proper oral vacuum (velopharyngeal insufficiency) for removing milk.

       c. Check the baby's oral-motor function.

         i. Correct sucking motion versus abnormal sucking motion.

         ii. Correct sucking pressure versus abnormal sucking pressure.

2. Tongue function: ability of tongue to cup, extend, lift, and lateralize (tight frenulum, a tongue-tie, may restrict tongue motion) (ABM, 2007; Amir, James, & Beatty, 2005; Amir, James, & Donath, 2006; Ballard, Auer, & Khoury, 2002; Fernando, 1999; Griffiths, 2004; Hazelbaker, 2005; Hogan, Westcott, & Griffiths, 2005; LaLakea & Messner, 2003; Ricke et al., 2004; Ricke et al., 2005; Srinivasan et al., 2006; Wallace & Clarke, 2006).

3. Airway.
   a. Open nostrils so baby can breathe.
   b. Positions where baby can breathe (prone feeding position).
   c. Laryngomalacia: floppy laryngeal structures are pulled into the airway upon inspiration (strider is heard with inspiration).
   d. Tracheomalacia: softening of the cartilaginous ring surrounding the trachea (stridor is heard with expiration).

4. Baby's comfort. Is the baby in any pain?
   a. Fractured clavicle; other birth injuries; scalp or brain bleeds from vacuum extraction.

5. Baby's health.
   a. Any infant medical condition that can impact on weight gain.
   b. Inadequate caloric intake.
   c. Inability to properly utilize ingested nutrients, reduced absorption/excessive loss of nutrients, due to metabolic problems, obstructions, disease process.
   d. Excessive utilization of energy due to metabolic problems, disease process, etc.

D. Observe a feeding (Yurdakök, Ösmert, & Yalçin, 1997).

1. Positioning.

2. Good latch.

3. Audible swallowing, one per suck at the start of the feeding.

4. Rhythmic sucking; a baby should be able to sustain 10 to 30 suck:swallow:breathe patterns in a row for some of the feeding.

5. Satisfied baby at the end of the feeding.

6. Test feed weights (on electronic scale accurate to 2 grams).

V. Basic Management of Milk Insufficiency

A. Make sure the baby is getting enough milk by assessing output and weight gain.

B. Protect the mother's milk supply.

C. Provide as close to a breastfeeding relationship as possible.

1. Supplementer at the breast if the baby has the ability to transfer milk.

2. Alternative feeding while holding baby on the bare breast.

D. To determine the woman's milk production in 24 hours, she can pump every hour for four pumping sessions.

1. The first two expressions will yield more milk than the third and fourth.

2. Take the third and fourth expressions and add them together. Multiply by 12 to obtain her 24-hour milk production (Lai et al., 2004).

VI. Increasing Milk Production

A. Additional therapeutic interventions depend on the cause of the problem.

1. Mothers should be taught how to position their baby at the breast, what constitutes an effective latch-on, and how to know when the baby is swallowing milk.

2. Nipple pain during a feeding can indicate that the baby is not positioned correctly or is not suckling correctly; each increases the likelihood of poor milk transfer, less milk removed from the breast, and less milk synthesized to replace it.

3. Mothers should be taught infant behavioral feeding cues, be encouraged to eliminate watching the clock, and to feed the baby when he or she demonstrates feeding readiness.

a. Feeding cues include rapid eye movements under the eyelids, sucking movements of the mouth and tongue, hand-to-mouth movements, body movements, and small sounds; these indicate a light sleep state moving to alertness when the baby is more likely to feed efficiently; babies who are in a deep sleep state do not breastfeed; feeding at proscribed intervals might catch the baby repeatedly at times when he or she is not "available" to feed.

b. Babies should be fed 8–12 times each 24 hours; feedings should not be skipped, complemented, or supplemented unless medically indicated; mothers should manually express or pump milk if the baby cannot go to the breast.

c. Mothers should demonstrate an awareness of cluster or bunched feedings that typically occur in the late afternoon or early evening, but could also occur at other times.

d. Alternate massage or breast compressions can be used to initiate and sustain suckling at the breast; some babies require the presence of milk flow to regulate their sucking (Stutte, Bowles, & Morman, 1988).

e. A mother should know how to gauge whether her baby is getting enough milk; bowel movements can be an indicator (size and color change are important) but ultimately weight gain is the best indicator (regain birth weight before two weeks and thereafter at least 5 to 7 ounces per week during the first 3 months).

f. Larger than normal weight loss during the first three days in a baby whose mother had pitocin and/or large amounts of intravenous fluids during labor should not be confused with insufficient milk intake (Dahlenburg, Burnell, & Braybrook, 1980).

4. Increase number of feedings/pumpings. Pump the way the baby would have breastfed (10×/day with at least one at night between 12 midnight and 5 AM).

5. Pump after breastfeeding starting on the third day postpartum.

6. Massage the breast while breastfeeding/pumping.

7. Compress the breast while feeding or pumping (hand express while breastfeeding).

8. Hold the baby skin-to-skin for as many hours a day as possible.

9. Supplement the baby while the baby is breastfeeding.

10. Put the baby back to the same breast several times.

11. Imagery audiotapes (Feder et al., 1989).

12. Acupuncture/acupressure (Clavey, 1996).
   a. Acupuncture has been used in China for low milk production since 256 AD (Clavey, 1996).
   b. Reports indicate that acupuncture is most effective if started within 20 days post delivery; little to no results will be obtained if started after six months (Clavey, 1996).
   c. Milk production can start to increase as soon as two to four hours following treatment or as late as 72 hours; the faster the response, the better the outcome (Clavey, 1996).
   d. There seem to be few (if any) side effects.

B. Pharmacologic galactogogues.

1. No drug is manufactured specifically for the purpose of increasing milk production; all galactogogue drugs are "off-label" uses (in United States, not reviewed or approved by the Food and Drug Administration for this application).

2. Drugs in common use (ABM Protocol #9, 2004).
   a. Metoclopramide (Reglan and Maxeran) is used quite successfully to increase a faltering milk supply, especially in preterm birth situations; some mothers experience depression as a side effect; mothers who have a history of depression might not be good candidates for use of this medication; other mothers find significant benefits from its use.
   b. Domperidone (Motilium; not always available in the United States, but may sometimes be available from compounding pharmacies) is used for the treatment of certain gastrointestinal disorders; it is quite effective at increasing milk production without the side effects of metoclopramide (de Silva et al., 2001; Gabay, 2002). "Domperidone is the only galactogogue available that has been scientifically evaluated through a randomized, double-blind, placebo-controlled study" (ABM #9, 2004). Typical dosage is 10 to 20 mg, three to four times daily (Hale, 2005).

3. Drugs not commonly used.

    a. Major tranquilizers such as chlorpromazine (Largactil and Thorazine) and haloperidol (Haldol) typically increase milk production as a side effect; however, significant side effects of sedation, fatigue, and neurologic aberrations preclude their use for insufficient milk supply; sulpiride is used as an antipsychotic in some countries and also increases milk production, but its side effects are similar to tranquilizers, and it is used only in emergency or disaster situations.

    b. Thyrotropin-releasing hormone has been used successfully to increase prolactin levels and milk production; side effects can include hyperthyroidism in larger doses.

    c. Human growth hormone has been shown to significantly increase milk production in both term and preterm mothers; adverse effects have not been reported in either mothers or babies (Breier et al., 1993; Milsom et al., 1998; Milsom et al., 1992).

4. Other drugs.

    a. Oxytocin nasal spray to increase milk flow.

      i. Has been used successfully in past (Lawrence & Lawrence, 2005; Renfrew, Lang, & Woolridge, 2000; Ruis et al., 1981).

      ii. Some conflicting research (Fewtrell et al., 2006).

    b. Metformin, normally used to treat type 2 diabetes (Gabbay & Kelly, 2003) and PCOS, has helped increase milk production in some PCOS women (anecdotal evidence).

C. Herbal galactogogues (ABM Protocol #9, 2004; Ayers, 2000).

1. Have been used for millennia to support and increase a mother's milk supply, but more controversial in western world.

2. Limited formal research to validate effectiveness.

3. When effective, galactogogues work best in conjunction with good management (that is, frequent and effective milk removal).

4. Quality can vary between manufacturers.

5. Dosage is largely anecdotal due to lack of formal testing.

6. Common reputed herbal galactogogues (Humphrey, 2003).

    a. Fenugreek seed.

    b. Blessed thistle.

    c. Milk thistle.

    d. Nettle.

    e. Alfalfa.

    f. Fennel seed.

    g. Goat's rue.

    h. Anise seed.

    i. Caraway seed.

j. Coriander seed.

k. Dill seed.

l. Marshmallow root.

References

Abadie V, André A, Zaouche A, et al. Early feeding resistance: a possible consequence of neonatal oro-oesophageal dyskinesia. *Acta Paediatr.* 2001;90:738–745.

Academy of Breastfeeding Medicine (ABM). Clinical Protocol #9: Use of galactogogues in initiating or augmenting maternal milk supply. 2004. Available at: http://www. bfmed.org/ace-files/protocol/prot9galactogoguesEnglish.pdf. Accessed Feb. 19, 2007.

Academy of Breastfeeding Medicine (ABM). Clinical Protocol #11: Guidelines for the evaluation and management of neonatal ankyloglossia and its complications in the breastfeeding dyad. *ABM News and Views.* 2005;11:6–8. Available at: http://www. bfmed.org. Accessed February 9, 2007.

Agostoni C, Marangoni F, Grandi F, Lammardo AM, Giovannini M, Riva E, Galli C. Earlier smoking habits are associated with higher serum lipids and lower milk fat and polyunsaturated fatty acid content in the first 6 months of lactation. *Eur J Clin Nutr.* 2003;57:1466–1472.

Aljazaf K, Hale TW, Ilett KF, Hartmann PE, et al. Pseudoephedrine: effects on milk production in women and estimation of infant exposure via breastmilk. *Br J Clin Pharmacol.* 2003;56:18–24.

Amir L. Maternal smoking and reduced duration of breastfeeding: a review of possible mechanisms. *Early Hum Dev.* 2001;64:45–67.

Amir LH, Donath SM. Does maternal smoking have a negative physiological effect on breastfeeding? The epidemiological evidence. *Breastfeeding Rev.* 2003;11:19–29.

Amir LH, James JP, Beatty J. Review of tongue-tie release at a tertiary maternity hospital. *J Paediatr Child Health.* 2005;41:243–245.

Amir LH, James JP, Donath SM. Reliability of the Hazelbaker assessment tool for lingual frenulum function. *Intl Breastfeed J.* 2006;1:3.

Anderson AM. Disruption of lactogenesis by retained placental fragments. *J Hum Lact.* 2001;17:142–144.

Andersen A, Lund-Andersen C, Larsen J, et al. Suppressed prolactin but normal neurophysin levels in cigarette smoking breast-feeding women. *Clin Endocrinol.* (Oxf) 1982;17:363–368.

Arabin B, Ruttgers H, Kubli F. Effects of routine administration of methylergometrin during puerperium on involution, maternal morbidity and lactation. *Geburtshilfe Frauenheilkd.* April 1986;46(4):215–220.

Astley SJ, Little RE. Maternal marijuana use during lactation and infant development at one year. *Neurotoxicol Teratol.* March/April 1990;12(2):161–168.

Auerbach K. The effect of nipple shields on maternal milk volume. *J Obstet Gynecol Neonatal Nurs.* 1990;19:419–427.

Ayers JF. The use of alternative therapies in the support of breastfeeding. *J Hum Lact.* 2000;16:52–56.

Baker JL, Cichaelsen KF, Rasmussen KM, Sorensen TI. Maternal prepregnant body mass index, duration of breastfeeding, and timing of complementary food introduction are associated with infant weight gain. *Am J Clin Nutr.* 2004;80:1579–1588.

Ballard JL, Auer CE, Khoury JC. Ankyloglossia: assessment, incidence, and effect of frenuloplasty on the breastfeeding dyad. *Pediatrics.* 2002;110:e63.

Ball DE, Morrison P. Oestrogen transdermal patches for postpartum depression in lactating mothers—a case report. *Cent Afr J Med.* 1999;45:68–70.

Betzold CM, Hoover KL, Snyder CL. Delayed lactogenesis II: a comparison of four cases. *J Midwifery Women's Health.* 2004;49:132–137.

Botta R, Donatelli M, Bucalo M, et al. Placental lactogen, progesterone, total estriol and prolactin plasma levels in pregnant women with insulin-dependent diabetes mellitus. *Eur J Obstet Gynecol Reprod Biol.* 1984;16:393–401.

Bowles BC, Williamson BP. Pregnancy and lactation following anorexia and bulimia. *J Obstet Gynecol Neonatal Nurs.* 1990;19:243–248.

Breier BH, Milsom SR, Blum WF, et al. Insulin-like growth factors and their binding proteins in plasma and milk after growth hormone-stimulated galactopoiesis in normally lactating women. *Acta Endocrinol.* 1993;129:427–435.

Burke-Snyder J. Bubble palate and failure to thrive: a case report. *J Hum Lact.* 1997; 13:139–143.

Butte NF. Energy requirements of infants. *Public Health Nutr.* 2005;8:953–967.

Caglar MK, Ozer I, Altugan FS. Risk factors for excess weight loss and hypernatremia in exclusively breast-fed infants. *Brazilian Journal of Medical and Biological Research.* 2006;39:539–544.

Chapman D, Perez-Escamilla R. Does delayed perception of the onset of lactation shorten breastfeeding duration? *J Hum Lact.* 1999;15:107–110.

Clavey S. The use of acupuncture for the treatment of insufficient lactation (Que Ru). *Am J Acupunct.* 1996;24:35–46.

Cobo E. Effect of different doses of ethanol on the milk-ejecting reflex in lactating women. *Am J Obstet Gynecol.* March 15, 1973;115(6):817–821.

Cooper W, Atherton H, Kahana M, Kotagal U. Increased incidence of severe breastfeeding malnutrition and hypernatremia in a metropolitan area. *Pediatrics.* 1995;96:957–960.

Cowley K. Psychogenic and pharmacologic induction of the let-down reflex can facilitate breastfeeding by tetraplegic women: a report of 3 cases. *Arch Phys Med Rehabil.* 2005;86:1261–1264.

Cox D, Kent J, Casey T, et al. Breast growth and the urinary excretion of lactose during human pregnancy and early lactation: endocrine relationships. *Exp Physiol.* 1999; 84:421–434.

Cregan MD. Complicating influences upon the initiation of lactation following premature birth (abstract A14). *JHL.* 2007;23(1):77.

Dahlenburg GW, Burnell RH, Braybrook R. The relationship between cord serum sodium levels in newborn infants and maternal intravenous therapy during labour. *Br J Obstet Gynaecol.* 1980;87:519–522.

de Araujo Burgos MG, Bion FM, Campos F. Lactation and alcohol: clinical and nutritional effects. *Arch Latinoam Nutr.* March 2004;54(1):25–35.

de Carvalho M, Robertson S, Merkatz R, Klaus M. Milk intake and frequency of feeding in breastfed infants. *Early Hum Dev.* 1982;7:155–163.

de Mello PR, Pinto GR, Botelho C. The influence of smoking on fertility, pregnancy and lactation. *J Pediatr* (Rio J). 2001;77:257–264.

de Silva OP, Knoppert DC, Angeline MM, Forret PA. Effect of Domperidone on milk production in mothers of premature newborns: a randomized, double blind, placebo-controlled trial. *Can Med Assoc J.* 2001;164:17–21.

Dewey K, Nommsen-Rivers L, Heinig M, et al. Risk factors for suboptimal infant breastfeeding behavior, delayed onset of lactation, and excess neonatal weight loss. *Pediatrics.* 2003;112:607–619.

Djulus J, Moretti M, Koren G. Marijuana use and breastfeeding. *Can Fam Physician.* 2005;51(3):349–350.

Elliott KG, Kjolhede CL, Gournis E, Rasmussen KM. Duration of breastfeeding associated with obesity during adolescence. *Obes Res.* 1997;5:538–541.

Engstrom JL, Meier PP, Jegier BJ. Factors associated with milk output differences from the right and left breasts. *J Hum Lact.* 2007;23(1):80.

Escobar GJ, Gonzales VM, Armstrong MA, et al. Rehospitalization for neonatal dehydration. *Arch Pediatr Adolesc Med.* 2002;156:155–161.

Feder SD, Berger LR, Johnson JD, Wilde JB. Increasing breast milk production for premature infants with a relaxation/imagery audiotape. *Pediatrics.* 1989;83:57–60.

Fenton SE, Hamm JT, Birnbaum LS, Youngblood GL. Persistent abnormalities in the rat mammary gland following gestational and lactational exposure to 2,3,7,8-Tetrachlorodibenzo-*p*-dioxin (TCDD). *Toxicol Sci.* 2002;67:63–74.

Fernando C. *Tongue-Tie: From Confusion to Clarity.* Sydney, Australia: Tandem Publications; 1999.

Ferris AM, Reece EA. Nutritional consequences of chronic maternal conditions during pregnancy and lactation: lupus and diabetes. *Am J Clin Nutr.* 1994;59(suppl): 465S–473S.

Fewtrell MS, Loh KL, Blake A, et al. Randomised, double blind trial of oxytocin nasal spray in mothers expressing breast milk for preterm infants. *Arch Dis Child Fetal Neonatal.* 2006; 91:F169–F174.

Fussy, S. The skinny on gastric bypass: what pharmacists need to know. *US Pharm.* 2005;2:HS3–HS12. Available at: http://www.uspharmacist.com/index.asp?show= article&page=8_1438.htm. Accessed February 6, 2007.

Gabay MP. Galactogogues: medications that induce lactation. *J Hum Lact.* 2002;18: 274–279.

Gabbay M, Kelly H. Use of metformin to increase breastmilk production in women with insulin resistance: a case series. *ABM News and Views*. 2003;9:20–21.

Gallas PR, Stolk RP, Bakker K, et al. Thyroid dysfunction in pregnancy and the first postpartum year in women with diabetes mellitus type 1. *Eur J Endocrinol*. 2002; 147:443–451.

Glenny AM, Hooper L, Shaw WC, et al. Feeding interventions for growth and development in infants with cleft lip, cleft palate or cleft lip and palate. *Cochrane Database of Systemic Reviews*. Issue 3, 2005.

Grange DK, Finlay JL. Nutritional vitamin B_{12} deficiency in a breastfed infant following maternal gastric bypass. *Pediatr Hematol Oncol*. 1994;11:311–318.

Griffiths DM. Do tongue ties affect breastfeeding? *J Hum Lact*. 2004;20:409–414.

Guillette EA, Conrad C, Lares F, et al. Altered breast development in young girls from an agricultural environment. *Environ Health Perspect*. 2006;114:471–475.

Halbert L. Breastfeeding in the woman with a compromised nervous system. *J Hum Lact*. 1998;14:327–331.

Hale T, Ilett K, Hartmann P, et al. Pseudoephedrine effects on milk production in women and estimation of infant exposure via human milk. *Adv Exp Med Biol*. 2004;554: 437–438.

Hale TW. Drug therapy and breastfeeding. In: Riordan J. *Breastfeeding and Human Lactation*. 3rd ed. Sudbury, MA: Jones and Bartlett Publishers; 2005:137–166.

Hale TW. *Medications and Mothers' Milk*. 12th ed. Amarillo, TX: Hale Publishing; 2006: 753–754.

Hall RT, Mercer AM, Teasley SL, et al. A breastfeeding assessment score to evaluate the risk for cessation of breastfeeding by 7 to 10 days. *J Pediatr*. 2002;141: 659–664.

Hapon M, Simoncini M, Via G, et al. Effect of hypothyroidism on hormone profiles in virgin, pregnant and lactating rats, and on lactation. *Reproduction*. 2003;126: 371–382.

Hapon M, Varas S, Jahn G, Gimenez M. Effects of hypothyroidism on mammary and liver lipid metabolism in virgin and late-pregnant rats. *J of Lipid Research*. 2005;46:1320–1330.

Hartmann P, Cregan M. Lactogenesis and the effects of insulin-dependent diabetes mellitus and prematurity. *J Nutr*. 2001;131(11):3016S–3020S.

Hartmann PE, Owens RA, Cox DB, Kent JC. Establishing lactation: breast development and control of milk synthesis. *Food Nutr Bull*. 1996;17. Available at: http://www. unu.edu/unupress/food/8F174e/8F174E00.htm#Contents.

Hazelbaker AK. *The Assessment Tool for Lingual Frenulum Function: Use in a Lactation Consultant Private Practice*. Columbus, OH: Alison Kay Hazelbaker; 1993.

Hazelbaker AK. Newborn tongue-tie and breastfeeding. *J Am Board Fam Pract*. 2005; 18:326–327.

Henderson JJ, Dickinson JE, Evans SF, et al. Impact of intrapartum epidural analgesia on breastfeeding duration. *Aust N Z J Obstet Gynaecol*. 2003;43:372–377.

Henly SJ, Anderson CM, Avery MD, et al. Anemia and insufficient milk in first-time mothers. *Birth.* 1995;22:87–92.

Hill PD, Aldag JC, Chatterton RT. Initiation and frequency of pumping and milk production in mothers of nonnursing preterm infants. *J Hum Lact.* 2001;17:9–13.

Hilson JA, Rasmussen KM, Kjolhede CL. Maternal obesity and breastfeeding success in a rural population of white women. *Am J Clin Nutr.* 1997;66:1371–1378.

Hilson JA, Rasmussen KM, Kjolhede CL. High prepregnant body mass index is associated with poor lactation outcomes among white, rural women independent of psychosocial and demographic correlates. *J Hum Lact.* 2004;20:18–29.

Hogan M, Westcott C, Griffiths M. Randomized, controlled trial of division of tongue-tie in infants with feeding problems. *J Paediatr Child Health.* 2005;41:246–250.

Hond ED, Roels HA, Hoppenbrouwers K, et al. Sexual maturation in relation to polychlorinated aromatic hydrocarbons: Sharpe and Skakkebaek's hypothesis revisited. *Environ Health Perspect.* 2002;8:771–776.

Hoover KL, Barbalinardo LH, Platia MP. Delayed lactogenesis II secondary to gestational ovarian theca lutein cysts in two normal singleton pregnancies. *J Hum Lact.* 2002; 18:264–268.

Hopkinson J, Schanler R, Fraley J, et al. Milk production by mothers of premature infants: influence of cigarette smoking. *Pediatrics.* 1992;90:934–938.

Huggins KE, Petok ES, Mireles O. Markers of lactation insufficiency: a study of 34 mothers. In: Auerbach K, ed. *Current Issues in Clinical Lactation 2000.* Sudbury, MA: Jones and Bartlett Publishers; 2000:25–35.

Hurst NM. Lactation after augmentation mammoplasty. *Obstet Gynecol.* 1996;87:30–34.

Humphrey S. *The Nursing Mother's Herbal.* Minneapolis, MN: Fairview Press; 2003.

Institute of Medicine (IoM). Nutrition During Lactation. Washington, DC: National Academy Press; 1991.

Janssen O, Mehlmauer N, Hahn S, et al. High prevalence of autoimmune thyroiditis in patients with polycystic ovary syndrome. *Eur J Endocrinol.* 2004;150:363–369.

Kennedy KI, Short RV, Tully MR. Premature introduction of progestin-only contraceptive methods during lactation. *Contraception.* 1997;55:347–350.

Kent J, Mitoulas L, Cox D, et al. Breast volume and milk production during extended lactation in women. *Exp Physiol.* 1999;84:435–447.

Kent KC, Mitoulas LR, Cregan MD, et al. Volume and frequency of breastfeedings and fat content of breast milk throughout the day. *Pediatrics.* 2006;117:387–395.

Knight CH, Sorenson A. Windows in early mammary development: critical or not? *Reproduction.* 2001;122;337–345.

Kugyelka JG, Rasmussen KM, Frongillo EA. Maternal obesity is negatively associated with breastfeeding success among Hispanic but not Black women. *J Nutr.* 2004;134: 1746–1753.

Lai CT, Hale T, Kent J, et al. Hourly Rate of Milk Synthesis in Women. Cambridge, UK: International Society for Research into Human Milk and Lactation (ISRHML); 2004.

LaLakea M, Messner A. Ankyloglossia: does it matter? *Pediatr Clin North Am.* 2003;50: 381–387.

Lau C, Sullivan M, Hazelwood R. Effects of diabetes mellitus on lactation in the rat. *Proc Soc Exp Biol Med.* 1993;204:81–89.

Lawrence RA, Lawrence RM. *Breastfeeding: A Guide for the Medical Profession.* 6th ed. Philadelphia: Elsevier Mosby; 2005.

Leung GM, Lam T-H, Ho L-M. Breastfeeding and its relation to smoking and mode of delivery. *Am Coll Obstet Gynec.* 2002;99:785–794.

Lewis BC, Hudgins S, Lewis A, et al. In utero and lactation treatment with 2,3,7,8-tetrachlorodibenzo-*p*-dioxin impairs mammary gland differentiation but does not block the response to exogenous estrogen in the postpubertal female rat. *Toxicol Sci.* 2001;62:46–53.

Livingstone VH, Willis CE, Abdel-Wareth LO, et al. Neonatal hypernatremic dehydration associated with breast-feeding malnutrition: a retrospective survey. *CMAJ.* 2000;162: 647–652.

Lovelady CA. Is maternal obesity a cause of poor lactation performance. *Nutr Rev.* 2005;63:352–355.

Marasco L. The impact of thyroid dysfunction on lactation. *Breastfeeding Abstr.* 2006; 25:9, 11–12.

Marasco L, Marmet C, Shell E. Polycystic ovary syndrome: a connection to insufficient milk supply? *J Hum Lact.* 2000;16:143–148.

Markey C, Rubin B, Soto A, Sonnenschein C. Endocrine disruptors: from Wingspread to environmental developmental biology. *J Steroid Biochem Mol Biol.* 2003;83:235–244.

Martens WS 2nd, Martin LF, Berlin CM Jr. Failure of a nursing infant to thrive after the mother's gastric bypass for morbid obesity. *Pediatrics.* 1990;86:777–778.

Mennella JA. Regulation of milk intake after exposure to alcohol in mothers' milk. *Alcohol Clin Exp Res.* 2001a;25(4):590–593.

Mennella JA. Alcohol's effect on lactation. *Alcohol Res Health.* 2001b;25(3):230–234.

Mennella JA, Pepino MY, Teff KL. Acute alcohol consumption disrupts the hormonal milieu of lactating women. *J Clin Endocrinol Metab.* April 2005;90(4):1979–1985.

Milsom SR, Breier BH, Gallaher BW, et al. Growth hormone stimulates galactopoiesis in healthy lactating women. *Acta Endocrinol.* 1992;127:337–343.

Milsom SR, Rabone DL, Gunn AJ, Gluckman PD. Potential role for growth hormone in human lactation insufficiency. *Horm Res.*1998;50:147–150.

Miyake A, Tahara M, Koike K, Tanizawa O. Decrease in neonatal suckled milk volume in diabetic women. *Eur J Obstet Gynecol Reprod Biol.* 1989;33:49–53.

Monteleone P, Brambilla F, Bortolotti F, et al. Plasma prolactin response to D-fenfluramine is blunted in bulimic patients with frequent binge episodes. *Psychol Med.* 1998;28:975–983.

Motil KJ, Sheng H-P, Montandon CM. Case report: failure to thrive in a breastfed infant is associated with maternal dietary protein and energy restriction. *J Am Coll Nutr.* 1994;13:203–208.

Neifert MR, McDonough SL, Neville MC. Failure of lactogenesis associated with placental retention. *Am J Obstet Gynecol.* 1981;140:477–478.

Neifert MR, Seacat JM. Lactation insufficiency; a rational approach. *Birth.* 1987;14: 182–190.

Neifert MR, Seacat JM, Jobe WE. Lactation failure due to insufficient glandular development of the breast. *Pediatrics.* 1985;76:823–828.

Neifert M, DeMarzo S, Seacat J, et al. The influence of breast surgery, breast appearance, and pregnancy-induced breast changes on lactation sufficiency as measured by infant weight gain. *Birth.* 1990;17:31–38.

Neubauer SH, Ferris AM, Chase CG, et al. Delayed lactogenesis in women with insulin-dependent diabetes mellitus. *Am J Clin Nutr.* 1993;58:54–60.

Neville M, Morton J. Physiology and endocrine changes underlying human lactogenesis II. *J Nutr.* 2001;131:3005S-3008S.

O'Brien LM, Heycock EG, Hanna M, et al. Postnatal depression and faltering growth: a community study. *Pediatrics.* 2004;113:1242–1247.

Ostrom KM, Ferris AM. Prolactin concentrations in serum and milk of mothers with and without insulin-dependent diabetes mellitus. *Am J Clin Nutr.* 1993;58:49–53.

Paul AA, Muller EM, Whitehead RG. The quantitative effects of maternal dietary energy intake on pregnancy and lactation in rural Gambian women. *Trans R Soc Trop Med Hyg.* 1979;73:686–692.

Picciano MF. Pregnancy and lactation: physiological adjustments, nutritional requirements and the role of dietary supplements. *J Nutr.* 2003;133:1997S-2002S.

Rainer C, Gardetto A, Frühwirth M, et al. Breast deformity in adolescence as a result of pneumothorax drainage during neonatal intensive care. *Pediatrics.* 2003;111:80–86.

Rasmussen KM, Lee VE, Ledkovsky TB, Kjolhede CL. A description of lactation counseling practices that are used with obese mothers. *J Hum Lact.* 2006;22:322–327.

Rasmussen KM, Kjolhede CL. Prepregnant overweight and obesity diminish the prolactin response to suckling in the first week postpartum. *Pediatrics.* 2004;113:e465–e471.

Rasmussen KM, Hilson JA, Kjolhede CL. Obesity may impair lactogenesis II. *J Nutr.* 2001;131:3009S-3011S.

Renfrew MJ, Lang S, Woolridge M. Oxytocin for promoting successful lactation. *Cochrane Database Syst Rev.* 2000;(2):CD000156.

Ricke LA, Baker NJ, Madlon-Kay DJ, DeFor TA. Newborn tongue-tie: prevalence and effect on breastfeeding. *J Am Board Fam Pract.* 2005;18:1–7.

Ricke LA, Madlon-Kay DJ, Baker NJ, et al. Newborn tongue-tie: incidence and effect on breastfeeding. *ABM News and Views.* 2004;10:27.

Rosato R, Gimenez M, Jahn G. Effects of chronic thyroid hormone administration on pregnancy, lactogenesis, and lactation in the rat. *Acta Endocrinol.* (Copenh) 1992; 127:547–554.

Ruis H, Rolland R, Doesburg W, et al. Oxytocin enhances onset of lactation among mothers delivering prematurely. *Br Med J.* (Clin Res Ed). 1981;283:340–342.

Saint L, Maggiore P, Hartmann PE. Yield and nutrient content of milk in eight women breastfeeding twins and one woman breastfeeding triplets. *Br J Nutr.* 1986;56:49–58.

Sheehan HL, Murdoch R. Post-partum necrosis of the anterior pituitary: pathological and clinical aspects. *J Obstet Gynaecol Br Emp.* 1938;45:456–489.

Smith C, Valentine C. Early hormonal contraception associated with increased galactogogue use. *JHL.* 2006;22(4):469–470.

Souto GC, Giugliani ERJ, Giugliani C, Schneider MA. The impact of breast reduction surgery on breastfeeding performance. *J Hum Lact.* 2003;19:43–49.

Srinivasan A, Dobrich C, Mitnick H, Feldman P. Ankyloglossia in breastfeeding infants: the effect of frenotomy on maternal nipple pain and latch. *J of Breastfeeding Medicine.* 2006;1(4):216–224.

Stagnaro-Green, A. Postpartum thyroiditis. *J Clin Endocrinol Metab.* 2002;87:4042–4047.

Stefanski J. Breastfeeding after bariatric surgery. *Today's Dietitian.* 2006;8(1):47–50. Available at: http://www.todaysdietitian.com/newarchives/jan2006pg47.shtml.

Stein M. Failure to thrive in a four-month-old nursing infant. *Dev Behav Pediatr.* 2002; 23:S69–S73.

Stutte P, Bowles B, Morman G. The effects of breast massage on volume and fat content of human milk. *Genesis.* 1988;10:22–25.

Vio F, Salazar G, Infante C. Smoking during pregnancy and lactation and its effects on breast-milk volume. *Am J Clin Nutr.* 1991;54;1011–1016.

Vorderstrasse B, Fenton S, Bohn A, et al. A novel effect of dioxin: exposure during pregnancy severely impairs mammary gland differentiation. *Toxicol Sci.* 2004;78: 248–257.

Wall V, Glass R. Mandibular asymmetry and breastfeeding problems: Experience from 11 cases. *J Hum Lact.* 2006;22:328–334.

Wallace H, Clarke S. Tongue tie division in infants with breastfeeding difficulties. *Int J Pediatr Otorhinolaryngol.* 2006;70:1257–1261.

Wardinsky TD, Montes RG, Friederich RL, et al. Vitamin B_{12} deficiency associated with low breast-milk vitamin B_{12} concentration in an infant following maternal gastric bypass surgery. *Arch Pediatr Adolesc Med.* 1995;149:1281–1284.

Weltzin T, McConaha C, MeKee M, et al. Circadian patterns of cortisol, prolactin, and growth hormone secretion during bingeing and vomiting in normal weight bulimic patients. *Biol Psychiatry.* 1991;30:37–48.

Wight NE. Breastfeeding the borderline (near-term) preterm infant. *Pediatric Ann.* 2003;32:329–336.

Wilde CJ, Addey CV, Boddy LM, Peaker M. Autocrine regulation of milk secretion by a protein in milk. *Biochem J.* 1995;305:51–58.

Willis C, Livingstone V. Infant insufficient milk syndrome associated with maternal postpartum hemorrhage. *J Hum Lact.* 1995;11:123–126.

Wilson-Clay B, Hoover K. *The Breastfeeding Atlas.* 3rd ed. Austin, TX: LactNews Press; 2005.

Wilson-Clay B, Maloney BM. A reporting tool to facilitate community-based follow-up for at-risk breastfeeding dyads at hospital discharge. In: Auerbach KG. *Current Issues in Clinical Lactation*. Austin, TX: LactNews Press; 2002:59–67.

Wilton JM. Cleft palates and breastfeeding. *AWHONN Lifelines*. 1998;2:11.

Woolridge, M. Problems of establishing lactation. *Food Nutr Bull*. 1996;17:316–323.

Woolridge MW, Baum JD, Drewett RF. Effect of a traditional and of a new nipple shield on sucking patterns and milk flow. *Early Hum Dev*. 1980;4:357–364.

Woolridge MW. Problems in Establishing Lactation. The United Nations University Press Food and Nutrition Bulletin 1996;17(4). Available at: http://www.unu.edu/unupress/food/8F174e/8F174E00.htm#Contents.

Yaseen H, Salem M, Darwich M. Clinical presentation of hypernatremic dehydration in exclusively breast-fed neonates. *Indian J Pediatr*. 2004;71:1059–1062.

Yurdakök K, Özmert E, Yalçin SS. Physical examination of breast-fed infants. *Arch Pediatr Adolesc Med*. 1997;151:429–430.

Zargar AH, Masoodl SR, Laway BA, et al. Familial puerperal alactogenesis: possibility of a genetically transmitted isolated prolactin deficiency. *Br J Obstet Gynaecol*. 1997;104:629–631.

Zargar AH, Salahuddin M, Laway BA, Masoodi SR, Ganie MA, Bhat MH. Puerperal alactogenesis with normal prolactin dynamics: is prolactin resistance the cause? *Fertil Steril*. September 2000;74(3):598–600.

Suggested Reading

Hale T, Ilett K, Hartmann P, et al. Pseudoephedrine effects on milk production in women and estimation of infant exposure via human milk. *Adv Exp Med Biol*. 2004;554:437–438.

Hill PD, Aldag JC, Chatterton RT, Zinaman M. Comparison of milk output between mothers of preterm and term infants: the first 6 weeks after birth. *J Hum Lact*. 2005;21:22–30.

Shrago LC. The neonatal bowel output study: indicators of adequate breast milk intake in neonates. *Pediatr Nurs*. 2006;32:195–201.

Williams N. Supporting the mother coming to terms with persistent insufficient milk supply: the role of the lactation consultant. *J Hum Lact*. 2002;18:262–263.

SLOW WEIGHT GAIN AND FAILURE TO THRIVE

Elsa Regina Justo Giugliani, MD, PhD, IBCLC

OBJECTIVES

- Distinguish between slow weight gain and failure to thrive.
- List the main causes of slow weight gain and failure to thrive.
- Discuss and assess parameters for an infant who is slow to gain weight.
- Develop appropriate management strategies according to the etiology of the slow weight gain.

Introduction

Inadequate weight gain in the breastfed infant is a condition that occasionally occurs, mainly in infants who are younger than six months of age. In most cases, it can be reversed when the problem(s) causing it is identified and promptly corrected. True failure to thrive is potentially dangerous, requiring early recognition and action.

I. Definitions

A. Slow weight gain.

1. When infants and children gain weight consistently, although slowly; this condition is usually familial or genetic.

2. It can become problematic when (Powers, 2001):

a. A newborn infant who is less than 2 weeks of age is more than 10% below birth weight.

b. An infant's weight at two weeks is less than birth weight.

c. An infant has no urine output in any given 24-hour period.

d. An infant has stools that have not changed to a yellow color by the end of the first week.

e. An infant has clinical signs of dehydration.

B. Failure to thrive.

1. Rate of weight gain is less than the −2 SD (standard deviation) value during an interval of two months or longer for infants less than six months of age, or three months or longer for infants over six months of age, and the weight for length is less than the 5th percentile (Fomon & Nelson, 1993).

2. Use of a percentage of the median values for the age on the growth chart.
   a. Normal is greater than 90% of median weight.
   b. Mild problem is 75% to 90%.
   c. Moderate problem is 60% to 74%.
   d. Severe is less than 60% of median weight.

3. Definition according to Lawrence and Lawrence (2005).
   a. Infant continues to lose weight after 10 days of life.
   b. Does not regain birth weight by three weeks of age.
   c. Gains at a rate below the tenth percentile for weight beyond one month of age.

II. Growth of Breastfed Children Differs from That of Artificially Fed Infants

A. The World Health Organization (WHO) Growth Standard for Children (2007) establishes the breastfed infant as the standard for measuring healthy growth. The International Growth Reference from the National Center for Health Statistics, which is based on predominantly formula-fed infants, is inadequate for the breastfed infant.

B. A key characteristic of the new standard is that it shows how children *should* grow when their needs are properly met (including full breastfeeding at least in the first four months and complemented until at least one year), rather than merely describing *how* they grew at a particular time and place.

1. According to the new WHO references, a fully breastfed girl gains an average of 1000 g in the first month, 900 g in the second month, 700 g in the third month, and 600 g in the fourth month of life.

2. A fully breastfed boy gains an average of 1200 g in the first month, 1100 g in the second month, 800 g in the third month, and 600 g in the fourth month.

III. Distinction Between Slow Weight Gain and Failure to Thrive

A. Slow weight gain.

1. Alert, responsive, and a healthy appearance.

2. Normal muscle tone and skin turgor.

3. Dilute urine, six or more times/day.

4. Frequent stools (or infrequent, but large amount).

5. Good suck with swallowing heard for the majority of the feeding.

6. Eight or more breastfeeds/day with infant determining length of feeding (Lawrence & Lawrence, 2005).

7. Efficient milk ejection reflex.

8. Weight gain slow, but consistent.

B. Failure to thrive.

1. Apathetic or weakly crying infant.

2. Poor muscle tone and skin turgor.

3. Concentrated urine, a few times/day.

4. Infrequent, scanty stools.

5. Fewer than eight breastfeeds/day, usually brief.

6. No or erratic signs of milk ejection reflex.

7. Poor and erratic weight gain or no weight gain.

8. Swallowing only with the milk ejection reflex or sporadic swallowing.

IV. Conditions Associated with Infant Weight Gain Problems (Table 40-1)

A. Poor intake.

1. Poor suckling.

2. Physical and/or structural factors.
   a. Cleft lip/palate.
   b. Short frenulum.
   c. Micrognathia.
   d. Macroglossia.
   e. Choanal atresia.

3. Preterm (Lucas et al., 1997), near-term, postterm, small for gestational age (SGA), intrauterine growth restriction (IUGR), large for gestational age (LGA) (may lack mature feeding skills).

B. Iatrogenic conditions.

1. Maternal analgesia/anesthesia can diminish the infant's alertness and ability to suck; may affect discrete parts of the feeding process.

2. Bottles and pacifiers can decrease suckling stimulation and cause nipple confusion.

3. Peripartum factors such as vacuum extraction, urgent cesarean, separation, nonmedical supplementation.

4. Mismanagement of early breastfeeding.

5. Cesarean delivery (Evans et al, 2003).

Table 40-1 Infant Factors That May Contribute to Slow Weight Gain

Factor	Effect
Gestational age and growth	Preterm, near-term, postterm, SGA, IUGR, and LGA infants may lack mature feeding skills. Provision of breast milk is especially important for SGA infants because it promotes better catch-up growth in head circumference (brain growth) than supplementing with a standard formula (Lucas et al., 1997).
Alterations in oral anatomy	Alterations such as ankyloglossia, cleft lip, cleft of hard or soft palate, bubble palate, facial growth anomalies such as micrognathia, or congenital syndromes that affect the oral structure may contribute to poor milk intake.
Alterations in oral functioning	Hypotonia, hypertonia, neurologic pathology or physiology that may interfere with the performance, strength, or stamina of the structures involved in the suck, swallow, breathe cycling.
High energy requirements	Cardiac disease, respiratory involvement (bronchopulmonary dysplasia–BPD), metabolic disorders that create a need for increased caloric intake or volume restriction that place limits on intake.
Known illness	Infection, trisomy 21, cystic fibrosis, or cardiac defects often put the infant at risk for poor growth because of the combination of a low endurance for feeding and high metabolic demands. Growth faltering may be apparent in the early months due to atopic dermatitis (Agostoni et al., 2000).
Maternal medications	Certain prenatal prescription medications or recreational drugs may interfere with normal sucking physiology.
Intrapartum factors	Cesarean delivery, hypoxia, anoxia, labor medications, state control difficulties, epidural analgesia, forceps, and vacuum extraction that affect brain function, anatomical structures, and nerves, contributing to ineffective milk transfer.
Iatrogenic factors	Hospital routines that separate mothers and infants, provide inappropriate supplementation, offer pacifiers, or provide conflicting or poor breastfeeding instruction leave both mothers and infants lacking needed feeding skills.
Gastrointestinal or metabolic/malabsorption problems	Gastroesophageal reflux or other conditions that limit nutrient intake or metabolism.

C. Medical conditions.

    1. Anoxia/hypoxia.

    2. Preterm.

    3. Neonatal jaundice can make infants lethargic.

    4. Trisomy 13, 15, or 21.

    5. Hypothyroidism.

    6. Neuromuscular dysfunction.

    7. Central nervous system impairment.

    8. Abnormal suckling patterns.

    9. Allergies (Agostoni et al., 2000).

D. Infrequent/less feeds.

    1. Mother-infant separation.

    2. Pacifiers.

    3. Water/juice supplementation.

    4. Early solids.

    5. Baby "training" programs that inhibit ability to breastfeed on cue.

E. Low net milk intake.

    1. Vomiting and diarrhea.

    2. Malabsorption such as with cystic fibrosis.

    3. Infection.

F. Infants with high energy requirements.

    1. SGA infant.

    2. Central nervous system.

    3. Stimulants in the milk.

    4. Neurologic disorders.

    5. Severe congenital heart disease.

V. Maternal Factors (Table 40-2)

A. Inadequate milk production.

    1. Severe postpartum hemorrhage.

    2. Mismanagement, a common cause of slow weight gain/failure to thrive.
       a. Improper positioning.
       b. Low frequency/duration of feedings.
       c. Rigid feeding schedules.
       d. Absence of night feedings.

Table 40-2 Maternal Factors That May Contribute to Slow Infant Weight Gain

Factors	Effect
Breast abnormalities	Previous breast surgery, insufficient glandular development, augmentation, reduction, and trauma may influence the ultimate volume of milk that the breasts will produce but do not preclude breastfeeding.
Nipple anomalies	Flat, retracted, inverted, oddly shaped, or dimpled nipples may make latching more difficult and reduce milk intake. Improper suckling on nipples may also damage them, further reducing infant milk intake.
Ineffective or insufficient milk removal	Improperly positioned/latched infant, ineffective suckling, unresolved engorgement leaves residual milk and reduces supply, making less milk available to the infant.
Delayed lactogenesis II	Mother who is overweight, obese, or diabetic may experience an initial delay in lactogenesis II. With copious milk production delayed, frequency of feedings must increase to offset volume deficit.
Poor breastfeeding management	Delayed or disrupted early feeding opportunities, separation, too few feedings, and illness reduce feeding opportunities at breast. Failure to pump milk in the absence of an infant suckling at breast may interfere with proliferation and sensitivity of prolactin receptors.
Medications/drugs	Prescription or recreational drugs, labor medications, and IV fluids may delay lactogenesis II or interfere with infant suckling. Oral contraceptives can reduce lactose content and overall milk volume (Hale, 2006). Smoking may also decrease volume (Vio, Salazar, & Infante, 1991) and fat content of milk (Hopkinson et al., 1992).
Hormonal alterations	Hypothyroid, retained placenta, superimposed pregnancy, pituitary disorders, polycystic ovarian syndrome, theta lutein cysts (Hoover, Barbalinardo, & Platia, 2002), oral contraceptives, diabetes insipidus, assisted reproduction/difficulty conceiving, or other endocrine-related problems may interfere with the normal progression of milk production.
Milk ejection problems	Drugs, alcohol, smoking, stress, pain, or other factors that inhibit the let-down reflex reduce the amount of milk available to the infant.
Miscellaneous factors	Lack of vitamin B_{12} in a vegetarian diet, parenting programs that limit feedings, ineffective breast pump or pumping schedule, inadequate weight gain during pregnancy, postpartum hemorrhage, anemia, cesarean delivery (Evans et al., 2003).

e. "Switch nurse" technique (sometimes leads to short duration of feedings or decreased intake of hindmilk).

f. Use of nipple shields.

g. Engorgement.

h. Non-graspable nipples.

3. Insufficient glandular development.

a. The mother experiences no or minimal breast changes during pregnancy and no postpartum breast fullness.

b. Often, there are marked differences in the shape and size of the breasts.

4. Other maternal physical factors.

a. Illness/infection.

b. Hypothyroidism.

c. Untreated diabetes.

d. Sheehan's syndrome.

e. Pituitary tumors.

f. Mental illness.

g. Retained placenta.

h. History of infertility or polycystic ovary syndrome.

i. Fatigue.

j. Emotional disturbance.

k. Other less frequently seen conditions (Hoover, Barbalinardo, & Platia, 2002).

5. Drugs (Hale, 2006).

a. Estrogen.

b. Antihistamine.

c. Pseudophedrine.

d. Sedatives.

e. Diuretics.

f. Large doses of vitamin B_6.

6. Severe diet restriction.

7. Breast reduction surgery.

8. Smoking (can decrease fat content of milk and inhibit the milk ejection reflex) (Hopkinson et al., 1992; Vio, Salazar, & Infante, 1991).

9. Pregnancy.

10. Impaired milk ejection reflex.

a. Psychological inhibition.

b. Stress.

c. Pain.

11. Breast surgery.

12. Smoking.

13. Alcohol.

14. Abnormal milk composition.

   a. Very low fat diet.

   b. Strict vegan vegetarian without vitamin B_{12} supplementation.

   c. Stimulants in the milk (coffee, tea, cola) may increase infant metabolic rate (Lawrence & Lawrence, 2005).

15. Assessment.

   a. Listening attentively to the mother and helping her express her feelings is an important aspect of the assessment.

VI. History (Powers, 2001; Powers, 2005)

A. Details of the breastfeeds/feedings.

   1. Frequency of breastfeeds.

      a. Usually an exclusively breastfed baby feeds at least eight times per 24 hours and before 12 weeks of life, most babies do not sleep for more than a six-hour stretch.

   2. Duration.

      a. Infant should breastfeed on one breast until he/she comes off spontaneously; then can be placed on the other side. "The duration of the feeding should be determined by the infant's response and not by time. Enough time must be spent on a single breast to assure getting the fat-rich, calorie-rich hindmilk" (Lawrence & Lawrence, 2005).

      b. Babies are finished with the first side when they will no longer suck and swallow when the breast is compressed.

   3. Signs of the milk ejection reflex.

      a. Leaking or spraying of milk.

      b. Tingling or burning sensations within the breast.

      c. Does the baby consistently swallow or is swallowing seen only when the milk release occurs?

   4. Use of nipple shields.

   5. Supplementation of other liquids and foods.

   6. Use of bottles.

B. Infant's aspects.

   1. General health.

   2. Birth weight/adequacy for gestational age.

   3. Lowest weight after birth and the age at that time.

   4. Sleep pattern.

   5. Fussiness.

6. Number of diapers.

   a. An infant is usually getting enough milk if there are at least six soaking wet diapers a day after day 4, and three or more bowels movements per day in infants younger than six weeks of age (Table 40–3).

   b. An infant can be well hydrated but calorically deprived.

7. Use of pacifiers.

C. Mother's aspects.

  1. General health.

  2. Psychological aspects.

  3. Presence of relatives or friends criticizing her for breastfeeding.

  4. The mother's level of commitment to breastfeeding.

  5. Dietary habits including herbal use.

   a. Some herbs are said to decrease milk supply, such as sage, parsley, and borage.

   b. Others containing caffeine may increase infant metabolic rate.

  6. Workload.

   a. Is the mother overextended or stressed?

   b. Constraints on milk expression in the workplace.

  7. Sleep patterns.

  8. Smoking.

  9. Alcohol consumption.

  10. Medications.

VII. Physical Assessment of the Infant Relative to Breastfeeding

A. Assess the hydration status.

  1. Number of wet diapers each 24 hours.

  2. Moist mucous membranes.

  3. Anterior fontanelle that is not depressed.

  4. Skin turgor.

B. Compare the infant's weight, length, and head circumference with previous measurements and determine the baby's pattern of weight gain.

C. Observe anatomical abnormalities of the mouth and major neurologic disturbances.

  1. Observe the ability to root, suck, and swallow.

  2. Observe muscle tone and mouth, tongue, and facial movements.

Table 40-3 Signs of Sufficient Breast Milk Intake

Age	Wet Diapers	Color	Urates	Stools	Color	Volume	Consistency	Weight Gain
Day 1	1	pale	possible	1	black	≥15 gm	tarry/ sticky	<5% loss
Day 2	2–3	pale	possible	1–2	greenish/ black	≥15 gm	changing	<5% loss
Day 3	3–4	pale	possible	3–4	greenish/ yellow	≥15 gm	soft	≤8–10% loss
Day 4	≥4–6 disposable ≥6–8 cloth	pale	none	4 large 10 small	yellow/ seedy	≥15 gm	soft/ liquidy	15–30 gm/day

Sources: Adapted from Powers NG, Slusser W. Breastfeeding update 2: clinical lactation management. *Pediatr Rev.* 1997;18:147–161; Black LS. Incorporating breastfeeding care into daily newborn rounds and pediatric office practice. *Ped Clin N Am.* 2001;48:299–319; Neifert MR. Prevention of breastfeeding tragedies. *Ped Clin N Am.* 2001;48:273–297.

VIII. Assessment of the Maternal Breast

A. Condition of breast/nipples/areolae.

B. Presence of scars.

C. Symmetry.

D. Signs of mastitis.

IX. Observation of the Feeding

A. Typical breast fullness-to-softness changes during feeding.

B. Positioning.

C. Latch-on.

D. Infant suck.

  1. Degree of vigor.

  2. Coordination.

  3. Rhythmic sucking and swallowing.

E. Signs of adequate milk "release."

  1. Milk flows from the opposite breast.

  2. Milk flows when feeding is interrupted abruptly.

  3. Baby's sucking pattern changes from 2 sucks per second to 1 per second with deep jaw excursions.

F. Interaction between mother and baby.

G. Duration of the feeding in each breast.

X. Laboratory Tests (Desmarais & Browne, 1990)

A. In specific situations, some specialized tests might be of help.

  1. Prolactin levels.
    a. Used to rule out inadequate glandular tissue or a primary prolactin secretion defect.
    b. Intrafeeding (after 15 minutes of breastfeeding) value should be at least twice that of the baseline (Lawrence & Lawrence, 2005).

  2. Creamtocrit (level of fat in the milk).
    a. Used to rule out poor milk ejection reflex or poor maternal nutrition (Lawrence & Lawrence, 2005).

  3. Sodium, chloride, potassium, pH, blood urea, nitrogen, and hematocrit when the infant is dehydrated.
    a. When electrolyte levels are abnormal, sodium, chloride, and potassium should be measured in the mother's milk (Lawrence & Lawrence, 2005).

B. Management (Frantz, 1992).

1. All infants who experience failure to thrive should be seen by their primary care providers.

2. If an underlying medical condition is suspected, the lactation consultant will refer the mother and/or baby for medical/surgical assessment.

3. The management of slow weight gain and failure to thrive is based on etiology (see related chapters).

4. When the mother's milk supply is low:
   a. Be sure that the baby is correctly positioned and latched on.
   b. Suggest to the mother the following actions:
      i. Increase the number of breastfeeds.
      ii. Offer both breasts at each feeding.
      iii. Give enough time for the baby to remove hindmilk (usually at least 20 minutes on the first side).
      iv. Breast compression when the baby no longer seems to be getting milk and is sucking, if the baby is sleepy or not sucking actively (Powers, 2001).
      v. Avoid bottles, pacifiers, and nipple shields.
      vi. Give only mother's milk in the first six months.
      vii. Eat a well balanced diet, drink enough fluids, and rest.

5. Supplementary feeding might be necessary (Academy of Breastfeeding Medicine, 2001).
   a. Temporary or permanent.
   b. Recommendations on the type and mode of these feedings depends on motivation and conditions (physical and emotional) of the mother.

6. When the mother's supply is adequate, the first choice is to supplement the child with her own fresh milk.
   a. Expressed hindmilk can be used as a high calorie supplement.
   b. Mothers can skim off the cream layer of milk that has sat in a refrigerator for 24 hours.
   c. In many circumstances, when the infant has neuromuscular or central nervous system disorders, physical therapy might be necessary.

7. In some selected cases, when routine methods fail, maternal medications (metoclopramide, domperidone) may be helpful and should be discussed with the primary care provider.

8. When no obvious cause is identified, a positive attitude to breastfeeding is helpful: a positive plan for the number and length of feedings, a good diet, and rest for the mother.

C. Evaluation.

   1. Is the infant gaining weight within the normal limits?

   2. Is the infant correctly positioned and latched on?

   3. Have possible causes of failure to thrive been removed?

   4. Has the infant had a medical/surgical assessment?

References

Academy of Breastfeeding Medicine. Clinical Protocol Number 3: Hospital guidelines for the use of complementary feeding in the healthy breastfed neonate. *ABM News and Views* [newsletter] 2001;7:2. Available at: http://www.bfmed.org. Accessed February 5, 2007.

Agostoni C, Grandi F, Scaglioni S, et al. Growth pattern of breastfed and nonbreastfed infants with atopic dermatitis in the first year of life. *Pediatrics.* 2000;106:e73.

Desmarais L, Browne S. Inadequate weight gain in breastfeeding infants: assessments and resolutions. Lactation Consultant Series No 8. New York: Avery Publishing Grouping Inc.; 1990.

Evans KC, Evans RG, Royal R, et al. Effect of cesarean section on breast milk transfer to the normal term newborn over the first week of life. *Arch Dis Child Fetal Neonatal Ed.* 2003;88:F380–F382.

Fomon SJ, Nelson SE. Size and growth. In: Foman SJ, ed. *Nutrition of Normal Infants.* St. Louis: Mosby Yearbook; 1993.

Frantz KB. The slow-gaining breastfeeding infant. NAACOG's clinical issues in perinatal and women's health nursing. 1992;3:647–655.

Hale TW. *Medications and Mother's Milk.* 12th ed. Amarillo, TX: Hale Publishing; 2006.

Hoover KL, Barbalinardo LH, Platia MP. Delayed lactogenesis II secondary to gestational ovarian theca lutein cysts in two normal singleton pregnancies. *J Hum Lact.* 2002;18:264–268.

Hopkinson JM, Schanler RJ, Fraley JK, Garza C. Milk production by mothers of premature infants: influence of cigarette smoking. *Pediatrics.* 1992;90:934–938.

Lawrence RA, Lawrence RM. *Breastfeeding: A Guide for the Medical Profession.* 6th ed. St. Louis: Mosby, Inc.; 2005.

Lucas A, Fewtrell MS, Davies PSW, et al. Breastfeeding and catch-up growth in infants born small for gestational age. *Acta Paediatr.* 1997;86:564–569.

Powers NG. How to assess slow growth in the breastfed infant. Birth to 3 months. *Pediatr Clin North Am.* 2001;48:345–363.

Powers NG. Low intake in the breastfed infant: maternal and infant considerations. In: Riordan J, ed. *Breastfeeding and Human Lactation.* 3rd ed. Sudbury, MA: Jones and Bartlett Publishers; 2005:277–309.

Vio F, Salazar G, Infante C. Smoking during pregnancy and lactation and its effects on breast milk volume. *Am J Clin Nutr.* 1991;54:1011–1016.

Walker M. *Breastfeeding Management for the Clinician: Using the Evidence.* Sudbury, MA: Jones and Bartlett Publishers; 2006.

World Health Organization (WHO). The WHO Child Growth Standard, 2007. Available at: http://www.who.int/childgrowth. Accessed February 5, 2007.

Appendix A

STANDARDS OF PRACTICE FOR INTERNATIONAL BOARD CERTIFIED LACTATION CONSULTANTS

International Lactation Consultant Association

Introduction

This is the third edition of *Standards of Practice for International Board Certified Lactation Consultants* (IBCLCs) published by the International Lactation Consultant Association (ILCA). All individuals practicing as a currently certified IBCLC should adhere to ILCA's *Standards of Practice* and the International Board of Lactation Consultant Examiners (IBLCE) *Code of Ethics for International Board Certified Lactation Consultants* in all interactions with clients, families, and other health care professionals. ILCA recognizes the certification conferred by the IBLCE as the worldwide professional credential for lactation consultants.

Quality practice and service are the core responsibilities of a profession to the public. Standards of practice are stated measures or levels of quality that are models for the conduct and evaluation of practice. Standards of practice:

- Promote consistency by encouraging a common systematic approach.
- Are sufficiently specific in content to guide daily practice.
- Provide a recommended framework for the development of policies and protocols, educational programs, and quality improvement efforts.
- Are intended for use in diverse practice settings and cultural contexts.

Standard 1. Professional Responsibilities

The IBCLC has a responsibility to maintain professional conduct and to practice in an ethical manner, accountable for professional actions and legal responsibilities.

1.1 Adhere to these ILCA *Standards of Practice* and the IBLCE *Code of Ethics*.

1.2 Practice within the scope of the *International Code of Marketing of Breast-milk Substitutes* and all subsequent World Health Association resolutions.

1.3 Maintain an awareness of conflict of interest in all aspects of work, especially when profiting from the rental or sale of breastfeeding equipment and services.

1.4 Act as an advocate for breastfeeding women, infants, and children.

1.5 Assist the mother in maintaining a breastfeeding relationship with her child.

1.6 Maintain and expand knowledge and skills for lactation consultant practice by participating in continuing education.

1.7 Undertake periodic and systematic evaluation of one's clinical practice.

1.8 Support and promote well-designed research in human lactation and breastfeeding, and base clinical practice, whenever possible, on such research.

Standard 2. Legal Considerations

The IBCLC is obligated to practice within the laws of the geopolitical region and setting in which she/he works. The IBCLC must practice with consideration for rights of privacy and with respect for matters of a confidential nature.

2.1 Work within the policies and procedures of the institution where employed, or if self-employed, have identifiable policies and procedures to follow.

2.2 Clearly state applicable fees prior to providing care.

2.3 Obtain informed consent from all clients prior to:

- assessing or intervening.

- reporting relevant information to other health care professional(s).

- taking photographs for any purpose.

- seeking publication of information associated with the consultation.

2.4 Protect client confidentiality at all times.

2.5 Maintain records according to legal and ethical practices within the work setting.

Standard 3. Clinical Practice

The clinical practice of the IBCLC focuses on providing clinical lactation care and management. This is best accomplished by promoting optimal health, through collaboration and problem solving with the client and other members of the health care team. The role of the IBCLC includes:

- Assessment, planning, intervention, and evaluation of care in a variety of situations.

- Anticipatory guidance and prevention of problems.

- Complete, accurate, and timely documentation of care.
- Communication and collaboration with other health care professionals.

3.1 Assessment.
    3.1.1 Obtain and document an appropriate history of the breastfeeding mother and child.
    3.1.2 Systematically collect objective and subjective information.
    3.1.3 Discuss with the mother and document as appropriate all assessment information.

3.2 Plan.
    3.2.1 Analyze assessment information to identify issues and/or problems.
    3.2.2 Develop a plan of care based on identified issues.
    3.2.3 Arrange for follow-up evaluation where indicated.

3.3 Implementation.
    3.3.1 Implement the plan of care in a manner appropriate to the situation and acceptable to the mother.
    3.3.2 Utilize translators as needed.
    3.3.3 Exercise principles of optimal health, safety, and universal precautions.
    3.3.4 Provide appropriate oral and written instructions and/or demonstration of interventions, procedures, and techniques.
    3.3.5 Facilitate referral to other health care professionals, community services, and support groups as needed.
    3.3.6 Use equipment appropriately.
- Refrain from unnecessary or excessive use.
- Assure cleanliness and good operating condition.
- Discuss the risks and benefits of recommended equipment including financial considerations.
- Demonstrate the correct use and care of equipment.
- Evaluate safety and effectiveness of use.

    3.3.7 Document and communicate to health care providers as appropriate.
- Assessment information.
- Suggested interventions.
- Instructions provided.
- Evaluations of outcomes.
- Modifications of the plan of care.
- Follow-up strategies.

3.4 Evaluation.
    3.4.1 Evaluate outcomes of planned interventions.
    3.4.2 Modify the care plan based on the evaluation of outcomes.

Standard 4. Breastfeeding Education and Counseling

Breastfeeding education and counseling are integral parts of the care provided by the IBCLC.

4.1 Educate parents and families to encourage informed decision-making about infant and child feeding.

4.2 Utilize a pragmatic problem-solving approach, sensitive to the learner's culture, questions and concerns.

4.3 Provide anticipatory guidance (teaching).
   4.3.1 Promote optimal breastfeeding practices.
   4.3.2 Minimize the potential for breastfeeding problems or complications.

4.4 Provide positive feedback and emotional support for continued breastfeeding, especially in difficult or complicated circumstances.

4.5 Share current evidence-based information and clinical skills in collaboration with other health care providers.

Appendix B

SUMMARY OF THE INTERNATIONAL CODE OF MARKETING OF BREAST MILK SUBSTITUTES AND SUBSEQUENT WORLD HEALTH ASSEMBLY RESOLUTIONS

Summary

"Inappropriate feeding practices lead to infant malnutrition, morbidity, and mortality in all countries, and improper practices in the marketing of breast milk substitutes and related products can contribute to these major public health problems" (Code Preamble).

The International Code was adopted by the World Health Assembly on May 21, 1981. The code is intended to be adopted as a minimum requirement by all governments and aims to protect infant health by preventing the inappropriate marketing of breast milk substitutes.

Scope

The code covers the marketing of all breast milk substitutes (Article 2), and these include the following:

- Infant formula (including so-called "hypo-allergenic" formula, preterm milks, and other "special" baby milks).
- Follow-up milks.
- Complementary foods such as cereals, teas and juices, water, and other baby foods that are marketed for use before the baby is six months old.
- The code also covers feeding bottles and teats.

Provision of Clear Information

Informational and educational materials dealing with the feeding of infants that is intended to reach health professionals, pregnant women, and mothers of infants and young children should include clear information about all of the following points:

- The benefits and superiority of breastfeeding.

- Maternal nutrition and the preparation for and maintenance of breastfeeding.
- The negative effect on breastfeeding of introducing partial bottle feeding.
- The difficulty of reversing the decision not to breastfeed.
- Where needed, the proper use of infant formula.

When such materials contain information about the use of infant formula, they should include the following points:

- Social and financial implications of its use.
- Health hazards of inappropriate foods or feeding methods.
- Health hazards of unnecessary or improper use of infant formula and other breastmilk substitutes.
- Such materials should not use pictures or text that might idealize the use of breastmilk substitutes (Articles 4.2, 7.2).

No Promotion to the Public

There should be no advertising or other form of promotion to the general public of products that are within the scope of the code. There should be no point-of-sale advertising, giving of samples, or giving any other promotional device in order to induce sales directly to the consumer at the retail level, such as special displays, discount coupons, premiums, special sales, loss-leaders, and tie-in sales. Marketing personnel should not seek direct or indirect contact with pregnant women or with mothers of infants and young children (Article 5).

No Gifts to Mothers or Health Workers

Manufacturers and distributors should not distribute to pregnant women or mothers of infants and young children any gifts of articles or utensils that might promote the use of breastmilk substitutes or bottle feeding. No financial or material inducements to promote products within the scope of the code should be offered to healthcare workers or members of their families. Financial support for professionals who are working in infant and young-child health professions should not create conflicts of interest (Articles 5.4 and 7.3, WHA 49.15 [1996]).

No Promotion to Healthcare Facilities

Facilities of healthcare systems should not be used to promote infant formula or other products within the scope of the code, nor should they be used for the display of products, placards, or posters concerning such products, or for the distribution of material bearing the brand name of products covered by the code (Articles 6.2, 6.3, and 4.3).

No Promotion to Health Workers

Information provided to health professionals by manufacturers and distributors regarding products covered by the code should be restricted to scientific and factual matters and should not imply or create a belief that bottle feeding is equivalent or superior to breastfeeding. Samples of products covered by the code, or equipment or utensils for their preparation or use, should not be provided to healthcare workers except where necessary for the professional evaluation or research at the institutional level (Articles 7.2 and 7.4).

No Free Samples or Supplies

Neither manufacturers nor healthcare workers should give pregnant women or mothers of infants and young children samples of products covered by the code. Free or low-cost supplies of breastmilk substitutes should not be given to any part of the healthcare system (which includes maternity wards, hospitals, nurseries, and child care institutions). Donated supplies in support of emergency-relief operations should only be given for infants who have to be fed on breastmilk substitutes and should continue for as long as the infants who are concerned need them. Supplies should not be used as a sales inducement (Articles 5.2 and 7.4). Note: Articles 6.6 and 6.7 of the code have been superseded (WHA Resolutions 39.28; 1986, WHA 45.34; 1992, and WHA 47.5; 1994).

No Promotion of Complementary Foods Before They Are Needed

It is important for infants to receive appropriate complementary foods at about six months of age. Every effort should be made to use locally available foods. Any food or drink given before complementary feeding is nutritionally required might interfere with the initiation or maintenance of breastfeeding and therefore should not be promoted for use by infants during this period. Complementary foods should not be marketed in ways that undermine exclusive and sustained breastfeeding (Code Preamble; WHA Resolution 39.28, 1986, WHA 45.34, 1992, WHA 47.5, 1994, and WHA 49.15, 1996).

Adequate Labels: Clear Information, No Promotion, and No Baby Pictures

Labels should provide the necessary information about the appropriate use of the product and should not discourage breastfeeding. Infant formula manufacturers should ensure that each container has a clear, conspicuous, and easily readable message in an appropriate language that includes all of the following points:

- The words "Important Notice" or their equivalent.
- A statement about the superiority of breastfeeding.

- A statement that the product should only be used on the advice of a health-care worker as to the need for its use and the proper method of use.

- Instructions for appropriate preparation and a warning of the health hazards of inappropriate preparation.

Neither the container nor the label should have pictures of infants or other pictures or text that might idealize the use of infant formula. The terms "humanized," "maternalized," or similar terms should not be used (Articles 9.1 and 9.2).

Companies Must Comply with the International Code

Monitoring the application of the international code and subsequent resolutions should be carried out in a transparent, independent manner, free from commercial influence (WHA 49.15, 1996).

Independently of any other measures taken for implementation of the code, manufacturers and distributors of products covered by the code should regard themselves as responsible for monitoring their marketing practices according to the principles and aim of the code.

Manufacturers should take steps to ensure that their conduct at every level conforms to all provisions above (Article 11.3).

Appendix C

UNIVERSAL PRECAUTIONS AND BREAST MILK

The Centers for Disease Control and Prevention (CDC) maintains a detailed database on the topic of breastfeeding. The following is reprinted with permission from a section in a monograph entitled, "Frequently Asked Questions (FAQs)" (http://www.cdc.gov/breastfeeding/faq/index.htm).

Are special precautions needed for handling breast milk?

CDC does not list human breast milk as a body fluid for which most health care personnel should use special handling precautions. Occupational exposure to human breast milk has not been shown to lead to transmission of HIV or HBV infection. However, because human breast milk has been implicated in transmitting HIV from mother to infant, gloves may be worn as a precaution by health care workers who are frequently exposed to breast milk (e.g., persons working in human milk banks).

For additional information regarding universal precautions as they apply to breast milk in the transmission of HIV and hepatitis B infections, visit the following resources:

- Perspectives in Disease Prevention and Health Promotion Update: Universal Precautions for Prevention of Transmission of Human Immunodeficiency Virus, Hepatitis B Virus, and Other Bloodborne Pathogens in Health-Care Settings. *MMWR* 1988; 37(24):377–388.

- CDC. Recommendations for prevention of HIV transmission in health-care settings. *MMWR* 1987; 36(suppl 2S):1S–18S.

The letter below is reprinted from The Department of Labor, Occupational Safety and Health Administration and is available on the Internet (http://www.osha.gov/pls/oshaweb/owadisp.show_document?p_table=INTERPRETATIONS&tp_id=20952). With regards to Standard Number 1910.1030, "Breast milk does not constitute occupational exposure as defined by standard."

December 14, 1992

Ms. Marjorie P. Alloy
Reed, Smith, Shaw & McClay
8251 Greensboro Drive
Suite 1100
McLean, Virginia 22102-3844

Dear Ms. Alloy:

This is in response to your letter of November 23, addressed to the Acting Assistant Secretary, Dorothy L. Strunk. You wrote on behalf of the International Lactation Consultants Association and inquired into the applicability of the Occupational Safety and Health Administration (OSHA) regulation 29 CFR 1910.1030, "Occupational Exposure to Bloodborne Pathogens," to breast milk.

Breast milk is not included in the standard's definition of "other potentially infectious materials." Therefore contact with breast milk does not constitute occupational exposure, as defined by the standard. This determination was based on the Centers for Disease Control's findings that human breast milk has not been implicated in the transmission of the human immunodeficiency virus (HIV) or the hepatitis B virus (HBV) to workers although it has been implicated in perinatal transmission of HIV and the hepatitis surface antigen has been found in the milk of mothers infected with HBV. For this reason, gloves should be worn by health-care workers in situations where exposures to breast milk might be frequent, for example, in milk banking.

We hope this information is responsive to your concerns and thank you for your interest in worker safety and health.

Sincerely,

Roger A. Clark,

Director
Directorate of Compliance Programs

INDEX

Page numbers followed by t denote tables; those followed by f denote figures